SECOND EDITION

SPORT NUTRITION

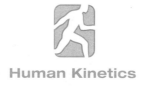

An Introduction to Energy Production and Performance

Asker Jeukendrup, MSc, PhD
University of Birmingham

Michael Gleeson, BSc, PhD
Loughborough University

Human Kinetics

Library of Congress Cataloging-in-Publication Data

Jeukendrup, Asker E., 1969-
  Sport nutrition : an introduction to energy production and performance / Asker Jeukendrup, Michael Gleeson. -- 2nd ed.
      p. ; cm.
  Includes bibliographical references and index.
  ISBN-13: 978-0-7360-7962-4 (print)
  ISBN-10: 0-7360-7962-9 (print)
  1. Athletes--Nutrition. I. Gleeson, Michael, 1956- II. Title.
[DNLM: 1. Nutritional Physiological Phenomena. 2. Sports Medicine--methods. 3. Exercise--physiology. 4. Food. 5. Physical Fitness--physiology. QT 261 J58s 2010]
  TX361.A8J48 2010
  613.2'024796--dc22

                          2009034956

ISBN-10: 0-7360-7962-9 (print)
ISBN-13: 978-0-7360-7962-4 (print)

Permission notices for material reprinted in this book from other sources can be found on page xi.

The Web addresses cited in this text were current as of August, 2009, unless otherwise noted.

Acquisitions Editor: Michael S. Bahrke, PhD; **Developmental Editor:** Judy Park; **Assistant Editors:** Lee Alexander, Casey A. Gentis, Christine Bryant Cohen, Dena P. Mumm, and Steven Calderwood; **Copyeditor:** Bob Replinger; **Indexer:** Marie Rizzo; **Permission Manager:** Dalene Reeder; **Graphic Designer:** Bob Reuther; **Graphic Artist:** Dawn Sills; **Cover Designer:** Keith Blomberg; **Photographer (cover):** Stefan Eisend; **Photo Asset Manager:** Laura Fitch; **Photo Production Manager:** Jason Allen; **Art Manager:** Kelly Hendren; **Associate Art Manager:** Alan L. Wilborn; **Illustrators:** Argosy and Denise Lowry; **Printer:** Versa Press

Printed in the United States of America   10 9 8 7 6 5 4 3 2 1

The paper in this book is certified under a sustainable forestry program.

Human Kinetics
Web site: www.HumanKinetics.com

United States: Human Kinetics
P.O. Box 5076
Champaign, IL 61825-5076
800-747-4457
e-mail: humank@hkusa.com

Canada: Human Kinetics
475 Devonshire Road Unit 100
Windsor, ON N8Y 2L5
800-465-7301 (in Canada only)
e-mail: info@hkcanada.com

Europe: Human Kinetics
107 Bradford Road
Stanningley
Leeds LS28 6AT, United Kingdom
+44 (0) 113 255 5665
e-mail: hk@hkeurope.com

Australia: Human Kinetics
57A Price Avenue
Lower Mitcham, South Australia 5062
08 8372 0999
e-mail: info@hkaustralia.com

New Zealand: Human Kinetics
P.O. Box 80
Torrens Park, South Australia 5062
0800 222 062
e-mail: info@hknewzealand.com

E4690

Contents

15 Eating Disorders in Athletes 347

16 Nutrition and Immune Function in Athletes 361

Preface

Sport and exercise nutrition is a relatively new discipline that is rapidly gaining importance and recognition. Only a few years ago sport nutrition was a topic that was covered in exercise physiology textbooks. In some of those books it received a mention in only one of the chapters. But in recent years sport and exercise nutrition has developed into a mature discipline with its own scientific journals and textbooks. The role of nutrition in exercise and sport will become increasingly important because it plays a crucial role in the adaptations to physical activity and exercise, in weight maintenance, and in the performance of exercise, whether by professional athletes or by those who are physically active for health reasons.

Indeed, nutrition influences nearly every process in the body involved in energy production and recovery from exercise. To understand and apply the principles of sport nutrition, some basic understanding of nutrition is necessary, as is some knowledge of the biochemical and physiological processes that occur in cells and tissues and the way in which those processes are integrated throughout the body.

When we wrote the first edition of this book we aimed it primarily at undergraduate students of sports science, exercise physiology, and other sport-related or exercise-related degree programs. Many degree courses in sports-related subjects now include some coverage of nutrition, and the aim of this book is to introduce students, as well as athletes and coaches, to the principles that underpin sport nutrition and its relation to sports performance. Because this background information is often lacking in current texts, an understanding of the reasoning behind particular nutritional guidelines can be difficult. Indeed, the wide range of sport nutrition products on the market and manufacturers' claims (often based on selective evidence or pseudoscience) can be confusing. In contrast, with a few notable exceptions, little confusion exists among scientists in most areas of sport nutrition, which perhaps emphasizes the importance of providing accurate and adequate information to students, athletes, and coaches. Thus, a book is needed that provides a scientific underpinning of sport nutrition guidelines and advice at a level appropriate for undergraduate study. In this book, we attempt to provide a scientific basis for sport nutrition that covers the principles, background, and rationale for current nutrition guidelines for athletes.

Readers of this book do not need a deep understanding of biochemistry, biology, chemistry, or physiology, but they should be familiar with some of the main concepts because the physical, chemical, and biochemical properties of cells and tissues determine the physiological responses to exercise and the effect that nutrition has on these responses. This book aims to develop the knowledge of these disciplines from a basic level to a relatively advanced level. Readers who are unfamiliar with or a bit rusty on fundamental concepts are advised to study appendix A before starting to read the chapters of the book. Appendix A contains a brief explanation of the basic physical, chemical, and biological processes and the structures of molecules, membranes, cells, and the organelles that they contain. Any confusion over terms used in this book can be overcome by reference to the extensive glossary, which defines many of the terms and commonly used abbreviations in nutrition, physiology, and metabolism.

How This Book Is Organized

In each chapter, we have tried to explain the specific role of nutrition in enhancing exercise performance and to provide the reader with up-to-date findings from the most current research. Topics discussed in this book include the following:

- General principles of nutrition and nutrient requirements
- Fuel sources for muscle and exercise metabolism
- Energy requirements of different sports
- Digestion and absorption of food
- The macronutrients: carbohydrates, fats, and proteins
- Water requirements and fluid balance
- The micronutrients: vitamins and minerals
- Nutrition supplements
- Body composition
- Weight management and eating disorders in athletes

- Effects of nutrition on the adaptation to training
- Nutrition and immune function in athletes

In the first chapters we explain some of the important principles of nutrition, including definitions and descriptions of the various terms used to describe such appropriate intakes as the recommended dietary allowance (RDA). Second, we cover the biochemistry of exercise, emphasizing the metabolic pathways that provide muscles with energy to perform physical work. This topic is followed by consideration of how the energy content of foods and the energy needs of athletes in different sports can be estimated. A full chapter, chapter 5, is devoted to explaining how food is digested and absorbed in the gastrointestinal tract and how exercise can influence these processes. The role of each of the major macronutrients—carbohydrate, fat, and protein—and the importance of adequate fluid intake in relation to exercise performance is discussed in the chapters that follow.

Nutrition supplements are sometimes considered synonymous with sport nutrition. But as the name suggests, they should only supplement a normal diet, not replace it. This topic is surrounded by much confusion and many questions. The chapter on supplements gives some guidance on how to distinguish fact from fallacy and discusses the claims and the scientific evidence that either supports or refutes the claims of a large number of supplements. The book also contains several specialized chapters that delve into other nutrition-related issues that are important for athletes, including weight management, eating disorders, and the effects of nutrition and exercise on immune function. This new edition focuses a bit more on body composition and weight management, which are now separate chapters. A new chapter covers the effects of nutrition on adaptations to training.

The material presented follows a logical sequence. For example, to understand the importance of carbohydrate intake for endurance performance, we first describe what carbohydrates are, how they are stored in the body, how they are broken down to supply energy, and how they are obtained from the diet through the gastrointestinal tract. The micronutrients—vitamins and minerals—are combined into functional groupings (e.g., those that are important in forming tissues, in transporting oxygen, as essential factors in energy metabolism and immune function, and as body fluid electrolytes) that provide a framework for understanding why they are needed for exercise performance and maintenance of health.

Special Chapter Elements

Each chapter begins with a list of objectives that explain what students should learn from the chapter. These objectives can be used to preview the chapter and to check whether students have met those objectives after reading the chapter. Key terms are previewed at the start of each chapter with page references. Terms, in blue, that may not be familiar to readers without a science background are defined in the glossary. Chapters are organized to promote learning of concepts and ideas rather than simple memorization of facts and figures. The illustrations and tables used in each chapter help accomplish this goal, as do occasional sidebars, which provide more detailed or in-depth coverage of selected topics.

At the end of every chapter, a listing of the key points reemphasizes the important facts that students should take away from each chapter. The appendixes provide useful definitions of units and tables that students can use to convert one system of measure to another (e.g., from kilojoules to kilocalories, from grams to ounces, and from liters into fluid ounces) and provide at-a-glance information on the RDAs or their equivalents in the United States, the United Kingdom, and Australia.

After reading this book, you should have a comprehensive understanding of the basics of nutrition as it relates to sport. You should also have an excellent grasp of how nutrition can influence exercise performance, training, and recovery from exercise. Thus, you should be able to explain the background to current sport nutrition advice given to athletes or coaches. The book should also encourage you to be critical toward information that is published in magazines, on the Internet, or even in scientific publications. Rather than accepting claims that are often made, you should think about underlying mechanisms and the strength of the evidence that supports those claims. Of course, every sport has specific nutritional requirements, and furthermore these requirements may be influenced by environmental factors and differences among individuals (e.g., gender, body mass). To offer a few examples, this book will help you understand why endurance athletes benefit from carbohydrate feedings during competition whereas weightlifters do not. On the other hand, you will also be able to explain why creatine supplements benefit games players and athletes in strength sports, whereas in endurance sports, creatine supplements may have no effect on performance. In addition, you will be able to appreciate why, in prolonged exercise, fluid intake

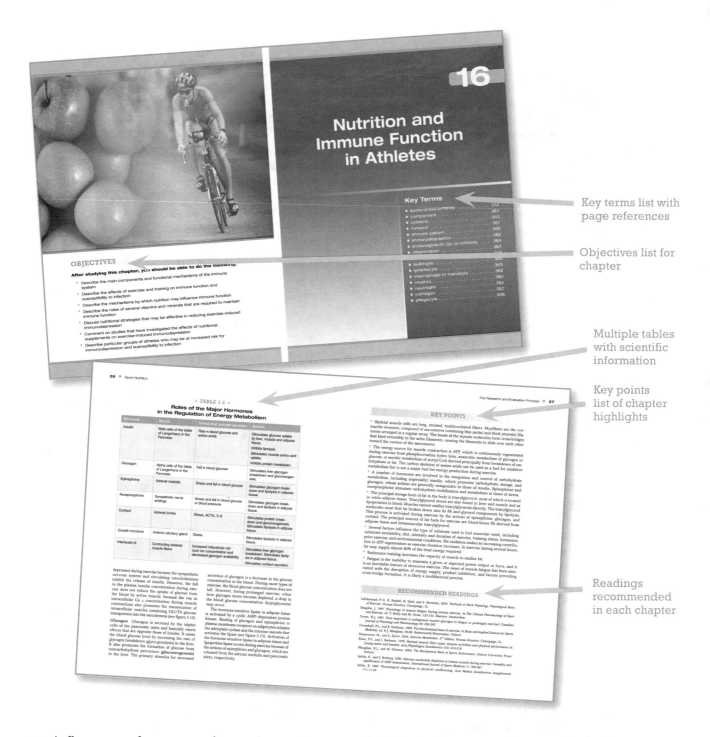

can influence performance, whereas in events lasting less than 30 minutes, fluid intake during exercise is unlikely to affect performance.

New to This Edition

This new edition contains a complete update of the nutrition guidelines, which have changed considerably since the last edition of this book. Two separate chapters now focus on nutrients and recommendations. Some areas have developed significantly in the last few years. For example, developments in the field of carbohydrate metabolism have altered the recommendations given to athletes. The role of protein has been studied more extensively, and our understanding has improved significantly. The chapter on protein was improved with many updates and a completely new structure. Another rapidly developing field is immunonutrition, and the chapter devoted to that topic has been updated and expanded. An important new area of study examines adaptations to training and how they can be altered by nutrition. Major advances in this area have occurred, mostly because of developments within molecular biology. To understand the role of nutrition on adaptations to exercise training, it is essential to understand the underlying molecular changes. For example, how is it possible that resistance exercise results in more muscle whereas endurance training does not change muscle mass but may improve the quality of the muscle (e.g., its capacity to oxidize fat)? Molecular processes underlie these distinctly different adaptations to exercise. We have incorporated a bit more basic knowledge of the regulation of protein synthesis in appendix A and discuss the molecular and cellular changes to exercise training in chapter 12. Because weight management is one of the most debated topics in sport nutrition, we have added more detail on weight management, and we discuss the possible role of various diets, the role of appetite regulation, and the effects of exercise. We have also added more detail on body composition—how it is measured and what the limitations are.

In brief, this new edition has been updated in all areas and has been significantly expanded in areas that are most important in sport nutrition. Parts of chapters that were less important have been reduced, and the text has been enlivened with sidebars and special elements to make the book more user friendly.

Notes for Instructors

The ancillaries should make adopting this book to teach a quality sport nutrition course easy. The Instructor Guide includes a detailed outline of each chapter, which could form the structure of a lecture. For each lecture the key points are indicated so that those can be stressed. In addition, suggestions are offered for practical lab activities. The Image Bank contains of most of the figures, content photos, and tables from the text. Easy-to-follow instructions are included so instructors can easily use these items to develop customized presentations for each chapters' material. The Test Package is a large question bank (with answers) that contains over 600 multiple choice and true–false questions that could be used as tests for students or in an exam. In addition, a large number of open-ended questions are provided, which could be used in seminars or as exam questions. All chapters have been updated, and students will learn not only about the basics but also about rapidly developing areas where cutting-edge research is performed. So with these extensive updates and the ancillaries provided, course instructors should easily be able to put together an informative and successful course from which students will gain both knowledge and enjoyment. In the many years that we have been teaching this subject, with similar materials, we have learned that this course has been one of those that students most appreciate.

Our approach in writing this book comes from years of experience in teaching sport nutrition at the university level. Thus, we have been conscious of the needs of course instructors. Above all, we wanted to create a book that will be a useful resource to students and instructors alike. Hence, the chapters of the book are constructed in the way that we would deliver a lecture on the subject matter of each chapter. The diagrams, figures, and tables that we present in the book are similar to the ones we use in our own lectures and tutorials to illustrate important concepts, methods, and research findings.

The content of the book provides broad coverage of nutrition as it relates to sport, including some unique aspects, such as the issue of nutrition, exercise, and immunity. We have attempted to provide an appropriate depth of content for students at the undergraduate level; thus, we describe the main findings of influential research studies without going into too much detail (except where absolutely necessary) about experimental protocols, and we critique the limitations of these studies. Although most of the text is based on appropriate scientific studies, not every statement is referenced by a bibliographic source because too many citations tend to interrupt the flow of the text. We have used references selectively so that students can be directed to look at appropriate primary sources of information to find more details about the experimental studies for themselves, without being overwhelmed by extensive reference lists.

The sequence of the chapters also follows the design of courses that we have adopted to teach modules in sport nutrition that take place over one or two semesters. These unique features of our book, we hope, will help instructors deliver a better course and expend less time in preparing lectures and tutorials.

We hope that this book inspires instructors as well as students, coaches, and athletes to achieve their potential in many ways, be it academic or athletic. Most of all, we hope that you enjoy reading our book on this fascinating subject.

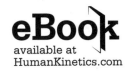

eBook available at HumanKinetics.com

Acknowledgments

For many years we have worked with students, athletes, coaches, industrial partners, governing bodies, and scientists. These interactions have not only shaped this book but also inspired us in our careers and our own sport participation.

We are very grateful to many people who have contributed to this book. First I would like to thank Trent and Hillary Stellingwerff, who were perfect hosts when I spent a significant amount of time in their house in Switzerland writing this book. It was the perfect way to write a second edition of this book—while removed from the busy office and in an inspiring environment. Both Trent, as a researcher, and Hilary, as a world-class 1,500-meter runner, contributed to this book in more than one way and provided valuable input and comments. I would also like to acknowledge the expertise and assistance of Dr. Stuart Phillips and Dr. Kevin Tipton in the writing of the chapter on protein and amino acid metabolism. Similarly, we thank Dr. Stella Volpe for her input into this book.

We acknowledge the discussions with many of our colleagues who have inspired us to write this book and with whom we had the pleasure to interact both socially and academically: Keith Baar, Louise Burke, Martin Gibala, Bret Goodpaster, Mark Hargreaves, John Hawley, Jorn Helge, Peter Hespel, Hans Hoppeler, David Jones, Luc van Loon, David Martin, Ronald Maughan, Romain Meeusen, Sam Mettler, David Nieman, Timothy Noakes, Stuart Phillips, David Rowlands, Bengt Saltin, Susan Shirreffs, Lawrence Spriet, Mark Tarnopolsky, Kevin Tipton, Anton Wagenmakers, and Clyde Williams.

We also thank the dedicated team at Human Kinetics, in particular Mike Bahrke and Judy Park, who have been very professional, patient, and helpful throughout the editorial process. Finally, we thank our partners, Joanne and Laura, for their love, continuing support, and patience during the many hours we spent writing this book.

Credits

Credits for the chapter opening photos are as follows:

Chapter 1: © RubberBall Productions and © Human Kinetics

Chapter 2: © RubberBall Productions and © PhotoDisc

Chapter 3: © Dan Galic/Blue Moon Stock and © Human Kinetics

Chapter 4: © PhotoDisc and © RubberBall Productions

Chapter 5: © Jean-Yves Ahern/Icon SMI and © PhotoDisc

Chapter 6: © PhotoDisc and © Human Kinetics

Chapter 7: © DPPI/Icon SMI and © dreambigphotos - Fotolia.com

Chapter 8: © RubberBall Productions and © PhotoDisc

Chapter 9: © RubberBall Productions and © PhotoDisc

Chapter 10: © PhotoDisc and © RubberBall Productions

Chapter 11: © PhotoDisc and © RubberBall Productions

Chapter 12: © PhotoDisc and © Human Kinetics

Chapter 13: © PhotoDisc and © PhotoDisc

Chapter 14: © PhotoDisc and © AFLO SPORT/ICON SMI

Chapter 15: © Corbis. All Rights Reserved. and © PhotoDisc

Chapter 16: © PhotoDisc and © Human Kinetics

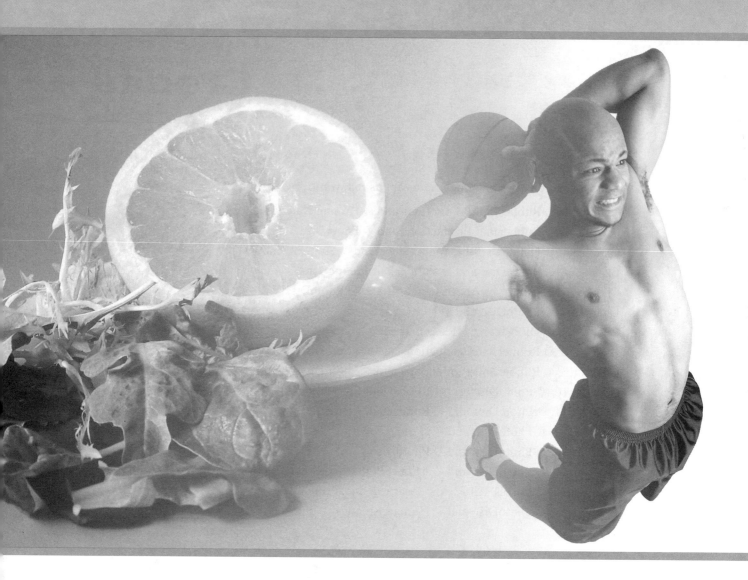

OBJECTIVES

After studying this chapter, you should be able to do the following:

- Describe the main classes of nutrients
- Describe the different types of carbohydrates (monosaccharides, disaccharides, polysaccharides, and dietary fiber)
- Describe the main composition of the average Western diet
- Describe the chemical properties of various lipids (fats), including the differences between saturated and unsaturated fatty acids and between *cis* and *trans* fatty acids, and the functions of dietary lipids
- Describe the chemical properties of amino acids and proteins and the functions of protein in the body
- Describe the general role of water in the human body
- Describe the different classes and the general role of micronutrients in the human body

1

Nutrients

Key Terms

Nutrition is often defined as the total of the processes of ingestion, digestion, absorption, and metabolism of food and the subsequent assimilation of nutrient materials into the tissues. A nutrient is a substance found in food that performs one or more specific functions in the body.

This chapter discusses the properties and functions of various components of the diet, and subsequent chapters discuss the recommended intakes of various nutrients and the specific nutritional needs of athletes and other physically active people. These needs are often higher than those for relatively sedentary individuals, and, in preparation for and during competition, different nutrition guidelines apply to athletes compared with the general public. But in principle, the guidelines for healthy nutrition apply to both the public and athletes. In a few cases or situations, guidelines for athletes and the public will not match, although during periods of training, guidelines will be similar. To optimize athletic performance, however, the guidelines may be modified somewhat. This is where sport nutrition recommendations deviate from general recommendations. For example, a high fiber intake is often recommended because it protects against cardiovascular disease and possibly against some forms of cancer. But the consumption of dietary fiber in the hours before or during prolonged endurance exercise may reduce gastric emptying, increase the risk of gastrointestinal problems, and impair athletic performance. Therefore, fiber should be consumed on training days, when performance is usually less critical, and may best be avoided before and during a race. Another example of different recommendations for the public and the athlete is sodium intake. A low-sodium diet is usually recommended to the public (see chapter 2), but as will be discussed in chapter 11, sodium requirements of endurance athletes competing in hot conditions may be substantially elevated. Therefore, relatively high intakes of sodium would be recommended. Similarly, although the general population likely consumes too much sugar, athletes can benefit from the ingestion of sugars during exercise or during recovery from exercise.

Function of Nutrients

Food provides nutrients that have one or more physiological or biochemical functions in the body. Nutrients are usually divided into six different categories: carbohydrates, fats, proteins, vitamins, minerals, and water. The functions of nutrients are often divided into three main categories:

■ *Promotion of growth and development.* This function is mainly performed by proteins. Muscle, soft tissues, and organs consist largely of protein, and protein is required for any tissue growth or repair. In addition, calcium and phosphorus are important building blocks for the skeleton.

■ *Provision of energy.* This function is predominantly performed by carbohydrates and fats. Although protein can also function as a fuel, its contribution to energy expenditure is usually limited, and energy provision is not a primary function of protein.

■ *Regulation of metabolism.* Nutrients used in this function are vitamins, minerals, and proteins. Enzymes are proteins that play an important role as catalysts, allowing metabolic reactions to proceed at far higher rates than they would spontaneously. An example of an enzyme is phosphorylase, which breaks down carbohydrate stores in the liver and muscles. Another important protein is hemoglobin, which is found in erythrocytes (red blood cells). Erythrocytes are essential for the transport of oxygen from the lungs to the tissues, and the hemoglobin molecule acts as an oxygen carrier. The hemoglobin molecule is a complex of protein (polypeptide chains) and nonprotein groups (porphyrin rings) that hold iron (to which oxygen molecules can be bound). For the synthesis of this complex, other enzymes, minerals, and vitamins are required. Thus, the interaction between vitamins, minerals, and proteins in the regulation of metabolism can be complex.

Categories of Nutrients

Macronutrients are present in relatively large amounts in the human diet, whereas micronutrients are present in minuscule amounts.

Macronutrients

- Carbohydrate
- Fat
- Protein
- Water

Micronutrients

- Vitamins
- Minerals
- Trace elements

The body requires substantial amounts of certain nutrients every day, whereas other nutrients may be ingested only in small amounts. Nutrients for which the daily intake is more than a few grams are usually referred to as macronutrients. Macronutrients are carbohydrates, fats, proteins, and water. Nutrients that are needed in only small amounts (less than 1 g/day) are referred to as micronutrients. Most nutrients are micronutrients, and they consist of vitamins, minerals, and trace elements.

Carbohydrate

The name carbohydrate indicates molecules built of carbon (carbo) and hydrogen (hydrate; water). The general formula of carbohydrate is CH_2O. In other words, the molar ratio of carbon, hydrogen, and oxygen is 1:2:1 in all carbohydrates. A carbohydrate can be one or a combination of many of these CH_2O units, and this is often written as $(CH_2O)n$, where n is the number of CH_2O units. For example, in glucose, n = 6; thus, a molecule of glucose contains 6 carbon atoms, 12 hydrogen atoms, and 6 oxygen atoms ($C_6H_{12}O_6$). The chemical structure glucose is depicted in figure 1.1. Glucose is formed during photosynthesis, and we obtain almost all our carbohydrates from plants. Carbohydrates, however, can be found in all living cells.

Carbohydrate is an important fuel during exercise and is a crucial component of the athlete's diet. In preparation for competition it becomes even more important (as discussed in chapter 7), and it is crucial as well in the recovery phase postexercise. Carbohydrate-rich foods include grains, potatoes, pasta, and rice, which contain mostly starches and fiber, but a large percentage of carbohydrate in the Western world is obtained from sugar (for examples of carbohydrate sources see table 1.1). The most important carbohydrates in our diet are glucose, fructose, sucrose, glucose polymers (maltodextrins), and starch (amylopectin). Glucose and glucose polymers are usually the main ingredients of sports drinks. Carbohydrates are typically divided into monosaccharides, disaccharides, polysaccharides, and fiber. Saccharide means "sugar" or "sweet." For an overview of the different classes of carbohydrate see table 1.2.

■ The monosaccharides represent the basic unit of a carbohydrate, and three monosaccharides—glucose, fructose, and galactose—are present in our diet. Glucose is often called dextrose or grape sugar, and fructose is often referred to as fruit sugar. Galactose is usually present in only small amounts in our diet, but relatively large amounts are released after the digestion of the disaccharide milk sugar (lactose). The monosaccharides glucose, fructose, and galactose have a similar structure and an identical number of carbon, hydrogen, and oxygen atoms, but slightly different carbon–hydrogen–oxygen linkages give these molecules different biochemical characteristics (see figure 1.1). Glucose is the only carbohydrate that can be oxidized in muscle. Fructose and galactose must be converted into glucose (or lactate) before they can be oxidized. The conversion of fructose and galactose into glucose occurs in the liver at relatively slow rates.

■ Disaccharides are a combination of two monosaccharides. Disaccharides and monosaccharides are collectively called sugars, simple sugars, or simple carbohydrates. The most important disaccharides are sucrose, lactose, and maltose. Sucrose, by far the most abundant dietary disaccharide, provides about 20% to 25% of the daily energy intake in the Western world. Sucrose is composed of a glucose molecule and a fructose molecule. Foods that contain sucrose include beet and cane sugar, brown sugar, table sugar, maple syrup, and honey. Lactose, or milk sugar, is found in milk and consists of glucose and galactose. Maltose, or malt sugar, is present in beer, in cereals, and in germinating seeds and consists of two glucose molecules. Maltose is present in only small amounts in our diet.

■ Oligosaccharides are 3 to 9 monosaccharides combined and can be found in most vegetables. Polysaccharides contain 10 or more monosaccharides combined in one molecule. Polysaccharides can contain 10 to 20 monosaccharides (often referred to as glucose polymers or maltodextrins) or up to thousands of monosaccharides (starch, glycogen, or fiber). Starch, glycogen, and fiber are the predominant forms of polysaccharides. Essentially, these polysaccharides are the storage forms of carbohydrate.

– Starch, or complex carbohydrates, is present in seeds, rice, corn, and various grains that make bread, cereal, pasta, and pastries. Starch is the storage form of carbohydrates in plants. The two apparently different forms of starch are amylopectin and amylose. Amylopectin is a highly branched molecule consisting of a large number of glucose molecules, whereas amylose is a long chain of glucose molecules (200–4,000) twisted into a helical coil. Starches

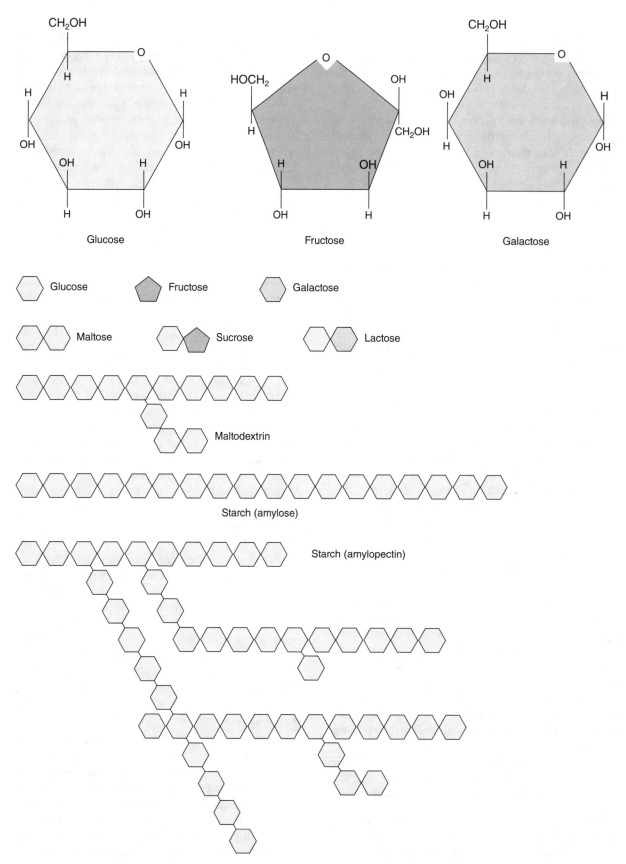

Figure 1.1 Carbohydrates and their structures. Human nutrition requires three monosaccharides (glucose, fructose, and galactose) and three disaccharides (maltose, sucrose, and lactose). Glucose polymers (maltodextrins) and starch are a series of coupled glucose molecules.

From Jeukendrup and Jentjens 2000.

with a relatively large amount of amylopectin are rapidly digested and absorbed, whereas those with high amylose content are digested more slowly. Most starches contain both amylase and amylopectin, and the relative contribution determines the properties of the food. For example, the quantity of amylose in rice kernels has a big effect on the properties of cooked rice kernels. That is, rice with little amylose will be sticky and soft, whereas rice with a large amount of amylose will be harder and not sticky. Approximately 50% of our total daily carbohydrate intake is in the form of starch.

– Glycogen is the storage form of carbohydrate in animals, including humans. It is stored in the liver (80 to 100 g) and in skeletal muscles (300 to 900 g), and its structure is comparable to amylopectin (see chapters 3 and 6 for detailed discussions).

– Dietary fiber used to be known as roughage. It comprises the edible parts of plants that are not broken down and absorbed in the human gastrointestinal tract. Fiber consists of structural plant polysaccharides such as cellulose. The human small intestine has no enzymes to break down these polysaccharides (and thus they cannot be digested). Although cellulose may be the most common type of fiber, there are many other types of fiber including gums, hemicellulose, beta-glucans, and pectin.

The National Academy of Sciences in the United States assembled a panel that came up with the following definitions that were published (Food and Nutrition Board 2005) in a report on dietary reference intakes:

■ Dietary fiber consists of nondigestible carbohydrates and lignin that are intrinsic and intact in plants.

■ Functional fiber consists of isolated, nondigestible carbohydrates that have beneficial physiological effects in humans.

■ Total fiber is the sum of dietary fiber and functional fiber. Differentiating between the forms of these fibers that are in the diet is not important. The total fiber is what matters.

Dietary fiber is also often divided into soluble and insoluble fiber. Soluble fiber dissolves well in water, whereas insoluble does not. Both types of fiber are present in plant foods. Some plants contain more soluble fiber, and others have more

■ **TABLE 1.1** ■

Types of Carbohydrates and Their Food Sources

Carbohydrate	Carbohydrate-rich foods
Sugars (simple carbohydrates)	Fruit juices, fruits, sweetened cereals and baked goods, jam, sweets, most sports drinks, beet and cane sugar, brown sugar, table sugar, maple syrup, honey
Starches	Cereal, potatoes, pasta, macaroni, rice, bread
Fiber	Whole-grain cereals and breads, oats, dried beans and peas, fruits and vegetables

■ **TABLE 1.2** ■

Classes of Carbohydrates

Carbohydrate	Carbohydrate-rich foods
Mono-saccharides	Glucose or dextrose (grape sugar)
	Fructose or levulose (fruit sugar)
	Galactose (brain sugar)
Disaccharides	Maltose (malt sugar)
	Sucrose (table sugar, cane sugar, saccharose, or beet sugar)
	Lactose (milk sugar)
	Trehalose or mycose
	Isomaltulose
Polysaccharides	Maltodextrin
	Starch
	Plant starch
	Amylose
	Amylopectin
	Resistant starch
	Animal starch
	Glycogen
Fiber	Dietary fiber
	Some forms of resistant starch
	Functional fiber
	Hemicellulose
	Resistant starch (some forms)
	Dietary and functional fiber
	Cellulose
	Beta-glucans
	Gums
	Pectins

insoluble fiber. Insoluble fiber possesses water-attracting properties that help to increase bulk, soften stool, and shorten transit time through the intestinal tract. Soluble fiber undergoes metabolic processing through fermentation, yielding end products with broad, significant health effects. For example, plums have a thick skin covering a juicy pulp. The skin is an example of an insoluble fiber source, whereas the pulp contains soluble fiber sources. Good sources of fiber are listed in table 1.3.

Dietitians and nutritionists commonly classify carbohydrates as simple (sugars) or complex carbohydrates (starches). The term *complex carbohydrate* was first used in the Senate Select Committee publication *Dietary Goals for the United States* (1977), where it denoted "fruit, vegetables and whole grains." Dietary guidelines generally recommend that complex carbohydrates and nutrient-rich simple carbohydrates such as fruit and dairy products make up the bulk of carbohydrate consumption (see chapter 2). Since its introduction, the term *complex carbohydrate* has been used to describe either starch alone or the combination of all polysaccharides, sometimes including dietary fiber and sometimes excluding it. Originally, the term *complex carbohydrate* was used to encourage consumption of what were considered healthy foods, such as whole-grain cereals. But the term becomes meaningless when it is used to describe fruit and vegetables, which are low in starch. In addition, we now realize that different starches, which by definition are all complex carbohydrates, can have different metabolic effects. Some forms can be rapidly absorbed and have a high glycemic index, whereas others are resistant to digestion. As a substitute term for starch, the term *complex carbohydrate* seems to have little merit, and in principle it is better to discuss carbohydrate components by using their common chemical names. The United States Department of Agriculture's (USDA) *Dietary Guidelines for Americans, 2005* dismissed the simple–complex distinction and instead recommended fiber-rich foods and whole grains.

The glycemic index and glycemic load systems are popular alternative classification methods that rank carbohydrate-rich foods based on their effect on blood glucose levels. The insulin index is a similar, more recent classification method that ranks foods based on their effects on blood insulin levels. More on the glycemic index and glycemic load can be found in chapter 6.

Functions of Carbohydrate

Carbohydrates have an important role in energy provision and exercise performance. They are the predominant fuel during high-intensity exercise (see chapter 3). Muscle glycogen and blood-borne glucose can provide more than 130 kJ/min (32 kcal/min) during very high-intensity exercise. Carbohydrate is stored in relatively small amounts in muscle and liver and can become completely depleted after prolonged strenuous exercise. Ingestion of carbohydrate will rapidly replenish carbohydrate stores, and excess carbohydrate is converted into fat and stored in adipose tissue.

■ **TABLE 1.3** ■

Dietary Fiber and Food Sources

Type of fiber	Food sources
Soluble fiber	Legumes (peas, soybeans, and other beans)
	Oats, rye, barley
	Some fruits and fruit juices (particularly prune juice, plums, and berries)
	Certain vegetables such as broccoli and carrots
	Root vegetables such as potatoes, sweet potatoes, and onions (skins of these vegetables are sources of insoluble fiber)
	Psyllium seed husk
Insoluble fiber	Whole-grain foods
	Bran
	Nuts and seeds
	Vegetables such as green beans, cauliflower, zucchini (courgette), and celery
	Skins of some fruits, including tomatoes

In normal conditions, blood glucose is the only fuel used by the cells of the central nervous system. After prolonged fasting (about 3 days), ketone bodies are produced by the liver (from fatty acids), which can serve as an alternative fuel for the central nervous system (especially after prolonged starvation). The central nervous system functions optimally when the blood glucose concentration is maintained above 4 mmol/L. Normal blood glucose concentration is about 5.5 mmol/L. At concentrations below 3 mmol/L, symptoms of hypoglycemia (low blood sugar) may develop, including weakness, hunger, dizziness, and shivering. Prolonged and severe hypoglycemia can result in unconsciousness and irreversible brain damage. Therefore, tight control of blood glucose concentration is crucial. Blood glucose also provides fuel for the red and white blood cells. New dietary guidelines for children and adults state that an intake of at least 130 g of carbohydrate each day should be achieved. This recommendation is based on the minimum amount of carbohydrate needed to produce sufficient glucose for the brain to function. Most people, however, consume far more than 130 g per day.

Functions of Fiber

The functions of a specific type of fiber are determined by whether the fiber is classified as soluble or insoluble. Insoluble fiber has its effects mainly in the colon, where it adds bulk and helps to retain water, resulting in a softer and larger stool. Fiber decreases the transit time of fecal matter through the intestines. So, a diet high in insoluble fiber is most often used in treatment of constipation resulting from poor dietary habits and is known to promote bowel regularity. On the other hand, soluble fiber lowers blood cholesterol concentrations and normalizes blood glucose.

In addition, most soluble fiber is highly fermentable, and fermentable fibers help maintain healthy populations of friendly bacteria. Besides producing necessary short-chain fatty acids, these bacteria play an important role in the immune system by preventing pathogenic (disease-causing) bacteria from surviving in the intestinal tract. Fiber also has several effects on nutrient digestion and absorption. It reduces the rate of gastric emptying and can influence the absorption of various micronutrients. Fiber

increases food bulk, which increases satiety, and it can reduce energy intake by 400 to 600 kJ/day (100 to 200 kcal/day). Fiber is associated with various health effects that will be discussed in more detail later.

Carbohydrate Intake and Health Effects

Carbohydrate intake varies enormously in different parts of the world. For instance, in many parts of Africa, a typical diet consists of 80% carbohydrate, whereas in the Western world, carbohydrate intake is often 40% to 50%. In Caribbean countries, carbohydrate intake averages 65%, which is closer to the recommended daily carbohydrate intake. A carbohydrate intake of 40% to 50% is about 300 g of carbohydrate a day in a relatively sedentary person. An athlete in a strenuous training program may consume as much as 1,000 g of carbohydrate a day. Athletes are usually encouraged to consume more than 60% of their total energy intake as carbohydrate. But (as will be discussed in chapter 6) carbohydrate needs of athletes are usually best expressed in relation to their body weight (grams of carbohydrate per kilogram of body weight). Expressing carbohydrate intake relative to body weight is most specific to an athlete's needs for training and competition.

In the Western diet, about 50% of the carbohydrate intake is in the form of sugars, especially sucrose and high-fructose corn syrups. Over the past century, the yearly intake of simple sugars has increased dramatically to approximately 50 kg per person—25 times more than 100 years ago. Most of this increase is due to increased consumption of soft drinks, but candy, cookies, cakes, and pies have also contributed to the increase (figure 1.2).

Evidence is accumulating that the intake of large amounts of simple sugars is linked to increased risk of obesity and cardiovascular disease. But considerable debate exists about this topic (Gibson 1996), and the results of studies are not conclusive either way. Generally, diets low in fiber and high in

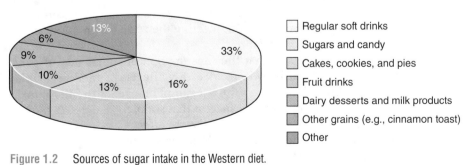

Figure 1.2 Sources of sugar intake in the Western diet.

Journal of the American Dietetic Association, 100 (1), J.F. Guthrie and J.F. Morton, "Food sources of added sweeteners in the diets of Americans," pgs. 43-51, Copyright 2000, with permission from Elsevier.

simple sugars are associated with increased risk of non-insulin-dependent diabetes mellitus (NIDDM), or type 2 diabetes. This disease is characterized by resistance of different tissues to insulin, resulting in various metabolic and related complications. For example, insulin-stimulated glucose uptake into tissues is disturbed, and fasting blood glucose concentrations are often extremely high. Fat mobilization is normally inhibited by insulin, and reduced insulin action will therefore result in increased fatty acid concentrations in the blood. This reduced insulin sensitivity (or increased insulin resistance) has far-reaching consequences and may result in many serious clinical complications. A high intake of fiber-rich foods seems to protect against this disease (American Dietetic Association 1997).

Concern has been raised about the dramatic increase in the intake of added sugar over the past 30 years—that is, sugars used as ingredients in processed and prepared foods such as bread, cake, soft drinks, jam, and ice cream—as well as sugars eaten separately. Fruit drinks and other soft drinks (e.g., cola) are the most important sources of added sugars. Soft drinks commonly contain sugar in amounts of 10 to 20 g/100 ml. Soft drink consumption in the United States among children 2 to 17 years of age increased from 198 g a day in 1989 through 1991 to 279 g a day in 1994 through 1995 (Morton & Guthrie 1998). Based on another survey, consumption of soft drinks increased 130% from 144 g to 332 g between 1977 and 1996 (Tippett & Cleveland 1999). Although the body's response to sugars is the same whether they are naturally present in a food or added to the food, added sugars supply calories but few or no nutrients. People who consume foods or beverages high in added sugars tend to consume more calories than those who choose to consume foods or beverages low in added sugars. Some studies have also shown an association between consumption of calorically sweetened beverages and weight gain. Another problem with this increased intake of soft drinks is that it is inversely related to the intake of milk. This problem has already resulted in an increased proportion of the population not meeting the recommended intake for calcium.

It has been suggested that the consumption of a diet high in total carbohydrate adversely affects insulin sensitivity compared with consumption of a high-fat diet. Animal studies suggest that simple sugars, particularly fructose, have adverse effects on insulin action, and evidence in humans seems to confirm this. Note, however, that these findings apply to a population with extremely low levels of physical activity, and therefore the observations may not relate to the carbohydrate intake per se. Endurance athletes, who generally consume diets with large amounts of carbohydrate in a relative as well as an absolute sense, also display high insulin sensitivity. Furthermore, increased intake of dietary fiber appears to improve insulin action and may offer protection against type 2 diabetes.

Another adverse effect of certain carbohydrates (primarily glucose, fructose, and sucrose but also starches) is on dental caries (bacterial tooth decay) by providing a substrate for bacterial fermentation. Sucrose in particular increases the prevalence and progression of dental caries (Depaola et al. 1999). Sugars are most detrimental if they are consumed between meals and in a form that is retained in the mouth for a long time. For example, sweets often consist of sucrose and have a relatively long contact time with teeth (Kandelman 1997). If sugar is consumed in beverages with low pH (such as soft drinks or sports drinks), the risk of dental caries and teeth erosion is further increased. Risks can be decreased by drinking fluoridated water, brushing or flossing teeth, and reducing frequency and duration of contact with these carbohydrates.

Fiber Intake and Health Effects

In the United States and Canada, a fiber intake of 10 to 13 g/4,200 kJ (1,000 kcal) of dietary energy intake is recommended (see chapter 2). For most people, this intake would equal 20 to 35 g of fiber a day. The typical fiber intake in Western countries, however, is about 14 to 15 g a day (American Dietetic Association 1997). Again, in African countries, the intake of fiber is much higher, about 40 to 150 g a day. High consumption of fruit and vegetables has been suggested to reduce the risk of numerous forms of cancer. This reduction has been linked to high fiber intake of these foods. Although earlier studies may have been confounded by the fact that populations with a high fiber intake generally were also poorer and had different nutritional habits (e.g., less meat intake), these findings seem to be confirmed by more recent studies that suggest that low fiber intake is associated with increased risk of cardiovascular disease. The reduced incidence of cancer with high consumption of fruit and vegetables, however, may be related not only to fiber intake but also to intake of folic acid (Willett 2000) and other phytonutrients (see later in this chapter).

Nevertheless, increasing dietary fiber intake is often recommended because it can decrease the risk of cardiovascular diseases, improves laxation, and has been associated with lower risk of type 2 diabetes (see chapter 2). Furthermore, it has been suggested that diets with high fiber content protect against colon cancer. The evidence, however, is not conclusive. Potential mechanisms include reduced transit time of food (the time that food spends in the gut) because of fiber intake, which could reduce the uptake of carcinogenic substances. A second possible mechanism would be that the fiber itself absorbs some of these carcinogenic substances. In addition, a change in fiber intake may be the result of an alteration of nutritional habits that reduce the presence of carcinogenic substances (i.e., an increase in fiber intake is often accompanied by decreased fat intake). Higher fiber intake has also been associated with better weight maintenance.

Fat

Lipids are compounds that are soluble in organic solvents such as acetone, ether, and chloroform. The term *lipid,* derived from the Greek word *lipos* (meaning fat), is a general name for oils, fats, waxes, and related compounds. Oils are liquid at room temperature, whereas fats are solid. Lipid molecules contain the same structural elements as carbohydrates: carbon, hydrogen, and oxygen. Lipids, however, have little oxygen relative to carbon and hydrogen. A typical structure of a fatty acid is $CH_3(CH_2)_{14}COOH$ (palmitic acid or palmitate): 16 carbons, 32 hydrogens, and only 2 oxygens.

Fatty acids have a carboxylic acid (COOH) at one end of the molecule and a methyl group at the other end, separated by a hydrocarbon chain that can vary in length (see figure 1.3). The carboxylic acid group can bind to glycerol to form a mono-, di-, or triacylglycerol.

Although the solubility of the different lipids varies considerably, they generally dissolve poorly in water. The three classes of lipids most commonly recognized are simple lipids, compound lipids, and derived lipids (see table 1.4). An overview of various lipids and their structure is provided in figure 1.3. Triacylglycerols, or triglycerides, are the most abundant dietary lipids consumed by humans. They are composed of a three-carbon glycerol backbone esterified with three fatty acids. Triacylglycerols differ in their fatty acid composition.

In humans, the chain length of fatty acids typically varies from C14 to C24, although shorter or longer chains may occur (see table 1.5). Fatty acids with a chain length of C8 or C10 are medium-chain fatty acids (MCFAs), and those with a chain length of C6 or less are short-chain fatty acids (SCFAs). The most abundant fatty acids are the long-chain fatty acids (LCFAs), which have a chain length of C12 or more. Of the long-chain fatty acids, palmitic acid (C16) and oleic acid (C18, one double bond) are the most abundant. Fatty acids with no double bonds in their hydrocarbon chains are called saturated fatty acids (SFA). Those with one or more double bonds are unsaturated fatty acids (UFA). Fatty acids are usually described with numbers that indicate the length of the fatty acid (the number of carbons), the number of double bonds in the molecule, and the location of the first double bond. For example, C18:3 (*n*-3) is an 18-carbon fatty acid with three double bonds. The

■ **TABLE 1.4** ■

Three Classes of Lipids

Lipid class	Lipid type	Examples
Simple lipids	Neutral fat	Triacylglycerol (triglyceride)
	Waxes	Beeswax
Compound lipids	Phospholipids	Lecithins, cephalins, lipositols
	Glycolipids	Cerebrosides, gangliosides
	Lipoproteins	Chylomicrons, very low-density lipoproteins (VLDL), low-density lipoproteins (LDL), high-density lipoproteins (HDL)
Derived lipids	Fatty acids	Palmitic acid, oleic acid, stearic acid, linoleic acid
	Steroids	Cholesterol, ergosterol, cortisol, bile acids, vitamin D, estrogens, progesterone, androgens
	Hydrocarbons	Terpenes

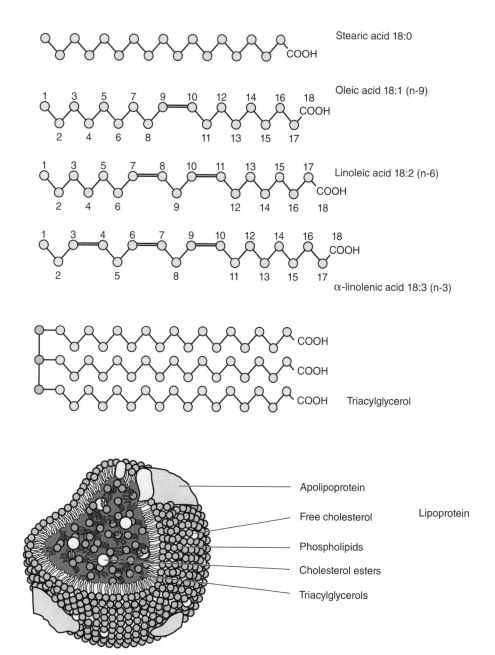

Figure 1.3   Lipids in the human body include fatty acids, triacylglycerols, lipoproteins, and phospholipids. Fatty acids differ in their chain length (number of carbons) and the number and location of double bonds.

first double bond starts at the third carbon counting from the terminal methyl (COOH) group (see figure 1.3). Another way of indicating the fatty acid and the position of the double bond is C20:4 ω3. The latter is called an omega-3 fatty acid.

Monounsaturated fatty acids (MUFA) have one double bond, and the hydrogen atoms are present on the same side of the double bond. Typically, plant sources rich in monounsaturated fatty acids (e.g., canola oil, olive oil, and safflower and sunflower oils) are liquid at room temperature. Mono-

unsaturated fatty acids are present in foods with a double bond located at 7 (n-7) or 9 (n-9) carbon atoms from the methyl end. Monounsaturated fatty acids that are present in the diet include 18:1n-9 oleic acid, 16:1n-7 palmitoleic acid, 20:1n-9 eicosenoic acid, and 22:1n-9 erucic acid. Oleic acid accounts for more than 90% of dietary monounsaturated fatty acids. Monounsaturated fatty acids, including oleic acid and nervonic acid (24:1n-9), are important in membrane structural lipids, particularly nervous tissue myelin. Other monounsaturated fatty acids, such as palmitoleic acid, are present in minor amounts in the diet.

The polyunsaturated fatty acids have two or more double bonds and can be roughly divided into two categories: n-6 and n-3 fatty acids. The most important n-6 polyunsaturated fatty acids are 18:2 linoleic acid, 18:3 γ-linolenic acid, 20:3 dihomo-γ-linolenic acid, 20:4 arachidonic acid, 22:4 adrenic acid, and 22:5 docosapentaenoic acid.

Humans cannot synthesize linoleic acid, and a lack of it results in adverse clinical symptoms, including a scaly rash and reduced growth. Linoleic acid is also the precursor to arachidonic acid, which is the substrate for eicosanoid production in tissues, is a component of membrane structural lipids and is important in cell signaling pathways. n-6 polyunsaturated fatty acids also play critical roles in normal epithelial cell function. n-3 polyunsaturated fatty acids tend to be highly unsaturated, and one of the double bonds is located at 3 carbon atoms from the methyl end. n-3 polyunsaturated fatty acids include 18:3 α-linolenic acid, 20:5 eicosapentaenoic acid, 22:5 docosapentaenoic acid, and 22:6 docosahexaenoic acid. Humans do not synthesize α-linolenic acid, and a lack of it results in adverse clinical symptoms, including

■ TABLE 1.5 ■

Overview of Different Fatty Acids (FA) and Their Nomenclature

FA	Double bonds	Common name	Chemical formula
2:0	–	Acetic	CH_3COO^-
4:0	–	Butyric	$CH_3(CH_2)_2COO^-$
6:0	–	Capronic	$CH_3(CH_2)_4COO^-$
8:0	–	Caprylic	$CH_3(CH_2)_6COO^-$
10:0	–	Caprynic	$CH_3(CH_2)_8COO^-$
12:0	–	Lauric	$CH_3(CH_2)_{10}COO^-$
14:0	–	Myristic	$CH_3(CH_2)_{12}COO^-$
16:0	–	Palmitic	$CH_3(CH_2)_{14}COO^-$
16:1	n-6	Palmitoleic	$CH_3(CH_2)_5CH=CH(CH_2)_7COO^-$
18:0	–	Stearic	$CH_3(CH_2)_{16}COO^-$
18:1	n-9	Oleic	$CH_3(CH_2)_7CH=CH(CH_2)_7COO^-$
18:2	n-6	Linoleic	$CH_3(CH_2)_4(CH=CHCH_2)_2(CH_2)_6COO^-$
18:3	n-6	γ-linolenic	$CH_3(CH_2)_4(CH=CHCH_2)_3(CH_2)_3COO^-$
18:3	n-3	α-linolenic	$CH_3(CH_2)(CH=CHCH_2)_3(CH_2)_6COO^-$
20:0	–	Arachidonic	$CH_3(CH_2)_{18}COO^-$
20:2	n-6	Eicosadinoic	$CH_3(CH_2)_4(CH=CHCH_2)_2(CH_2)_8COO^-$
20:3	n-6	Eicosatrinoic	$CH_3(CH_2)_4(CH=CHCH_2)_3(CH_2)_5COO^-$
20:4	n-6	Arachidonic	$CH_3(CH_2)_4(CH=CHCH_2)_4(CH_2)_2COO^-$
20:5	n-3	Eicosapentaenoic (EPA)	$CH_3(CH_2)(CH=CHCH_2)_5(CH_2)_2COO^-$
22:0	–	Behenic	$CH_3(CH_2)_{20}COO^-$
22:5	n-3	Docosapentaenoic	$CH_3(CH_2)(CH=CHCH_2)_5(CH_2)_4COO^-$
22:6	n-3	Docosahexaenoic (DHA)	$CH_3(CH_2)(CH=CHCH_2)_6(CH_2)COO^-$
24:0	–	Lignoceratic	$CH_3(CH_2)_{22}COO^-$

neurological abnormalities and poor growth. It is also the precursor for synthesis of eicosapentaenoic acid (EPA) and docosahexaenoic acid (DHA). EPA is the precursor of n-3 eicosanoids, which have been shown to have beneficial effects in preventing coronary heart disease, arrhythmias, and thrombosis. All the fatty acids listed have a so-called *cis* configuration, which refers to the arrangement of the double bond (see figure 1.4). Fatty acids that have a *trans* configuration are called the *trans* fatty acids.

Trans fatty acids are unsaturated fatty acids that contain at least one double bond in the *trans* configuration. The *trans* double-bond configuration results in a larger bond angle than the *cis* configuration, which in turn results in a more extended fatty acid carbon chain more similar to that of saturated fatty acids rather than that of *cis* unsaturated, double-bond–containing fatty acids. The conformation of the double bond affects the physical properties of the fatty acid. Fatty acids containing a *trans* double bond have the potential for closer packing or aligning of acyl chains, resulting in decreased mobility; hence fluidity is reduced when compared with fatty acids containing a *cis*

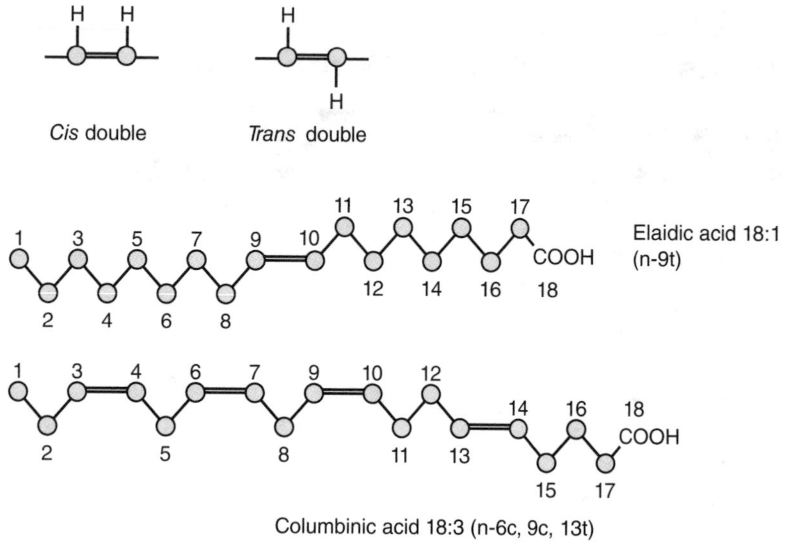

H   H   H
Cis double   Trans double
                  H

Elaidic acid 18:1 (n-9t)

Columbinic acid 18:3 (n-6c, 9c, 13t)

Figure 1.4 *Trans* fatty acids have a slightly different chemical configuration than *cis* fatty acids and are recognized as a cardiovascular risk factor.

Nomenclature

In the literature, various nomenclature is used with regard to fatty acids. To avoid misunderstandings or misinterpretations, the nomenclature in this book will be explained. Distinction must be made between fatty acids that are incorporated into triacylglycerols or other particles and fatty acids that are not incorporated into triacylglycerols. The fatty acids that are not esterified to form a monoacylglycerol, diacylglycerol, or triacylglycerol are so-called nonesterified fatty acids (NEFAs), or free fatty acids (FFAs). The term *free fatty acid* might be somewhat ambiguous because, for example, in plasma, these fatty acids are bound to albumin and are not "free." Only a minuscule fraction of fatty acids (less than 0.01% of the plasma fatty acid pool) is not bound to any other compound (non-protein-bound fatty acids).

In this book, the term *fatty acid* (not free fatty acid) is used to designate fatty acids that are not esterified to monoacylglycerols, diacylglycerols, or triacylglycerols but might be bound to albumin or fatty-acid-binding proteins.

double bond. Partial hydrogenation of polyunsaturated oils causes isomerization of some of the remaining double bonds and migration of others, resulting in an increase in *trans* fatty acid content and hardening of fat. Hydrogenation of oils, such as corn oil, can result in both *cis* and *trans* double bonds anywhere between carbon 4 and carbon 16. A major *trans* fatty acid is elaidic acid (9-*trans* 18:1) (figure 1.4). Production of hydrogenated fats increased steadily until the 1960s as processed vegetable fats replaced animal fats in the United States and other Western countries. These more saturated fats have a higher melting point, which makes them attractive for baking and extends their shelf life. Unlike other dietary fats, *trans* fats are neither essential nor salubrious and, in fact, the consumption of *trans* fats increases the risk of coronary heart disease by raising levels of "bad" LDL cholesterol and lowering levels of "good" HDL cholesterol (see chapter 2).

During hydrogenation of polyunsaturated fatty acids, small amounts of several other *trans* fatty acids (9-*trans*, 12-*cis* 18:2; 9-*cis*, 12-*trans* 18:2) are produced. In addition to these isomers, dairy fat and meats contain 9-*trans* 16:1 and conjugated dienes (9-*cis*, 11-*trans* 18:2). The *trans* fatty acid content in foods tends to be higher in foods containing hydrogenated oils.

Cholesterol is a lipid found in the cell membranes of all animal tissues, and it is transported in the blood plasma. Cholesterol, also considered a sterol (a combination steroid and alcohol), is required to build and maintain cell membranes; it regulates membrane fluidity over a wide range of temperatures. Cholesterol aids in the manufacture of bile (which is stored in the gallbladder and helps digest fats), is important for the metabolism of fat soluble vitamins, and is the major precursor for the synthesis of vitamin D and various steroid hormones.

Triacylglycerols (and cholesterol esters) found in plasma are usually incorporated into the core of a lipoprotein with phospholipids, free cholesterol, and apolipoproteins surrounding it. Apoprotein is a general name given to a protein that combines with another type of molecule to form a complex conjugated protein. Apolipoproteins are proteins that combine with lipids to form a complex as in the various lipoprotein particles. Various lipoproteins differ in their density, triacylglycerol content, and cholesterol content, but they also fulfill different functions. Examples of such lipoproteins are chylomicrons, very low-density lipoproteins (VLDLs), low-density lipoproteins (LDLs), intermediate-density lipoproteins (IDLs), and high-density lipoproteins (HDLs) (see figure 1.5).

Functions of Lipids

Lipids are an important energy source, especially during prolonged exercise. Large amounts of fat can be stored in the body, mainly in subcutaneous adipose tissue, from which it is mobilized and transported to the organ that uses it. Skeletal muscle contains a directly accessible store of fat (intramuscular triacylglycerol). Lipids have many other important functions, including the following:

- It is a fuel to most cells and an important fuel for the contracting muscle.

- Fat protects vital organs such as the heart, liver, spleen, kidneys, brain, and spinal cord. A layer of adipose tissue covers these organs to protect them against trauma. About 2% to 4% of total body fat is stored around vital organs.

- The intake of fat-soluble vitamins A, D, E, and K and carotenoids depends on daily fat intake, and fats provide the transport medium in the body.

- Phospholipids and cholesterol are important constituents of cell membranes.

- Cholesterol is also an important precursor in the formation of bile and is itself an important component of bile.

- Cholesterol is a precursor for important hormones, in particular steroids such as testosterone.

- Linoleic acid plays an important role in the formation of eicosanoids, hormonelike substances formed in cells with a regulatory function. Eicosanoids play a role in the maintenance of blood pressure, platelet aggregation, intestinal motility, and immune function.

- Fat often makes food more tasty and attractive. It carries many aromatic substances and makes food more creamy and appetizing.

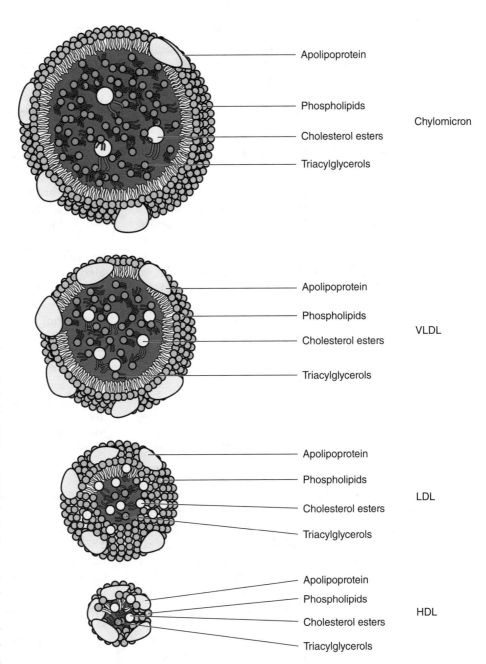

Figure 1.5 Various lipoproteins. The various shades of blue represent different types of apolipoproteins.

Lipids as Fuel

Only some of the lipid forms can be used as a fuel. Oxidizable lipid fuels include fatty acids, intramuscular triacylglycerols (IMTG), and circulating plasma triacylglycerols (chylomicrons and VLDLs). VLDL, for instance, is the main transport of triacylglycerols from the liver to adipose tissue and muscle while HDL is transporting cholesterol from the peripheral tissues to the liver. Therefore, chylomicrons and VLDL may play a role in energy metabolism during exercise, but LDL,

IDL, and HDL probably do not play a significant role in energy provision for muscle. In addition, fat-derived compounds such as ketone bodies (acetoacetate and β-hydroxybutyrate) can serve as a fuel, and glycerol can be converted into glucose in gluconeogenesis in the liver and subsequently oxidized.

Fat Intake in Western Countries

According to a large nutrition survey in the United States called National Health and Nutrition Examination Survey (NHANES), fat intake has declined from 36.9% to 33.5% for men and from 36.1% to 33.9% for women in the period 1971 through 2004. Although the percentage of fat in the diet decreased, the actual fat intake (in grams) increased slightly because of an increase in energy intake. Few people in Western countries have a fat intake below 20%. Over 95% of the daily fat intake is in the form of triacylglycerols; phospholipids, fatty acids, cholesterol, and plant sterols make up the remainder. The daily triacylglycerol intake in the North American diet is about 100 to 150 g/day. The average person in the United States consumes about a third of fat from plant origin (vegetables) and two-thirds from animal sources. Saturated fatty acids typically represent 11% of the total energy intake (NHANES 2003–2004).

Most of the cholesterol in the body is synthesized in the liver, and only a small percentage is obtained by diet (about 4%). Cholesterol is found in eggs, red meat, organ meat (heart, liver, and kidney), shellfish, and dairy products such as whole milk, butter, cheese, and cream. Foods of plant origin contain no cholesterol. But even if a cholesterol-free diet is consumed, the liver synthesizes 0.5 to 2.9 g of cholesterol a day.

Epidemiological research has shown that populations that consume diets high in saturated fats have relatively high levels of blood cholesterol and suffer a high prevalence of coronary heart disease. Particularly, LDL cholesterol promotes the development of arteriosclerosis and predisposes to cardiovascular disease. HDL cholesterol, on the other hand, seems to protect against cardiovascular disease. Reducing blood LDL cholesterol decreases the risk for coronary heart disease, thus providing evidence for a direct causal relationship. Various ways by which LDL cholesterol in the blood can be lowered seem effective in reducing the risk of cardiovascular disease, such as reducing the intake of saturated fat, increasing physical activity, and consuming cholesterol-lowering drugs (Gould et al. 1998). For example, Gordon (1995 a, b) analyzed

the results of six studies in a meta-analysis (a large-scale statistical analysis based on data from studies available in the literature) and concluded that decreasing the intake of saturated fat reduces the incidence of coronary heart disease by 24% and decreases coronary mortality by 21%.

A large body of evidence indicates that *trans* fatty acid intake raises blood LDL cholesterol levels and lowers HDL cholesterol levels (Mensink & Katan 1990; Lichtenstein et al. 1999). Most naturally occurring fatty acids contain *cis* double bonds, but *trans* fatty acids occur in processed foods (e.g., margarine). *Trans* fatty acids resemble saturated fatty acids more closely than do *cis* fatty acids.

Controversy exists over the health risks associated with regular consumption of butter compared with margarine. Although butter and margarine cannot be distinguished by their energy density or fat content, they can be distinguished by the composition of their fatty acids. Margarine is manufactured from plant-derived unsaturated fatty acids that are hydrogenated to convert the lipids into a hardened form (although not as hard as butter). About 20% of the fatty acids in margarine are *trans* fatty acids compared with 7% in butter. Margarine does not contain cholesterol, because it is manufactured from vegetable oil, whereas each gram of butter contains 10 to 15 mg of cholesterol.

The issue of butter versus margarine is controversial because *trans* unsaturated fatty acids will increase blood LDL cholesterol concentrations while decreasing HDL cholesterol concentrations. The saturated fatty acids in butter will also raise LDL cholesterol but will not lower HDL cholesterol. High intake of *trans* fatty acids is known to increase the risk of cardiovascular disease. Reducing total fat intake will reduce the intake of saturated fat and *trans* fatty acids, which may also reduce the risk of several forms of cancer.

High fat intake (along with low fiber intake) has been linked with increased incidence of colon and prostate cancer and with increased body weight. Studies have suggested a correlation between high dietary fat intake and obesity. But other studies seem to raise questions about the effect of the percentage of energy from dietary fat on body weight. Thus, the evidence that high fat intake contributes to obesity is insufficient to make definitive recommendations for a very low-fat diet. Therefore, the most recent version of *Dietary Guidelines for Americans* (USDA 2005) states that fat intake should be moderate (rather than low) (see chapter 2).

In fact, a very low-fat, high-carbohydrate intake may have adverse health effects. Reducing dietary fat to below 20% of energy intake results in elevated plasma triacylglycerols, increased LDL cholesterol, and decreased HDL cholesterol. As discussed earlier this lipoprotein pattern has been shown to predispose to coronary heart disease.

Epidemiological studies suggest that, as with cardiovascular diseases, the type of fat is important to cancer risk. The associations between high fat intake and cancer may be due to the intake of animal fat (saturated fat), not vegetable fat (unsaturated fat), raising the possibility that fat per se is not the most important factor (Willett 2000). Omega-3-(n-3) fatty acids from fish seem to protect against cancer. For example, native Eskimos of Alaska and populations in Japan, who rely heavily on fish and thus have a relatively high intake of fish oil, have lower incidences of cancer.

Protein

Amino acids are the building blocks of all proteins. Amino acids are bound by so-called peptide bonds, and once connected they are called a peptide. Most proteins are polypeptides combining up to 300 amino acids. Some examples of proteins are actin, tropomyosin, troponin, and myosin, which together make up the contractile apparatus in the muscle (see chapter 3 for a detailed discussion). Because muscle is mostly protein, meat is a good source of protein. Twenty different amino acids are commonly found in proteins. Each amino acid consists of a carbon atom bound to four chemical groups: a hydrogen atom; an amino group, which contains nitrogen; a carboxylic acid group; and a fourth group called a side chain, which varies in length and structure (see figure 1.6). Different side chains give different properties to the amino acid.

Of the 20 amino acids normally found in dietary protein, humans can synthesize 11. The human body cannot manufacture the other 9 amino acids. Those that can be synthesized are called nonessential amino acids. Those that cannot be synthesized and must be derived from the diet are called the essential amino acids (see the highlight box). Figure 1.6 lists the various amino acids and their structures.

Amino acids have central roles in the metabolism of many organs and tissues. Amino acids are not only precursors for the synthesis of body proteins but also precursors and regulators of the synthesis of important metabolic mediators and compounds with a regulatory biological activity (e.g., neurotransmitters, hormones, DNA, and RNA).

Nonessential and Essential Amino Acids

Dispensable (nonessential) amino acids
- Alanine
- Arginine
- Asparagine
- Aspartate
- Cysteine
- Glutamate
- Glutamine
- Glycine
- Proline
- Serine
- Tyrosine

Indispensable (essential) amino acids
- Histidine
- Isoleucine
- Leucine
- Lysine
- Methionine
- Phenylalanine
- Threonine
- Tryptophan
- Valine

Proteins provide structure to all cells in the human body. They are an integral part of the cell membrane, the cytoplasm, and the organelles. Muscle, skin, and hair are composed largely of protein. Bones and teeth are composed of minerals embedded in a protein framework. When a diet is deficient in protein, these structures break down, resulting in reduced muscle mass, loss of skin elasticity, and thinning hair. Many proteins are enzymes that increase the rate of metabolic reactions.

Unlike fat and carbohydrate, protein is not usually linked with diseases such as cancer, tooth caries, or arteriosclerosis. For this reason protein is often associated with health, and many companies use this association in their marketing strategies (e.g., protein shampoo). Indeed, in the developed world, where protein deficiency is uncommon, dietary protein intake is less critical and not related to disease. But in developing countries, protein

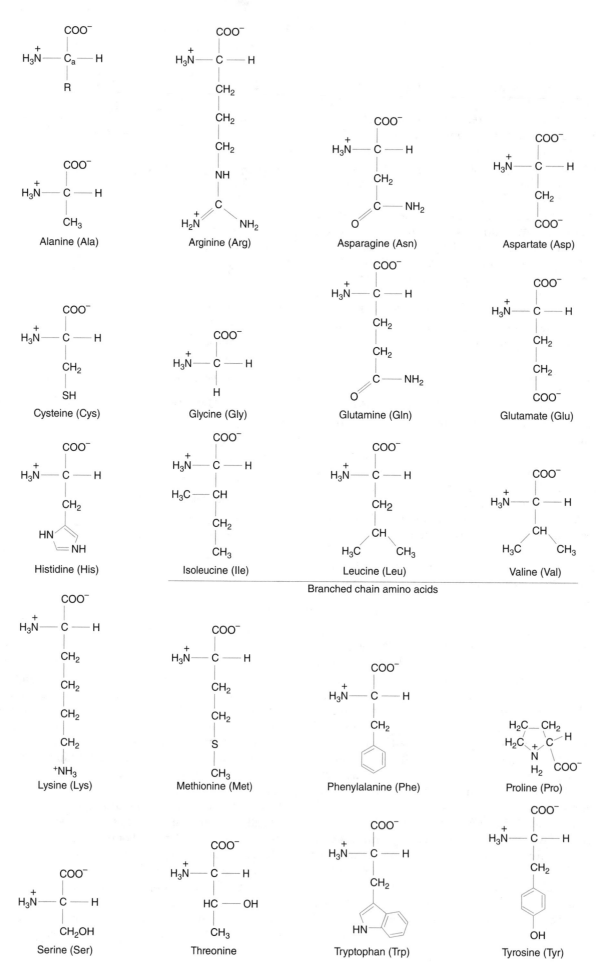

Figure 1.6 Chemical structures and abbreviations of amino acids.

deficiency is more common and can result in kwashiorkor (a pure protein deficiency, mainly in children, characterized by a bloated belly) or marasmus (a protein deficiency resulting from a total dietary energy deficiency, characterized by extreme muscle wasting).

Although it has sometimes been suggested that long-term consumption of a high-protein diet may result in impaired kidney function, evidence for this is nonexistent. In cases of preexisting kidney problems this circumstance may be different. The amino acids are broken down, and the resulting (toxic) ammonia nitrogen is excreted mainly as urea by the kidneys.

Recommended intakes are generally based on data from nitrogen balance studies (see chapter 9). Recommended protein intake varies worldwide from 0.8 to 1.2 g/kg of body weight. Protein intake in the Western world is usually well in excess of the recommendations, averaging about 80 to 100 g/day. Because meat and fish are the most common sources of protein, vegetarians could be at risk for marginal protein intake. Vegetarians often compensate by eating more grains and legumes, which both are excellent protein sources. But grains and legumes do not contain all essential amino acids. Grains lack the essential amino acid lysine, and legumes lack methionine. An exception may be well-processed soybean protein, which is a high-quality protein comparable to protein from animal sources. Many cultures have an extremely high protein intake, and most Western countries have protein intakes between 10% and 15% of the total daily energy intake.

The data on which recommendations are based are typically obtained from studies in sedentary

Quality of Proteins

The quality of a protein relates to the degree to which that protein contributes to daily requirements. Proteins that contain all the essential amino acids are called complete proteins or high-quality proteins. Proteins that are deficient in one or more amino acids are called incomplete proteins, and they are commonly referred to as low-quality proteins. To produce a measure of the protein quality of a food, various methods have been proposed. The most recent method is the protein digestibility corrected amino acid score (PDCAAS). PDCAAS is a method of evaluating the protein quality based on the amino acid requirements of humans. Using the PDCAAS method, protein quality rankings are determined by comparing the amino acid profile of the specific food protein against a standard amino acid profile. The maximum score of 1.0 means that after digestion of the protein, it provides, per unit of protein, 100% or more of the indispensable amino acids required. Although this classification was adopted by the U.S. Food and Drug Administration (FDA) and the Food and Agricultural Organization of the United Nations–World Health Organization (FAO–WHO) in 1993 as "the preferred best" method to determine protein quality, it has received much criticism. People rarely eat a single source of protein, and therefore having the information of the individual components does not give information about the overall diet. In addition, the fact that most common proteins, all with different amino acid profiles, receive identical scores of 1.0 limits its usefulness as a comparative tool. But in the absence of a better method the PDCAAS is frequently used.

A PDCAAS value of 1.0 is the highest and 0.0 is the lowest, as demonstrated in the following ratings of common foods:

Whey protein	1.0
Egg white protein	1.0
Casein protein	1.0
Milk protein	1.0
Soy protein isolate	1.0
Beef	0.92
Soybean	0.91
Kidney beans	0.68
Rye	0.68
Whole wheat	0.54

people. Are protein requirements greater for athletes involved in strenuous training programs? Although many national committees recognize the possibility that strenuous daily activity may increase protein needs, most experts do not suggest increased protein intake for active people. It has also been observed that after a period of training, the efficiency of protein utilization increases. Therefore, protein requirements to maintain muscle mass may not increase. The requirements are discussed in more detail in chapter 8. Note, however, that the diet of endurance-trained people often contains twice the recommended amounts, mainly because the increased energy intake also increases the protein intake.

As mentioned earlier, both the amount and the quality of protein are important. Proteins that contain all the essential amino acids are called complete proteins or high-quality proteins. Proteins that are deficient in one or more amino acids are called incomplete proteins, and they are commonly referred to as low-quality proteins. Incomplete proteins are unable to support human life and growth. Animal proteins are generally of higher quality than plant proteins, although the individual amino acids found in animal proteins and plant proteins are identical and of equal quality. The quality of the protein therefore depends purely on the kinds of amino acids present in the protein. Animal protein is considered of higher quality not only because all essential amino acids are present but also because they are present in larger quantities and in proper proportion.

Because the metabolism of all amino acid is integrated, all 20 amino acids must be obtained by dietary intake. A short supply of any amino acid can interfere with normal protein synthesis. An appropriate selection of plant protein sources can provide an adequate supply of amino acids, but consumption of animal protein is more likely to ensure a balanced intake. By combining plant foods such as rice and beans, obtaining a balanced intake of amino acids is possible. Essential amino acids that are deficient in one food can be obtained from another, so that in the overall diet, all amino acids are obtained. Proteins from sources that balance the amino acid intake are called complementary proteins.

Water

Water (H_2O), the most abundant molecule on the surface of the Earth, is essential for the survival of all known forms of life. One molecule of water has two hydrogen atoms covalently bonded to a single oxygen atom. Oxygen attracts electrons much more strongly than hydrogen does, resulting in a net positive charge on the hydrogen atoms and a net negative charge on the oxygen atom. The presence of a charge on each of these atoms gives each water molecule a net dipole moment and explains many of the properties of water.

The adult body is about 60% water by weight. So a 70 kg person consists of approximately 40 kg of water. The percentage of water is highest in infants and generally decreases with age. Water content varies among different tissues of the body. Blood is about 90% water, muscle is about 75%, bone is about 25%, and adipose tissue is about 5%. The proportion of water in various body compartments also varies. About two-thirds of body water is found inside cells as intracellular fluid. The remaining one-third is found outside cells as extracellular fluid. Extracellular fluid includes water in the blood, lymph, and cerebrospinal fluid as well as in the fluid found between cells, which is called interstitial fluid (see appendix A for detailed explanations).

Water transports nutrients, provides protection, helps regulate body temperature, participates in biochemical reactions, and provides the medium in which these reactions take place (blood transports nutrients and oxygen to the tissues and transports carbon dioxide and waste products away from the tissues). Water in urine transports waste products such as urea, excess salt, and ketones out of the body.

The protective functions of water are lubrication, cleansing, and cushioning. Tears lubricate the eyes and wash away dirt. Synovial fluid lubricates the joints. Saliva lubricates the mouth, making chewing and swallowing food possible. Water inside the eyeballs and spinal cord acts as a cushion against shock. During pregnancy, water in the amniotic fluid provides a protective cushion for the fetus.

An important role of water during exercise is regulating body temperature (see chapter 9). When body temperature starts to rise above the normal temperature of around 37 °C (98.6 °F), the blood vessels in the skin dilate, causing blood to flow close to the surface of the body and release some of the heat. This release occurs with fever, with an increase in the environmental temperature, and with exercise. In a cold environment, blood vessels in the skin constrict, restricting blood flow near the surface and conserving body heat. The most obvious way that water helps regulate body temperature is through sweat. When body temperature increases, the sweat glands in the skin secrete sweat. As the sweat evaporates, heat is removed from the body surface.

Water also acts in the body as a solvent, a fluid in which solutes dissolve to form a solution. Water is an ideal solvent for some substances because it is polar, which means that the two sides, or poles, of the water molecule have different electrical charges. The oxygen side of a water molecule has a slightly negative charge, and the hydrogen side has a slightly positive charge. This polarity allows water to surround other charged molecules and disperse them. Table salt, which dissolves well in water, consists of a positively charged sodium ion bound to a negatively charged chloride ion. In water, the sodium and chloride ions dissociate because the positively charged sodium ion is attracted to the negative pole of the water molecule and the negatively charged chloride ion is attracted to the positive pole. Substances like sodium chloride, which dissociate in water to form positively and negatively charged ions, are known as electrolytes, so named because they can conduct an electrical current when dissolved in water.

As with all other nutrients, a regular and sufficient water intake is required to maintain health and good physical performance. The hydration status of the body is determined by the balance between water intake and water loss. Loss of water (through diarrhea or sweating) may result in dehydration; a failure to drink fluid for more than only a few days can result in death. With a water loss of 3% of total body weight, blood volume decreases and exercise performance deteriorates (see chapter 9). A 5% loss can result in confusion and disorientation, and a loss greater than 10% can be life threatening. Dehydration is a frequently occurring problem in certain sports (see chapter 9 for a detailed discussion).

Water intake of an adult is typically 2.0 to 2.8 L/day. Because water requirements are highly dependent on sweat rates and sweat rates are dependent on energy expenditure, as a rule of thumb, fluid requirements are 1 ml for every 4 kJ of energy expended, or 1 ml/kcal. Of the daily 2.0 to 2.8 L consumed, 1.0 to 1.5 L is usually in the form of fluids, and the remainder is obtained from foods. Athletes who train and compete in hot conditions may have fluid requirements greater than 15 L/day.

Vitamins, Minerals, and Trace Elements

Vitamins are organic compounds, and minerals and trace elements are inorganic compounds. Collectively known as micronutrients, these essential compounds have many biological functions. They serve as regulators and links in the processes of energy release from food. They are important cofactors in various chemical reactions and as such are important in maintaining homeostasis (relatively constant internal conditions). The public often considers vitamin intake synonymous with good health (e.g., folic acid prevents birth defects, vitamin E protects the heart, and vitamin A prevents cancer), and some minerals are reputed to have strong relations to health (e.g., calcium helps to prevent osteoporosis).

All of the 13 known vitamins have important functions in most metabolic processes in the body. Vitamins must be obtained from the diet, except vitamin D, which can be synthesized from sunlight, and vitamin K, which is synthesized by bacteria in the intestine. When a vitamin becomes unavailable in the diet, a deficiency may develop within 3 to 4 weeks. Vitamins are either water soluble or fat soluble (see the highlight box). Water-soluble vitamins dissolve in water; fat-soluble vitamins dissolve in organic solvents and are usually ingested with fats. Minerals can be divided into macrominerals, requiring a daily intake of more than 100 mg or presence in the body in amounts greater than 0.01% of the body weight, and microminerals (trace elements), requiring a daily intake of less than 100 mg or presence in the

---

Fat-Soluble and Water-Soluble Vitamins

The asterisk (*) indicates that choline is not classed as an essential vitamin.

- Vitamin B_1 (thiamine)
- Vitamin B_2 (riboflavin)
- Vitamin B_3 (niacin)
- Vitamin B_6 (pyridoxine)
- Vitamin B_{12}
- Biotin
- Pantothenic acid
- Folic acid
- Choline*
- Vitamin C (ascorbic acid)
- Vitamin A
- Vitamin D
- Vitamin E (alpha-tocopherol)
- Vitamin K

body in amounts less than 0.01% of body weight (see chapter 10 for a detailed discussion).

Sodium, often ingested as sodium chloride (table salt), has various functions in the body, including some related to muscle contraction (see chapter 10). Excess sodium intake, however, is related to the development of high blood pressure (hypertension). Normal blood pressure (normotension) is below 120 mmHg (systolic) and below 80 mmHg (diastolic). Blood pressure is largely regulated by the degree of constriction of blood vessels and by sodium and water retention in the kidney. When blood volume is increased or blood vessels are narrowed, blood pressure rises. If blood pressure is chronically above 140/90 mmHg (hypertension), risk of arteriosclerosis, heart attack, stroke, kidney disease, and early death increases. Blood pressure between 120 and 139 mmHg systolic and 80 and 89 mmHg diastolic is referred to as prehypertension and may indicate increased risk for the diseases mentioned earlier.

Epidemiological studies (Carvalho et al. 1989) have shown that high sodium intake (more than 5.8 g/day) is associated with high blood pressure, and based on these studies a low-sodium diet has been recommended. But controversy surrounds this recommendation. Whether increased salt intake elevates blood pressure in people without existing hypertension is unclear. Salt reduction in normotensive individuals has little or no effect on blood pressure, and high sodium intake does not affect blood pressure in all people (Graudal et al. 1998). About 50% of people may be "salt sensitive," and the other half may be unaffected by increased sodium intake. Because targeting only those who are salt sensitive would be difficult, and because moderate salt intake has no reported negative effects (Kumanyika & Cutler 1997), dietary guidelines recommend that people choose and prepare foods with less salt (USDA 2000). Low potassium intake (because of not eating enough fruits and vegetables) can also increase blood pressure.

Phytonutrients

Another component of foods are the so called **phytonutrients.** Phytonutrients (*phyto* is Greek for plant) are certain organic components of plants that are thought to promote human health but are non-nutrients. They differ from vitamins because they are not considered an essential nutrient, meaning that without them people will not develop a nutritional deficiency.

The many types of phytonutrients can be divided into different classes (see the highlight box). The most well known and most researched of these are probably the carotenoids, found in carrots, broccoli, leafy green and yellow vegetables, spinach, and other vegetables; and polyphenols, found in various berries, fruits, and wine.

Of all the phytonutrients, carotenoids are the ones that receive the most attention and are the

---

Alcohol

Alcohol, or ethanol, is a nutrient that provides 28 kJ of energy per gram (7 kcal/g) but is not essential in our diet. Average alcohol intake in the United States is about 2 to 3% of daily energy intake. Alcohol is the most widely abused addictive drug and causes specific liver damage and other organ damage. It is responsible for approximately 1 in 20 deaths in the United States (McGinnis & Foege 1993). But alcohol may have health benefits when ingested in moderation. Moderate alcohol consumption reduces stress and raises levels of HDL cholesterol, which has a protective effect against cardiovascular diseases. Protection may also be provided by phenols in red wine, antioxidant compounds that reduce lipoprotein oxidation and thereby prevent or reduce the formation of atherosclerotic plaques. A large intake of alcohol, however, increases blood pressure, which outweighs the positive effects of alcohol consumption. Consumption of alcohol in any amount has been shown to increase the risk of oropharygeal, esophageal, and breast cancers.

Common Classes of Phytonutrients

- Carotenoids
- Flavonoids (polyphenols) including isoflavones (phytoestrogens)
- Inositol phosphates (phytates)
- Lignans (phytoestrogens)
- Isothiocyanates and indoles
- Phenols and cyclic compounds
- Saponins
- Sulfides and thiols
- Terpenes

most researched. Carotenoids are the red, orange, and yellow pigments in fruits and vegetables. The carotenoids most commonly found in vegetables are listed in table 1.6 along with common sources of these compounds. Fruits and vegetables that are high in carotenoids appear to protect humans against certain cancers, heart disease, and age-related macular degeneration.

Polyphenolic compounds are natural components of a wide variety of plants. Food sources rich in polyphenols include onions, apples, tea, red wine, red grapes, grape juice, strawberries, raspberries, blueberries, cranberries, and certain nuts (table 1.7). The average polyphenol intake in most countries has not been determined with precision, largely because no food database currently exists for these compounds. It has been estimated that in the Dutch diet a subset of flavonoids (flavonols and flavones) provide 23 mg per day. These small amounts, however, may have significant effects.

Polyphenols can be classified as nonflavonoids and flavonoids. The flavonoids quercetin and catechins are the most extensively studied polyphenols relative to absorption and metabolism. Green tea is a good source of catechins.

Phytonutrient Intake and Health Effects

Several mechanisms have been proposed by which phytonutrients may protect human health. More research is needed to establish the mechanisms of action of the various phytochemicals. Among the possible mechanisms are the following:

- Serve as antioxidants
- Enhance immune response
- Enhance cell-to-cell communication
- Alter estrogen metabolism
- Convert to vitamin A (by metabolizing beta-carotene)
- Cause cancer cells to die (apoptosis)
- Repair DNA damage caused by smoking and other toxic exposures

Evidence that fruit and vegetable consumption protects human health is accumulating from large-population (epidemiological) studies, human feeding studies, and cell culture studies. At least some of these effects are thought to be caused by phytonutrients. The following are results of a few selected population studies from the literature that link fruit and vegetable consumption to health. For example, fruit and vegetable consumption has been linked to decreased risk of stroke. Each increment

■ TABLE 1.6 ■
Carotenoids and Their Food Sources

Carotenoid	Common food source
Alpha-carotene	Carrots
Beta-carotene	Leafy green and yellow vegetables (e.g., broccoli, sweet potato, pumpkin, carrots)
Beta-cryptoxanthin	Citrus, peaches, apricots
Lutein	Leafy greens such as kale, spinach, turnip greens
Lycopene	Tomato products, pink grapefruit, watermelon, guava
Zeaxanthin	Green vegetables, eggs, citrus

■ TABLE 1.7 ■
Polyphenols and Their Food Sources

Nonflavonoids	Sources
Ellagic acid	Strawberries, blueberries, raspberries
Coumarins	Bell peppers, bok choi, cereal grains, broccoli
Flavonoids	**Sources**
Anthocyanins	Fruits
Catechins	Tea, wine
Flavanones	Citrus
Flavones	Fruits and vegetables
Flavonols	Fruits, vegetables, tea, wine
Isoflavones	Soybeans

of three daily servings of fruits and vegetables equated to a 22% decrease in risk of stroke, including transient ischemic attack.

- Older men who had the highest intake of dark green and deep yellow vegetables had about a 46% decrease in risk of heart disease relative to men with the lowest intake. Men with the highest intake had about a 70% lower risk of cancer than did their counterparts with the lowest intake. The differences in vegetable consumption between high and low intake rankings were not striking. Men with the highest intake consumed more than two (between 2.05 and 2.2) servings of dark green or deep yellow vegetables a day; those with the lowest intake consumed less than one (between 0.7 and 0.8) serving daily. This evidence suggests that small, consistent changes in vegetable consumption can make important changes in health outcomes.

■ Consumption of tomato products has been linked to decreased risk of prostate cancer. Men with the highest intake of tomato products (10 or more servings a week) had about a 35% decrease in risk of prostate cancer compared with counterparts with the lowest intake (1.5 or fewer servings of tomato products a week).

■ People with the highest intake of spinach or collard greens, plants high in the carotenoid lutein, had a 46% decrease in risk of age-related macular degeneration compared with those who consumed these vegetables less than once per month.

■ Flavonoid consumption has been linked to lower risk of heart disease in some, but not all, studies. Older Dutch men with the highest flavonoid intake had a risk of heart disease that was about 58% lower than that of counterparts with the lowest intake. Similarly, Finnish subjects with the highest flavonoid intake had a risk of mortality from heart disease that was about 27% lower for women and 33% lower for men than that of subjects with the lowest intake.

But other studies could not confirm the protective effect of flavonoids. In one study, flavonol intake did not predict a lower rate of ischemic heart disease and was weakly and positively associated with ischemic heart disease mortality. In another study in U.S. male individuals, data did not support a strong link between intake of flavonoids and coronary heart disease.

Although large studies have linked fruit and vegetable consumption with lowering the risk for chronic diseases including specific cancers and heart disease, claims made in the media about phytonutrients and functional foods seem far ahead of established proof that documents the health benefits of these foods or food components for humans. But our knowledge of phytonutrients and their effects is improving, and more specific information on phytonutrient consumption and human health will be forthcoming in the near future.

Fruit and Vegetable Intake

On average, Americans consume 3.3 servings of vegetables a day (NHANES). But dark green vegetables and deep yellow vegetables each represent only 0.2 daily servings. On any given day, about half the population does not consume the minimum number of servings of vegetables recommended (three servings per day). About 10% of the population consumes less than one serving of vegetables per day. On any given day about 71% of the population does not consume the minimum number of servings of fruit recommended (two servings per day). About half the population consumes less than one serving of fruit a day. This trend seems to be worldwide; a recent study showed that 77.6% of men and 78.4% of women from 52 mainly low- and middle-income countries consumed less than the minimum recommended five daily servings of fruits and vegetables (Hall et al. 2009).

KEY POINTS

■ Food provides nutrients that have one or more physiological or biochemical functions in the body.

■ Nutrients are usually divided into six different categories: carbohydrates, fats, proteins, vitamins, minerals, and water.

■ Functions of nutrients include promotion of growth and development, provision of energy, and regulation of metabolism.

■ Among the several different classes of carbohydrates are sugars, starches, and fiber.

■ Fiber, although it is not absorbed, has several important functions including maintaining normal gut function. For most people, the recommended intake would be 20 to 35 g of fiber a day, but the typical fiber intake in Western countries is only 14 to 15 g a day.

■ There are several classes of fats, including fatty acids, triacylglycerols, and lipoproteins. Triacylglycerol is the main storage form.

■ Epidemiological studies suggest that the type of fat in the diet is important to cancer risk and cardiovascular diseases.

■ Amino acids are the building blocks of proteins. Of the 20 amino acids normally found in dietary protein, humans can synthesize 11. Those that can be synthesized are called nonessential amino acids. Those that cannot be synthesized and must be derived from the diet are called the essential amino acids.

■ Proteins that contain all the essential amino acids are called complete proteins or high-quality proteins. Proteins that are deficient in one or more amino acids are called incomplete proteins, and they are commonly referred to as low-quality proteins.

■ Water is an extremely important nutrient. The adult body is about 60% water by weight. Two-thirds of the water is intracellular fluid, and the remaining one-third is extracellular fluid.

■ Vitamins, minerals, and trace elements are micronutrients. Vitamins are organic compounds, and minerals and trace elements are inorganic compounds.

■ Phytonutrients are certain organic components of plants which are thought to promote human health but are non-nutrients. They differ from vitamins because they are not considered an essential nutrient, meaning that people who lack them will not develop a nutritional deficiency.

RECOMMENDED READINGS

Bender, D.A., and A.E. Bender. 1997. *Nutrition. A reference handbook.* Oxford: Oxford University Press.

Food and Nutrition Board. 2005. *Dietary reference intakes for energy, carbohydrate, fiber, fat, fatty acids, cholesterol, protein, and amino acids (macronutrients).* Washington, DC: National Academies Press.

Gibney, M.J., I. Macdonald, and H. Roche, eds. 2008. *Nutrition and metabolism (the Nutrition Society textbook).* Oxford: Blackwell Science.

Mann, J., and A.S. Truswell. 2002. *Essentials of human nutrition.* Oxford: Oxford University Press.

Shils, M.E., J.A. Olson, M. Shike, A.C. Ross, B. Caballero, and R.J. Cousins, eds. 2005. *Modern nutrition in health and disease.* Baltimore: Williams and Wilkins.

USDA. 2005. *Dietary guidelines for Americans.* www.health.gov/DietaryGuidelines. Chapter 7, Carbohydrate.

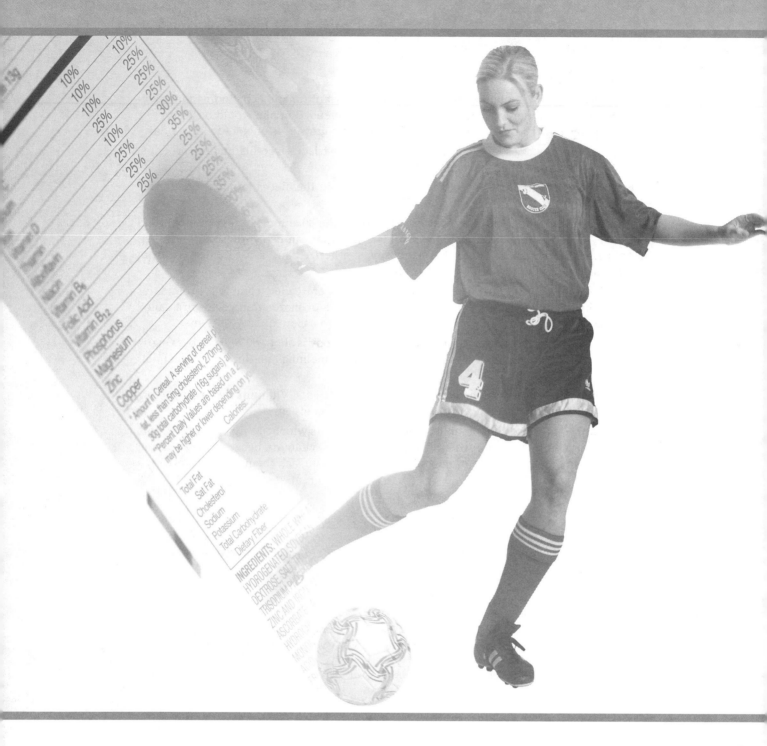

OBJECTIVES

After studying this chapter, you should be able to do the following:

- Discuss the differences between essential and nonessential nutrients
- Discuss the basis of recommended daily intakes of nutrients
- Discuss the basis of the guidelines for establishing a balanced healthy diet
- Understand the effects of food processing
- Discuss the differences in the various methods to assess food intake and diet composition and their advantages and disadvantages

Nutrients and Recommended Intakes

2

Key Terms

In the previous chapter we described the various nutrients and their functions. When people sit down for a meal, however, they eat food, not nutrients. Most people do not think about the nutrients. Instead, they are concerned about the flavor, the texture, and the smell of the food. Although many people recognize the importance and nutritional value of food, food choices are based on many factors, including availability, cost, and convenience. Advice is offered about foods or combinations of foods that will deliver certain amounts of nutrients. This chapter explores the recommendations given to people in various countries. We discuss how recommendations for certain nutrients are established and how these are translated into practical advice for the public. We discuss as well nutrition in the general population, assuming relatively low physical activity levels. In subsequent chapters, we will discuss the energy requirements of exercise and the specific needs for macronutrients and micronutrients in the athletic population. The chapter also discusses how to assess whether an individual or group is achieving the recommendations.

As discussed in chapter 1, nutrients can be divided into nonessential and essential nutrients; the former can be synthesized within the body and the latter cannot. This terminology is sometimes confusing because a nutrient that is essential for the body can be classified as a nonessential nutrient because it can be synthesized within the body. To avoid confusion, nutritionists often prefer the terms indispensable (essential) and dispensable (nonessential). In this book we continue to use the terms *essential* and *nonessential*. In the next section we will discuss the definition of essential nutrients in more detail.

Essential Nutrients

Although Hippocrates practiced a form of dietetic medicine in 400 BC, this area has evolved exponentially over the past 200 to 250 years. In ancient times people were already aware that certain food components could prevent disease or be used to treat diseases. But only during the past two centuries have some nutrients been recognized as essential for human life. Scurvy was a disease common among sailors, pirates, and others aboard ships at sea longer than perishable fruits and vegetables could be stored. In 1740 a British naval surgeon named James Lind discovered that the consumption of citrus fruits by sailors could prevent and cure scurvy. Other shipboard foods and medicine did not have this effect. Although scurvy was not

attributed to a deficiency in vitamin C at that time, the essentiality of certain nutrients for the maintenance of health was established.

Tragic studies with prisoners in Nazi death camps have revealed the importance of various vitamins and minerals. The prisoners received a diet deficient in a certain vitamin or mineral, and their health status was recorded. With diets deficient in certain nutrients, specific diseases developed and ultimately resulted in death. In early studies with rats, diets deficient in one or more nutrients retarded growth, and the animals experienced specific disease symptoms. But when the animals were subsequently fed with the missing nutrient, they recovered completely and growth was promoted. The nutrients that exhibited these health effects were classified as essential. According to more recent definitions (Harper 1999) a nutrient is considered essential if it meets the following criteria:

■ The substance is required in the diet for growth, health, and survival.

■ Absence of the substance from the diet or inadequate intake results in characteristic signs of a deficiency disease and ultimately death.

■ Growth failure and characteristic signs of deficiency are prevented only by the nutrient or a specific precursor of it and not by other substances.

■ Below some critical level of intake of the nutrient, growth response and severity of signs of deficiency are proportional to the amount consumed.

■ The substance is not synthesized in the body and is therefore required for some critical function throughout life.

Some nutrients are classified as conditionally essential or conditionally indispensable. The term was introduced in 1984 because some nutrients that were normally not essential seemed to become essential under certain conditions. Conditionally essential nutrients must be supplied exogenously to specific populations that do not synthesize them in adequate amounts. The deficiency can be the result of a defect in the synthesis of a certain nutrient or (temporarily) an increased need for that nutrient. An example of the former condition (defect in synthesis) is the genetic defect in the synthesis of carnitine. Without carnitine supplementation, people with this condition experience muscle-wasting disease (myopathy). When carnitine is supplemented, however, the condition is corrected. The latter condition (increased need) may occur in surgical patients in an intensive care unit who usually have lower than normal plasma and muscle glutamine concentrations. This deficit is associated with a negative nitrogen balance, decreased protein synthesis, and increased protein breakdown, resulting in muscle wasting. The patients improve when glutamine is supplemented. Thus, glutamine is classified as conditionally essential.

Development of Recommended Intakes

Nowadays, the list of nutrients classified as essential or indispensable is quite extensive (see the highlight box). More than 40 nutrients meet the criteria. For many centuries people have tried to define the minimum and optimum intakes of various nutrients. In 1941 the first Food and Nutrition Board was formed in the United States. In 1943 dietary standards for evaluating nutritional intakes of large populations and for planning of agricultural production were published. Since then, the guidelines have been revised several times. Initially, reference values for only 10 nutrients were established. Current guidelines in the United States and Canada, established between 1997 and 2004, cover 46 nutrients.

When the first set of recommendations (the recommended dietary allowance, or RDA) was created in 1941, its primary goal was to prevent diseases caused by nutrient deficiencies. They were originally intended to evaluate and plan for the nutritional adequacy of groups, for example, the armed forces and children in school lunch programs, rather than to determine individuals' nutrient needs.

But because the RDAs were essentially the only nutrient values available, they began to be used in ways other than the intended use. Health professionals often used RDAs to size up the diets of

Essential (Indispensable) Nutrients

Water

Amino acids
- Histidine
- Isoleucine
- Leucine
- Lysine
- Methionine
- Phenylalanine
- Threonine
- Tryptophan
- Valine

Fatty acids
- Linoleic
- α-linoleic (linolenic acid)

Minerals
- Calcium
- Phosphorus
- Magnesium
- Iron

Trace Minerals
- Zinc
- Copper
- Manganese

- Iodine
- Selenium
- Molybdenum
- Chromium

Electrolytes
- Sodium
- Potassium
- Chloride

Vitamins
- Ascorbic acid
- Vitamin A
- Vitamin D
- Vitamin E
- Vitamin K
- Thiamin
- Riboflavin
- Niacin
- Vitamin B_6 (pyridoxine)
- Panthotenic acid
- Folic acid
- Biotin
- Vitamin B_{12} (cobalamin)

Ultratrace Elements

individual patients or clients. Statistically speaking, RDAs would prevent deficiency diseases in 97% of a population, but there was no scientific basis that RDAs would meet the needs of a single person.

It was evident that the RDAs were not addressing individual needs, and new science needed to be included. Therefore, the Food and Nutrition Board sought to redefine nutrient requirements and develop specific nutrient recommendations for individuals as well as groups. Along with these changes, concepts such as tolerable upper intakes and adequate intakes emerged to meet individuals' needs.

For the first time, the RDAs are no longer focused only on preventing deficiency diseases such as scurvy or beriberi. Now they are also aimed at reducing the risk of diet-related chronic conditions such as heart disease, diabetes, hypertension, and osteoporosis. After the initial guidelines were formulated, guidelines have also become more specific and have been developed for various sex and age groups (and for pregnant and lactating women). Groups will have different reference values.

Current Recommended Intakes

The framework for a set of new recommendations is the dietary reference intake, or DRI. The DRI has been released in stages over the past few years. Under the umbrella of DRI, four standards have been developed: the estimated average requirement (EAR), the recommended dietary allowance (RDA), the adequate intake (AI), and the tolerable upper intake level (UL).

Establishment of these reference values requires that a criterion of nutritional adequacy be carefully chosen for each nutrient and that the population for whom these values apply be carefully defined.

The estimated average requirement (EAR) represents the amount of a nutrient that is deemed sufficient to meet the needs of the average individual in a certain age and gender group (see figure 2.1). At an intake level equal to the EAR, half of a specified group would *not* have their nutritional needs met. This is equivalent to saying that randomly chosen individuals from the population

---

Definitions

Dietary Reference Intake (DRI)

The new standards for nutrient recommendations that can be used to plan and assess diets for healthy people. Think of DRI as the umbrella term that includes the following values.

Estimated Average Requirement (EAR)

The EAR is a nutrient intake value that is estimated to meet the requirement of half of the healthy individuals in a group. It is used to assess nutritional adequacy of intakes of population groups. In addition, EARs are used to calculate RDAs.

Recommended Dietary Allowance (RDA)

This value is a goal for individuals and is based on the EAR. It is the daily dietary intake level that is sufficient to meet the nutrient requirement of 97 to 98% of all healthy people in a group. If an EAR cannot be set, no RDA value can be proposed.

Adequate Intake (AI)

This value is used when a RDA cannot be determined. A recommended daily intake level based on an observed or experimentally determined approximation of nutrient intake for a group (or groups) of healthy people.

Tolerable Upper Intake Level (UL)

The UL is the highest level of daily nutrient intake that is likely to pose no risks of adverse health effects to almost all individuals in the general population. As intake increases above the UL, the risk of adverse effects increases.

would have a 50:50 chance of having their requirement met at this intake level.

The recommended dietary allowance (RDA) is an estimate of the minimum daily average dietary intake level that meets the nutrient requirements of nearly all (97 to 98%) healthy individuals in a particular life stage and gender group. The RDA is intended to be used as a goal for daily intake by individuals as this value estimates an intake level that has a high probability of meeting the requirement of a randomly chosen individual (about 97.5%). The process for setting the RDA is described below; it depends on being able to set an EAR and estimating the variance of the requirement itself. Note that if an EAR cannot be set due to limitations of the data available, no RDA will be set.

The RDA is a safe excess of nutrients that prevents nutritional deficiencies in the majority of the population. When the distribution of a requirement among individuals in a group can be assumed to be approximately normal (or symmetrical), and a standard deviation (SD) of requirement ($SD_{requirement}$) can be determined, the EAR can be used to set the RDA as follows (see figure 2.1):

$$RDA = EAR + 2 \times SD_{requirement}$$

The RDA is intended to be used as a goal for daily intake by individuals. Meals in institutions (groups of people) will, generally speaking, be considered adequate if they achieve vitamin and mineral levels between the RDA and the EAR. These recommendations vary depending on how old the person is, what gender the person is, and whether a woman is pregnant or lactating; they do not apply to other populations or to conditions that may have specific requirements. The RDA is based on the median heights and weights of a population, and thus groups of adults who weigh more or less than this median may have a slightly higher or lower requirement, respectively, than the RDA. Also, stress, disease, injuries, and total energy expenditure can influence the needs for certain nutrients. RDAs are currently available for energy intake, protein, 11 vitamins, and 7 minerals (see appendixes C, D, and E).

When scientific evidence available to estimate an EAR is insufficient, an AI (adequate intake) will be set. People should use the AI as a goal for intake where no RDAs exist. The AI is derived through experimental or observational data that show a mean intake that appears to sustain a desired indicator of health, such as calcium retention in bone for most members of a population. The AI has been set for two B vitamins, the vitamin-like choline, vitamin D, and some minerals such as calcium and fluoride (see appendix C).

UL is the maximum level of daily nutrient intake that is unlikely to pose health risks to the greatest number of individuals in the group for whom it is designed (see figure 2.1). The UL is not intended to be a recommended level of intake; no benefit has been established for individuals to consume nutrients at levels above the RDA or AI. For most nutrients, the upper limit (**UL**) refers to total intakes from food, fortified food, and nutrient supplements. The need for setting the UL grew out of the increased practice of fortifying foods with nutrients and of the popularity of dietary supplements resulting in high intakes of some nutrients. In excess some nutrients can be toxic.

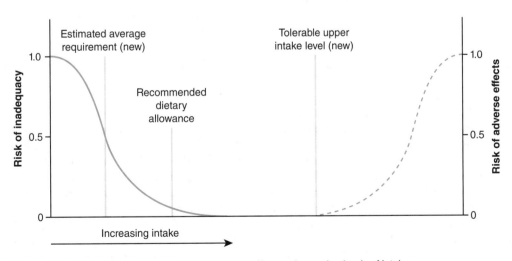

Figure 2.1 Risk of inadequacy and risk of adverse effects at increasing levels of intake.

DRIs are mainly intended for diet planning. Specifically, a diet should aim to meet any RDA (or AI) set and not exceed the UL. DRIs are based on averages of large populations and thus are not designed to detect nutrient deficiencies in individuals. So someone below the recommendations for a particular nutrient may not be deficient in that nutrient. Only a clinical and biochemical examination can determine whether an individual has a nutritional deficiency. Comparison of an individual's intake to the RDA, however, can help determine whether the person is *at risk* for a deficiency. To determine whether an individual's nutrient intake meets the RDA, it should be calculated over a period of 5 to 8 days. A person whose diet does not contain the full RDA on one day is not necessarily at risk for deficiencies because the inadequacy can be compensated the next day. Note that the RDA does not reflect the minimum requirements, but a safe excess intake. Of course, people who do not consistently take in near or at the RDA for a number of nutrients have a chance of becoming deficient over time.

RDAs do not account for unusual requirements caused by disease or environmental stress. In addition, the data used to determine the RDAs often did not include athletes, or the activity levels of the subjects were not reported. Therefore, the RDAs may not be an accurate means of evaluating the nutritional needs of people engaged in regular strenuous exercise.

Simplifying Food Label Recommendations

The reference values used to determine RDAs are age specific and gender specific, and for food-labeling purposes, an additional set of reference values had to be produced. Packages must be the same for men and women and for children and adults, so the RDA values had to be condensed into an acceptable recommendation for all groups. Originally, the labels contained the U.S. recommended dietary allowances (U.S. RDA). The U.S. RDA has been replaced by daily values (DV).

The U.S. RDA, which was based on RDAs, was developed by the Food and Drug Administration (FDA) in 1973 for use in food labeling. The U.S. RDA is a single number that does not vary with age and gender, except for children under 4 years of age and pregnant or lactating women, where the RDA is still the standard. The FDA usually picked the highest RDA level needed by age or gender group to determine the U.S. RDA. This value was adopted not only for the sake of simplicity in food packaging but also to reflect advances in scientific knowledge since 1968 with respect to essential nutrient requirements.

The DV is based on two sets of references: (1) the reference daily intakes, or RDI, which is a new name for the U.S. RDA, which makes up most of the DVs and provides a set of dietary references for essential vitamins and minerals, and (2) the daily reference value (DRV), a standard for proteins and various dietary components that have no RDA or other established nutrient standard (e.g., cholesterol, total fat, carbohydrate, dietary fiber, sodium, and potassium) (see figure 2.1 and table 2.1). On food labels all reference values are listed as DV although they can be either DRV or RDI. On current food labeling, the "% Daily Value" is the percentage of RDI or DRV available in a single serving.

Differences Between Countries

Some countries have formulated recommendations with respect to the amount of each nutrient that should be consumed. Therefore, definitions of RDA differ slightly in different countries (see appendixes C, D, and E). The United Nations and the European Union have formulated their own reference intakes, as have many individual countries. In the United Kingdom (appendix D) and Germany, the RDA has been redefined as the reference nutrient intake (RNI), and in Australia it has been redefined as the recommended daily intake (RDI) (appendix E). Canada now uses the same system as the United States, and Canada's RNI is being replaced by the DRI.

United Kingdom In the United Kingdom, the RNI, similar to the original RDA, is the level of intake required to meet the known nutritional needs of more than 97.5% of healthy persons. The estimated average requirement (EAR) in the United Kingdom is similar to the EAR in the United States, but unlike the United States, the United Kingdom also has a lower reference nutrient intake (LRNI) value. The LRNI represents an amount of a nutrient that is virtually certain to be inadequate. (Notably, the average intake of the trace element selenium in the United Kingdom falls well below the LRNI.). In the United Kingdom, estimated requirements for particular groups of the population are based on advice that was given by the Committee on Medical Aspects of Food and Nutrition Policy (COMA) back in the early 1990s. COMA examined the available scientific evidence and estimated nutritional requirements

■ TABLE 2.1 ■
Daily Reference Values

Food component	DRV
Total fat	Less than 65 g (30% of energy intake)
Saturated fat	Less than 20 g (10% of energy intake)
Cholesterol	Less than 300 mg
Total carbohydrate	300 g (60% of energy intake)
Dietary fiber	25 g (11.5 g/1,000 kcal)
Sodium	Less than 2,400 mg
Potassium	3,500 mg
Protein	50 g (10% of energy intake)

DRV based on 8 MJ (2,000 kcal) guideline.

of various groups within the UK population. These were published in the 1991 report *Dietary Reference Values for Food Energy and Nutrients for the United Kingdom*. Since this time, COMA has been superseded by the Scientific Advisory Committee on Nutrition (SACN). SACN will likely review the UK nutritional requirements in the near future because they are now over 10 years old. Meanwhile, SACN is focusing on nutrients about which there is cause for concern (e.g., iron, folate, and selenium).

Australia In Australia a set of guidelines was developed over the years that was referred to as the recommended dietary intakes for use in Australia. The last version of the RDIs was published in 1991 by the National Health and Medical Research Council in Australia, which was later also adopted in New Zealand. In July 1997 a workshop of invited experts, including representatives from New Zealand, was held in Sydney to discuss the need for a revision of the 1991 recommended dietary intakes for use in Australia. This was the beginning of the development of a new set of reference values for each nutrient, which would be referred to as nutrient reference values (NRVs). The NRVs were further updated in 2005.

The RDI was defined as "the levels of intake of essential nutrients considered, in the judgement of the National Health and Medical Research Council (NHMRC), on the basis of available scientific knowledge, to be adequate to meet the known nutritional needs of practically all healthy people." They therefore apply to group needs. RDIs exceed the actual nutrient requirements of practically all

healthy persons and are not synonymous with requirements.

Despite the emphasis on the population basis of the RDI, the RDIs were often misused in assessing dietary adequacy of individuals, or even foods. To overcome this misuse, many countries have moved to a system of reference values that retains the concept of the RDI while attempting to identify the average requirements needed by individuals. In Australia it was decided to retain the term *recommended dietary intake (RDI)* rather than use the term *RDA* for the average daily dietary intake level that is sufficient to meet the nutrient requirements of nearly all (97–98%) healthy people in a particular life stage and gender group.

In contrast to the U.S. and Canadian approach, the method used by the Australia and New Zealand working party retained the traditional concept of adequate physiological or metabolic function or avoidance of deficiency states as the prime reference point for establishing the EAR and RDIs and dealt separately with the issue of chronic disease prevention.

World Health Organization This approach differs somewhat from that used by the World Health Organization, Food and Agriculture Organization, and International Atomic Energy Agency (WHO–FAO–IAEA) Expert Consultation in *Trace Elements in Human Nutrition and Health* (WHO 1996). That publication uses the term *basal requirement* to indicate the level of intake needed to prevent pathologically relevant and clinically detectable signs of a dietary inadequacy.

Practical Guidelines for a Balanced Healthy Diet

Although the recommendations like the DRI may provide guidance on nutrient requirements, they are not a practical way of informing people about appropriate food choices. For example, how does someone know whether he or she is consuming about 0.8 g/kg of body weight of protein per day? A healthy diet is often referred to as a balanced diet that stresses variety and moderation. But how do we achieve a balanced diet? Nutritionists addressed this question early in the 20th century and developed several simple and comprehensive food guides, the most important of which is the food guide pyramid. The food guide pyramid has six categories of foods (see table 2.2).

As mentioned earlier, more than 40 nutrients are considered essential and the concept of a balanced diet refers to eating a variety of foods in moderation to support normal or optimal functioning. In the United States a food guide called **MyPyramid** was developed (see figure 2.2), based on a previous version called the food guide pyramid. The new guide distinguishes six food groups:

- Milk, yogurt, and cheese
- Meat, poultry, fish, eggs, dry beans, and nuts
- Bread, cereal, rice, and pasta
- Vegetables
- Fruits
- Fats, oils, and sweets

The foods in each category make a similar nutrient contribution. In previous versions of the guide, the only macronutrient with an RDA was protein. The latest version, however, includes recommendations for carbohydrate and fat to minimize the risk of chronic diseases. For adults the recommendation is that 45 to 65% of energy intake should be from carbohydrate, 20 to 35% from fat, and 10 to 35% from protein. Carbohydrates are found in the bread, cereal, rice, and pasta category as well as in the vegetable category and fruit category. But carbohydrates can also be found in the beans category and sweets category. Proteins and fats are found mostly in the meat, poultry, fish, eggs, dry beans, and nuts category. Solid fats are a major component of the oils and sweets category.

MyPyramid was developed by the United States Department of Agriculture (USDA) and represents the 2005 *Dietary Guidelines for Americans* (www.healthierus.gov/dietaryguidelines).

Many countries have developed their own guidelines. Canada has its own food guide (www.hc-sc.gc.ca/fn-an/food-guide-aliment/index_e.html). In the United Kingdom the food guide is depicted as a plate and is called the Eatwell Plate (figure 2.3). In Australia the food selection guide is called the Healthy Eating Pyramid.

MyPyramid is unique in that it includes advice about physical activity. In addition, the model stresses variety, proportionality, moderation, and individualization. Variety is symbolized by the six color bands, representing the five food groups (in orange, green, red, blue, and purple) and oils (yellow; not regarded as a separate food group). The figure illustrates that having all food groups in the diet is important. Proportionality, or balance, is shown by the different widths of the food groups. The width of each food group band serves as a general guideline to how much of each of the food groups should be consumed (the grains food group is relatively large, the meat and beans food group is relatively small, and oils should be used sparingly).

Moderation is represented by the narrowing of each food group from bottom to top. Some foods in each food group should be eaten in larger amounts than others. For example, in the grain group, whole-wheat, high-fiber foods should be consumed in larger quantities and refined grains should be

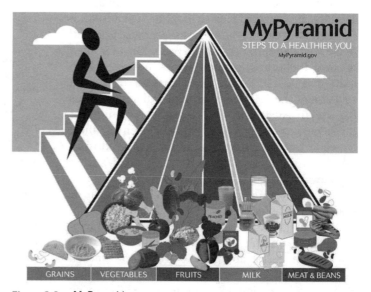

Figure 2.2 MyPyramid.

U.S. Department of Agriculture and the U.S. Department of Health and Human Services or USDA and DHHS.

■ **TABLE 2.2** ■

Major Nutrients in the Six Categories of the Food Guide Pyramid and the Most Important Nutrients That They Provide

Food categories	Essential nutrients
Breads, cereals, rice, pasta	Thiamin, niacin, riboflavin, iron
Dairy products: milk, yogurt, cheese	Calcium, protein, riboflavin, vitamin A
Meat, poultry, fish, eggs, dry beans, nuts	Protein, thiamin, niacin, iron
Vegetables	Vitamin A, vitamin C
Fruit	Vitamin A, vitamin C
Fats, oils, sweets*	Vitamin A, vitamin D, vitamin E

The asterisk (*) indicates a component that mainly adds to energy intake and does not provide micronutrients.

consumed in smaller quantities. The more active a person is, the more of these foods she or he can fit in the diet.

Personalization is shown by the person on the steps as well as by the slogan (Steps to a healthier you). The slogan also encourages gradual improvement. Physical activity, represented by the steps and the person climbing them, is included in the nutrition guidelines for the first time to remind people of the importance of daily physical activity. MyPyramid has a Web site that will help to develop an individualized food plan. The Web site also contains MyPyramid tracker (www.mypyramidtracker.gov/), a database containing more than 8,000 foods and 600 physical activities that will help people develop a specific plan.

Although the new MyPyramid may be an improvement over the previous version, it has also been criticized. Some have argued that the new MyPyramid lacks clarity and does not give information about what foods may be healthier or less healthy, requires people to be computer literate, and does not use height and weight to calculate energy needs. Overall, however, it provides a good guide for healthy nutrition. The American Dietetic Association (ADA) does not support the concept that a food is healthy or unhealthy. In a position stand the ADA warns that the value of food should be determined in the context of the total diet because classifying foods as good or bad may foster unhealthy eating behaviors. If consumed in moderation all foods can fit into a healthful diet (Nitzke et al. 2007).

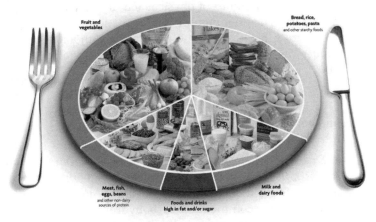

Figure 2.3 The Eatwell Plate in the United Kingdom.
© Crown copyright material is reproduced with the permission of the Controller of HMSO and Queen's Printer for Scotland.

Recommendations for healthy eating can be drawn up based on MyPyramid, *Dietary Guidelines for Americans*, and recommendations published by organizations and institutions in various countries. These guidelines are based on the status of research and may be helpful in the prevention of chronic diseases, including cardiovascular disease and cancer. The guidelines that follow are drawn from a variety of sources including (among others) MyPyramid, *Dietary Guidelines for Americans*, American Heart Association, American Dietetic Association, American Diabetes Association, and the Eatwell Plate.

■ *Balance food intake with physical activity to maintain a healthy weight.* Consuming moderate food portions and being physically active are important steps toward the prevention of obesity. Methods of regulating body weight will be discussed in detail in chapter 14.

■ *Be physically active.* People should aim to do at least 30 minutes of physical activity on most, if not all, days. The American College of Sports Medicine (ACSM) and the American Heart Association (AHA) have recently updated their physical activity guidelines. They recommend moderately intense aerobic exercise 30 minutes a day, 5 days a week or vigorously intense aerobic exercise 20 minutes a day, 3 days a week. Alternatively, people can undertake resistance exercise by performing 8 to 12 repetitions of each of 8 to 10 strength-training exercises twice a week.

Moderate-intensity physical activity means working hard enough to raise the heart rate and break a sweat yet still be able to carry on a conversation. Note that to lose weight or maintain weight loss, 60 to 90 minutes of physical activity may be necessary. The 30-minute recommendation is for the average healthy adult to maintain health and reduce the risk for chronic disease (Haskell et al. 2007).

■ *Eat a wide variety of nutrient-rich foods.* By eating a variety of foods from within each food group and between food groups, people will likely ingest adequate amounts of all essential nutrients.

■ *Eat a diet rich in vegetables, fruits, and whole-grain and high-fiber foods.* Consuming vegetables, fruits, and whole-grain and high-fiber foods will help to achieve the recommended carbohydrate intake and increase fiber intake. In addition, these foods contain relatively large amounts of phytonutrients, which have some beneficial health effects. Epidemiological studies have generally shown that diets high in whole-grain products (bread and cereals), legumes (beans and peas), fruits, and vegetables have significant health benefits. People should eat at least five portions of fruit and vegetables daily.

■ *Choose a diet moderate in total fat but low in saturated fat, trans fats, and cholesterol.* Apart from the essential fatty acids linoleic and alpha-linolenic acid, there is no specific requirement for fats. But fats are needed to help with the intake of fat-soluble vitamins. Because most foods contain some fats, the intake of these vitamins is usually not a problem. To lower total fat intake, dairy products that are fat free or low in fat are recommended.

The standard recommendation is to have an intake of saturated fatty acids below 10% of total energy intake and to limit cholesterol intake to 300 mg or less per day. People should eat fewer commercially prepared baked goods and avoid fast foods. These foods are generally high in fat and contain a significant amount of *trans* fatty acids. Epidemiological evidence based on up to 20 years of follow-up in prospective studies has consistently reported an adverse effect of *trans* fatty acids on coronary heart disease risk, although estimates of the size of the effect are smaller than originally thought. In addition, the evidence for cardioprotective effects of HDL cholesterol has strengthened the last few years, resulting in greater recognition of the potential hazards of *trans* fatty acids because of their unique properties in reducing HDL cholesterol compared with other fatty acid classes. The reduction in risk of coronary heart disease if all the population were to reduce *trans* fatty acid intake to less than 1% of total energy intake has been estimated to be about 7.5%. Based on this evidence *trans* fats have already been banned in some places. New York City, for example, passed a *trans* fat ban in July 2008.

■ *Cut back on beverages and foods high in calories and low in nutrition.* Beverages such as soft drinks and foods with added sugar contribute significantly to energy intake while not adding nutrients. The National Academy of Sciences recently advised that added sugars should make up no more than 25% of the total daily energy intake but that reducing this to 10% may be a healthier alternative. As discussed in chapter 1, added sugar intake has been associated with high blood triglyceride concentrations, dental cavities, and obesity.

■ *Use less sodium and salt.* Healthy adults are generally advised to reduce sodium intake to 2,300 mg of sodium per day or less. Most people consume 2,300 to 6,900 mg per day. One teaspoon of salt contains 2,000 mg of sodium. People should choose foods with little salt and prepare food with minimal amounts of salt. At the same time, they should consume potassium-rich foods, such as fruits and vegetables.

■ *Those who drink alcohol should drink in moderation.* Alcohol is a non-nutrient but contains 28 kJ per gram (7 kcal/g). Excessive alcohol consumption is one of the greatest health threats in today's society, and it can add significant energy to total daily intake without adding nutrients. Current evidence suggests that light to moderate alcohol intake (one drink per day) will cause no negative health effects for healthy adults. During pregnancy alcohol should be avoided. Current guidelines recommend drinking up to one drink per day for women and up to two drinks per day for men. A drink is defined as 360 ml (12 oz) of regular strength beer (5% alcohol), 150 ml (5 oz) of wine (12% alcohol), or 45 ml (1.5 oz) of spirits (40% alcohol). In the United Kingdom alcohol intake is measured in units. One unit is 8 g or 10 ml of pure alcohol, regardless of the type of alcohol being consumed (beer, wine, or spirit). British recommendations are two to three units of alcohol a day for women and three to four units for men. Units are often defined as being one small glass of wine, half a pint of beer, or one pub measure of spirits. But the alcohol content of different products varies. Some stronger beers and lagers may contain as many as five units of alcohol per 500 ml.

■ *Practice food hygiene and safety.* Food should be stored to avoid accumulation of bacteria. This practice often means refrigerating perishable foods and not storing foods for too long. Food should be cooked to a safe temperature to kill microorganisms, but people should be aware that excess grilling of meat can produce carcinogenic substances (heterocyclic amines). To avoid microbial foodborne illness, people should clean hands, food-contact surfaces, and fruits and vegetables. Meat and poultry should not be washed or rinsed. People should avoid raw (unpasteurized) milk or any products made from unpasteurized milk, raw or partially cooked eggs or foods containing raw eggs, raw or undercooked meat and poultry, unpasteurized juices, and raw sprouts.

■ *Avoid excessive intake of questionable food additives and nutrition supplements.* Although most food additives used in processed foods are safe, it is often recommended to avoid these additives. In addition, nutritional supplements are often claimed to have various positive health effects or performance benefits, but negative effects may occur. Nutrition supplements are not under strict regulation, may contain substances that are not

listed on the label, and therefore form a greater risk. Nutrition supplements will be discussed in detail in chapter 11.

Food Labels

Food labels are another useful tool for diet planning or nutritional assessment (see figure 2.4). Food labels help consumers make choices by providing detailed information about the nutrient content of food and the way in which that food fits into the overall diet. In the United States, food labeling is standardized as specified by the Nutrition

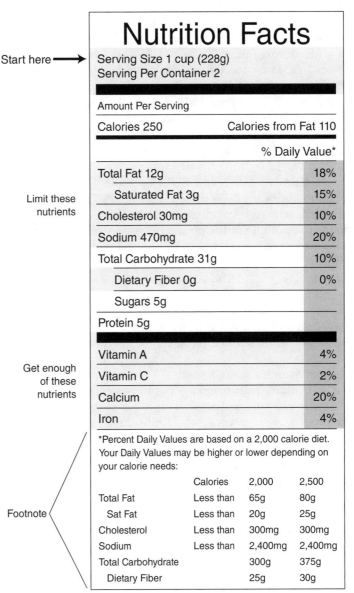

Figure 2.4 How to read a food label.

Labeling and Education Act of 1990. All packaged foods, except those produced by small businesses and those in packages too small to fit the labeling information, must be labeled. Serving size and the format of the food labels are identical on all products to make comparing foods easier. In Canada, nutrition labeling is voluntary but standardized. In other parts of the world, labels are not yet standardized. Food labeling laws regulate about 75% of all food consumed in the United States.

Two sets of reference values are used for reporting nutrients in nutrition labeling: (1) daily reference values (DRVs) and (2) reference daily intakes (RDIs). These values assist consumers in interpreting information about the amount of a nutrient that is present in a food and in comparing nutritional values of food products. DRVs are established for adults and children 4 or more years of age, as are RDIs, with the exception of protein. DRVs are provided for total fat, saturated fat, cholesterol, total carbohydrate, dietary fiber, sodium, potassium, and protein. RDIs are provided for vitamins and minerals and for protein for children less than 4 years of age and for pregnant and lactating women. To limit consumer confusion, however, the label includes a single term (i.e., daily value [DV]), to designate both the DRVs and RDIs. Specifically, the label includes the %DV, except that the %DV for protein is not required unless a protein claim is made for the product or the product is to be used by infants or children under 4 years of age. Figure 2.4 shows the DVs based on a daily energy intake of 2,000 kcal (8.4 MJ) for adults and children 4 or more years of age.

The information on food labels usually includes the name of the product; the name and contact details of the manufacturer, packager, or distributor; the net contents or weight of the package; and the date by which the product must be sold. The label also contains information about the ingredients in the food, expressed per unit of weight of the whole product. For instance, whole milk contains 3.5 g of fat, 3.2 g of protein, 4.7 g of carbohydrate (all sugars), 120 mg of calcium, 0.4 µg of vitamin B_{12}, and 270 kJ (65 kcal) per 100 g of milk. In the United States, the ingredients are expressed per serving; in Europe, they are expressed per serving as well as per 100 g. In the United States, the ingredients are also expressed as a percentage of the daily recommended value.

The nutrition facts label in the United States has a main top section that includes information that can vary with each product (serving size, energy content, and nutrition information). The lower part contains footnote information with daily values per 2,000 and 2,500 kcal diets. The place to start when looking at the nutrition facts label is the serving size and number of servings per package. Serving sizes are expressed in familiar terms like cups and pieces followed by the metric amount (grams). The next line on the label indicates the energy content and the energy from fat. The label then informs the consumer about key nutrients and the percentage of daily value. The nutrients are categorized by those whose intake should be limited, such as total grams of fat, saturated fats, *trans* fats, cholesterol, and sodium. Next are total carbohydrate and protein.

The carbohydrate entry is divided into sugars (which should be limited) and fiber (which should be encouraged). The nutrients are expressed in grams or milligrams per serving size but also as a percentage of daily value. The percent daily value (%DV) is based on the 2,000 kcal diet and expresses the content as a percentage of the recommended daily value. No %DV is given for sugar because no such value has been established. Keep in mind that the sugars on the label include the natural sugars in the product as well as the added sugars.

Labels often contain information that might be of interest to the consumer such as "low fat," "reduced fat," "fat free," "light," and "lean." The use of these and other terms is also regulated, and definitions of these terms have been established (see table 2.3). A consumer who buys a product with "low fat" on the label can be sure that it meets the definition established by the FDA (less than 3 g of fat per serving).

Many of the foods that we buy have statements on the label about their beneficial effects on the body, such as "Helps maintain a healthy heart" or "Aids digestion." These are examples of health claims. Previously, the rules on claims were extremely general, making it difficult for people to know what certain terms meant. In most countries specific rules now help protect consumers from misleading claims, which means that any claims made about the nutritional and health benefits of a food will be allowed only if they are based on good science. In Europe new rules came into effect on July 1, 2007, but the food industry has been given additional time to change its processes and comply with the new rules. Therefore, changes on products in shops in Europe will not occur for some time. The Food Standards Agency has collated a list of claims that will need to be approved in Europe, and in the future only claims that have been approved will be allowed on food.

■ TABLE 2.3 ■
Definitions of Nutrient Content Claims

Nutrient	Calories	Total fat	Sugars
Free (zero, no, without, trivial source of, negligible source of)	Calorie free: Less than 5 cal per reference amount and per labeled serving	Fat free: Less than 0.5 g per reference amount and per labeled serving (or for meals and main dishes, less than 0.5 g per labeled serving)	Sugar free: Less than 0.5 g sugars per reference amount and per labeled serving (or for meals and main dishes, less than 0.5 g per labeled serving)
Low (little, few for calories, contains a small amount of, low source of)	Few calories: 40 cal or less per reference amount (and per 50 g if reference amount is small); meals and main dishes: 120 cal or less per 100 g	Low fat: 3 g or less per reference amount (and per 50 g if reference amount is small); meals and main dishes: 3 g or less per 100 g and not more than 30% of calories from fat	Not defined; no basis for recommended intake
Reduced or less (lower, fewer for calories)	Fewer calories: At least 25% fewer calories per reference amount than an appropriate reference food; reference food may not be low calorie	Reduced fat: At least 25% less fat per reference amount than an appropriate reference food; reference food may not be low fat	Reduced sugar: At least 25% less sugars per reference amount than an appropriate reference food
Comments	Light or lite: If 50% or more of the calories are from fat, fat must be reduced by at least 50% per reference amount; if less than 50% of calories are from fat, fat must be reduced by at least 50% or calories must be reduced by at least 1/3 per reference amount	__% fat free: Allowed if food meets the requirements for low fat; 100% fat free: food must be fat free	No added sugars, or without added sugars: Allowed if no sugar or sugar-containing ingredient is added during processing; state if food is not low-calorie or reduced-calorie

Reference amount = reference amount customarily consumed. Small reference amount = reference amount of 30 g or less or 2 tbsp or less (for dehydrated foods that are typically consumed when rehydrated with water or a diluent containing an insignificant amount).

General claims about benefits to overall good health, such as "Healthy" or "Good for you," will be allowed only if accompanied by an appropriate and approved claim. This rule means that general claims must be backed up by an explanation about why the food is "healthy" or what makes it a "superfood." Labels cannot claim that a food can treat, prevent, or cure any disease or medical condition. These sorts of claims can only be made for licensed medicines.

For instance, calcium-rich products such as milk may reasonably claim to protect against osteoporosis. But no such claims are allowed on food labels. Only the claims summarized in table 2.4 are legal (detailed information on health claims can be found on the FDA Web site). Health claims can be used only when a certain percentage of the DV is present in the food product, and the claims must be backed up by scientific evidence, usually derived from epidemiological studies. In the United States, health claims must be accompanied by a disclaimer or otherwise qualified.

Processed Food and Additives

The term *processed food* refers to food treated to extend storage life or to improve taste, nutrition, color, or texture. Processing includes adding preservatives, colorings, or flavorings; fortifying, enriching, dehydrating, smoking, drying, or freezing; and a number of other treatments. Concern has been expressed that the nutritional quality of food has declined during recent years because the amount of processing has increased. Indeed, modern foods contain greater amounts of refined

■ **TABLE 2.4** ■

Health Claims Allowed on Food Labels

Health issue	Claim
Calcium and osteoporosis	Adequate calcium intake throughout life helps maintain bone health and reduce the risk of osteoporosis. A food must contain 20% or more of the DV for calcium.
Sodium and hypertension	Diets high in sodium may increase the risk of high blood pressure in some people; hence, a diet low in sodium may protect against hypertension.
Dietary fat and cancer	Diets high in fat increase the risk of some types of cancer; hence, low-fat diets may be protective.
Saturated fat and cholesterol and risk of coronary heart disease	Diets high in saturated fat and cholesterol increase blood cholesterol and thus the risk of heart disease. A diet low in saturated fat may therefore reduce this risk.
Foods high in fiber and cancer	Diets low in fat and rich in fiber-containing grain products, fruits, and vegetables may reduce the risk of some types of cancer.
Foods high in fiber and risk of coronary heart disease	Diets low in saturated fat and cholesterol and rich in fruits, vegetables, and grain products that contain fiber, particularly soluble fiber, may reduce the risk of coronary heart disease.
Folic acid and birth defects	Adequate folic acid intake by the mother reduces the risk of birth defects of the brain or spinal cord in her baby.
Dietary sugar and dental caries	Sugar-free foods that are sweetened with sugar alcohols do not promote tooth decay and may reduce the risk of dental caries.

A food carrying a health claim must be a naturally good source (10% or more of the daily value) for one of six nutrients (vitamin A, vitamin C, protein, calcium, iron, or fiber) and must not contain more than 20% of the daily value for fat, saturated fat, cholesterol, or sodium.

sugar, extracted oils, and white flour, products from which nutrients are lost in the refinement process. For example, in the bleaching of flour, 22 known essential nutrients are lost. Artificially ripened fruit contains much smaller amounts of micronutrients than naturally ripened fruit.

Many products are completely artificial, such as synthetic fruit juices, soft drinks, and nondairy creamers. Refined or artificial products may contain few or no nutrients but have the same energy content as their natural counterparts. Thus, the nutrient density (the amount of essential nutrients per unit of energy) of refined or artificial products is extremely low. However, although some nutrients are lost during processing, modern techniques used by most food manufacturers prevent major losses of nutrients. Frozen and canned vegetables, for example, contain amounts of essential nutrients similar to those in fresh vegetables. So although food processing can reduce nutrient density, the problem seems to be relatively small. In fact, most nutrients may be lost when the food is prepared at home. When vegetables are boiled or steamed, vitamins and minerals may end up in the water. With other cooking methods, heat-labile vitamins may be lost because of overcooking. The increased use of refined sugar, oils, unenriched white flour, salt,

and questionable additives is a greater concern. Food labels can help consumers make decisions about the quality of processed foods.

Food additives lengthen shelf lives; enhance color, texture, or taste; facilitate food preparation; or otherwise make food products more marketable. Certain additives, such as sugar, are derived from natural sources. Other additives, such as the artificial sweetener aspartame, are made synthetically. Although artificial sweeteners have been said to cause cancer, concrete evidence to support such claims has not been found. A selection of common artificial sweeteners is listed in table 2.5 (see also chapter 14 on weight management).

The color of food is an integral part of our culture. Even early civilizations such as Rome recognized that people "eat with their eyes" as well as their palates. Saffron was often used to provide a rich yellow color to various foods. Butter was colored yellow as far back as the 1300s. Today, the FDA carefully regulates all food color additives to ensure that foods with such additives are accurately labeled and safe to eat. Food colorants are both natural and synthetic. Natural colorants include beta-carotene, beet powder, carrot oil, carmine, fruit juice, paprika, riboflavin, saffron, and turmeric.

■ **TABLE 2.5** ■

Artificial Sweeteners and Their Characteristics

Sweetener	Sweetness × sucrose	Characteristics	Can be found in
Saccharin	300–500	• Not metabolized in the human body and is excreted in urine. • Fairly strong aftertaste.	Soft drinks, tabletop sweeteners, and a wide variety of foods (Sweet 'n Low).
Aspartame	180	• Derived from the two amino acids: phenylalanine and aspartate. • Contains 16 kJ (4 kcal) per g, but because such small amounts are needed it adds virtually no energy. • Aspartame is metabolized to its amino acids, phenylalanine and aspartate. • The taste of aspartame can be quite pleasant, and it is therefore sometimes added to foods to improve taste.	Although aspartame is used in a wide variety of food products, the disadvantage of aspartame is that it cannot be used in foods that need to be heated. At high temperatures aspartame will denature. Aspartame also has limited stability in foods with a low pH such as soft drinks. Aspartame is sold under the brand name Nutrasweet.
Acesulfame potassium	200	• Not metabolized in the body and is excreted in urine (noncaloric sweetener).	Sold under the brand name Sunnet.
Sorbitol	0.5–0.7	• Is produced from sugar but contains only 10.4 kJ (2.6 kcal) per g compared with 16 kJ (4 kcal) for sucrose. • Excessive consumption of sorbitol (more than 50 g) can cause gastrointestinal problems.	Various food products.
Sucralose	300–1000	• Discovered in 1976 and approved by the FDA in 1998. • A relatively new artificial sweetener synthesized from sucrose. • Sucralose is absorbed only in small quantities, and the small amounts that are absorbed are excreted in urine.	Various food products.
Xylitol	1	• Contains slightly less energy than sucrose (2.4 kcal per g).	Chewing gum, candy, and oral health products.
Stevia	200	• Stevia sweetener is a natural sweetener made from a herbal plant extract (Stevia rebaudiana). • High stability at low pH and high temperature. • Can provide long shelf life; cooking and baking resistant.	Chewing gum, candy, ice cream, yogurt, and soft drinks.

Fat Substitutes

Fat substitutes have one or more of the technical effects of fat in food but are not absorbed or metabolized as fat. The three types of fat substitutes include carbohydrate-based fat substitutes, which use plant polysaccharides in place of fat; proteins and microparticulated proteins, which block fat absorption; and fat-based fat substitutes, which also block fat absorption.

Examples of carbohydrate-based fat replacements are corn syrup solids, dextrin, maltodextrin, and modified food starch. These fat substitutes have little or no taste and contain less energy than fat does. Dietary fibers such as cellulose gel, cellulose gum, guar gum, insulin, and pectin have some of the properties of fat but minimal absorption. A protein-based fat substitute sold under the name Simplesse is approved for use in low-temperature foods such as ice cream. It contains 4 to 8 kJ/g (1 to 2 kcal/g).

Probably the most studied fat substitute is Olestra (Olean). Olestra looks like fat, cooks like fat, and gives foods all the rich taste and "mouth feel" of ordinary fat. But unlike ordinary fats and oils, Olestra is not digested or absorbed in the body and therefore contributes no fat or calories to the diet. Olestra is made from sucrose polyester, which is composed of sucrose with six to eight fatty acids bound to it. These fatty acids are from vegetable oils such as soybean or corn oil. Because the Olestra molecule is large in comparison with a fat molecule, it is not hydrolyzed by the body's digestive enzymes. It passes through the digestive system unchanged. Olestra is currently approved for snack foods such as chips and crackers. Because Olestra is not absorbed, the absorption of fat-soluble vitamins is reduced. Therefore, products containing Olestra are enriched with vitamins A, D, E, and K. It has been argued, however, that this enrichment may not solve nutrient-depletion problems. Olestra also has several side effects including diarrhea-like symptoms. Although the FDA considers the fat substitutes already on the market safe, their long-term or cumulative health effects are unknown.

Analyzing Dietary Intake

As discussed in this chapter, a list of recommended nutrient intakes and guidelines for the population is available, but the only way that people can get a good idea of whether their intake is within these recommendations is to analyze their diet. This section deals with methods to analyze the diet in more detail.

Analyzing dietary intake can be useful for several reasons. The average intake in a group of athletes can be studied, and the data can be used in conjunction with biochemical or anthropometric data to inform them of the adequacy of their diet. Dietary intake data can also be used in conjunction with a medical report or to explain the incidence or prevalence of health problems. Such measurements can also be used for educational purposes, and the efficacy of nutritional advice or intervention programs can be investigated. Several methods

have been developed to measure dietary intake (see table 2.6), and each method has advantages and disadvantages.

After the nutrient intake information is obtained, it can be compared with the recommendations. A simple but not especially accurate comparison is with a guide such as the food guide pyramid. When a 3-day to 7-day dietary survey is completed, however, the intake can be analyzed in detail. To calculate the intake of specific nutrients, food labels or one of many food composition databases can be used. In the United States the major source of information is the USDA Nutrient Database, which is available online (USDA 2003). Various software packages and some online programs use this database or other databases to calculate food intake. In all cases, the exact amount and kind of food must be entered in the computer program. If a food is not included in the database, an appropriate substitute should be chosen. Most such programs allow the user to add new products to the database, which can be done using information on the food label. The software will usually produce an average intake over 24 hours for all macronutrients and micronutrients. These values can then be compared with the recommended amounts.

Three-Day Food Record

The 3-day dietary survey, or diet record, is a relatively simple and reasonably accurate way to determine the total daily energy intake and the quality of food. The 3-day log should represent a normal eating pattern. Inclusion of 2 weekdays and 1 day during a weekend is recommended. Calculations of energy intake from records of daily food consumption are usually within 10% of the actual energy intake. This method provides reliable results for the intake of some nutrients such as carbohydrate and water, but longer periods may be required to get a more reliable classification of individual intake for nutrients such as cholesterol and fat and some of the micronutrients.

To obtain an accurate measure of food, common measuring tools may be used, including a ruler to measure the length, width, and height of food; standard measuring cups, teaspoons, and tablespoons to determine volume; and a balance to determine weight to the nearest gram. A weighed food intake is an accurate measurement, but individuals must be motivated to perform this activity. Poor compliance has been reported with weighed food records, and the use of household measuring devices is often the preferred method. Weighed food records,

Methods to Estimate Nutrient Intake

Method	Short description	Advantages	Disadvantages
PROSPECTIVE METHODS			
3-day dietary survey	Recording all foods consumed for 3 days	• Fairly accurate • Inexpensive • Provides detailed information • Provides information about eating habits	• May not represent normal diet • Tends to underestimate energy intake
3-day weighed food record	Weighing and recording all foods consumed for 3 days	• Accurate • Inexpensive • Provides detailed information • Provides information about eating habits	• Demanding for respondent • Potential compliance problems • May not represent normal diet • Tends to underestimate energy intake
7-day dietary survey	Recording all foods consumed for 7 days	• Fairly accurate • Inexpensive • Provides detailed information • Provides information about eating habits	• Demanding for respondent • Compliance may diminish after 4 days • May not represent normal diet • Tends to underestimate energy intake
7-day weighed food record	Weighing and recording all foods consumed for 7 days	• Accurate • Inexpensive • Provides detailed information • Provides information about eating habits	• Highly demanding for respondent • Compliance may diminish after 4 days • May not represent normal diet • Tends to underestimate energy intake
Duplicate food collections	Saving a duplicate of each food for chemical analysis	• Probably the most accurate method • Provides detailed information	• Expensive (analysis) • Time consuming • May affect food choice • Demanding for respondent • Likely to underestimate food intake
RETROSPECTIVE METHODS			
24-hour recall	Questionnaire or interview to assess dietary intake in the previous 24 hours	• Good response rate • Relatively easy • Inexpensive • Can be used to rank nutrient intakes in groups of people	• May not represent usual food intake • Memory bias • Underestimates total energy intake • Does not provide quantitative data
Food frequency	Questionnaire or interview with questions about the frequency of intake of certain foods	• Good response rate • Relatively easy • Inexpensive • Can be used to rank nutrient intakes in groups of people in qualitative terms	• Memory bias • Underestimates total energy intake • Does not provide quantitative data • Overestimates at low energy intake and underestimates at high energy intake • May not represent normal food intake
Diet history	Combination of 24-hour recall and food frequency questionnaire	• Can be used to rank nutrient intakes in groups of people	• Requires trained interviewer • Takes longer to complete than 24-hour recall or food frequency questionnaire

however, may be the method of choice for use with highly motivated athletes.

All foods consumed, including beverages, should be recorded using the blank 3-day food logs on the pages of the diary (see table 2.7). When completing a diet record, the person should always keep the sheets nearby and record the food intake while consuming the food. When the food log is completed, the energy intake and nutrient intakes can be calculated using either a software package or a food table. People should use a software package or food table of the country in which they live because many products are specific to particular countries.

Most people are only vaguely aware of what they eat. Without instruction, food records lack sufficient detail to be useful for most research purposes. Errors occur mainly because of memory failures. In general, the common foods are recorded accurately, but the uncommon foods are sometimes poorly registered. Most errors are made in reporting the frequency of consumption. Errors in estimating portion size are common as well. If food is not weighed, the mass of various foods may be considerably under- or overestimated. Errors are sometimes as large as 50% for foods and 20% for particular nutrients (Burke and Deakin 2000; Shils et al. 1999). Training and instructing the persons who are registering their food intake can reduce errors, but the instructions should be repeated several times. On an individual level, the 3-day food survey is generally accepted as one of the best methods to assess nutritional intake. But this method also has disadvantages. Overweight people tend to underestimate their portion sizes, whereas underweight people tend to overestimate portions (Johansson et al. 1998). People may not report their food intake accurately, which makes coding of the specific food type difficult. For example, writing "four potatoes" is not sufficiently informative. Were the potatoes large or small? Were they boiled, baked, fried, or raw? Were the skins removed?

Some food records may be illegible, introducing more coding errors. Therefore, people must be carefully instructed and asked to provide as much detail as possible.

Seven-Day Food Record

The 7-day dietary survey is identical to the 3-day survey, except for the duration of the recording period. The extended recording time may allow a more reliable classification of a person's normal diet and nutrient intake. The 7-day survey includes all weekdays and the 2 days of the weekend. The disadvantage of this method is that with a long period of recording, people may become tired of recording and forget to write down foods consumed, resulting in a less-accurate nutritional assessment. Often, lack of compliance is reported after about 4 days. Besides the 3-day and 7-day dietary surveys, other alternatives have been used, such as 4, 5, or 6 days of recording and even up to 12 months of continuous recording.

Duplicate Food Collections

A highly accurate method is the duplicate food collections method, which involves preparing two portions of food and saving a duplicate of everything that is eaten. These portions are then collected and put in a blender for chemical analysis of the nutrient content. This method, used mainly for research purposes, is extremely expensive because of the costs of the chemical analyses, especially when a wide range of nutrients is investigated. The method also places a burden on the individual and is likely to affect food choices. This method may result in underreporting of food intake.

Twenty-Four-Hour Recall

The most common technique of assessing food intake is the 24-hour recall. A trained interviewer asks participants on one or more occasions to

■ **TABLE 2.7** ■
Sample of an Accurate Food Diary

Time	Place	Kind or brand	How prepared?	Amount
7:00 a.m.	Home	Cornflakes, Kellogg's		1 small bowl
9:00 a.m.	Office	Whole milk		1 glass (200 ml)
		Coffee	Filter	1 cup
		Sugar		1 teaspoon

describe the food, drinks, and dietary supplements that they have consumed during the previous 24 hours. The data obtained may include information about the time of food intake, preparation of the food, and the eating environment.

The advantages of the 24-hour recall technique are that it is easy to administer, time efficient, and inexpensive. Disadvantages include the likelihood of underreporting, even when participants are interviewed by a skilled dietitian; the underestimation of energy and nutrient intake, sometimes by as much as 20%; and the tendency of overweight people to underestimate their portions (underweight persons tend to overestimate portions) (Johansson et al. 1998). In addition, this technique relies heavily on memory, which makes it unsuitable for certain groups, such as the elderly.

The data obtained from 24-hour recalls are more accurate when they are repeated several times at random. This approach also corrects somewhat for the day-to-day variation in food intake. The 24-hour recall method is a reasonably good way to estimate nutrient intake in a group of people, but it is less valuable for individual use. But it can give a foundation for pursuing a more detailed picture of someone's nutrient intake. Obtaining more than one 24-hour recall within a week and including at least one weekend day is the preferred method. One recall per week is unlikely to represent usual intake.

Food Frequency Questionnaire

A food frequency questionnaire (see table 2.8) is often used to get a general picture of someone's patterns of food intake. Individuals respond to a series of questions about the frequency of their food intake: How often do you eat red meat? How often do you eat fruit? How often do you drink milk? Questions about portion size, food preparation, and supplement use can be included, but their use is not a standard procedure. A problem with this method is that the products mentioned in the questionnaire may not represent the respondent's actual food intake.

The food frequency questionnaire is a relatively easy and quick method, but it does not itemize intake on a specific day. The information obtained is qualitative rather than quantitative. The food frequency questionnaire is regularly used in clinical or research settings. If investigators are interested only in one particular food item or food group, the food frequency questionnaire can be extremely

■ TABLE 2.8 ■
Food Frequency Questionnaire

	Once a day	Twice or more a day	Once a week	Twice or more a week	Once a month	Twice or more a month
Milk Whole Reduced fat Nonfat		✓	✓			
Yogurt Whole Reduced fat Nonfat					✓	
Cheese Hard Soft Reduced fat		✓		✓		
Ice cream Regular Reduced fat					✓	

useful. Food frequency questionnaires have been developed for specific populations to address the intakes in various cultures and populations with differing age (e.g., children).

Diet History

A diet history provides general information about dietary habits and patterns. This technique was originally described by Burke in 1947 and combines the 24-hour recall with a food frequency questionnaire. Combining these different methods usually gives a better view of a person's dietary habits by asking questions of the following type: Do you always have breakfast? Do you skip lunch? Did you drink milk as an adolescent? Diet history can provide information about changes in dietary habits, including seasonal changes. A diet history takes about 20 minutes to complete. This method also requires substantial skill from the interviewer, who must be a well-trained dietitian.

KEY POINTS

■ Essential nutrients cannot be synthesized in the body and are therefore required for some critical functions throughout life, and they are required in the diet for growth, health, and survival. Absence from the diet or inadequate intake results in characteristic signs of a deficiency, disease, and ultimately death.

■ Nonessential nutrients can be synthesized in the body from their precursors.

■ Humans have an essential requirement for over 40 nutrients.

■ General guidelines for healthy eating include balancing food intake with physical activity to maintain a healthy body weight; being physically active; eating a wide variety of nutrient-rich foods; eating a diet rich in vegetables, fruits, whole-grain foods, and high-fiber foods; selecting a diet that is moderate in total fat but low in saturated fat, *trans* fat, and cholesterol; cutting back on beverages and foods that are high in energy but low in nutrients; using less sodium and salt; drinking alcohol in moderation; practicing food hygiene and safety; and avoiding excessive intake of food additives and supplements.

■ The term *processed food* refers to food treated to extend storage life or to improve taste, nutrition, color, or texture. Processing includes adding preservatives, colorings, or flavorings; fortifying, enriching, dehydrating, smoking, drying, or freezing; and a number of other treatments. Concern has been expressed that the nutritional quality of food has declined during recent years because the amount of processing has increased.

■ Several methods are used to assess food intake and diet composition. These methods include diet history, 24-hour recalls, food frequency questionnaires, self-reported food records, and weighed food records. The methods differ substantially in their accuracy and practicality.

RECOMMENDED READINGS

Bender, D.A., and A.E. Bender. 1997. *Nutrition. A reference handbook.* Oxford: Oxford University Press.

Food and Nutrition Board. 2005. *Dietary reference intakes for energy, carbohydrate, fiber, fat, fatty acids, cholesterol, protein, and amino acids (macronutrients).* Washington, DC: National Academies Press.

Gibney, M.J., I. Macdonald, & H. Roche, eds. 2008. *Nutrition and metabolism (the Nutrition Society textbook).* Oxford: Blackwell Science.

Mann, J., and A.S. Truswell. 2002. *Essentials of human nutrition.* Oxford: Oxford University Press.

Shils, M.E., J.A. Olson, M. Shike, A.C. Ross, B. Caballero, and R.J. Cousins, eds. 2005. *Modern nutrition in health and disease.* Baltimore: Williams and Wilkins.

USDA. 2005. *Dietary guidelines for Americans.* www.health.gov/DietaryGuidelines/.

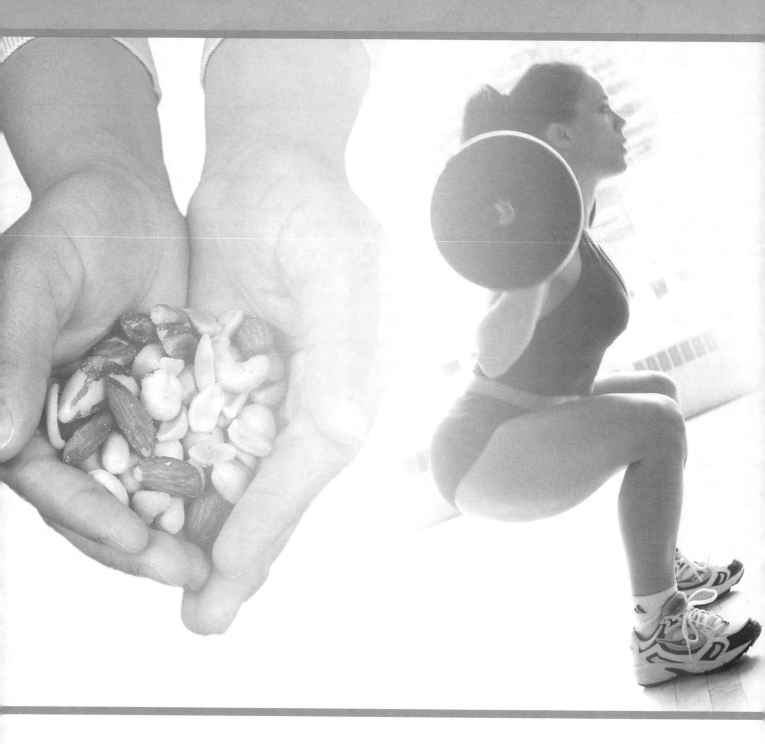

OBJECTIVES

After studying this chapter, you should be able to do the following:

- Describe the structure of skeletal muscle and explain the process of muscle contraction

- Describe the characteristics of the various muscle fiber types

- Describe the metabolic pathways that supply energy for muscle contraction

- Describe the nature and size of body fuel stores

- Describe the factors involved in the control of fuel mobilization and utilization

- Describe the metabolic responses and main causes of fatigue in moderate- and high-intensity exercise

3

Fuel Sources for Muscle and Exercise Metabolism

Key Terms

An in-depth understanding of sport nutrition requires some knowledge of biochemistry, which usually refers to the study of events such as reactions, energy transfer, and transport processes at the subcellular and molecular levels. Those who lack a basic understanding of biochemistry and cell biology should refer to appendix A, which explains some of the basic principles. This chapter describes the sources of energy available for muscle force generation and explains how acute exercise modifies energy metabolism through intracellular effects and the action of hormones (for further details see the books by Maughan and Gleeson 2004 and Hargreaves and Spriet 2006). The diet before exercise and feeding during exercise influence the hormonal and metabolic responses to exercise. Training also modifies the metabolic response to exercise, and training-induced adaptations encompass both biochemical responses (e.g., changes in enzyme activities in trained muscles) and physiological responses (e.g., changes in maximal cardiac output and maximal oxygen uptake, $\dot{V}O_2$max). These influences are also described in this chapter.

Subcellular Skeletal Muscle Structure

Muscles are composed of long, cylindrical cells called fibers. These fibers contain the internal organelles and structures that allow muscle to contract and relax. Individual muscles are made up of many parallel fibers that may extend the entire length of the muscle. Inside the muscle fiber is the sarcoplasm (muscle cell cytoplasm), a red viscous fluid containing nuclei, mitochondria, myoglobin, and about 500 threadlike 1 to 3 mm thick myofibrils that are continuous from end to end in the muscle fiber. The red color is caused by myoglobin, an intracellular respiratory pigment. Surrounding the myofibrils is an elaborate baglike membranous structure called the sarcoplasmic reticulum. Its interconnecting membranous tubules lie in the narrow spaces between the myofibrils, surrounding and running parallel to them. Energy is stored in the sarcoplasm as fat (triacylglycerol droplets), **glycogen,** phosphocreatine (PCr), and adenosine triphosphate (ATP).

The myofibrils are composed of overlapping thin and thick filaments made of protein, and the arrangement of these filaments gives skeletal muscle its striated appearance when viewed through a microscope. The thick filaments are composed of myosin molecules, each of which consists of a rodlike tail and a globular head. The latter contains adenosine triphosphatase (ATPase) activity sites and actin-binding sites. ATP is the energy currency of the cell. The breakdown of ATP to adenosine diphosphate (ADP) and inorganic phosphate (Pi) by the myosin ATPase provides the energy for muscle contraction. The thin filaments are composed of actin molecules and several regulatory proteins. Globular actin (G-actin) monomers are polymerized into long strands of fibrous actin (F-actin). Two F-actin strands twisted together in ropelike fashion form the backbone of each thin filament. Rod-shaped tropomyosin molecules spiral about the F-actin chains. The other main protein present in the thin filaments is troponin, which contains three subunits. One of these subunits, troponin-I, binds to actin; another subunit, troponin-T, binds to tropomyosin; and the third subunit, troponin-C, binds to calcium ions. A sarcomere is the smallest contractile unit, or segment, of a muscle fiber and is the region between two Z-lines (see figure 3.1).

Force Generation in Skeletal Muscle

When calcium and ATP are present in sufficient quantities, the filaments form actomyosin and

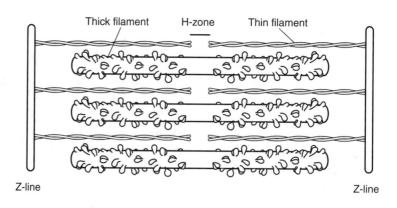

Figure 3.1 *(a)* Longitudinal cross section of a sarcomere shows the molecular components of the myofilaments and the arrangement of the thick and thin filaments between two Z-lines in a myofibril.

shorten by sliding over each other. Sliding begins when the myosin heads form cross-bridges attached to active sites on the actin subunits of the thin filaments. Each cross-bridge attaches and detaches several times during a contraction, pulling the thin filaments toward the center of the sarcomere in a ratchetlike action. When a muscle fiber contracts, its sarcomeres shorten throughout the cell, and the whole muscle fiber shortens.

The attachment of the myosin cross-bridges requires the presence of calcium ions. In the relaxed muscle, calcium is sequestered in the sarcoplasmic reticulum. Without calcium, the myosin binding sites on actin are physically blocked by the tropomyosin rods, as illustrated in figure 3.1. Electrical excitation passing as an action potential along the muscle cell membrane (sarcolemma) and down the T-tubules releases calcium from the sarcoplasmic reticulum into the sarcoplasm, subsequently causing activation and contraction of the filament array. The calcium ions bind to troponin, causing a change in its shape that physically moves tropomyosin away from the myosin binding sites on the underlying actin chain.

Excitation is initiated by the arrival of a nerve impulse at the muscle membrane via the motor end plate. Activated, or "cocked," myosin heads now bind to the actin, and the myosin head changes from its activated configuration to its bent shape, which causes the head to pull on the thin filament, sliding it toward the center of the sarcomere. This action represents the power stroke of the cross-bridge cycle, and simultaneously ADP and inorganic phosphate (Pi) are released from the myosin head. As a new ATP molecule binds to the myosin head at the ATPase activity site, the myosin cross-bridge detaches from the actin. Hydrolysis of the ATP to ADP and Pi by the ATPase provides the energy required to return the myosin to its activated state, giving it the potential energy needed for the next cross-bridge cycle. ATP is the only source of energy that can be used directly not only for muscle contraction but also for other energy-requiring processes in the cell.

While the myosin is in the activated state, the ADP and Pi remain attached to the myosin head. The myosin head can attach to another actin unit farther along the thin filament, and the cross-bridge cycle is repeated. Sliding of the filaments continues as long as calcium is present in the sarcoplasm at a concentration in excess of 10 μmol/L. Removal and sequestration of the calcium by the ATP-dependent calcium pump (ATPase) of the sarcoplasmic reticulum restore the tropomyosin inhibition of cross-bridge formation and the muscle fiber relaxes.

Fiber Types

The existence of different fiber types in skeletal muscle has long been recognized. On the basis of their contraction speed and metabolic characteristics, muscle fibers can be broadly classified as type I fibers or type II fibers. The physiological and biochemical bases for these differences and their functional significance have only recently been established. Much of the impetus for investigating these differences has come from the realization that success in athletic activities that require the ability to generate either high power output or great endurance is related to the

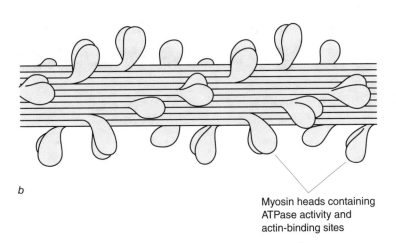

b

Myosin heads containing ATPase activity and actin-binding sites

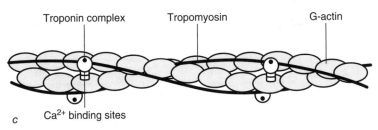

Troponin complex   Tropomyosin   G-actin

c   Ca²⁺ binding sites

Figure 3.1   *(b)* The thick filaments are composed of myosin molecules. Each myosin molecule consists of a rodlike tail and a globular head. The latter contains ATPase activity sites and actin-binding sites. *(c)* The thin filaments are composed of actin molecules and the regulatory proteins tropomyosin and tropinin.

proportions of the fiber types in the muscles. The muscle fibers are, however, extremely plastic (i.e., adaptable), and although the distribution of fiber type is genetically determined and not easily altered, an appropriate training program will have a major effect on the metabolic potential of the muscle, regardless of the proportion of fiber types.

Human muscle fibers are commonly divided into types I, IIa, and IIX, which are analogous to animal muscle fibers that have been classified on the basis of direct observation as slow-twitch fibers, fast-twitch fatigue-resistant fibers, and fast-twitch fatigable fibers, respectively. The myosin of the different fiber types exists in different molecular forms (isoforms), and the myofibrillar ATPase activity of the different isoforms displays differential pH sensitivity that provides the basis for the differential chemical staining and identification of fiber types. The biochemical characteristics of the three fiber types are summarized in table 3.1.

Type I Fibers

Type I fibers are small-diameter red cells that contain relatively slow-acting myosin ATPases and hence contract slowly. The red color is caused by myoglobin, which is capable of binding oxygen and releasing it only at very low partial pressures. Type I fibers have numerous energy-producing mitochondria, mostly located close to the periphery of the fiber, near the blood capillaries that provide a rich supply of oxygen and nutrients. Type I fibers possess a high capacity for oxidative metabolism, are extremely fatigue resistant, and are specialized for repeated contractions over prolonged periods.

Type II Fibers

Type IIX fibers contain little myoglobin. They possess rapidly acting myosin ATPases; therefore, their contraction (and relaxation) time is relatively fast. These fibers have fewer mitochondria and a poorer capillary supply, but they have greater glycogen and phosphocreatine stores compared with the type I fibers. High glycogenolytic and glycolytic enzyme activity gives type IIX fibers a high capacity for rapid (but relatively short-lived) ATP production in the absence of oxygen (anaerobic capacity). Lactic acid accumulates quickly in these fibers, and they fatigue rapidly. Thus, these

■ TABLE 3.1 ■

Biochemical Characteristics of Human Muscle Fiber Types

Characteristic	Type I	Type IIa	Type IIX
Nomenclature	Slow, red Fatigue resistant Oxidative	Fast, red Fatigue resistant Oxidative/glycolytic	Fast, white Fatigable Glycolytic
Capillary density	1.0	0.8	0.6
Mitochondrial density	1.0	0.7	0.4
Myoglobin content	1.0	0.6	0.3
Phosphorylase activity	1.0	2.1	3.1
PFK activity	1.0	1.8	2.3
Citrate synthase activity	1.0	0.8	0.6
SDH activity	1.0	0.7	0.4
Glycogen content	1.0	1.3	1.5
Triacylglycerol content	1.0	0.4	0.2
Phosphocreatine content	1.0	1.2	1.2
Myosin ATPase activity	1.0	>2	>2

Values of metabolic characteristics of type II fibers are shown relative to those found in type I fibers. PFK = phosphofructokinase; SDH = succinate dehydrogenase.

fibers are best suited for delivering rapid, powerful contractions for brief periods. The metabolic characteristics of type IIa fibers lie between the extreme properties of type I and type IIX fibers. Type IIa fibers contain fast-acting myosin ATPases like the type IIX fibers but have an oxidative capacity more like that of type I fibers.

The differences in activation threshold of the motor neurons supplying the different fiber types determine the order in which fibers are recruited during exercise and in turn influence the metabolic response to exercise. During most forms of movement, an orderly hierarchy of motor unit recruitment occurs that roughly corresponds with a progression from type I to type IIa to type IIX. Light exercise uses mostly type I fibers, moderate exercise uses both type I and type IIa fibers, and severe exercise uses all fiber types.

Muscle Fiber Composition

Muscles contain a mixture of the three different fiber types, although the proportions in which the types are found differ substantially among muscles and can also differ among individuals. For example, muscles involved in maintaining posture (e.g., soleus in the leg) have a high proportion (usually >70%) of type I fibers, which is in keeping with their function of maintaining prolonged but relatively weak contractions. Type II fibers, however, predominate in muscles that produce rapid movements, such as the muscles of the hand and the eye. Muscles such as the quadriceps group in the leg contain a variable mixture of fiber types. The vastus lateralis muscle in the quadriceps muscle group of successful marathon runners has a high percentage (about 80%) of type I fibers, whereas the same muscle in elite sprinters contains a higher percentage (about 60%) of type II fibers. The fiber type composition of muscles is genetically determined and is not pliable to any significant degree by training. Hence, athletic capabilities are mostly inborn (assuming that the person realizes her or his genetic potential through appropriate nutrition and training).

Energy for Muscle Force Generation

Energy is the potential for performing work or producing force. In muscle, energy from the hydrolysis of ATP by myosin ATPase activates specific sites on the contractile elements, as described previously, causing the muscle fiber to shorten.

The hydrolysis of ATP yields approximately 31 kJ (7 kcal) of free energy per mole of ATP (a mole is equivalent to molecular weight in grams) degraded to ADP and Pi:

$$ATP + H_2O \rightarrow ADP + H^+ + Pi - 31 \text{ kJ per mole of ATP}$$

Active reuptake of calcium ions by the sarcoplasmic reticulum also requires ATP, as does the restoration of the membrane potential of the muscle cell through the action of the Na^+–K^+–ATPase (commonly known as the sodium pump).

Three mechanisms are involved in the resynthesis of ATP for muscle force generation: (1) PCr hydrolysis, (2) glycolysis, which involves metabolism of glucose-6-phosphate, derived from muscle glycogen or blood-borne glucose, and produces ATP by substrate-level phosphorylation reactions, and (3) the products of carbohydrate, fat, protein, and alcohol metabolism enter the tricarboxylic acid (TCA) cycle in the mitochondria and are oxidized to carbon dioxide and water; this process is known as oxidative phosphorylation and yields energy for the synthesis of ATP.

These mechanisms regenerate ATP at sufficient rates to prevent a significant fall in the intramuscular ATP concentration. The resting concentration of ATP in skeletal muscle is about 4 to 5 mmol/kg wet weight (w.w.) of muscle, which can only provide enough energy to sustain a few seconds of intense exercise. PCr breakdown and glycolysis are anaerobic mechanisms that occur in the sarcoplasm. Each uses only one specific substrate for energy production: PCr and glucose-6-phosphate, respectively. The aerobic processes in the mitochondria utilize a variety of different substrates, and the sarcoplasm contains a variety of enzymes that can convert carbohydrates, fats, and proteins into usable substrate, primarily a two-carbon acetyl group linked to coenzyme A (acetyl-CoA), which can be completely oxidized in the mitochondria with the resultant production of ATP. A general summary of the main energy sources and pathways of energy metabolism is presented in figure 3.2.

Phosphocreatine in Anaerobic Metabolism

Some of the energy for ATP resynthesis is supplied rapidly and without the need for oxygen. Within the muscle fiber, the concentration of PCr is three to four times greater than that of ATP. When PCr is broken down to creatine and Pi by the action of the enzyme creatine kinase (CK), a large amount of free energy is released (43 kJ [10.3 kcal] per mole of PCr). Because PCr has a higher free energy of hydrolysis than ATP, its phosphate is donated directly to the ADP molecule to re-form ATP. When the ATP content begins to fall during exercise, PCr

is broken down, releasing energy for restoration of ATP. During extremely intense exercise, PCr can be almost completely depleted. The reactions of ATP and PCr hydrolysis are reversible, however, and when energy is readily available from other sources (oxidative phosphorylation), creatine and phosphate can be rejoined to form PCr:

$$ADP + PCr + H^+ \rightarrow ATP + Cr - 43 \text{ kJ per mole of PCr}$$

Note that the resynthesis of ATP through the breakdown of PCr buffers some of the hydrogen ions formed as a result of ATP hydrolysis. This action helps to prevent a rapid acidification of the muscle sarcoplasm, which could induce premature failure of the contractile mechanism.

The PCr in muscle is immediately available at the onset of exercise and can be used to resynthesize ATP quickly. This rapid energy transfer corresponds to the ability to produce high power output (see table 3.2). The major disadvantage of this process compared with other means of regenerating ATP is its limited capacity. The total amount of energy available is small (see table 3.3).

An additional pathway to regenerate ATP when ATP and PCr stores are depleted is through a kinase

---

Sources of ATP for Muscle Force Generation

1. **PCr hydrolysis:** Rapid energy release without the need for oxygen (anaerobic metabolism); occurs in the sarcoplasm.

2. **Glycolysis:** Energy available from the breakdown of glucose (anaerobic metabolism) through uptake from the blood, muscle glycogen breakdown, the glycolytic pathway (figure 3.3, p. 55); occurs in the sarcoplasm.

3. **Oxidative phosphorylation:** Carbohydrates, fats, and proteins are oxidized (aerobic metabolism); occurs in the mitochondrion. See figures 3.4 through 3.8 (p. 56-60).

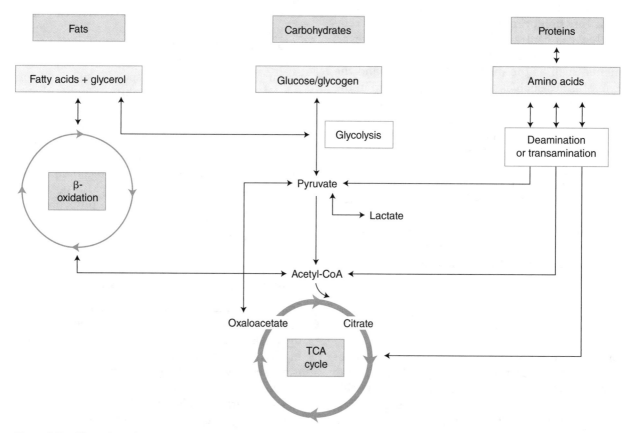

Figure 3.2   The main pathways of energy metabolism using carbohydrates, lipids, and proteins as energy sources.

reaction that utilizes two molecules of ADP to generate one molecule of ATP (and one molecule of adenosine monophosphate [AMP]). This reaction is catalyzed by the enzyme myokinase:

$$ADP + ADP \rightarrow ATP + AMP - 31 \text{ kJ per mole of ADP}$$

This reaction becomes important only during high-intensity exercise. Even then, the amount of energy available in the form of ATP is extremely limited, and the real importance of the reaction may be the formation of AMP, which is a potent activator of a number of enzymes involved in energy metabolism.

The total adenylate pool can decline rapidly if the AMP concentration of the cell rises during muscle force generation. This decline occurs principally by deamination of AMP to inosine monophosphate (IMP), but it also occurs by the dephosphorylation of AMP to adenosine. The loss of AMP may initially appear counterproductive because of the reduction in the total adenylate pool. But the deamination of AMP to IMP occurs only under low ATP:ADP ratio conditions, and, by preventing excessive accumulation of ADP and AMP, it enables the adenylate kinase reactions to

continue, resulting in an increase in the ATP:ADP ratio and continuing muscle force generation. Furthermore, the free energy of ATP hydrolysis possibly decreases when ADP and Pi accumulate, which could further impair muscle force generation. For these reasons, adenine nucleotide loss is important to muscle function during conditions of metabolic crisis, such as during maximal exercise or in the later stages of prolonged submaximal exercise when glycogen stores become depleted.

Glycolysis in Anaerobic Metabolism

Under normal conditions, muscle does not fatigue after only a few seconds of effort, so a source of energy other than ATP and PCr must be available. The source is glycolysis, which involves the breakdown of glucose (or glycogen) in a series of chemical reactions that yield pyruvate. This process does not require oxygen but does result in ATP being available to the muscle from reactions involving substrate-level phosphorylation. But the pyruvate must be removed for the reactions to proceed. In low-intensity exercise, when adequate oxygen is available to the muscle, pyruvate is converted to

■ **TABLE 3.2** ■

Anaerobic Production of ATP

	Capacity (mmol ATP/kg w.w.)	Power (mmol ATP · kg w.w.$^{-1}$ · s^{-1})
Phosphagen system	14–24	2.3
Glycolytic system	48–75	1.1
Combined	62–93	2.8

Values are expressed per kilogram of wet weight (w.w.) of muscle and are based on estimates of ATP provision during high-intensity exercise of human vastus lateralis muscle.

■ **TABLE 3.3** ■

ATP Resynthesis From Anaerobic and Aerobic Metabolism

	Max rate of ATP resynthesis (mmol ATP · kg w.w.$^{-1}$ · s^{-1})	Delay time*
PCr breakdown	2.25	Instantaneous
Glycolysis	1.10	5-10 seconds
Glycogen oxidation	0.70	1–3 minutes
Glucose (from blood) oxidation	0.35	~ 90 minutes
Fat oxidation	0.25	>2 hours

*Approximate delay time before maximal rates are attained after onset of exercise.

carbon dioxide and water by oxidative metabolism in the mitochondria. In some situations when oxygen availability is limited (e.g., isometric exercise) or the rate of formation of pyruvate is extremely high (e.g., sprinting), the pyruvate can also be removed by conversion to lactate, a reaction that does not involve oxygen.

Muscle Uptake of Glucose From the Blood A specific transporter protein, GLUT4, carries glucose molecules across the cell membrane. After the glucose molecule is inside the muscle cell, an irreversible phosphorylation (addition of a phosphate group), catalyzed by the enzyme hexokinase, occurs to prevent the loss of glucose from the cell. The glucose is converted to glucose-6-phosphate (G6P). Skeletal muscles lack the enzyme glucose-6-phosphatase and so are not able to re-form free glucose following the formation of G6P. Thus, the addition of a phosphate group to glucose ensures that the glucose is effectively trapped inside the cell. Note that this is an important difference between skeletal muscle and the liver. In the liver, which contains glucose-6-phosphatase, G6P can be broken down to form free glucose that can be released into the blood. In this way the liver plays an important role in the maintenance of the blood glucose concentration, whereas muscle tissue cannot do so directly. The hexokinase reaction is an energy-consuming reaction, requiring the investment of one molecule of ATP for each molecule of glucose. This reaction also ensures a concentration gradient for glucose across the cell membrane, down which transport can occur. Hexokinase is inhibited by an accumulation of G6P, and during high-intensity exercise, the increasing concentration of G6P limits the contribution that the blood glucose can make to carbohydrate metabolism in the active muscles.

Values are expressed per kilogram of wet weight (w.w.) of muscle and are based on estimates of ATP provision during high-intensity exercise of human vastus lateralis muscle.

Muscle Glycogen Breakdown If glycogen, rather than blood glucose, is the substrate for glycolysis, a single glucose molecule is split off by the enzyme glycogen phosphorylase, and the products are glucose-1-phosphate and a glycogen molecule that is one glucose residue shorter than the original. The substrates are glycogen and inorganic phosphate, so, unlike the hexokinase reaction, no breakdown of ATP occurs. Phosphorylase acts on the α-1,4 carbon bonds at the free ends of the glycogen molecule but cannot break the α-1,6 bonds

forming the branch points. These bonds are hydrolyzed by the combined actions of a debranching enzyme and amylo-1,6-glucosidase, releasing free glucose, which is quickly phosphorylated to G6P by hexokinase. Free glucose accumulates within the muscle cell only in very high-intensity exercise, where glycogenolysis is proceeding rapidly. Because relatively few α-1,6 bonds exist, no more than about 10% of the glucose residues appear as free glucose.

Glycolytic Pathway From Glucose-6-Phosphate to Pyruvate The enzyme phosphoglucomutase rapidly converts the glucose-1-phosphate formed by the action of phosphorylase on glycogen to G6P, which then proceeds down the glycolytic pathway (see figure 3.3). After a further phosphorylation, the glucose molecule is cleaved to form two molecules of the three-carbon sugar glyceraldehyde-3-phosphate. The second stage of glycolysis is the conversion of glyceraldehyde-3-phosphate into pyruvate, accompanied by the formation of ATP and reduction of nicotinamide adenine dinucleotide (NAD^+) to NADH.

The net effect of glycolysis is the conversion of one molecule of glucose to three molecules of pyruvate, with the formation of two molecules of ATP and the conversion of two molecules of NAD^+ to NADH. If glycogen rather than glucose is the starting substrate, three molecules of ATP are produced because no initial investment of ATP is made when the first phosphorylation step occurs. Although this net energy yield appears small, the relatively large carbohydrate store available and the rapid rate at which glycolysis proceeds make energy supplied in this way crucial for the performance of intense exercise. The 800 m runner, for example, obtains about 60% of the total energy requirement from anaerobic metabolism and may convert about 100 g of carbohydrate (mostly glycogen and equivalent to about 550 mmol of glucose) to lactate in less than 2 minutes. The amount of ATP released in this way (three ATP molecules per glucose molecule degraded, about 1,667 mmol of ATP in total) far exceeds the ATP available from PCr hydrolysis. This high rate of anaerobic metabolism not only allows a faster "steady state" speed than is possible with aerobic metabolism alone but also allows a faster pace in the early stages, before the cardiovascular system has adjusted to the demands and before the delivery and utilization of oxygen have increased in response to the exercise stimulus.

The reactions of glycolysis occur in the cytoplasm of the muscle cell, and some pyruvate will escape from active muscle tissues when the rate of glycolysis is high, but most is further metabolized. The fate of the pyruvate produced depends not only on factors such as exercise intensity but also on the metabolic capacity of the tissue. When glycolysis proceeds rapidly, the availability of NAD⁺, which is necessary as a cofactor in the glyceraldehyde 3-phosphate dehydrogenase reaction, becomes limiting. Reduction of pyruvate to lactate will regenerate NAD⁺ in muscle, and this reaction can proceed in the absence of oxygen. That is not to say, however, that lactate formation occurs only in the absence of oxygen. Even at low exercise intensities, such as when walking, some

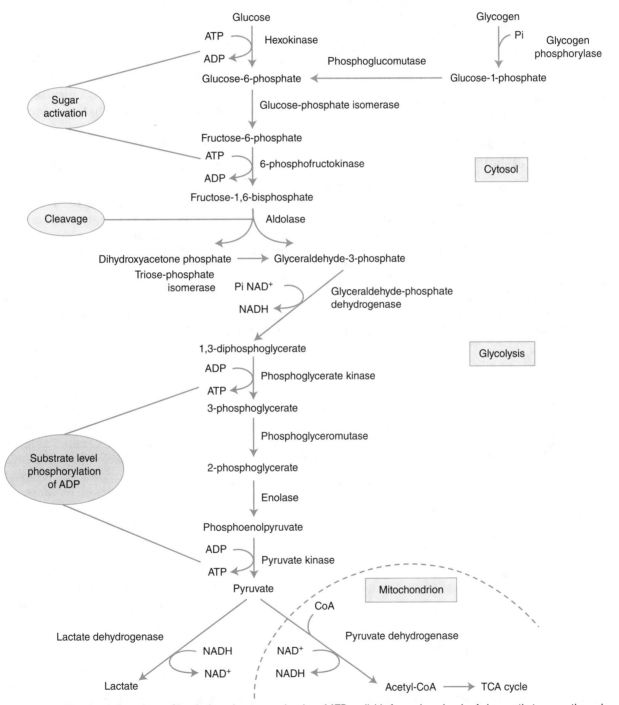

Figure 3.3 The glycolytic pathway. Glycolysis makes two molecules of ATP available for each molecule of glucose that passes through the pathway, or three molecules of ATP if muscle glycogen is the starting substrate.

lactate formation occurs. Lactate can accumulate within the muscle fibers, reaching much higher concentrations than those reached by any of the glycolytic intermediates including pyruvate. But when lactate accumulates in high concentrations, the associated hydrogen ions cause intracellular pH to fall, inhibiting some enzymes such as phosphorylase and phosphofructokinase, and the contractile mechanism begins to fail. A low pH also stimulates free nerve endings in the muscle, causing the perception of pain. Although the negative effects of the acidosis resulting from lactate accumulation are often stressed, the energy made available by anaerobic glycolysis allows the performance of high-intensity exercise that would otherwise not be possible.

Carbohydrate Oxidation in Aerobic Metabolism

Pyruvate may also undergo oxidative metabolism to carbon dioxide (CO_2) and water. This process occurs within the mitochondrion, and pyruvate that is produced in the sarcoplasm is transported across the mitochondrial membrane by a specific carrier protein (monocarboxylic acid transporter). The three-carbon pyruvate is converted by oxidative decarboxylation into a two-carbon acetate group, which is linked by a thio-ester bond to coenzyme A (CoA) to form acetyl-CoA. This reaction, in which NAD^+ is converted to NADH, is catalyzed by the pyruvate dehydrogenase enzyme complex. Acetyl-CoA is also formed from the metabolism of fatty acids (FAs) within the mitochondria, in a metabolic process called **β-oxidation.** These processes are summarized in figure 3.4. Note that this figure builds on figure 3.2 by including the products of the TCA cycle and the subcellular locations of the pathways involved.

Tricarboxylic Acid Cycle Acetyl-CoA is oxidized to CO_2 in the TCA cycle (also known as the Krebs cycle and the citric acid cycle). The reactions involve a combination of acetyl-CoA with oxaloacetate to form citrate, a six-carbon tricarboxylic acid. A series of reactions lead to the sequential loss of hydrogen atoms and CO_2, resulting in the regeneration of oxaloacetate.

$$\text{acetyl-CoA} + \text{ADP} + \text{Pi} + 3\text{NAD}^+ + \text{FAD} + 3\text{H}_2\text{O} \rightarrow 2\text{CO}_2 + \text{CoA} + \text{ATP} + 3\text{NADH} + 3\text{H}^+ + \text{FADH}_2$$

Because acetyl-CoA is also a product of FA oxidation, the final steps of oxidative degradation are common to both fat and carbohydrate. The hydrogen atoms are carried by the reduced coenzymes NADH and flavin adenine dinucleotide ($FADH_2$). These coenzymes act as carriers and donate pairs of electrons to the electron-transport chain, allowing oxidative phosphorylation with the subsequent regeneration of ATP from ADP.

The reactions involved in the TCA cycle are shown in figure 3.5. The two-carbon acetate units of acetyl-CoA are combined with the four-carbon oxaloactate to form six-carbon citrate. The latter undergoes two successive decarboxylations (removal of CO_2) to yield four-carbon succinate, which, in subsequent reactions, is converted to oxaloacetate, completing the TCA cycle. Molecular oxygen (O_2) does not participate directly in these reactions. The most important function of the TCA cycle is to generate hydrogen atoms for subsequent passage to the electron-transport chain by means of NADH and $FADH_2$ (see figure 3.6).

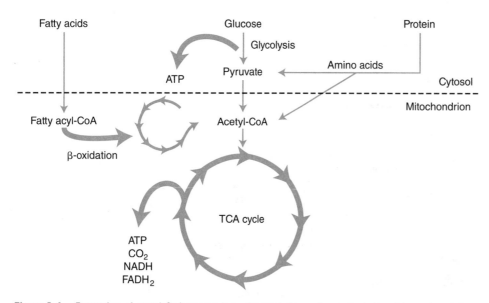

Figure 3.4 Formation of acetyl-CoA occurs from the catabolism of carbohydrates, fats, and proteins. Acetyl-CoA is oxidized in the tricarboxylic acid (TCA) cycle, generating CO_2, reduced coenzymes, and ATP.

Electron-Transport Chain and Oxidative Phosphorylation   The aerobic process of electron transport and oxidative phosphorylation regenerates ATP from ADP, thus conserving some of the chemical energy contained within the original substrates in the form of high-energy phosphates. As long as the O_2 supply is adequate and substrate is available, NAD^+ and FAD are continuously regenerated and TCA metabolism proceeds. This process cannot occur without oxygen. For each molecule of NADH that enters the electron-transport chain, 3 molecules of ATP are generated, and for each molecule of $FADH_2$, 2 molecules of ATP are formed. Thus, for each molecule of acetyl-CoA undergoing complete oxidation in the TCA cycle, a total of 12 ATP molecules are formed.

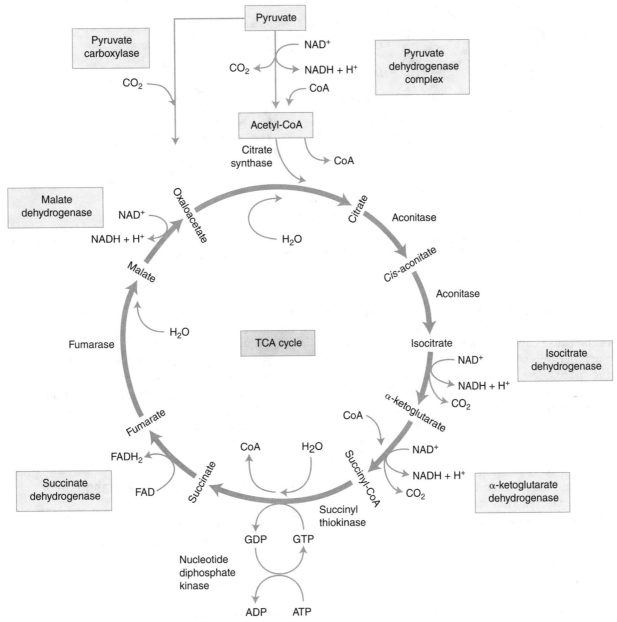

Figure 3.5   The reactions of the tricarboxylic acid (TCA) cycle showing sites of substrate-level phosphorylation and NAD^+ and FAD reduction.

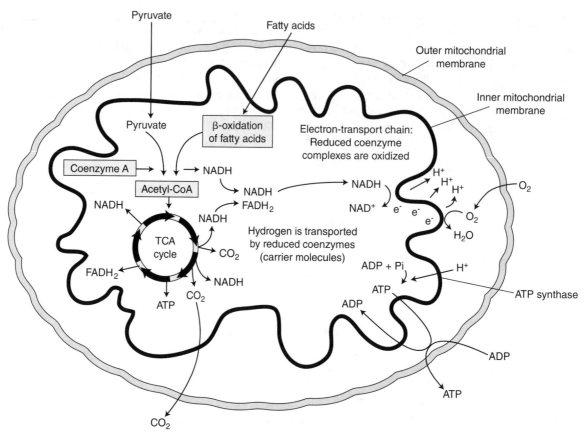

Figure 3.6 The TCA cycle generates the reduced coenzymes NADH and FADH$_2$. Oxidation of these coenzymes in the electron-transport chain releases energy that is used for the resynthesis of ATP. This process is called oxidative phosphorylation.

The transfer of electrons through the transport chain located on the inner mitochondrial membrane causes hydrogen ions, or protons (H$^+$), from the inner mitochondrial matrix to be pumped into the space between the inner and outer mitochondrial membranes. The high concentration of positively charged hydrogen ions in this outer chamber causes H$^+$ to flow back into the mitochondrial matrix through an ATP synthase protein complex embedded in the inner mitochondrial membrane. The flow of H$^+$ through this complex constitutes a proton-motive force that drives ATP synthesis. The overall reaction starting with glucose as the fuel can be summarized as follows:

Glucose + 6O$_2$ + 38ADP + 38Pi → 6CO$_2$ + 6H$_2$O + 38ATP

The total ATP synthesis of 38 moles per mole of glucose oxidized is primarily from oxidation of reduced coenzymes in the terminal respiratory system as shown in table 3.4.

The reactions of oxidative phosphorylation occur within the mitochondria, whereas glycolysis takes place in the cytoplasm, and the inner mitochondrial membrane is impermeable to NADH and to NAD$^+$.

Without regeneration of the NAD$^+$ in the cytoplasm, glycolysis will stop. Therefore, a mechanism must exist for the effective oxidation of the NADH formed during glycolysis. This mechanism is provided by a number of substrate shuttles that transfer reducing equivalents into the mitochondrion.

Fat Oxidation in Aerobic Metabolism

Fat and carbohydrate are the major nutrients that provide energy for muscular contraction. Because acetyl-CoA is also a product of fat oxidation, the sequence of reactions involving the TCA cycle and oxidative phosphorylation is common to both fat and carbohydrate.

Lipolysis To generate the two-carbon acetyl groups from fat, several metabolic steps must occur. The first step involves the breakdown of the storage

■ TABLE 3.4 ■

ATP Resynthesis in the Complete Oxidation of Glucose

ATP synthesized	Source	
2		In glycolysis
6	NADH	In glycolysis
24	NADH	In TCA cycle
4	FADH$_2$	In TCA cycle
2	GTP	In TCA cycle
38	*Total*	

form of fat, triacylglycerol, into its FA and glycerol components. This process is called lipolysis, and it begins with the hydrolytic removal of an FA molecule from the glycerol backbone at either position 1 or position 3. This step is catalyzed by a hormone-sensitive lipase (see figure 3.7). Insulin promotes triacylglycerol synthesis and inhibits lipolysis, whereas catecholamines (epinephrine and norepinephrine), glucagon, growth hormone, and cortisol stimulate lipolysis by activating the hormone-sensitive lipase. A specific lipase for the remaining diacylglycerol removes another FA, and another specific lipase removes the last FA from the monoacylglycerol. Thus, from each molecule of triacylglycerol, one molecule of glycerol and three molecules of FA are produced. Glycerol may diffuse, and FAs are transported out of the adipose cells and into the circulation.

Both the rate of lipolysis and the rate of adipose tissue blood flow influence the rate of entry of FA and glycerol into the circulation. During prolonged exercise at about 50% of $\dot{V}O_2$max, adipose tissue blood flow increases. During intense exercise, however, sympathetic vasoconstriction causes a fall in adipose tissue blood flow, resulting in accumulation of FA within adipose tissue and effectively limiting the entry of FA (and glycerol) into the circu-

lation. Another factor that limits fat mobilization during high-intensity exercise is the accumulation of lactate in the blood. Lactate promotes the reesterification of FA back into triacylglycerol (see figure 3.7) and therefore limits the entry of FA into the bloodstream.

Glycerol in plasma can be taken up by the liver and phosphorylated to glycerol-3-phosphate, which can be used to form triacylglycerol as described earlier, or, alternatively, can be oxidized to dihydroxyacetone phosphate, which can enter the glycolytic pathway or be converted to glucose. FAs are poorly soluble in water, and most of the FAs in plasma are transported loosely bound to albumin, the most abundant protein in plasma. The usual resting plasma concentration of FA is 0.2 to 0.4 mM. However, during (or shortly after) prolonged exercise, the plasma FA concentration may increase to about 2.0 mM.

FA Uptake Into Muscle Uptake of FA by muscle is directly related to the plasma FA concentration, and, hence, the mobilization of fat stores is an important step in ensuring an adequate nutrient supply for prolonged muscular work. The normal plasma albumin concentration is about 45 g/L (approximately 0.7 mM). Each albumin molecule contains three high-affinity binding sites for FA (and seven other low-affinity binding sites). When the three high-affinity binding sites are full (at an FA concentration of 2.0 mM or more), the concentration of FA not bound to albumin (i.e., FFAs) increases markedly, forming fatty-acid micelles,

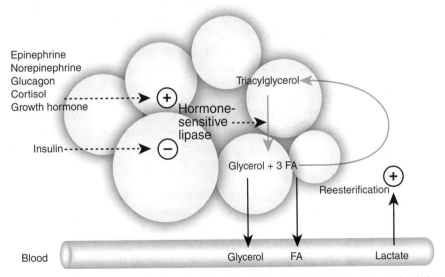

Figure 3.7   Lipolysis in adipose tissue mobilizes free fatty acids (FAs), which enter the circulation and thus become available for muscle to use as a fuel for exercise.

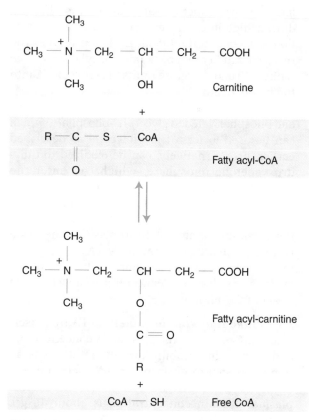

Figure 3.8 In the carnitine–fatty acyl-CoA transferase reaction, carnitine is linked to a FA.

which are potentially damaging to tissues because of their detergent-like properties.

FA transport across the sarcolemmal membrane into the muscle fiber occurs by a carrier-mediated transport mechanism that becomes saturated at high-plasma unbound FA concentration (approximately equivalent to 1.5 mM total FA concentration). FA uptake into muscle will occur only if the intracellular FA concentration is less than that in true aqueous solution in the extracellular fluid (that is, < 10 μM). The low intracellular FA concentration is probably maintained by the presence of a FA-binding protein inside the cell, perhaps similar to the ones found in the cells of the small intestine and liver. Also, the rate of uptake of FA into muscle fibers will be proportional to the difference in their concentrations inside and outside the cell, until the plasma membrane transport mechanism becomes saturated. After the FAs enter the muscle cell, they are converted into a CoA derivative by the action of ATP-linked fatty acyl-CoA synthetase (also known as thiokinase), in preparation for β-oxidation, the major pathway for FA breakdown. Hence, the

priming (activation) of each FA molecule requires the utilization of one molecule of ATP:

$$RCOOH + ATP + CoA\text{-}SH$$
$$\rightarrow R\text{-}C(=O)\text{-}S\text{-}CoA + AMP + PPi$$

β-Oxidation of Fatty Acids The process of β-oxidation occurs in the mitochondria and is the sequential removal of two-carbon units from the FA chain in the form of acetyl-CoA, which can then enter the TCA cycle. Fatty acyl-CoA molecules in the muscle sarcoplasm are transported into the mitochondria through formation of an ester of the FA with carnitine, as illustrated in figure 3.8. The latter is synthesized in the liver and is normally abundant in tissues able to oxidize FAs. Concentrations of about 1.0 mM are found in muscle. The enzyme regulating the transport of FA by carnitine is carnitine acyl-transferase (CAT), two forms of which exist in muscle. One form (CAT-I) is located on the outer surface of the membrane (to generate acyl-carnitine), and the other form (CAT-II) is located on the inner surface of the inner mitochondrial membrane and regenerates the acyl-CoA and free carnitine (see figure 3.9). CAT-I and CAT-II are also often referred to as CPT I and CPT II (carnitine palmitoyl tranferase I and II). This transport process may be the main rate-limiting step in the utilization of FAs for energy production in muscle.

At high exercise intensities (above about 60% of $\dot{V}O_2$max) the rate of fat oxidation cannot provide sufficient ATP for muscle contraction, and, increasingly, ATP is derived from carbohydrate oxidation and anaerobic glycolysis. Energy cannot be derived from fat through anaerobic pathways. After its release into the mitochondrial matrix, the fatty acyl-CoA is able to enter the β-oxidation pathway. Carnitine acyl-transferase is inhibited by malonyl-CoA, a precursor for FA synthesis. Hence, when the ATP supply is sufficient, surplus acetyl-CoA will be diverted away from the TCA cycle to malonyl-CoA, reducing catabolism of FAs and promoting their formation and subsequent triacylglycerol synthesis.

After it is inside the mitochondria, fatty acyl-CoA is oxidized through a series of reactions catalyzed by a multienzyme complex that releases a molecule of acetyl-CoA and a fatty acyl-CoA, which is now a 2-carbon unit shorter. This fatty acyl-CoA can now repeat the cycle, and the acetyl CoA formed can enter the TCA cycle. At each passage through the cycle, the FA chain loses a 2-carbon fragment as acetyl-CoA and 2 pairs of hydrogen atoms to

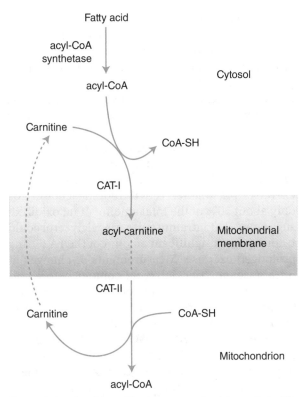

Fatty acid

acyl-CoA
synthetase

acyl-CoA

Cytosol

Carnitine

CoA-SH

CAT-I

acyl-carnitine

Mitochondrial
membrane

CAT-II

Carnitine

CoA-SH

Mitochondrion

acyl-CoA

Figure 3.9 Carnitine aids the transport of long-chain FAs across the mitochondrial membrane. Inside the mitochondrion, carnitine is removed, and fatty acyl-CoA is re-formed, freeing carnitine to diffuse back across the mitochondrial membrane into the cytoplasm.

specific acceptors. The 16-carbon palmitic acid thus undergoes a total of seven such cycles to yield in total eight molecules of acetyl-CoA and 14 pairs of hydrogen atoms. The palmitic acid only needs to be primed or activated with CoA once because at the end of each cycle, the shortened FA appears as its CoA ester. The most common FAs oxidized contain 16 (e.g., palmitic acid) or 18 (e.g., oleic acid) carbons in the acyl chain. The 14 pairs of hydrogen atoms removed during β-oxidation of palmitic acid enter the mitochondrial respiratory chain, 7 pairs in the form of the reduced flavin coenzyme of fatty acyl-CoA dehydrogenase and 7 pairs in the form of NADH. The passage of electrons from $FADH_2$ to oxygen and from NADH to oxygen leads to the expected number of oxidative phosphorylations of ADP (that is, two ATP molecules from each $FADH_2$ and three ATP molecules from each NADH). Hence, a total of five molecules of ATP are formed per molecule of acetyl-CoA cleaved:

$$\text{Palmitoyl-CoA} + 7 \text{ CoA} + 7 \text{ O}_2 + 35 \text{ ADP}$$
$$+ 35 \text{ Pi} \rightarrow 8 \text{ acetyl-CoA} + 35 \text{ ATP} + 42 \text{ H}_2\text{O}$$

The eight molecules of acetyl-CoA can enter the TCA cycle, and the following equation represents the result of their oxidation and the coupled phosphorylations:

$$8 \text{ acetyl-CoA} + 16 \text{ O}_2 + 96 \text{ ADP}$$
$$+ 96 \text{ Pi} \rightarrow 8 \text{ CoA} + 96 \text{ ATP} + 104 \text{ H}_2\text{O} + 16 \text{ CO}_2$$

Combining the two previous equations gives the overall equation:

$$\text{Palmitoyl-CoA} + 23 \text{ O}_2 + 131 \text{ ADP}$$
$$+ 131 \text{ Pi} \rightarrow \text{CoA} + 16 \text{ CO}_2 + 146 \text{ H}_2\text{O} + 131 \text{ ATP}$$

Because 1 molecule of ATP was required initially to activate the FA, the net yield for the complete oxidation of 1 molecule of palmitic acid is 130 molecules of ATP.

Protein Oxidation in Aerobic Metabolism

In most situations, carbohydrates and fats supply most of the energy required to regenerate ATP to fuel muscular work. Protein catabolism can provide up to 20 different amino acids, some of which may eventually be oxidized, but this normally contributes less than 5% of the energy provision for muscle contraction during physical activity. During starvation and when glycogen stores become depleted, protein catabolism may become an increasingly important source of energy for muscular work.

Before amino acids can be oxidized, the amino (-NH_2) group must be removed. Removal of the amino group can be achieved for some amino acids by transferring it to another molecule called a keto-acid, which results in the formation of a different amino acid. This process is called transamination and is catalyzed by enzymes called aminotransferases. A good example is the transfer of the amino group from the amino acid leucine to the keto-acid α-ketoglutarate forming α-ketoisocaproate (which can be further metabolized to form acetyl-CoA) and glutamate, respectively. Each amino acid has a unique corresponding keto-acid. Alternatively, the amino group can be removed from the amino acid to form free ammonia (NH_3), in a process called oxidative deamination. After the removal of the amino group from an amino acid, the remaining carbon skeleton (the keto-acid) is eventually oxidized to CO_2 and H_2O in the TCA cycle. The carbon skeleton of amino acids can enter the TCA cycle in several ways. Some can be converted to acetyl-CoA and enter the TCA cycle just like acetyl-CoA from carbohydrate or fat. They can also enter the TCA cycle as α-ketoglutarate or oxaloacetate as metabolites of glutamate and aspartate, respectively.

Although all carbon skeletons of amino acids can be used for oxidation, only 6 of the available 20 amino acids in protein are oxidized in significant amounts by muscle: asparagine, aspartate, glutamate, isoleucine, leucine, and valine. Amino acid oxidation has been estimated to contribute up to only about 15% to energy expenditure in resting conditions. During exercise, this relative contribution likely decreases to less than 5% because of an increasing importance of carbohydrate and fat as fuels. During prolonged exercise, when carbohydrate availability becomes limited, amino acid oxidation may increase somewhat but the contribution of protein to energy expenditure still does not exceed about 10% of total energy expenditure.

Fuel Stores in Skeletal Muscle

Carbohydrates are stored in the body as the glucose polymer glycogen. Skeletal muscle contains a significant store of glycogen in the sarcoplasm. The glycogen content of skeletal muscle at rest is approximately 13 to 18 g/kg w.w. (75 to 100 mmol glucosyl units/kg w.w.). For cycling and running, a total of about 300 g of glycogen is available in the leg muscles (see figure 3.10). About 100 g of glycogen are stored in the liver of an adult human in the postabsorptive state, which can be released into the circulation to maintain the blood glucose concentration at about 5 mmol/L (0.9 g/L). Fats are stored as triacylglycerol, mainly in white adipose tissue. Triacylglycerol molecules must be broken down by a lipase enzyme to release FA into the circulation for uptake by working muscle. Skeletal

muscle also contains some triacylglycerol that can be used as an energy source during exercise after lipolysis. Some of this intramuscular triacylglycerol may be contained in adipose cells dispersed among the muscle fibers in the tissue, but evidence from light and electron microscopy suggests the existence of triacylglycerol droplets located close to the mitochondria within the fibers themselves.

Early studies (Havel et al. 1967; Issekutz et al. 1964) of FA turnover during exercise using ^{14}C-labeled FAs showed that during prolonged exercise, plasma-derived FA could account for only about 50% of the total amount of fat oxidized, suggesting that intramuscular triacylglycerol could be providing a significant amount of the FA during prolonged exercise. Measurements of changes in intramuscular triacylglycerol content before and after exercise strongly support this view. Several studies have reported reductions of about 25% to 35% in triacylglycerol content after 1 to 2 hours of exercise at 55% to 70% of $\dot{V}O_2$max. These changes have been observed in several studies despite the unreliable nature of triacylglycerol measurement in small biopsy samples of skeletal muscle (Turcotte et al. 1995).

Human skeletal muscle contains approximately 12 g/kg w.w. of triacylglycerol, and type I fibers contain more triacylglycerol than type II fibers do. Between 12 and 20 MJ of chemical potential energy is estimated to be available for oxidation after intramuscular lipolysis. The lipolysis is probably mediated by an intracellular lipase similar to the hormone-sensitive lipase of adipose tissue; evidence suggests that catecholamines regulate the mobilization of intramuscular triacylglycerol stores.

Fat stores in the body are far larger than carbohydrate stores, and fat is a more efficient form of energy storage, releasing 37 kJ/g (9 kcal/g) compared with 16 kJ/g (4 kcal/g) from carbohydrate. Each gram of carbohydrate stored also retains about 3 g of water, further decreasing the efficiency of carbohydrate as an energy source. But the energy yield per liter of O_2 consumed during fat oxidation is about 8% to 10% less than for carbohydrate (about 19.5 kJ/L O_2 for fat compared with 20.9 kJ/L O_2 for carbohydrate). The energy cost of running a marathon is about 12,000 kJ (2,900 kcal); if this energy could be derived from the oxidation of fat alone, the total amount of fat required would be about 320 g, compared with 750 g of carbohydrate and an additional

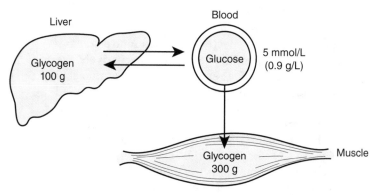

Figure 3.10 Carbohydrate availability in liver, blood, and muscle for two-legged exercise (e.g., cycling and running).

2.3 kg of associated water. Aside from the weight that would have to be carried, this amount of carbohydrate exceeds the total amount normally stored in the liver, muscles, and blood combined. The total storage capacity for fat is extremely large, and for most practical purposes, the amount of energy stored in the form of fat far exceeds that required for any exercise task (see table 3.5).

The main problem associated with the utilization of fat as a fuel for exercise is the rate at which it can be taken up by muscle and oxidized to provide energy. Fat oxidation can only supply ATP at a rate sufficient to maintain exercise at an intensity of about 60% of $\dot{V}O_2$max. To generate ATP to sustain higher exercise intensities, carbohydrate must be utilized. Both the oxidative pathway of carbohydrate utilization and the anaerobic pathway of glycolysis can supply ATP at a much faster rate than fat oxidation can. During most forms of submaximal exercise, a mixture of fat and carbohydrate is oxidized to provide energy for muscular contraction. Obviously, utilizing more fat allows greater sparing of the limited carbohydrate reserves, permitting exercise to be prolonged.

Unlike carbohydrate (as glycogen) and fat (as triacylglycerol), protein is stored only as functionally important molecules (e.g., structural proteins, enzymes, ion channels, receptors, and contractile proteins), and the concentration of free amino acids in most extracellular and intracellular body fluids is quite low (e.g., the total free amino acid concentration in muscle sarcoplasm is about 20 mmol/L). Hence, carbohydrate and fat are the preferred fuels for exercise, and the contribution of protein to energy expenditure during even prolonged exercise does not usually exceed a maximum of about 10% of total energy expenditure.

Regulation of Energy Metabolism

Experiments in which muscle biopsies were taken before and immediately after exercise indicate that the intramuscular ATP concentration remains fairly constant (Spriet 1995a). Thus, ATP is being continuously regenerated by other energy-liberating reactions at the same rate that it is being used. This situation provides a sensitive mechanism for the control of energy metabolism within the cell. This control is exerted through changes in a number of intracellular factors, and further control is effected through the actions of the sympathetic nervous system and hormones that can also bring about changes in the activities of some enzymes involved in fuel mobilization and utilization (see highlight box).

Intracellular Factors

Within the muscle fiber, several intracellular factors control the activity of key rate-limiting or flux-generating enzymes involved in energy metabolism, which allows rapid (virtually instantaneous) alteration in the rate of ATP resynthesis to occur when such an alteration is needed, such as at the onset of exercise.

Assume a body mass of 70 kg (154 lb), a fat content of 15% of body mass, and a protein content of about 12% of body mass. The value for blood glucose includes the glucose content of extracellular fluid. The exercise times are the approximate times

■ TABLE 3.5 ■

Energy Stores in the Average Man

Fuel type	Mass (kg)	Energy available (kJ) (kcal)		Exercise time (min)
Liver glycogen	0.10 (0.22 lb)	1,600	400	20
Muscle glycogen	0.40 (0.88 lb)	6,400	1,600	80
Blood glucose	0.01 (0.022 lb)	160	40	2
Fat	10.5 (22.0 lb)	390,000	93,000	4,900
Protein	8.5 (18.7 lb)	142,000	34,000	1,800

Assumes a body mass of 70 kg (154 lb), a fat content of 15% of body mass, and a protein content of about 12% of body mass. The value for blood glucose includes the glucose content of extracellular fluid. The exercise times are the approximate times that these stores would last if they were the only source of energy available during exercise at marathon-running pace (equivalent to an energy expenditure of about 80 kJ/min [19 kcal/min]).

Factors That Regulate the Mobilization of Fuels by Altering the Activities of Enzymes

Intramuscular factors
- ATP/ADP
- Pi
- AMP
- Ca2+

Sympathetic nervous system
- Norepinephrine (noradrenaline)

Hormones
- Epinephrine (adrenaline)
- Insulin
- Glucagon
- Cortisol
- Growth hormone

these stores would last if they were the only source of energy available during exercise at marathon-running pace (equivalent to an energy expenditure of about 80 kJ/min [19 kcal/min]).

The decline in cellular concentration of ATP at the onset of muscle force generation and parallel increases in ADP and AMP concentrations (i.e., a decline in the energy charge) directly stimulate anaerobic and oxidative ATP resynthesis. The relatively low concentration of ATP (and ADP) inside the cell means that any increase in the rate of hydrolysis of ATP (e.g., at the onset of exercise) produces a rapid change in the ratio of ATP to ADP (and also increases the intracellular concentration of AMP). These changes, in turn, activate enzymes that immediately stimulate the breakdown of intramuscular fuel stores to provide energy for ATP resynthesis. In this way, energy metabolism increases rapidly after the start of exercise.

ATP, ADP, and AMP are activators or inhibitors of the enzymatic reactions involved in PCr, carbohydrate, and fat degradation and utilization (see figure 3.11). For example, CK, the enzyme responsible for the rapid rephosphorylation of ATP at the initiation of muscle force generation, is rapidly activated by an increase in cytoplasmic ADP concentration and is inhibited by an increase

in cellular ATP concentration. Similarly, glycogen phosphorylase, the enzyme that catalyzes the conversion of glycogen to glucose-1-phosphate, is activated by increases in AMP and Pi (and calcium ion) concentration and is inhibited by an increase in ATP concentration.

The rate-limiting step in the glycolytic pathway is the conversion of fructose-6-phosphate to fructose-1,6-diphosphate, which is catalyzed by phosphofructokinase (PFK). The activity of this complex enzyme is affected by many intracellular factors, and it plays an important role in controlling flux through the pathway. The PFK reaction regulates the metabolism of both glucose and glycogen. The activity of PFK is stimulated by increased concentrations of ADP, AMP, Pi, ammonia, and fructose-6-phosphate and is inhibited by ATP, H^+, citrate, phosphoglycerate, and phosphoenolpyruvate. Thus, the rate of glycolysis is stimulated when ATP and glycogen breakdown are increased at the onset of exercise. Accumulation of citrate and, thus, inhibition of PFK may occur when the rate of the TCA cycle is high and provides a means whereby the limited stores of carbohydrate are spared when the availability of FAs is high. Inhibition of PFK also causes accumulation of G6P, which inhibits the activity of hexokinase and reduces the entry into the muscle of glucose, which is not needed.

Conversion of pyruvate to acetyl-CoA by the pyruvate dehydrogenase complex is the rate-limiting step in carbohydrate oxidation. It is stimulated by an increased intracellular concentration of calcium and decreased ratios of ATP/ADP, acetyl-CoA/free CoA, and NADH/NAD$^+$ and thus offers another site of regulation of the relative rates of fat and carbohydrate catabolism. If the rate of formation of acetyl-CoA from the β-oxidation of FAs is high, as after 1 to 2 hours of submaximal exercise, then this activity can reduce the amount of acetyl-CoA derived from pyruvate and cause accumulation of phosphoenolpyruvate and inhibition of PFK, thus slowing the rate of glycolysis and glycogenolysis. This process forms the basis of the glucose–fatty acid cycle proposed by Randle et al. (1963), which has for many years been accepted as the key regulatory mechanism in the control of carbohydrate and fat utilization by skeletal muscle. Recent work has challenged this hypothesis, however, and it seems likely that the regulation of the integration of fat and carbohydrate catabolism in exercising skeletal muscle must reside elsewhere; for example, at the level of glucose uptake into muscle, of glycogen breakdown by phosphorylase, or of the entry of FAs into the mitochondria (for

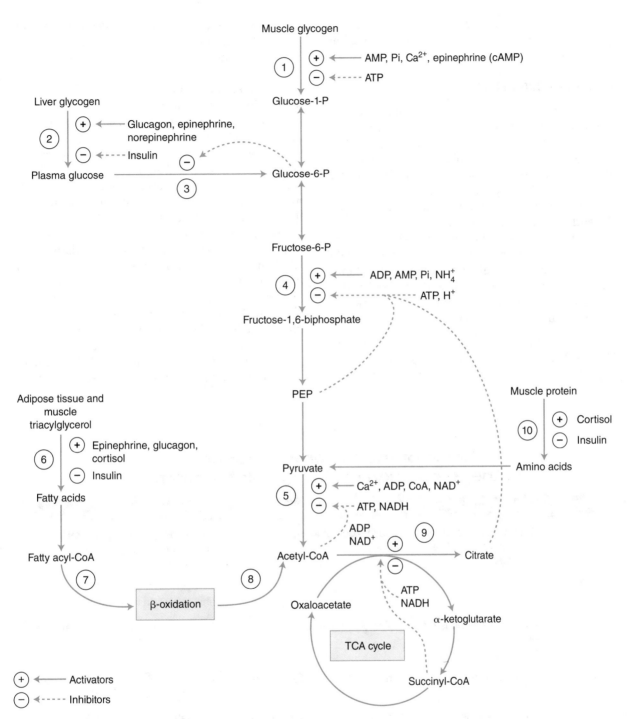

Figure 3.11 Metabolic pathways important to energy provision during exercise. The main sites of regulation and the principal hormone and allosteric activators and inhibitors are shown. 1 and 2 = phosphorylase; 3 = hexokinase; 4 = phosphofructokinase; 5 = pyruvate dehydrogenase; 6 = hormone-sensitive lipase; 7 = carnitine acyl transferase; 8 = fatty acyl-CoA dehydrogenase; 9 = citrate synthase; 10 = proteases.

further details see the books by Hargreaves 1995 and Maughan, Gleeson, and Greenhaff 1997).

A key regulatory point in the TCA cycle is the reaction catalyzed by citrate synthase. The activ-

ity of this enzyme is inhibited by ATP, NADH, succinyl-CoA and fatty acyl-CoA; the activity of the enzyme is also affected by citrate availability. Hence, when cellular energy levels are high, flux through the TCA cycle is relatively low but can be greatly increased when ATP and NADH utilization is increased, such as during exercise.

Hormones and Cytokines

Many hormones influence energy metabolism in the body (for a detailed review, see Galbo 1983). During exercise the interaction among insulin, glucagon, and the catecholamines (epinephrine and norepinephrine) is mostly responsible for fuel substrate availability and utilization; cortisol and growth hormone also have some significant effects. Recently, it has been recognized that a cytokine called interleukin-6, which is released from active skeletal muscle during exercise, also plays a role in the regulation of fuel mobilization and metabolism. The source, stimuli for secretion, and major actions of these various hormones and cytokines are summarized in table 3.6.

Insulin   Insulin is secreted by the β cells of the islets of Langerhans in the pancreas. Its basic biological effects are to inhibit lipolysis and increase the uptake of glucose from the blood by the tissues, especially skeletal muscle, liver, and adipose tissue. Cellular uptake of amino acids is also stimulated by insulin.

These effects reduce the plasma glucose concentration, inhibit the release of glucose from the liver, promote the synthesis of glycogen (in liver and muscle), promote synthesis of fat and inhibit FA release (in adipose tissue), increase muscle amino acid uptake, and enhance protein synthesis. The primary stimulus for increased insulin secretion is a rise in the blood glucose concentration (e.g., after a meal). Plasma insulin concentration is usually depressed during exercise because the sympathetic nervous system and circulating catecholamines inhibit the release of insulin. However, the fall in the plasma insulin concentration during exercise does not reduce the uptake of glucose from the blood by active muscle, because the rise in intracellular Ca^{2+} concentration during muscle contractions also promotes the translocation of intracellular vesicles containing GLUT4 glucose transporters into the sarcolemma (see figure 3.12).

■ **TABLE 3.6** ■

Roles of the Major Hormones in the Regulation of Energy Metabolism

Hormone	Source	Stimuli that activate secretion	Actions
Insulin	Beta cells of the islets of Langerhans in the pancreas	Rise in blood glucose and amino acids	Stimulates glucose uptake by liver, muscle, and adipose tissue. Inhibits lipolysis. Stimulates muscle amino acid uptake. Inhibits protein breakdown.
Glucagon	Alpha cells of the islets of Langerhans in the pancreas	Fall in blood glucose	Stimulates liver glycogen breakdown and gluconeogenesis.
Epinephrine	Adrenal medulla	Stress and fall in blood glucose	Stimulates glycogen breakdown and lipolysis in adipose tissue.
Norepinephrine	Sympathetic nerve endings	Stress and fall in blood glucose or blood pressure	Stimulates glycogen breakdown and lipolysis in adipose tissue.
Cortisol	Adrenal cortex	Stress, adrenocorticotrophic hormone, interleukin-6	Stimulates protein breakdown and gluconeogenesis. Stimulates lipolysis in adipose tissue.
Growth hormone	Anterior pituitary gland	Stress	Stimulates lipolysis in adipose tissue.
Interleukin-6	Contracting skeletal muscle fibers	Increased intracellular calcium ion concentration and decreased glycogen availability	Stimulates liver glycogen breakdown. Stimulates lipolysis in adipose tissue. Stimulates cortisol secretion.

Glucagon Glucagon is secreted by the α cells of the pancreatic islets and exerts effects that are opposite those of insulin. It raises the blood glucose level by increasing the rate of glycogen breakdown (glycogenolysis) in the liver. It also promotes the formation of glucose from noncarbohydrate precursors (**gluconeogenesis**) in the liver. The primary stimulus for increased secretion of glucagon is a decrease in the glucose concentration in the blood. During most types of exercise, the blood glucose concentration does not fall. But during prolonged exercise, when liver glycogen stores become depleted, a drop in the blood glucose concentration (hypoglycemia) may occur.

The hormone-sensitive lipase in adipose tissue is activated by a cyclic AMP-dependent protein kinase. Binding of glucagon and epinephrine to plasma membrane receptors on adipocytes initiates the adenylate cyclase and the enzyme cascade that activates the lipase (see figure 3.13). Activation of the hormone-sensitive lipase in adipose tissue and lipoprotein lipase occurs during exercise because of the actions of epinephrine and glucagon, which are released from the adrenal medulla and pancreatic islets, respectively. FAs thus released from triacylglycerols in the fat storage sites are delivered by the blood to muscle tissue, and additional FA can be provided from the breakdown of intramuscular fat depots. These FAs provide a readily usable source of energy that is liberated through the process of β-oxidation and contribute significantly to the energy requirements of exercise.

During brief periods of light to moderate exercise, energy is derived equally from oxidation of carbohydrate and fat. If exercise is continued for an hour or more and carbohydrates become depleted, the quantity of fat used for energy gradually increases. In very prolonged exercise, fat (mainly as FA) may supply almost 80% of total energy. This condition prob-

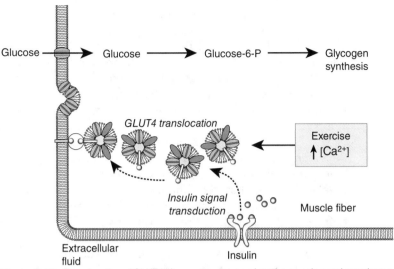

Figure 3.12 Translocation of GLUT4 glucose transporters into the sarcolemmal membrane under the influence of insulin (important during rest) and calcium ions (important during exercise).

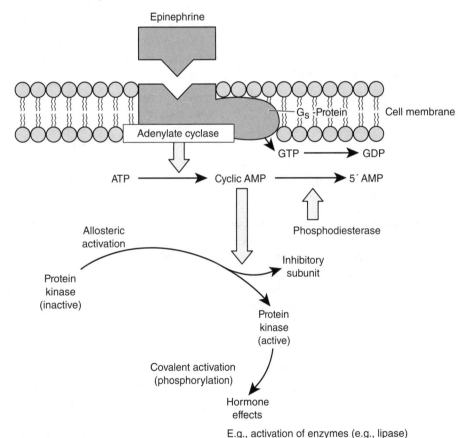

Figure 3.13 Mode of action of epinephrine (adrenaline).

ably arises because of a small fall in blood glucose concentration and a subsequent increase in glucagon (and decrease in insulin) release from the pancreas. Plasma concentrations of epinephrine and cortisol also increase as exercise progresses.

These hormonal changes stimulate the mobilization and subsequent utilization of fat stores (see figure 3.7). The uptake of FA by working muscle rises during 1 to 4 hours of continuous moderate exercise. Lipolysis is stimulated by exercise, but this process occurs only gradually. Furthermore, it does not cease immediately after exercise has stopped.

The FA concentration in blood plasma reflects the balance between the FA release into the circulation (mainly from adipose tissue depots) and FA uptake by various tissues. Although the concentration of FAs in blood plasma is low (usually in the range of 0.2 to 2.0 mM), their plasma half-life is extremely short, less than 2 minutes in fact, indicating a rapid rate of uptake by tissues. At the onset of exercise, muscle capillaries open up, facilitating FA uptake, and this process is reversed shortly after the end of exercise. Consequently, plasma FA concentrations commonly fall in the early stages of exercise and then gradually increase. At the end of exercise, when muscle uptake falls abruptly but stimulation of lipolysis continues, plasma FA concentration rises sharply, reaching up to 3 mM.

Catecholamines The catecholamines epinephrine (adrenaline) and norepinephrine (noradrenaline) are released from the adrenal medulla. Norepinephrine is also released from sympathetic nerve endings, and leakage from such synapses appears to be the main source of the norepinephrine in blood plasma. The catecholamines have many systemic effects, including stimulation of the heart rate and contractility and alteration of blood vessel diameters. These substances also influence substrate availability, with the effects of epinephrine being more important than those of norepinephrine. Epinephrine, like glucagon, promotes glycogenolysis in both liver and muscle. Epinephrine also promotes lipolysis in adipose tissue, increasing the availability of plasma FA, and inhibits insulin secretion. The primary stimulus for catecholamine secretion is the activation of the sympathetic nervous system by stressors such as exercise, hypotension, and hypoglycemia. Substantial increases in the plasma catecholamine concentration can occur within seconds of the onset of high-intensity exercise. But the relative exercise intensity must be above 50% of $\dot{V}O_2$max to elevate the plasma catecholamine concentration significantly.

Growth Hormone and Cortisol Growth hormone, secreted from the anterior pituitary gland, also stimulates mobilization of FA from adipose tissue, and increases in plasma growth hormone concen-

tration are related to exercise intensity. During prolonged strenuous exercise, cortisol secretion from the adrenal cortex increases. Cortisol, a steroid hormone, increases the effectiveness of catecholamines in some tissues (e.g., it promotes lipolysis in adipose tissue). But its main effects are to promote protein degradation and amino acid release from muscle and to stimulate gluconeogenesis in the liver. The primary stimulus to cortisol secretion is stress-induced release of adrenocorticotrophic hormone (ACTH) from the anterior pituitary gland. Cortisol is derived from cholesterol, and its high fat solubility allows it to diffuse across cell membranes. Cortisol receptors in the cell cytoplasm translocate the hormone to the nucleus of the cell. Interaction of the hormone-receptor complex with specific sections of DNA switches on the transcription of specific genes and thus stimulates the synthesis of new proteins in the cell (see figure 3.14). This activity is common to all the steroid hormones (e.g., testosterone, estrogen, and aldosterone).

Interleukin-6 Interleukin-6 (IL-6) is a cytokine (a peptide chemical messenger) produced by several different cells and tissues, although it is most well known for its actions in the regulation of immune function. Contracting skeletal muscle fibers also produce and release IL-6 into the circulation and, indeed, muscle secretion of IL-6 has been shown to be almost entirely responsible for the up to 100-fold rise in plasma IL-6 concentration during prolonged exercise such as marathon running. The release of IL-6 is primarily regulated by an altered intramuscular milieu in response to exercise: Changes in calcium homeostasis, impaired glucose availability (glycogen depletion), and increased formation of reactive oxygen species are all associated with exercise and capable of activating transcription factors known to regulate IL-6 synthesis. Acute IL-6 administration to humans increases lipolysis, fat oxidation, liver glycogenolysis, and insulin-mediated glucose disposal. IL-6 also has anti-inflammatory effects and may exert some of its biological effects through stimulation of cortisol secretion and inhibition of the proinflammatory cytokine tumor necrosis factor-alpha.

Metabolic Responses to Exercise

The most important factor influencing the metabolic response to exercise is exercise intensity. The physical fitness of the subject also modifies

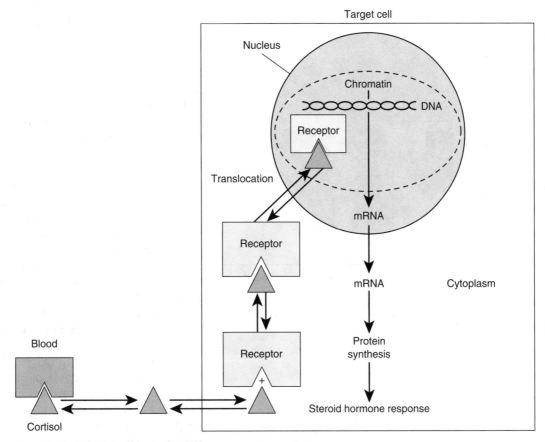

Figure 3.14   Mode of action of steroid hormones such as cortisol.

the metabolic response to exercise, and other factors—including exercise duration, substrate availability, nutritional status, diet, feeding during exercise, mode of exercise, previous exercise, drugs, environmental temperature, and altitude—are also important.

Causes of Fatigue in High-Intensity Exercise

ATP is the only fuel that can be used directly for skeletal muscle force generation, and the available ATP will fuel about 2 seconds of maximum-intensity exercise. Therefore, for muscle force generation to continue, ATP must be resynthesized rapidly from ADP. During high-intensity exercise, the relatively low rate of ATP resynthesis from oxidative phosphorylation stimulates rapid anaerobic energy production from PCr and glycogen hydrolysis. PCr breakdown begins at the onset of contraction to buffer the rapid accumulation of ADP from ATP hydrolysis. But the rate of PCr hydrolysis declines after only a few seconds of maximal force generation (see figure 3.15).

If high-intensity exercise is to continue beyond the first few seconds, a marked increase in the contribution from glycolysis to ATP resynthesis is necessary. Anaerobic glycolysis involves several more steps than PCr hydrolysis, although compared with oxidative phosphorylation, it is still extremely rapid. Anaerobic glycolysis starts at the onset of contraction, but unlike PCr hydrolysis, it does not reach a maximal rate until after 5 seconds of exercise, and it can be maintained at this level for several seconds during maximal muscle force generation (see figure 3.16). The mechanism or mechanisms responsible for the eventual decline in glycolysis during maximal exercise have not been determined. Exercise at an intensity equivalent to 95% to 100% of $\dot{V}O_2$max can be sustained for about 5 minutes before fatigue is experienced. Under these conditions, carbohydrate oxidation can make a significant contribution to ATP production, but its relative importance is often underestimated.

Fatigue, the inability to maintain a given or expected force or power output, is an inevitable feature of maximal exercise. Typically, the loss of power output or force production is likely to be in the region of 40% to 60% of the maximum observed during 30 seconds of all-out exercise. Many factors

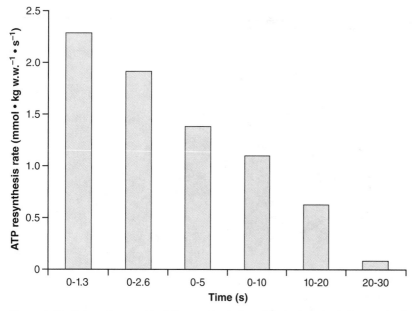

Figure 3.15 Rates of anaerobic ATP resynthesis from PCr hydrolysis during maximal isometric contraction in human skeletal muscle.

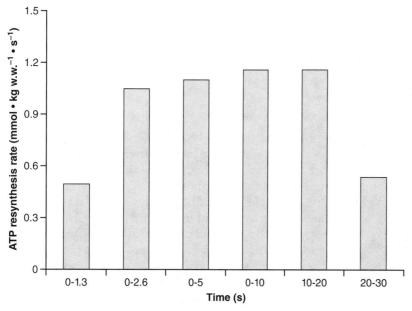

Figure 3.16 Rates of anaerobic ATP resynthesis from glycolysis during maximal isometric contraction in human skeletal muscle.

contribute to fatigue. But during maximal short-duration exercise, it will be caused primarily by a gradual decline in anaerobic ATP production or an increase in ADP accumulation caused by a depletion of PCr and a fall in the rate of glycolysis.

In high-intensity exercise lasting 1 to 5 minutes, lactic acid accumulation may contribute to the fatigue process. At physiological pH values, lactic acid almost completely dissociates into its constituent lactate and hydrogen ions, and studies using animal muscle preparations have demonstrated that direct inhibition of force production can be achieved by increasing hydrogen and lactate ion concentrations (Green 1995). Reduced muscle pH may cause some inhibition of PFK and phosphorylase, reducing the rate of ATP resynthesis from glycolysis. This development is unlikely to be important in exercising muscle, however, because the in vitro inhibition of PFK by a reduced pH is reversed in the presence of other activators such as AMP (Spriet 1991). Lactate and hydrogen ion accumulation also appear to result in muscle fatigue independent of one another, but the latter is the more commonly cited mechanism. However, although likely to be related to the fatigue process, it is unlikely that both lactate and hydrogen ion accumulation are wholly responsible for muscle fatigue. For example, studies involving human volunteers have demonstrated that muscle force generation after fatiguing exercise can recover rapidly, despite also having a very low muscle pH value. The consensus appears to be that the maintenance of force production during high-intensity exercise is pH dependent, but the initial force generation is more related to PCr availability.

One of the consequences of rapid PCr hydrolysis during high-intensity exercise is the accumulation of Pi, which inhibits muscle contraction coupling directly. But the simultaneous PCr depletion and Pi accumulation make in vivo separation of the effect of PCr depletion from the effect of Pi accumulation difficult. This problem is further confounded by the parallel increases in hydrogen and lactate ions that occur during high-intensity exercise. All these metabolites have been independently implicated in muscle fatigue.

Calcium release by the sarcoplasmic reticulum as a consequence of muscle depolarization is essential for the activation of muscle contraction coupling. During fatiguing contractions, calcium transport slows and calcium transients become progressively smaller, which has been attributed to a reduction in calcium reuptake by the sarcoplasmic reticulum or increased calcium binding. Strong evidence that a disruption of calcium handling is responsible for fatigue comes from studies showing that the stimulation of sarcoplasmic reticulum calcium release caused by the administration of caffeine to isolated muscle can improve muscle force production, even in the presence of a low muscle pH (Green 1995). Alternatively, fatigue during high-intensity exercise may be associated with an excitation-coupling failure and possibly a reduced nervous drive caused by reflex inhibition at the spinal level. In the latter hypothesis, accumulation of interstitial potassium in muscle may play a major role.

When repeated bouts of maximal exercise are performed, the rates of muscle PCr hydrolysis and lactate accumulation decline. In the case of PCr, this response is thought to occur because of incomplete PCr resynthesis during recovery between successive exercise bouts. But the mechanism or mechanisms responsible for the fall in the rate of lactate accumulation are unclear.

Causes of Fatigue in Prolonged Exercise

The term *prolonged exercise* is usually used to describe exercise intensities that can be sustained for 30 to 180 minutes. Because the rate of ATP demand is relatively low compared with high-intensity exercise, PCr, carbohydrate, and fat can all contribute to energy production. The various fuel sources available to resynthesize ATP are summarized in figure 3.17. The rates of PCr degradation and lactate production during the first minutes of prolonged exercise are closely related to the intensity of exercise performed, and energy production during this period would likely be compromised without this contribution from anaerobic metabolism. After a steady state has been reached, however, carbohydrate and fat oxidation become the principal means of resynthesizing ATP. Muscle glycogen is the principal fuel during the first 30 minutes of exercise at 60% to 80% of $\dot{V}O_2max$. The rate of muscle glycogen utilization depends on exercise intensity (see figure 3.18).

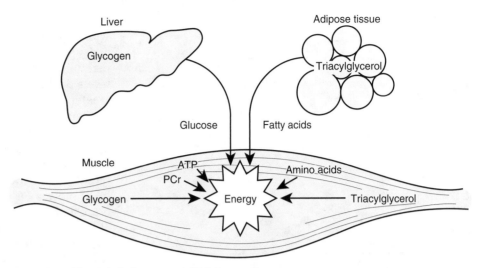

Figure 3.17 The main fuel sources available for exercise.

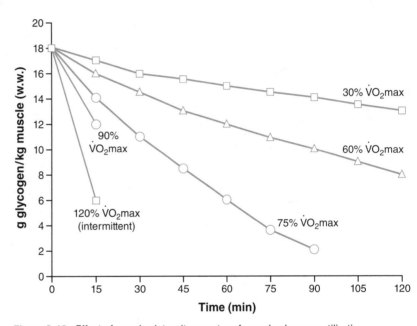

Figure 3.18 Effect of exercise intensity on rates of muscle glycogen utilization.

During the early stages of exercise, fat oxidation is limited by the delay in the mobilization of FAs from adipose tissue. At rest after an overnight fast, the plasma FA concentration is about 0.3 to 0.4 mmol/L. This concentration is commonly observed to fall during the first hour of moderate-intensity exercise, followed by a progressive increase (see figure 3.19) as lipolysis is stimulated by the actions of catecholamines, glucagon, and cortisol. During very prolonged exercise, the plasma FA concentration can reach 1.5 to 2.0 mmol/L, and muscle uptake of blood-borne FA is proportional to the plasma FA concentration.

The glycerol released from adipose tissue cannot be used directly by muscle, which lacks

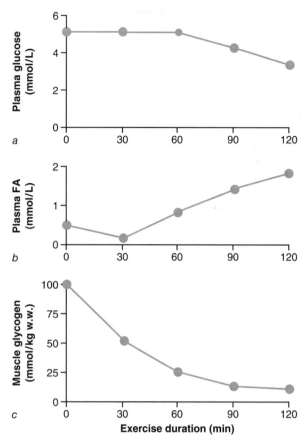

a

b

c

Figure 3.19 Changes in the concentrations of plasma glucose, plasma FAs, and muscle glycogen during continuous exercise at an intensity equivalent to 70% of $\dot{V}O_2$max.

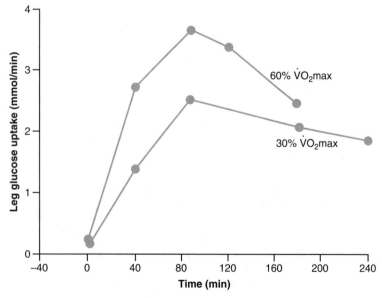

60% $\dot{V}O_2$max

30% $\dot{V}O_2$max

Figure 3.20 Rate of uptake of glucose from the blood by muscle during exercise at 30% of $\dot{V}O_2$max and 60% of $\dot{V}O_2$max. Peak uptake occurs after about 90 minutes of exercise.

the enzyme glycerol kinase. But glycerol (together with alanine and lactate) is taken up by the liver and used as a gluconeogenic precursor to help maintain liver glucose output as liver glycogen levels decline. The utilization of blood glucose is greater at higher work rates and increases during prolonged submaximal exercise. At an exercise intensity of 60% of $\dot{V}O_2$max, blood glucose uptake by muscle peaks after about 90 minutes (see figure 3.20). The decline in blood glucose uptake after 90 minutes is attributable to the increasing availability of plasma FA as fuel (which appears to inhibit muscle glucose uptake directly) and the depletion of liver glycogen stores.

At marathon-running pace, muscle carbohydrate stores alone can fuel about 80 minutes of exercise before depletion (see table 3.5). The simultaneous utilization of body fat and hepatic carbohydrate stores, however, enables ATP production to be maintained and exercise to continue. Figure 3.21 shows the contributions of fat oxidation, muscle glycogen, and blood glucose to energy expenditure during running at various speeds. At marathon-running pace, the muscle and hepatic carbohydrate stores will ultimately become depleted. At this point, ATP production becomes compromised because of the inability of fat oxidation to increase sufficiently to offset this deficit. The rate of ATP resynthesis from fat oxidation alone cannot meet the ATP requirement for exercise intensities higher than about 50% to 60% of $\dot{V}O_2$max. The factor that limits the maximal rate of fat oxidation during exercise (i.e., why it cannot increase to compensate for carbohydrate depletion) is currently unknown, but it must precede acetyl-CoA formation because from this point, fat and carbohydrate share the same fate. The limitation may reside in the rate of uptake of FA into muscle from blood or the transport of FA into the mitochondria, rather than in the rate of β-oxidation of FA in the mitochondria.

The glucose–FA cycle partly regulates the integration of carbohydrate and fat oxidation during prolonged exercise. But although this circumstance may be true of resting muscle, evidence (Dyck et al. 1993) suggests that the cycle does not operate in exercising muscle and that the site of regulation must reside elsewhere (e.g., at the level of phosphorylase or CAT-I). The integration of muscle carbohydrate and fat utilization during prolonged exercise is complex and unresolved.

During prolonged submaximal exercise, the main factors influencing the selection of fuel for muscular work are exercise intensity and duration. The effect of exercise duration on the contribution of different fuels during constant-load exercise at about 60% of $\dot{V}O_2$max is illustrated in figure 3.22, and the effect of exercise intensity is summarized in figure 3.23.

In sedentary people, the glycogen store in muscle is fairly resistant to change. The combination of exercise and dietary manipulation, however, can have a dramatic effect on muscle glycogen storage. A clear positive relationship exists between muscle glycogen content and subsequent endurance performance. Furthermore, the ingestion of carbohydrate during prolonged exercise decreases muscle glycogen utilization and fat mobilization and oxidation, and it increases the rate of ~~carbohydrate~~ oxidation and endurance ~~performance. There~~fore, the contribution of ~~carboh~~ydrate to total ATP ~~under th~~ese conditions must ~~differ from that~~ normally derived ~~from oxidation~~. The precise bio~~chemical mechani~~sm by which muscle ~~glycogen depletio~~n causes fatigue is cur~~rently unclear~~. However, the inabil~~ity of muscle to~~ maintain the rate of ATP sy~~nthesis i~~n the glycogen-depleted state possibly results in ADP and Pi accumulation and consequently fatigue. Of course, a substantial fall in intramuscular ATP concentration is unlikely in this form of exercise, because very low ATP concentrations cause rigor and irreversible damage to muscle fibers. Hence, some factor other than muscle glycogen depletion, probably linked to low muscle glycogen concentrations, must act to constrain the activity of glycogen-depleted muscle before rigor can develop.

Starvation rapidly depletes the liver of carbohydrate. The rate of hepatic glucose release in resting, postabsorptive individuals is sufficient to match the carbohydrate demands of only the central nervous system. Approximately 70% of this release is derived from liver carbohydrate stores, and the

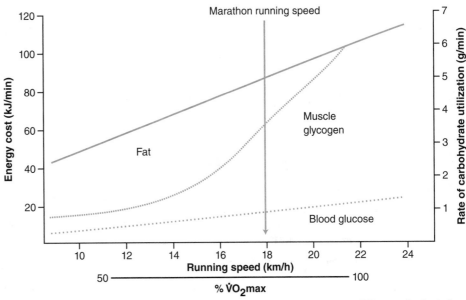

Figure 3.21 Changes in the relative contributions of the major fuel sources to ATP resynthesis during running at various speeds. At the marathon-running speed of an elite endurance athlete, the rate of carbohydrate oxidation is about 3.5 g/min.

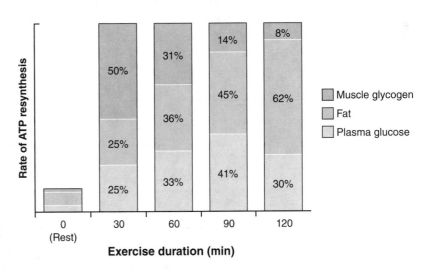

Figure 3.22 Changes in the relative contributions of the major fuel sources to ATP resynthesis during prolonged submaximal exercise at an intensity equivalent to about 60% of $\dot{V}O_2$max (approximately 10 times the resting metabolic rate).

remainder is derived from liver gluconeogenesis. During exercise, the rate of hepatic glucose release is related to exercise intensity. Liver carbohydrate stores contribute 90% of this release, ultimately resulting in liver glycogen depletion.

Prolonged exercise, particularly after a period of fasting or a diet low in carbohydrate results in hypoglycemia, which may be a direct cause of fatigue. Alterations in liver rather than muscle glycogen concentrations could possibly be the more important determinant of the marked difference in exercise capacity induced by high-carbohydrate

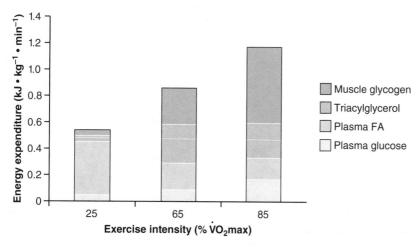

Figure 3.23 The contributions of different fuel sources to energy expenditure at three different exercise intensities.

From Romijn et al. 1995.

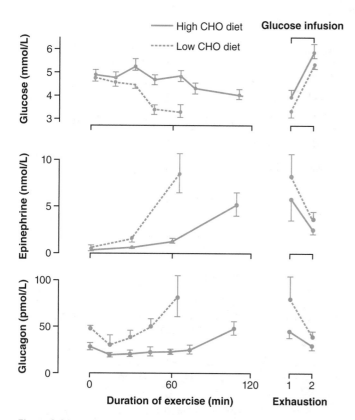

Figure 3.24 Influence of a high-carbohydrate or low-carbohydrate diet (for the preceding 3 days) on the hormonal response to prolonged exercise. Mean plasma hormone concentrations are shown for a group of seven subjects running at 70% of V̇O₂max after 4 days on a low-carbohydrate or high-carbohydrate diet. At exhaustion (1), the subjects were encouraged to run for 10 more minutes (2) with glucose infusion.

Reprinted, by permission, from H. Galbo et al., 1979, "Exercise physiology: Humoral function," *Sport Science Review* 1: 65-93; H. Galbo et al., 1979, "The effect of different diets and of insulin on the hormonal response to prolonged exercise," *Acta Physiologica Scandanavica* 107: 19-32.

and low-carbohydrate diets. Hypoglycemia is detected by the brain and causes symptoms of tiredness and dizziness. This central fatigue could then reduce the degree of skeletal muscle recruitment by the motor cortex, causing a fall in muscle force generation. Furthermore, afferent chemoreceptor information from both the hepatic portal system (monitoring hepatic portal blood glucose concentration) and the skeletal muscle (monitoring muscle glycogenolysis) possibly feeds back to the motor cortex. These signals increase as hypoglycemia develops, and the availability of muscle glycogen declines, inducing more central fatigue and causing athletes to reduce their exercise intensity.

Thus, carbohydrate ingestion during exercise can also delay fatigue development by slowing the rate of liver glycogen depletion and helping to maintain the blood glucose concentration. Central fatigue is certainly a possibility during prolonged exercise, and undoubtedly the development of hypoglycemia contributes to this. Fatigue is a protective mechanism designed to prevent irreversible muscle damage, and—even more important—to prevent neural damage by hypoglycemia.

When exercise is performed with high initial muscle and liver glycogen levels, the hormonal response to exercise is attenuated compared with when exercise is performed in a carbohydrate-depleted state (see figure 3.24). Similarly, carbohydrate feeding during exercise is associated with smaller rises in the plasma concentrations of epinephrine, norepinephrine, glucagon, and cortisol. Because these hormones are involved in the stimulation of lipolysis, fat mobilization is delayed and the rate of fat oxidation is less when carbohydrate is consumed during exercise.

Metabolic Adaptations to Exercise Training

Muscle adaptations to aerobic endurance training include increases in capillary density and mitochondrial size and number. The activity of the TCA cycle and of other oxidative enzymes increases, and a concomitant increase occurs in the capacity to oxidize both fat and carbohydrate. Training adaptations in muscle affect substrate utilization. Endurance training also increases the relative cross-sectional area of type I fibers, increases intramuscular content of triacylglycerol, and increases the capacity to use fat as an energy source during submaximal exercise. Trained subjects also demonstrate increased reliance on intramuscular triacylglycerol as an energy source. These effects and other physiological effects of training, including increased maximum cardiac output and $\dot{V}O_2$max, improved oxygen delivery to working muscle, and attenuated hormonal responses to exercise (see figure 3.25), decrease the rate of muscle glycogen and blood glucose utilization, and decrease the rate of lactate accumulation during submaximal exercise. These adaptations contribute to marked improvement in endurance capacity after training.

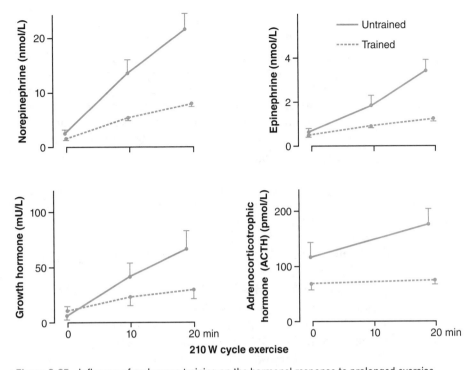

Figure 3.25 Influence of endurance training on the hormonal response to prolonged exercise.

Reprinted, by permission, from H. Galbo et al., 1979, "Exercise physiology: humoral function," *Sport Science Review* 1: 65-93; adapted from M. Kjaer et al., 1988, "Hormonal response to exercise in humans: Influence of hypoxia and physical training," *American Journal of Physiology* 254: R197-203.

Alterations in substrate use with endurance training could be caused, at least in part, by less disturbance to ATP homeostasis during exercise. With increased mitochondrial oxidative capacity after training, smaller decreases in ATP and PCr and smaller increases in ADP and Pi are needed to balance the rate of ATP synthesis with the rate of ATP utilization. In other words, with more mitochondria, the amount of oxygen as well as the ADP and Pi required per mitochondrion will be less after training than before training. The smaller increase in ADP concentration would result in formation of less AMP by the myokinase reaction, and also less IMP and ammonia would be formed by AMP deamination. Smaller increases in the concentrations of ADP, AMP, Pi, and ammonia could account for the slower rate of glycolysis and glycogenolysis in trained muscle compared with untrained muscle.

Training for strength, power, or speed has little if any effect on aerobic capacity. Heavy resistance training or sprinting brings about specific changes in the immediate (ATP and PCr) and short-term (glycolytic) energy delivery systems, increases in muscle buffering capacity, and improvements in strength or sprint performance. Several months of heavy resistance training cause hypertrophy of the muscle fibers, thus increasing total muscle mass and the possible maximum power output. Stretch, contraction, and damage to muscle fibers during exercise provide the stimuli for adaptation, which involves changes in the expression of different myosin isoforms.

KEY POINTS

- Skeletal muscle cells are long, striated, multinucleated fibers. Myofibers are the contractile elements, composed of sarcomeres containing thin (actin) and thick (myosin) filaments arranged in a regular array. The heads of the myosin molecules form cross-bridges that bind reversibly to the actin filaments, causing the filaments to slide over each other toward the centers of the sarcomeres.

- The energy source for muscle contraction is ATP, which is continuously regenerated during exercise from phosphocreatine hydrolysis, anaerobic metabolism of glycogen or glucose, or aerobic metabolism of acetyl-CoA derived principally from breakdown of carbohydrate or fat. The carbon skeleton of amino acids can be used as a fuel for oxidative metabolism but is not a major fuel for energy production during exercise.

■ Phosphocreatine is present in the sarcoplasm of muscle at about three times the concentration of ATP. Phosphocreatine hydrolysis is initiated at the immediate onset of contraction to buffer the rapid accumulation of ADP resulting from ATP hydrolysis. But the rate of phosphocreatine hydrolysis begins to decline after only a few seconds of maximal force generation. The importance of phosphocreatine to muscle energy production and function lies in the extremely rapid rate at which it can resynthesize ATP.

■ Carbohydrate provides energy by anaerobic metabolism, with lactate as the end product, or by complete oxidation to carbon dioxide and water. The net effect of glycolysis is conversion of one molecule of glucose to two molecules of pyruvate. This process makes two molecules of ATP available for each molecule of glucose that is broken down. If muscle glycogen is the starting substrate, three ATP molecules are generated for each glucose residue passing down the pathway.

■ Glycolysis involves the reduction of NAD to NADH, depleting the intracellular pool of NAD. Reduction of pyruvate to lactate allows the NAD to be regenerated from NADH. The alternative pathway for NAD regeneration involves conversion of pyruvate to acetyl-CoA for subsequent oxidation in the TCA cycle.

■ The TCA cycle and oxidative phosphorylation occur in the mitochondria. In the aerobic resynthesis of ATP, oxygen is the final electron acceptor in the electron-transport chain, and it combines with hydrogen to form water.

■ Carbohydrate stores are rapidly depleted during exercise (muscle glycogen) or during fasting (liver glycogen). Muscle glycogen stores are normally depleted after 1 to 2 hours of hard exercise. In very high-intensity exercise, muscle glycogen content falls rapidly but is not completely depleted at the point of fatigue.

■ Carbohydrate is the major fuel for muscle activity in high-intensity exercise: When muscle glycogen stores are depleted, only low-intensity exercise is possible. The time that a fixed exercise intensity can be sustained is related to the size of the preexercise glycogen store. The size of the store depends on the pattern of exercise and diet in the previous hours and days.

■ A number of hormones are involved in the integration and control of carbohydrate metabolism, including (especially) insulin, which promotes carbohydrate storage, and glucagon, whose actions are generally antagonistic to those of insulin. Epinephrine and norepinephrine stimulate carbohydrate mobilization and metabolism at times of stress.

■ The principal storage form of fat in the body is triacylglycerol, most of which is located in white adipose tissue. Triacylglycerol stores are also found in liver and muscle and as lipoproteins in blood. Muscles cannot oxidize triacylglycerols directly. The triacylglycerol molecules must first be broken down into its FA and glycerol components by lipolysis. This process is activated during exercise by the actions of epinephrine, glucagon, and cortisol. The principal sources of fat fuels for exercise are blood-borne FAs derived from adipose tissue and intramuscular triacylglycerol.

■ Several factors influence the type of substrate used to fuel muscular work, including substrate availability, diet, intensity and duration of exercise, training status, hormones, previous exercise, and environmental conditions. Fat oxidation makes an increasing contribution to ATP regeneration as exercise duration increases. In exercise lasting several hours, fat may supply almost 80% of the total energy required.

■ Endurance training increases the capacity of muscle to oxidize fat.

■ Fatigue is the inability to maintain a given or expected power output or force, and it is an inevitable feature of strenuous exercise. The onset of muscle fatigue has been associated with the disruption of energy supply, product inhibition, and factors preceding cross-bridge formation. It is likely a multifactorial process.

RECOMMENDED READINGS

Åstrand, P.-O., K. Rodahl, H. Dahl, and S. Stromme. 2003. *Textbook of work physiology. Physiological basis of exercise.* Champaign, IL: Human Kinetics.

Bangsbo, J. 1997. Physiology of muscle fatigue during intense exercise. In *The clinical pharmacology of sport and exercise,* ed. T. Reilly and M. Orme, 123–133. Amsterdam: Elsevier.

Green, H.J. 1991. How important is endogenous muscle glycogen to fatigue in prolonged exercise? *Canadian Journal of Physiology and Pharmacology* 69:290–297.

Greenhaff, P.L., and E. Hultman. 1999. The biochemical basis of exercise. In *Basic and applied sciences for sports medicine,* ed. R.J. Maughan, 69–89. Oxford: Butterworth-Heinemann.

Hargreaves, M., and L. Spriet. 2006. *Exercise metabolism,* 2nd ed. Champaign, IL: Human Kinetics.

Komi, P.V., and J. Karlsson. 1978. Skeletal muscle fibre types, enzyme activities and physical performance in young males and females. *Acta Physiologica Scandinavica* 103:210–218.

Maughan, R.J., and M. Gleeson. 2004. *The biochemical basis of sports performance,* 2nd ed. Oxford: Oxford University Press.

Sahlin, K., and S. Broberg. 1990. Adenine nucleotide depletion in human muscle during exercise: Causality and significance of AMP deamination. *International Journal of Sports Medicine* 11:S62–S67.

Saltin, B. 1985. Physiological adaptation to physical conditioning. *Acta Medica Scandinavica* 711 (supplement): 11–24.

Sjøgaard, G. 1991. Role of exercise-induced potassium fluxes underlying muscle fatigue: A brief review. *Canadian Journal of Physiology and Pharmacology* 69:238–245.

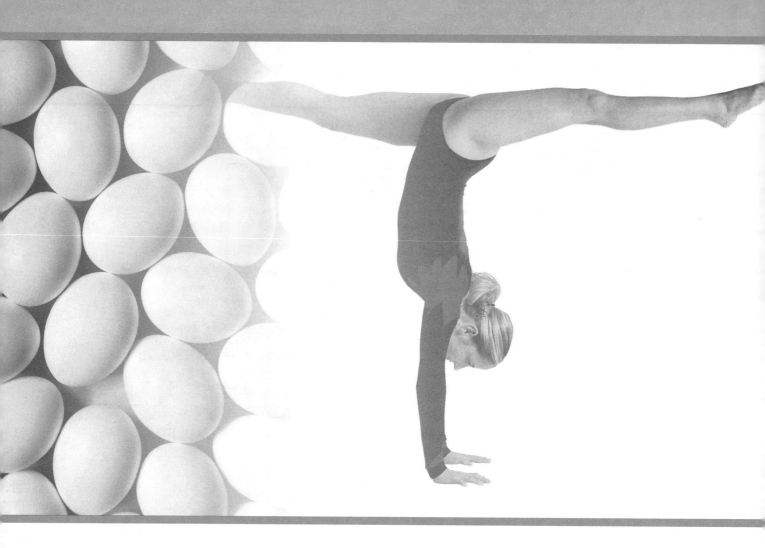

OBJECTIVES

After studying this chapter, you should be able to do the following:

- Describe what energy is and how it is expressed and give an overview of the different types of energy

- Define the terms *gross efficiency, net efficiency, delta efficiency,* and *economy*

- Describe various ways to measure energy expenditure and explain the advantages and disadvantages of these methods

- Describe the various components of human energy expenditure and their respective contributions to energy expenditure in active and inactive persons

- Discuss the concept of energy balance and how it relates to body weight and physical performance

- Discuss the upper and lower limits of human energy expenditure and the practical problems associated with these energy expenditures

4

Energy

Cells need energy to function, muscle fibers need energy to contract, and ionic pumps in membranes need energy to transport ions across cell membranes. Although the human body has some energy reserves, most of its energy must be obtained through nutrition. During exercise, energy requirements increase and energy provision can become critical. Persons with a defect in energy metabolism have problems performing vigorous physical exercise. For instance, a person with McArdle's disease lacks the enzyme glycogen phosphorylase and cannot break down muscle glycogen. Hence, that person's energy provision and exercise capacity are severely impaired. In athletes, energy provision can be crucial, and energy depletion (carbohydrate depletion) is one of the most common causes of fatigue. Different types of exercise and sports have different energy requirements. Therefore, athletes must adjust their food intake accordingly. This chapter describes the energy requirements and associated practical problems for some athletes.

Forms of energy range from light energy to chemical energy. Plants use light energy in the process of photosynthesis to produce carbohydrate, fat, or protein. The energy in food is stored in the chemical bonds of various molecules. Breaking these bonds releases the energy, and it becomes available for conversion into other forms of energy. For instance, when glucose is broken down during glycolysis, chemical energy is converted to another form of chemical energy (ATP) and ultimately transformed into mechanical energy (muscle contraction).

In physiology, energy represents the capacity to do work, which is often referred to as mechanical energy. Walking, running, throwing, and jumping require the production of mechanical energy. Work (energy) is the product of force times the vertical distance covered:

$$\text{work} = \text{force} \times \text{distance, or } W = F \times d$$

If work is expressed per unit of time, the term *power* (P) is used:

$$\text{power} = \text{work/time, or } P = W/t$$

Energy expenditure (EE) refers to energy expended (in **kiloJoules [kJ]** or kilocalories [kcal]) per unit of time to produce power. During conversion of one form of energy into another, no energy is lost. For example, in carbohydrate and fat combustion, chemical energy is converted into mechanical energy (muscle contraction) and heat energy.

The human body is not efficient in its use of energy from the breakdown of carbohydrate and fat. During cycling exercise, for instance, only 20% of that energy is converted to power. The remainder of the energy becomes heat. This heat can be partly used to maintain body temperature at 37 °C (98.6 °F), but during exercise heat production may be excessive. To prevent body temperature from rising too high, various heat-dissipating mechanisms must be activated (see chapter 10).

Energy is often expressed in calories (the English system) or joules (the metric system). One calorie expresses the quantity of energy (heat) needed to raise the temperature of 1 g (1 ml) of water by 1 °C (1.8 °F) (from 14.5 °C to 15.5 °C [58.1 °F to 59.9 °F]). Thus, food containing 200 kcal (kilocalories) has enough energy potential to raise the temperature of 200 L of water by 1 °C (1.8 °F). (In everyday language, kilocalories are often referred to as calories. Because this may be a source of confusion, we will stick to kilojoules or kilocalories in this book.)

The SI (International System of Units) unit for energy is the joule, named for the British scientist Sir Prescott Joule (1818–1889). One joule of energy moves a mass of 1 g at a velocity of 1 m/s. A joule is not a large amount of energy; therefore, kilojoules are more often used. To convert calories to joules or kilocalories to kilojoules, the calorie value must be multiplied by 4.186.

When discussing energy expenditure or intake over 24 hours, megajoules (MJ) are often used to avoid large numbers. Because joules are not yet part of everyday language, both units are often mentioned on food labels. In this book kJ will be used, with the equivalent in kcal given in parentheses.

Converting Kilocalories to Kilojoules

1 calorie (cal) = 4.186 J

1 kcal = 4.186 kJ

1 kcal = 1,000 cal

1 kJ = 1,000 J

1 MJ = 1,000 kJ

For example:

250 kcal = 250 × 4.186 = 1,047 kJ = 1.047 MJ

5,000 kJ = 5000/4.186 = 1,194 kcal

Energetic Efficiency

The effective work performed after muscle contraction, or **efficiency,** is expressed as the percentage of total work. As already mentioned, approximately 20% of all energy produced in the human body is used to accomplish work (movement). Therefore, humans are approximately 20% efficient. Most of the remaining 80% is used to maintain homeostasis and is wasted as heat. No system is 100% efficient. A gasoline engine is 20% to 30% efficient. A diesel engine is 30% to 40% efficient. An ordinary light bulb is about 20% efficient, and an energy-saving bulb is about 80% efficient.

The precise definition of efficiency can vary. For example, gross efficiency (GE) is the ratio of the total work to energy expended:

GE (%) = work accomplished/energy expended × 100%

As exercise intensity increases, however, the relative proportion of the energy expended as resting metabolism decreases, causing GE to increase with work rate. A solution for this problem is to subtract baseline energy expenditure from total energy expenditure. One way to calculate the baseline is to use net efficiency (NE), where the baseline is the energy expended at rest:

NE (%) = work accomplished/(energy expended
– resting energy expenditure) × 100%

The second way to calculate the baseline is to use work efficiency (WE), where the baseline is the energy cost of unloaded (0 W) work (for example, unloaded cycling):

WE (%) = work accomplished/(energy expended
– energy expended in unloaded condition) × 100%

Unfortunately, work efficiency is difficult or even impossible to determine reliably because of the unnatural nature of unloaded movements.

A fourth definition of efficiency is delta efficiency (DE), which expresses the change in energy expended per minute relative to the change in actual work accomplished per minute:

DE (%) = delta work accomplished/
delta energy expended × 100%

Delta efficiency may be the most accurate reflection of muscle efficiency, but it is more difficult to determine and is more variable. All four calculations of efficiency are commonly used in the literature, and all have their limitations.

The term *economy* is typically expressed as the oxygen uptake required to exercise at a certain intensity. For runners, it is the oxygen uptake at a speed of 16 km/h. Efficient runners are usually better runners because they "waste" less energy. In other sports, such as cycling, the relationship between efficiency and performance does not seem to be as strong.

When weight loss is the goal, low efficiency is probably desirable because the person is expending more energy for the same amount of work (see chapter 5).

Measuring the Energy Content of Food

Food contains energy in the form of carbohydrate, fat, and protein, which all have energy stored within their chemical bonds. To determine the energy content of food, we use a technique called direct calorimetry. The food is combusted (oxidized), and the resulting heat is used as a measure of the energy content. The measurement takes place in a bomb calorimeter (see figure 4.1).

A weighed amount of food (about 1 g) is placed in a sealed steel chamber with high oxygen pressure. The reaction is started through ignition by an electrical current. The food burns inside the chamber and produces heat, which is transferred through the metal walls of the chamber and heats the water that surrounds it. The rise in water

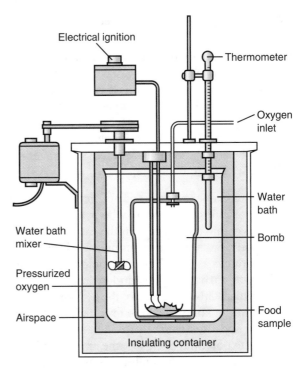

Figure 4.1 Bomb calorimeter.

temperature directly reflects the energy content of the food. If the water volume surrounding the chamber is 2 L and the temperature rises by 4.0 °C (7.2 °F), the energy content of that food is $2 \times 4 = 8$ kcal (or $8 \times 4.186 = 33.5$ kJ). If the weight of the food combusted was 1.2 g, the energy content of the food was $8/1.2 = 6.7$ kcal/g (27.9 kJ/g). This measure is the gross energy value, or total energy content of the food, and no distinction is made between carbohydrate, fat, and protein. Although the bomb calorimeter is probably the most accurate method of determining the energy content of food, it is expensive to run, and the results tend to overestimate actual calories absorbed because not all the energy eaten can be digested or absorbed.

■ Carbohydrates have varying energy content, depending on the type of carbohydrate and the arrangements of atoms within the carbohydrate. The combustion of glucose, for instance, gives 15.7 kJ/g (3.7 kcal/g), whereas the combustion of glycogen and starch is about 17.6 kJ/g (4.2 kcal/g). The latter figure is normally used as the energy value of carbohydrate (1 g carbohydrate = 17.6 kJ = 4.2 kcal).

■ The energy content of fat also depends on the structure of the triacylglycerol or FA. A medium-chain FA, such as octanoate (eight-carbon FA) may contain 36.0 kJ/g (8.6 kcal/g), whereas a long-chain FA may contain up to 40.2 kJ/g (9.6 kcal/g). The energy content of fat in the average diet is 39.3 kJ/g (9.4 kcal/g).

■ The energy content of protein depends on the type of protein and the nitrogen content. Nitrogen does not provide energy, and, therefore, proteins with a higher nitrogen density contain less energy per gram. Nitrogen content in foods may vary from 15% (whole milk) to approximately 19% (nuts and seeds). The energy content of protein in the average diet is 23.7 kJ/g (5.65 kcal/g).

The gross energy value is not necessarily the amount of energy that would be available if the food was eaten, particularly in the case of protein. In the body, the nitrogen in amino acids is excreted by the kidneys as urea. The urea molecule consists of nitrogen, carbon, oxygen, and hydrogen and has the formula $CO(NH_2)_2$. Some of the hydrogen atoms present in the amino acid are excreted along with nitrogen and thus cannot provide energy. About 20% of the potential energy of the amino acid will be lost. If a bomb calorimeter shows that protein contains 23.7 kJ/g (5.65 kcal/g), in the human body

only 19.3 kJ/g (4.6 kcal/g) is available. This value is the net energy of food.

Food is sometimes not completely absorbed. Incomplete digestion and absorption will, of course, result in decreased availability of energy. Wilbur Olin Atwater (1844–1907), one of the pioneers in studying human energy balance, determined this fact. After measuring many kinds of foods, Atwater came up with energy values for foods that accounted for differences in digestibility. Conveniently, these energy values were rounded to whole numbers. The energy contents of carbohydrate, fat, and protein were 4 kcal/g, 9 kcal/g, and 4 kcal/g, respectively (16 kJ/g, 36 kJ/g, and 16 kJ/g). These correction factors are often referred to as the Atwater factors or Atwater energy values.

The percentage of food energy that is absorbed is often expressed in a coefficient of digestibility. A coefficient of digestibility of 50 means that only half of the energy ingested is absorbed. Adding fiber to a meal generally reduces the coefficient of digestibility. Thus, a smaller amount of energy is available to the body from a food item high in fiber than from a food item with identical energy content but low in fiber. Fiber causes the food to move faster through the gastrointestinal system, leaving less time for absorption processes. On average, 97% of carbohydrate is completely digested and absorbed. For fat, this value is 95%, and for protein, it is 92% (see table 4.1). On the other hand, the coefficient of digestibility of wheat bran protein is only 40%, and its protein calorie contribution is just 7.62 kJ/g (1.82 kcal/g), significantly less than the 16 kJ/g (4 kcal/g) estimated by Atwater. Furthermore, the coefficient of digestibility of wheat bran carbohydrate is 56%, and its calorie contribution is only 9.84 kJ/g (2.35 kcal/g), again, far below the 16 kJ/g (4 kcal/g) used by Atwater.

Atwater had begun to analyze the composition and the energy content of food. Nowadays many extensive databases exist, usually compiled by governmental institutions. One of the largest and most comprehensible databases is the U.S. Nutrient Data Bank (USNDB), which is compiled by the U.S. Department of Agriculture's Consumer Nutrition Center and contains over 6,000 items. The UK database contains over 3,500 food items. The U.S. database can be downloaded from the USDA Nutrient Laboratory database (www.ars.usda.gov/main/site_main.htm?modecode=12354500). Software manufacturers base their programs on this database and comparable nutritional databases. Because each country has its specific products and brands, no one database covers all food items.

■ **TABLE 4.1** ■

■ TABLE 4.1 ■
Energy Content of Nutrients and the Availability of Energy in the Body

	Energy of combustion per gram in kJ (kcal)	Energy available per gram in kJ (kcal)	Coefficient of digestibility
PROTEIN			
Animal food	23.7 (5.65)	17.9 (4.27)	97
Meats, fish, and poultry	23.7 (5.65)	17.9 (4.27)	97
Eggs	24.1 (5.75)	18.3 (4.37)	97
Dairy products	23.7 (5.65)	17.9 (4.27)	97
Plant food	23.7 (5.65)	15.7 (3.74)	85
Cereals	24.3 (5.80)	16.2 (3.87)	85
Legumes	23.9 (5.70)	14.5 (3.47)	78
Vegetables	20.9 (5.00)	13.0 (3.11)	83
Fruits	21.8 (5.20)	14.1 (3.36)	83
Average protein	*23.7 (5.65)*	*17.0 (4.05)*	*92*
FAT			
Animal food	39.3 (9.40)	37.4 (8.93)	95
Meat and eggs	39.8 (9.50)	37.8 (9.03)	95
Dairy products	38.7 (9.25)	36.8 (8.79)	95
Vegetable food	38.9 (9.30)	35.0 (8.37)	90
Average lipid	*39.3 (9.40)*	*37.4 (8.93)*	*95*
CARBOHYDRATE			
Animal food	16.3 (3.90)	16.0 (3.82)	98
Vegetable food	17.4 (4.15)	16.9 (4.03)	97
Cereals	17.6 (4.20)	17.2 (4.11)	98
Legumes	17.6 (4.20)	17.0 (4.07)	97
Vegetables	17.6 (4.20)	16.7 (3.99)	95
Fruits	16.7 (4.00)	15.1 (3.60)	90
Sugars	16.5 (3.95)	16.2 (3.87)	98
Average carbohydrate	*17.4 (4.15)*	*16.9 (4.03)*	*97*

The coefficient of digestibility reflects the percentage of energy in a nutrient that is actually available.

Adapted from A.L. Merrill and B.K. Watt, 1973, Energy value of foods: Basis and derivation, revised. In *Agriculture Handbook 74*. U.S. Department of Agriculture.

Measuring Energy Expenditure

The methods of measuring or estimating human energy expenditure range from direct but complex measurements of heat production (direct calorimetry) to relatively simple indirect metabolic measurements (indirect calorimetry), and from expensive stable isotope tracer methods (doubly labeled water) to relatively cheap and convenient rough estimates (heart rate monitoring and

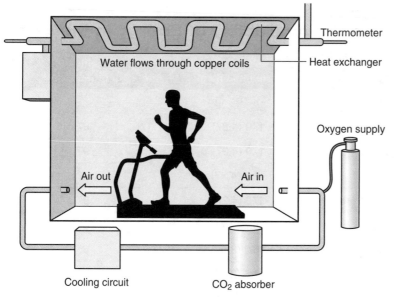

Figure 4.2 Direct calorimetry chamber.

accelerometry). Following are some of the methods used to measure human energy expenditure:

- Direct calorimetry
- Indirect calorimetry
- Closed-circuit spirometry
- Open-circuit spirometry
- Douglas bag technique
- Breath-by-breath technique
- Portable spirometry
- Doubly labeled water
- Labeled bicarbonate
- Heart rate monitoring
- Accelerometry
- Observations, records of physical activity, activity diaries, recall

Direct Calorimetry

Ultimately, all biochemical processes in the body result in heat production. This heat production can be measured in a similar manner as the heat production from combusting food. A human calorimeter is a small, well-insulated chamber with adequate ventilation (see figure 4.2). The top of the chamber consists of a series of coils through which a known amount of water flows. The water absorbs the heat radiated by the subject in the chamber, which reflects the metabolic rate of that person.

The air is recirculated, and carbon dioxide and water are filtered out of the air before it reenters the chamber, together with added oxygen. This process prevents heat being lost from the chamber in the form of expired gases.

Although the direct calorimeter is based on a simple principle, the actual engineering and operation of the chamber are complicated. Specially trained personnel are required to operate the device; therefore, it is not the most popular and most common way to measure energy expenditure. An important disadvantage of the direct calorimeter is that it is unsuitable for field studies and assessment of energy expenditure in most exercise and sport situations.

Direct Calorimeter Suit

To overcome some of the practical problems of the direct calorimeter chamber, a direct calorimeter suit was developed. This suit consists of a long plastic tube through which a known amount of water flows. The tubing touches the skin and absorbs body heat. Again, the rise in temperature of the water is directly related to the subject's heat production and thus to the metabolic rate. With this suit, measurements can be conducted outside the chamber, but the suit may impair movement. The suit has been shown to be useful for walking exercise, but because it is heavy and not very flexible, it might impede more vigorous activities or faster movements. Nevertheless, the suit has been used successfully for those purposes as well.

Indirect Calorimetry

The energy for all biochemical reactions ultimately depends on the oxygen supply. The term *indirect* refers to the measurement of O_2 uptake and CO_2 production rather than to the measurement of heat transfer. This measurement requires a steady state CO_2 production and respiratory exchange ratio (RER = VCO_2/VO_2) and subjects with a normal acid–base balance. Studies with the bomb calorimeter have shown that the amount of oxygen required to combust carbohydrate, fat, and protein is directly related to the energy content. In fact, for every kJ, 50 ml of O_2 is required, or for every kcal, 207 ml of O_2 is required. In other words, the energy equivalent of 1 L of O_2 is 20.2 kJ (4.82 kcal). This energy equivalent of oxygen is relatively stable and largely independent of the mixture of carbohydrate, fat, and protein oxidized. Indirect calorimetry is an indirect but accurate estimate of energy expenditure.

When $\dot{V}O_2$ is measured in L of O_2 at STPD (standard temperature [0 °C, or 32 °F], pressure [760 mm Hg], and dry) per minute, energy expenditure (EE) can be measured by

$$EE\ (kJ/min) = 20.2 \times \dot{V}O_2$$

Energy expenditure can be estimated even more accurately if the RER is known because the energy equivalent for oxygen is 19.6 kJ/L at an RER of 0.7 (when 100% fat is being oxidized), rising to 20.9 kJ/L at a RER of 1.0 (when carbohydrate is the only fuel being oxidized). For these calculations, the relatively small contribution of protein oxidation is ignored.

Closed-Circuit and Open-Circuit Spirometry

O_2 uptake and CO_2 production can be measured using closed-circuit and open-circuit methods. The closed-circuit method is used to measure resting energy expenditure (see figure 4.3). The technique was developed in the late 1800s and is routinely used in clinical settings. The subject breathes through a mouthpiece into a spirometer that is prefilled with 100% oxygen. During each inspiration, some of the oxygen in the chamber of gas is consumed. Expired gas is passed back into the spirometer, and the CO_2 produced is trapped in a filter. The residual oxygen in the chamber is available for the next inspiration. As oxygen is consumed, the volume of oxygen in the spirometer decreases, and this change in volume is measured. The oxygen taken up and energy expenditure can then be calculated. Closed-circuit spirometry is a good method in resting conditions, but it is not suitable during exercise, especially high-intensity exercise. When CO_2 production is high, the trap-

ping of CO_2 may become problematic. The subject breathes through a three-way valve from and into a spirometer, which is prefilled with 100% oxygen. A recorder is connected so that the changes in volume are accurately measured.

With open-circuit spirometry (for research purposes the most common method of estimating energy expenditure), the subject inhales ambient air (0.03% CO_2, 20.93% O_2, and 79.04% N_2). Energy expenditure is calculated from the difference in O_2 and CO_2 content between the inspired and expired gases and the ventilation rate. Such measurements can be made in a respiration chamber by so-called Douglas bags or online systems.

Respiration Chamber

For measurement of a complete energy balance, a respiration chamber was developed. The respiration chamber (see figure 4.4) is comparable to the chamber used for direct calorimetry but without the coils to measure heat exchange and the insulation. Sufficient airflow into the respiration chamber prevents the chamber air from falling much below 20% oxygen, and the ventilation rate is carefully measured. Flow of air into the chamber is continuous. This flow is carefully monitored. In addition, the oxygen and carbon dioxide concentrations at the inlet and outlet of the chamber are recorded, from which oxygen uptake and carbon dioxide production can be calculated. Respiration chambers are usually designed like small hotel rooms, with a bed, chair, television, radio, and telephone, and measurements can be performed over a period of several hours to several days.

The chamber is ideal for measurements of energy balance because food intake can be accurately controlled, and all food is prepared by the investigators and handed to the subject through special hatches.

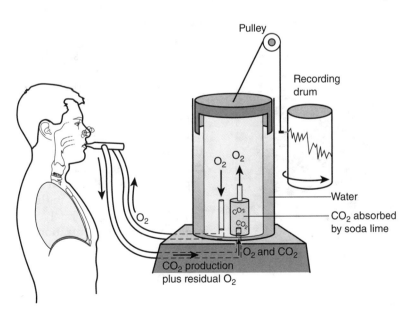

Figure 4.3 Closed-circuit spirometry.

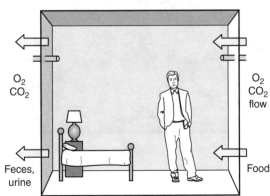

Figure 4.4 A respiration chamber.

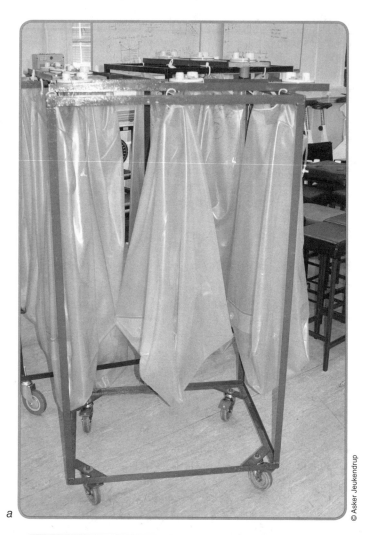

Urine and feces can also be collected for further analysis, which is often done when a complete energy and nitrogen balance is required.

The advantage of this technique is that, besides producing accurate information about gas exchange (and thus energy expenditure), it allows accurate control over energy intake and permits analysis of potential energy losses in feces and urine. The main disadvantages of this technique are that it requires highly trained personnel and is extremely expensive. In addition, the stay in the chamber interferes with everyday life because not all activities can be performed inside the chamber. Furthermore, most chambers are not adapted to high ventilation rates and are not suitable for vigorous exercise. But modern respiration chambers with fast-response analyzers are capable of measuring energy expenditure during very high-intensity exercise, and several studies have been performed of highly trained people performing vigorous exercise for prolonged periods.

Douglas Bag

A way to measure oxygen uptake and carbon dioxide production at the same time is by collecting the expired gases for a certain period and measuring the volume, O_2 concentration, and CO_2 concentration of this gas. The test subject inspires room air and expires through a mouthpiece connected to a high-flow, low-resistance valve into a large plastic bag. These Douglas bags are named after British scientist Claude Douglas (1882–1963), who was the first to use this method to measure gas exchange in humans (see figure 4.5).

After collection, the bags are closed until analysis. They are then emptied into a gas meter to measure the total volume. From the duration of collection (usually 1 minute) and the volume measurement, the ventilation rate can be calculated. A small sample of expired gas is collected from or in addition to the gas in this large Douglas bag for analysis of O_2 and CO_2 concentrations. From the difference between the inspired and expired O_2 and CO_2 concentrations and

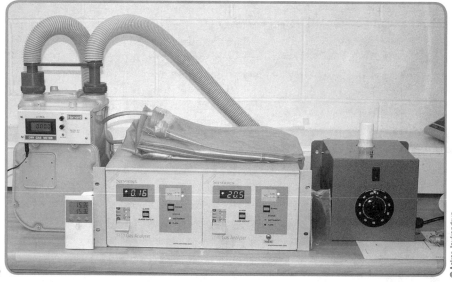

Figure 4.5 *(a)* Douglas bags and *(b)* dry gas meter (left) and oxygen and carbon dioxide analyzer (middle).

the ventilation rate, O_2 uptake and CO_2 production can be calculated. This relatively simple technique has been applied successfully for many years and is still used by exercise physiologists. Various versions of this technique are used, including methods in which flow is measured directly from the expired or inspired air.

Breath-by-Breath Systems

Respiratory physiologists have taken the Douglas bag technique one step further, and computers and fast-response O_2 and CO_2 analyzers have made it possible to develop an online breath-by-breath gas analysis system. This semiautomated or fully automated analyzer usually measures volume at the mouthpiece, and a small gas sample is collected every expiration for analysis of O_2 and CO_2 concentrations (see figure 4.6). This technique enables respiratory physiologists to look at the time course of changes in various ventilatory variables. When averaged over periods of 20 seconds to several

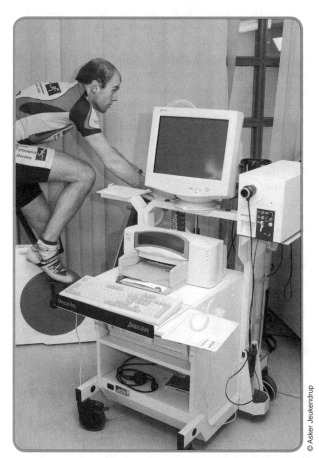

© Asker Jeukendrup

Figure 4.6 Automated breath-by-breath system.

minutes, this technique gives similar values to those obtained with the Douglas bag technique. The main advantage of the breath-by-breath systems is that they can analyze every breath and are therefore able to register rapid changes and give instant feedback. Breath-by-breath systems are convenient, and most systems give an accurate estimation of energy expenditure.

The measurements are restricted to a laboratory situation, however, because the bulky, sensitive equipment is difficult to move. Recently, manufacturers have developed smaller and portable breath-by-breath systems for measurements in free-living conditions. These attempts have been reasonably successful, and in the future smaller analyzers may replace some of the laboratory-based equipment.

Indirect Calorimetry and Substrate Utilization

Gas exchange measurements allow an estimation not only of the energy expenditure but also of the substrate mixture used. Krogh and Lindhard, in the beginning of the 20th century, used the inherent differences in chemical properties of carbohydrate, fat, and protein to obtain information about fuel utilization (Krogh et al. 1920). The complete oxidation of carbohydrate, fat, and protein requires different amounts of O_2 and produces different amounts of CO_2. The oxidation of 1 g of glucose requires 0.746 L of O_2 and produces 0.743 L of CO_2 and 3.868 kcal. The oxidation of 1 g of FA (palmitic acid) requires 2.009 L of O_2 and produces 1.414 L of CO_2 and 9.746 kcal. The substrate used, therefore, determines the total O_2 required and total CO_2 produced. The ratio of CO_2 production and O_2 consumption, or respiratory quotient (RQ), provides a convenient indication of the substrate that is being utilized during steady-state exercise.

$$RQ = VCO_2/VO_2$$

The complete oxidation of one molecule of glucose (1 mole = 180 g) requires six molecules of O_2 and produces six molecules of CO_2. The number of oxygen molecules equals the number of CO_2 molecules, and the RQ for carbohydrate is therefore 1.

$$C_6H_{12}O_6 + 6\,O_2 \rightarrow 6\,CO_2 + 6\,H_2O$$
$$RQ = 6\,CO_2/6\,O_2 = 1$$

Lipids contain significantly fewer oxygen atoms compared with carbohydrate and therefore require more oxygen in the oxidation process. Lipids can have different chemical compositions, unlike carbohydrate, whose biochemical formula is always the same ($C_6H_{12}O_6$). The O_2 required and the CO_2 produced, therefore, depend somewhat on the type of lipid oxidized. Complete oxidation of 1 molecule of a typical (and most abundant) FA (palmitic acid; 1 mole = 256 g) in the human body oxidizes to CO_2 and H_2O using 23 molecules of O_2. It produces 16 molecules of CO_2 and 16 molecules of H_2O. The RQ of palmitic acid is therefore 16/23 = 0.696. This RQ value, however, may vary from 0.727 (octanoic acid, C8:0) to 0.686 (lignoceric acid, C24:0), depending on the chain length of the FA oxidized:

$$C_{16}H_{32}O_2 + 23\ O_2 \rightarrow 16\ CO_2 + 16\ H_2O$$
$$RQ = 16\ CO_2/23\ O_2 = 0.696$$

In addition to carbon, oxygen, and hydrogen, proteins (amino acids) also contain nitrogen and sometimes sulfur, which cannot be oxidized. Proteins have to be deaminated (removal of nitrogen), and nitrogen (as urea) and sulfur will be excreted in urine and feces. The remaining carbon skeleton can be oxidized to CO_2 and H_2O in a similar manner to carbohydrate and fat. The O_2 required and the CO_2 produced depend somewhat on the type of protein. An example of the oxidation of a protein is the following:

$$\text{(albumin) } C_{72}H_{112}N_{18}O_{22}S + 77\ O_2 \rightarrow 63\ CO_2$$
$$+ 38\ H_2O + SO_3 + 9\ CO(NH_2)_2 \text{ (urea)}$$
$$RQ = 63\ CO_2/77\ O_2 = 0.818$$

If a mixture of carbohydrate and fat is oxidized, O_2 consumption will equal the sum of O_2 required to oxidize the carbohydrate plus that required for fat. Similarly, CO_2 production will be the sum of CO_2 production from carbohydrate and CO_2 production from fat. If, for instance, 100 g of carbohydrate and 50 g of fat is oxidized, O_2 consumption is (100 × 0.746) + (50 × 2.009) = 175 L. CO_2 production is (100 × 0.743) + (50 × 1.414) = 145 L. The RQ is 145/175 = 0.829.

When experiments are performed using indirect calorimetry and measures of $\dot{V}O_2$ and $\dot{V}CO_2$ are obtained, the reverse calculation is used:

Rate of carbohydrate oxidation (g/min) × O_2 (L/g) + rate of fat oxidation (g/min) × O_2 (L/g) = $\dot{V}O_2$ (L/min)

Rate of carbohydrate oxidation (g/min) × CO_2 (L/g) + rate of fat oxidation (g/min) × CO_2 (L/g) = $\dot{V}CO_2$ (L/min)

Using different assumptions for the composition of fat substrate (chain length of the fatty acids) will result in different equations (see highlight box). These calculations give two equations and two unknown variables, which can be solved:

Carbohydrate oxidation (g/min) = 4.585 $\dot{V}CO_2$ – 3.226 $\dot{V}O_2$

Fat oxidation (g/min) = 1.695 $\dot{V}O_2$ – 1.701 $\dot{V}CO_2$

Oxidation Rates

Carbohydrate oxidation (g/min) = 4.21 × $\dot{V}CO_2$ – 2.96 × $\dot{V}O_2$ – 2.37 × N

Fat oxidation (g/min) = 1.70 × $\dot{V}O_2$ – 1.70 × $\dot{V}CO_2$ – 1.77 × N

Protein oxidation (g) = 6.25 × N

Energy expenditure (kJ) = 16.18 × $\dot{V}O_2$ + 5.02 × $\dot{V}CO_2$ – 5.99 × N

Energy expenditure (kcal) = 0.55 × $\dot{V}CO_2$ – 4.47 × $\dot{V}O_2$ – 1.43 × N

Where N is the urinary nitrogen in grams.

If it is assumed that protein oxidation is negligible, then N should be substituted by 0. These equations are obtained from Jeukendrup and Wallis (2005).

Using different assumptions for the composition of fat substrate (chain length of the fatty acids) will result in different equations (see highlight box). These calculations assume that protein is not an important energy fuel. In some extreme conditions, protein may contribute up to 15% to the total energy expenditure (see chapter 8). In this case, correction for protein oxidation should be made. To make this correction, urine samples are collected, and protein oxidation is estimated from the nitrogen content. One gram of nitrogen in urine represents the oxidation of 6.25 g of protein. This result is subtracted from the fat and carbohydrate oxidation rates (see highlight box).

As mentioned previously, because the energy equivalent for oxygen is slightly different, depending on what substrate is utilized, measuring both O_2 consumption and CO_2 production increases the accuracy of the estimate of energy expenditure. For instance, if $\dot{V}O_2$ is 600 L/day, $\dot{V}CO_2$ is 500 L/day, and nitrogen excretion is 25 g/day, energy expenditure is 12,068 kJ (2,886 kcal). With the simple formula (i.e., ignoring protein oxidation) the result is 12,120 kJ (2,892 kcal), a difference of only 0.2%.

The application of RQ is based on the premise that exchange of O_2 and CO_2 at the mouth represents the processes that occur in the tissues that oxidize the fuels. This assumption is valid at rest and during light to fairly high-intensity exercise (up to about 85% of $\dot{V}O_2$max). But because RQ measured at the mouth does not always reflect the oxidation processes in cells, it is usually referred to as respiratory exchange ratio (RER, or R). For moderate to high exercise intensities where glycogen is an important fuel source (50% to 75% $\dot{V}O_2$max) the equations in the highlight box should be used.

One common condition in which RER is different from RQ is hyperventilation. During hyperventilation excess amounts of CO_2 are expired. This CO_2 is not derived from metabolic processes but is simply an extra excretion of body CO_2 stores. (CO_2 is mainly stored in the form of bicarbonate in the extracellular body fluids.) Because little change occurs in $\dot{V}O_2$ during hyperventilation, the RER increases, usually above 1.00, and clearly no longer reflects metabolism in the cells.

Another situation in which RER differs from RQ is during strenuous exercise at intensities above 80% of $\dot{V}O_2$max. At these high exercise intensities, high glycolytic rates in the muscle result in the production and accumulation of lactic acid. The hydrogen ions associated with this acid must be buffered. The body's bicarbonate buffer system neutralizes the acidity. Hydrogen ions bind with bicarbonate ions (HCO_3^-) to form H_2CO_3 and subsequently H_2O and CO_2:

$$H^+ + HCO_3^- \leftrightarrow H_2CO_3 \leftrightarrow H_2O + CO_2$$

This CO_2 is expired, and as a result the RER increases rapidly and can reach values between 1.00 and 1.30. This increase does not reflect the metabolism in the cell; therefore, calculation of energy expenditure or substrate utilization is only valid during steady-state exercise, when no accumulation of lactic acid occurs. Situations in which lipogenesis (i.e., the synthesis of fat from carbohydrate) and ketogenesis (the formation of ketone bodies) play a role are further examples of conditions in which RER may differ from RQ.

Doubly Labeled Water

The doubly labeled water technique is based on the administration of a bolus dose of two stable isotopes of water: ^2H_2O and $H_2{}^{18}O$. (For an explanation of stable isotopes, see appendix A.) These two isotopes are used as tracers, and the slightly heavier atoms ^2H and ^{18}O can be measured in various body fluids (e.g., urine). ^2H is lost from the body in water alone, and ^{18}O is lost in water and as $C^{18}O_2$ in breath. The difference between the two tracer excretion rates, therefore, represents the CO_2 production rate (see figure 4.7). With the knowledge of the fuel mixture oxidized, energy expenditure can be calculated.

The main advantage of this technique is that it does not interfere with everyday life, and unbiased measurements of a free-living situation can be obtained. In addition, measurements can be conducted over prolonged periods, and, therefore, the values can be used to estimate the typical daily energy expenditure and, in turn, the energy needs of a free-living person. The main disadvantages of the technique are the expense, the limited availability of the tracer, and the need for sophisticated equipment (mass spectrometer) to measure the isotopes. This method is only suitable for relatively long-term (days or weeks) estimation of energy expenditure.

Labeled Bicarbonate

Another method based on stable isotopes is the infusion of labeled bicarbonate (^{14}C or ^{13}C). When $H^{13}CO_3$ or $H^{14}CO_3$ (the latter is radioactive) is infused at a constant rate, it eventually reaches equilibrium with the body's CO_2 pool, after which any change in the body's CO_2 production will result in a change in the percentage of labeled CO_2. The change in this so-called enrichment is, therefore, a direct indication of total CO_2 production. This value can be used to calculate energy expenditure in a manner similar to the doubly labeled water technique. Samples are collected from expired gases, and tiny portions are needed for the analysis. Because $H^{13}CO_3$ has to be infused, this technique can be applied only for short periods (hours and, under some conditions, days). The bicarbonate labeling technique is relatively inexpensive but still requires sophisticated equipment and expertise.

Heart Rate Monitoring

To avoid some of the problems associated with the measurement of energy expenditure during free-living physical activity, various less complicated (and less accurate) methods have been developed. One of these methods is based on heart rate (HR), because of its linear relationship with oxygen uptake at submaximal exercise intensities. At very low and very high exercise

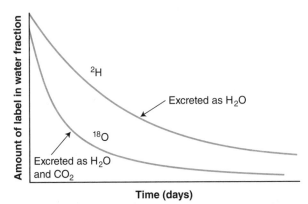

Figure 4.7   Doubly labeled water technique. Excretion of ^2H and ^{18}O occurs at different rates. The more rapid the drop in ^{18}O relative to the drop in ^2H, the higher the energy expenditure is.

intensities (supramaximal), this estimation is less reliable. To use HR for the estimation of energy expenditure, the relationship between HR and $\dot{V}O_2$ (and EE) must be determined. Measurements of oxygen uptake can then be used to calculate energy expenditure at several different HRs. The main limitation of the use of HR for measuring energy expenditure is the almost flat slope of the relationship at low levels of energy expenditure. At rest, slight movements can increase HR, while energy expenditure (i.e., oxygen consumption) remains almost the same. Emotions (e.g., anger or anxiety) may also cause HR to rise at rest with little or no change in oxygen uptake.

Although the HR method provides satisfactory estimates of average EE for a group, it is not necessarily accurate for individual subjects. For instance, Spurr et al. (1988) compared 24 hours of EE by calorimetry with EE by the HR method in 22 subjects. The maximum deviations of the values of EE between the two methods varied between +20% and –15% in individuals, but when the methods were compared statistically, no differences were found.

In addition, several factors influence the HR–$\dot{V}O_2$ relationship, including environmental conditions (temperature and humidity), altitude, body position, static (isometric) exercise, anxiety (at low work rates), and so on. Nevertheless, in some conditions HR can provide a convenient and relatively inexpensive estimate of energy expenditure.

Accelerometer

Another way of estimating activity level is through accelerometry. Accelerometers, small devices that can be attached to the body, register all accelerations that the body makes. The number and the degree of the accelerations give an indication of activity level. Accelerometers can record accelerations along one, two, or three axes. A single-axis, or single-plane, accelerometer measures acceleration only in the vertical direction. Triaxial accelerometers measure accelerations along three axes and are likely to be more accurate. Generally, accelerometer readings (usually expressed as activity counts or in kJ [kcal]) correlate well with energy expenditure. For some movements, however, especially those in free-living conditions, the accelerometer tends to underestimate true energy expenditure.

In the future, combined HR and accelerometer data may be used to estimate energy expenditure. Initial studies show promising results for simultaneous HR and motion measurements. Given the low weight and compactness of modern accelerometers, this instrument provides a convenient and easy method of getting an estimation of activity level in a free-living situation. The disadvantage, of course, is that the measurement provided is just a rough estimation (or indication) of energy expenditure.

Activity Records

Activity records, physical activity diaries, or physical activity recall instruments are used to record activities during a 24-hour period, and from this information a rough estimation of the daily energy expenditure is obtained. Most of the existing questionnaires measure only some types of activities and may therefore not always be accurate when used on an individual basis. Some people tend to overestimate their physical activity, whereas others underestimate it. Nevertheless, average physical activity scores reflecting a long-term period can be estimated satisfactorily using self-administered questionnaires.

Components of Energy Expenditure

Energy is needed for various processes in the body, including basal functions, digestion, absorption metabolism, and storage of food. In addition, active people expend energy during exercise. The three components, resting metabolic rate, diet-induced thermogenesis, and exercise-related energy expenditure, will be discussed in this section.

Resting Metabolic Rate

The largest component (60% to 75%) of daily energy expenditure (average daily metabolic rate, or ADMR) in a relatively inactive person is the resting metabolic rate (RMR), the energy required for the maintenance of normal body functions and homeostasis in resting conditions. Factors such as sympathetic nervous system activity, thyroid hormone activity, and sodium–potassium pump activity contribute to RMR. Another measure is the basal metabolic rate (BMR). This test was developed for patients with thyroid disease and aimed at measuring the lowest oxygen uptake in resting thermoneutral conditions. Measurements were performed in the morning after a 12-hour to 18-hour fast. This measurement was inconvenient for many patients, and metabolism was affected because patients were disturbed in their sleep. Therefore, RMR has become the more popular measure, and BMR is now rarely measured. The

RMR is primarily related to the fat-free mass (muscle mass) and is influenced by age, gender, body composition, and genetic factors.

Different body tissues have markedly different resting energy requirements. Organs that have large metabolic demands, such as the liver, gut, brain, kidney, and heart, have the highest energy requirements per gram of tissue. In a lean adult, these organs account for approximately 75% of resting energy expenditure, although they constitute only 10% of total body weight. In contrast, resting skeletal muscle consumes only 20% of resting metabolic rate, although it represents approximately 40% of total body weight. Adipose tissue consumes less than 5% of resting metabolic rate but usually accounts for approximately 20% of body weight. Resting energy expenditure (REE) correlates closely with fat-free mass. Although energy expenditure of metabolically active organs is responsible for a large component of REE, fat-free mass, which is composed primarily of skeletal muscle, accounts for most of the variability in energy expenditure between individuals.

RMR seems to decrease with age (2% to 3% per decade), and males generally have a higher RMR than females (because of their larger body size). See the highlight box for a glossary of the most common abbreviations used in relation to energy expenditure.

Diet-Induced Thermogenesis

The diet-induced thermogenesis (DIT), or thermic effect of food (TEF), is the increase in energy expenditure above RMR that occurs for several hours after ingestion of a meal. DIT is the result of digestion, absorption, metabolizing, and storage of food and normally represents about 10% of the total daily energy expenditure. The magnitude of DIT depends on several factors, including the energy content of the food and the size and composition of the meal. DIT also depends on the metabolic fate of the ingested substrate. The cost of storing fat in adipose tissue is approximately 3% of the energy of the ingested meal, whereas if carbohydrate is stored as glycogen, about 7% of the energy is lost. The energy cost for the synthesis and breakdown of protein is approximately 24% of the available energy. Energy expenditure can be increased up to 8 hours. The sympathetic nervous system seems to play an important role in DIT. When the effects of the sympathetic nervous system are reduced by administering a β-adrenergic blocker (for instance, propanolol), DIT is also reduced. With increasing age, a small decline occurs in DIT, possibly associated with a decrease in insulin sensitivity.

Thermic Effect of Exercise

The thermic effect of exercise (TEE), or energy expenditure for activity (EEA), is by far the most variable component of daily energy expenditure. It includes all energy expended above the RER and DIT. The TEE often has a voluntary component (exercise) and an involuntary component (shivering, fidgeting, or postural control). In highly trained, extremely active people, the TEE can be as much as 32 MJ/day (8,000 kcal/day). In sedentary people, the TEE may be as low as 400 kJ/day (100 kcal/day). Figure 4.8 compares the various components of daily energy expenditure in a sedentary

Energy Expenditure Common Abbreviations

ADMR—average daily metabolic rate

BMR—basal metabolic rate

RMR—resting metabolic rate

REE—resting energy expenditure (= RMR)

TEF—thermic effect of food

DIT—diet-induced thermogenesis

TEE—thermic effect of exercise

EEA—energy expenditure for physical activity

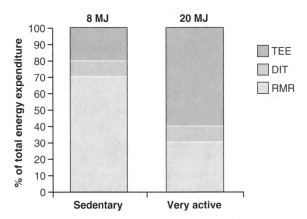

Figure 4.8   Energy expenditure and the relative contribution of its various components in a sedentary person (energy expenditure 8 MJ/day, or 2,000 kcal/day) and in an athlete involved in heavy training (energy expenditure 20 MJ/day, or 5,000 kcal/day). RMR = resting metabolic rate; DIT = diet-induced thermogenesis; TEE = energy expenditure during exercise.

person and in an endurance athlete involved in heavy training. TEE can vary from an average of 30% of the daily energy expenditure up to 80% in extreme conditions during heavy endurance training or competition. Exercise is therefore extremely important for the maintenance of the daily energy balance. It is not only the most variable component of 24-hour energy expenditure but also the component that can be controlled voluntarily.

Energy Balance

The energy balance is usually calculated over longer periods (days or weeks) and represents the difference between energy intake and energy expenditure. When energy intake exceeds energy expenditure, the energy balance is positive and weight gain will occur. When energy intake is below energy expenditure, the energy balance is negative and weight loss will result. Over the long term, energy balance is maintained in weight-stable individuals even though this balance may be either positive or negative on a day-to-day basis. People who want to lose weight should increase energy expenditure relative to energy intake.

In many activities in which body composition or body weight is believed to be important (gymnastics, dancing, bodybuilding, and weight category sports such as judo and boxing) participants often try to maintain a negative energy balance to lose weight. Thus, the energy intakes in these activities can be very low. At the other extreme are endurance sports such as triathlon, cycling, cross-country skiing, and ultraendurance running, which require extremely high energy expenditures and energy intakes. In these sports, maintaining energy balance on a day-to-day basis is crucial for performance. Both the upper and the lower limits of energy expenditure are discussed in the following sections.

Table 4.2 depicts the daily energy intake of a large number of Dutch elite female and male athletes in various sports. The data show that females generally have lower energy intake than males. For females, energy intake ranged between 5.1 MJ (1,600 kcal) and 10.2 MJ (3,200 kcal). For males, energy intake ranged between 12.1 MJ (2,900 kcal) and 24.7 MJ (5,900 kcal). These differences in energy intake may be related to body size and weight, to body composition, and to the number of hours spent training on a daily basis. Athletes in team sports have a moderate energy intake, whereas some endurance athletes have an extremely high energy intake. In fact, only in

endurance sports were energy intakes in excess of 12.6 MJ (3,000 kcal) for females and 16.7 MJ (4,000 kcal) for males.

Energy Balance in Different Activities

Some physical activities require higher energy outputs than others, as shown in tables 4.3 and 4.4. Tennis, for example, has relatively low energy expenditure if played recreationally. At this level of play, it could be classified as a light-to-moderate activity, although during a game the exercise can sometimes be extremely intense, requiring high rates of energy expenditure in short bursts. But because a longer period of low-intensity activity (walking or even standing) typically follows the high-intensity activity, the average energy expenditure for tennis is relatively low. Tennis played at a high level has shorter periods of rest, and the average intensity is much higher. On the other hand, in continuous sports such as cycling and running, which usually include little or no recovery during the activity, energy expenditures can be relatively high.

Lower Limits of Energy Expenditure

Female gymnasts, ballet dancers, and ice dancers often have energy intakes as low as 4 MJ (1,000 kcal) to 8 MJ (2,000 kcal). In some cases, this intake is only 1.2 to 1.4 times the RMR, which is lower than sedentary people who, on average, expend 1.4 to 1.6 times the RMR, despite the fact that these athletes and dancers may be involved in 3 to 4 hours of training a day. Although not all the time gymnasts and dancers spend in the gym or in the dance studio is high-intensity training, the metabolic rate is still expected to be higher than that of the average sedentary person.

The food records of members of this group, who are striving for low body weight, may not be accurate and may represent an underestimation of the true energy intake. But even when the reported intakes are corrected for this underestimation, the energy intakes are still very low. The lower limits of energy expenditure are determined by the sum of RMR, DIT, and a minimum of physical activity. DIT is directly affected by the amount of food consumed. Reducing food intake results in decreased DIT, and it may also indirectly influence the RMR. One of the problems associated with reducing energy intake to very low levels is the possibility of marginal nutrition, particularly of essential nutrients such as fat-soluble vitamins, calcium, iron, and essential FAs (see chapters 1 and 10).

▪ TABLE 4.2 ▪
Energy Intake in Various Sports

Sport	Gender	Body mass in kg (lb)	kJ/kg	kcal/kg	MJ	kcal
Tour de France	M	70.8 (155.8)	347	83	24.6	5,869
Tour de l'Avenir	M	73.7 (162.1)	316	75	23.3	5,564
Triathlon	M	70.2 (154.4)	272	65	19.1	4,561
Cycling, amateur	M	72.3 (159.1)	253	60	18.3	4,370
Marathon speed skating	M	72.3 (159.1)	222	53	16.1	3,834
Swimming	M	72.9 (160.4)	221	53	16.1	3,849
Rowing	M	77.2 (169.8)	189	45	14.6	3,486
Running	M	68.8 (151.4)	193	46	13.3	3,172
Rowing	F	69.8 (153.6)	186	44	13.0	3,101
Cycling, amateur	F	66.0 (145.2)	164	39	10.8	2,586
Running	F	52.1 (114.6)	168	40	8.8	2,091
Subtop swimming	F	43.6 (95.9)	200	48	8.7	2,083
Bodybuilding	M	87.3 (192.1)	157	38	13.7	3,274
Judo	M	82.5 (181.5)	157	38	13.0	3,094
Weightlifting	M	76.4 (168.1)	167	40	12.8	3,048
Judo	M	68.7 (151.1)	177	42	12.2	2,905
Top gymnastics	F	46.9 (103.2)	158	38	7.4	1,770
Subtop gymnastics	F	39.8 (87.6)	206	49	8.2	1,959
Bodybuilding	F	56.0 (123.2)	110	26	6.2	1,472
Water polo	M	85.5 (188.1)	194	46	16.6	3,962
Soccer	M	74.5 (163.9)	192	46	14.3	3,417
Hockey	M	75.0 (165.0)	181	43	13.6	3,243
Volleyball	F	66.0 (145.2)	140	33	9.2	2,207
Hockey	F	62.1 (136.6)	145	35	9.0	2,151
Handball	F	63.2 (139.0)	142	34	9.0	2,144

M = male; F = female.

International Journal of Sports Medicine: From A.M.J. van Erp-Baart, et al., 1989a, "Nationwide survey on nutritional habits in elite athletes. Part I: Energy carbohydrate, protein," 10 (suppl 1): S3-S10. Adapted by permission.

Upper Limits of Energy Expenditure

Energy-related problems in endurance sports are totally different from the problems discussed in the previous section. Well-trained endurance athletes can expend more than 4 MJ/h (1,000 kcal/h) for prolonged periods, resulting in extremely high daily energy expenditures. To maintain performance, energy stores must be replenished and energy balance must be restored, which means that these athletes must eat large amounts in periods of heavy training or competition.

■ TABLE 4.3 ■
Energy Cost of Various Activities

Activity	(kJ/min)	(kcal/min)	Examples
Resting	4	1	Sleeping, reclining while watching TV
Very light activities	12–20	3–5	Sitting and standing activities, driving, cooking, card playing, typing
Light activities	20–28	5–7	Walking (3 to 5 km/h), baseball, bowling, horseback riding, golf
Moderate activities	28–36	7–9	Jogging, basketball, badminton, soccer, tennis, volleyball, walking (7 to 8 km/h)
Strenuous activities	36–52	9–13	Running at 10 km/h to 13 km/h, cross-country skiing (8 to 10 km/h)
Very strenuous activities	>52	>13	Cycling at 35 km/h, running at >14 km/h, cross-country skiing at >12 km/h

■ TABLE 4.4 ■
Estimated Energy Cost of Activities
in Kilojoules per Minute (Kilocalories per Minute)

Activity	BODY WEIGHT				
	50 kg (110 lb)	60 kg (132 lb)	70 kg (154 lb)	80 kg (176 lb)	90 kg (198 lb)
Aerobics					
Beginners	22 (5.5)	26 (6.5)	30 (7.5)	34 (8.5)	39 (9.8)
Advanced	28 (7.0)	33 (8.3)	40 (10.0)	45 (11.3)	51 (12.8)
Badminton	20 (5.0)	24 (8.0)	28 (7.0)	33 (8.3)	37 (9.3)
Ballroom dancing	11 (2.8)	13 (3.3)	15 (3.8)	17 (4.3)	19 (4.8)
Basketball	29 (7.2)	35 (8.8)	40 (10.0)	46 (11.5)	52 (13.0)
Boxing	46 (11.5)	56 (14.0)	65 (16.3)	74 (18.5)	84 (21.0)
Sparring in ring	29 (7.2)	35 (8.8)	40 (10.0)	46 (11.5)	52 (13.0)
Canoeing					
Leisure	9 (2.3)	11 (2.8)	13 (3.3)	15 (3.8)	17 (4.3)
Racing	22 (5.5)	26 (6.5)	30 (7.5)	34 (8.5)	39 (9.8)
Circuit training	22 (5.5)	26 (6.5)	30 (7.5)	34 (8.5)	40 (10.0)
Cricket					
Batting	17 (4.3)	21 (5.3)	24 (6.0)	28 (7.0)	32 (8.0)
Bowling	19 (4.8)	22 (5.5)	26 (6.5)	30 (7.5)	34 (8.5)
Cycling					
9 km/h	13 (3.3)	16 (4.0)	18 (4.5)	21 (5.3)	24 (6.0)
15 km/h	21 (5.3)	24 (8.0)	28 (7.0)	33 (8.3)	38 (9.5)
Racing	35 (8.8)	42 (10.5)	49 (12.3)	56 (14.0)	63 (5.8)
Football	28 (7.0)	33 (8.3)	39 (9.8)	44 (11.0)	50 (12.5)
Golf	18 (4.5)	21 (5.5)	25 (6.3)	28 (7.0)	32 (8.0)
Gymnastics	14 (3.5)	16 (4.0)	19 (4.8)	22 (5.5)	25 (6.3)
Hockey	18 (4.5)	20 (5.0)	24 (6.0)	29 (7.3)	33 (8.3)

Activity	BODY WEIGHT				
	50 kg (110 lb)	60 kg (132 lb)	70 kg (154 lb)	80 kg (176 lb)	90 kg (198 lb)
Judo	41 (10.3)	49 (12.3)	57 (14.3)	65 (16.3)	73 (18.3)
Running					
5.5 min/km	40 (10.0)	49 (12.3)	57 (14.3)	65 (16.3)	73 (18.3)
5 min/km	44 (11.0)	52 (13.0)	61 (15.3)	70 (17.5)	78 (19.5)
4.5 min/km	48 (12.0)	55 (13.8)	65 (16.3)	75 (18.8)	85 (21.3)
4 min/km	54 (13.5)	65 (16.3)	76 (19.0)	87 (21.8)	98 (24.5)
Skiing					
Cross-country	35 (8.8)	42 (10.5)	49 (12.3)	56 (14.0)	63 (15.8)
Downhill (easy)	18 (4.5)	21 (5.5)	25 (6.3)	29 (7.3)	33 (8.3)
Downhill (hard)	29 (7.3)	35 (8.8)	40 (10.0)	49 (12.3)	55 (13.8)
Squash	44 (11.0)	53 (13.3)	62 (15.5)	71 (17.8)	79 (19.8)
Swimming					
Freestyle	33 (8.3)	40 (10.0)	46 (11.5)	52 (13.0)	59 (14.8)
Backstroke	36 (9.0)	43 (10.8)	49 (12.3)	56 (14.0)	63 (15.8)
Breaststroke	34 (8.5)	41 (10.3)	47 (11.8)	54 (13.5)	61 (15.3)
Table tennis	14 (3.5)	17 (4.3)	19 (4.8)	23 (5.8)	26 (6.5)
Tennis					
Social	15 (3.8)	17 (4.3)	20 (5.0)	23 (5.8)	26 (6.5)
Competitive	37 (9.3)	44 (11.0)	50 (12.5)	58 (14.5)	65 (16.3)
Volleyball	10 (2.5)	12 (3.0)	15 (3.6)	17 (4.3)	19 (4.8)
Walking					
10 min/km	21 (5.3)	26 (6.5)	30 (7.5)	35 (8.8)	39 (9.8)
8 min/km	25 (6.3)	30 (7.5)	35 (8.8)	40 (10.0)	45 (11.3)
5 min/km	44 (11.0)	52 (13.0)	61 (15.3)	70 (17.5)	78 (19.5)

Note: All figures are approximate values.

Adapted from van Erp-Baart et al. 1989a.

Scientists have studied whether an upper limit to human energy expenditure exists. The highest values reported are from sports such as cycling, triathlon, cross-country skiing, and ultraendurance running.

The Tour de France is a 3-week, 20-stage cycling event in which cyclists cover approximately 3,500 km (2,175 mi), including various mountain stages. On some days, the cyclists spend up to 8 hours on their bicycles. Average daily energy expenditure in the Tour de France reached values of 24 MJ (6,000 kcal) when measured in weekly intervals. The highest recorded average energy intake during the entire 3 weeks of the Tour de France was 36 MJ/day (9,000 kcal/day) (van Erp-Baart et al. 1989) (see figure 4.9). Athletes involved in sports with such extreme energy expenditures on a daily basis face the problem of consuming large quantities if they want to maintain their body weight and performance. Figure 4.9 shows that generally such consumption is possible, but on days with extremely high energy expenditures, the cyclists tend to have a negative energy balance of about 4 MJ (1,000 kcal).

These cyclists do not face an easy task because they have to consume an enormous amount of energy (mostly in the form of carbohydrate) to maintain energy balance. This requirement can be problematic for several reasons:

■ Time for eating is limited, making consumption of large amounts of food during the 3-hour to 7-hour race difficult.

■ Hunger feelings may be depressed for several hours after strenuous exercise.

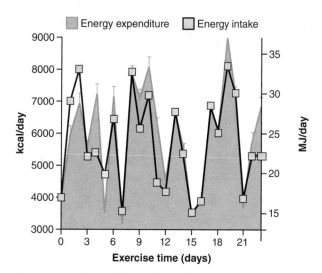

Figure 4.9 Energy balance during the Tour de France.

International Journal Sports Medicine: From W.H.M. Saris et al., 1989, "Study on food intake and energy expenditure during extreme sustained exercise: The Tour de France," 10 (1 suppl): S26-S31. Reprinted by permission.

■ Especially during the last week of the Tour de France, gastrointestinal problems often make absorbing large quantities of food difficult or even impossible.

Nevertheless, hardly any changes in body weight occur among participants during the Tour de France, indicating that these cyclists are indeed able to maintain energy balance (Jeukendrup et al. 2000). On the other hand, perhaps the cyclists who do not maintain their body weight drop out.

Although eating large amounts during the race is difficult, energy intake in the form of carbohydrate solutions has been shown to be crucial. During 2 days of high-intensity cycling, when 26 MJ (6,000 kcal) of energy expenditure were not supplemented with carbohydrate during the rides, cyclists were not able to maintain energy balance (5 to 10 MJ [1,200 to 2,400 kcal] negative energy balance). When the cyclists were given a 20% carbohydrate solution during exercise, from which they could drink as much as they liked, they maintained energy balance (Brouns et al. 1989).

In some sports, even higher 24-hour energy expenditures may be reached. Using doubly labeled water, similar estimates of energy expenditure were made in Norwegian cross-country skiers during training. Energy expenditure amounted up to 36 MJ/day (8,600 kcal/day) (Sjodin et al. 1994). A case report indicated that an ultraendurance runner expended 134 MJ (55,970 kcal) during a 1,000 km (600 mi) running race. The athlete ran for 5 days and 5 hours, during which he had an average energy expenditure of 45 MJ/day (10,750 kcal/day). In both cases, the athletes' food intake was extremely high and almost matched the energy expenditure. The greatest recorded human endurance performances occurred during the Antarctic sledding expeditions led by Robert Scott in 1911–12 and Ernest Shackleton in 1914–16. By man-hauling sleds for 10 hours daily for approximately 159 and 160 consecutive days respectively, members of those expeditions would have expended almost 1,000,000 kcal (Noakes 2007). Significant weight loss occurred because their energy intake was limited.

KEY POINTS

■ All biological functions require energy, and although the human body has some energy reserves most of the energy must be obtained through nutrition.

■ Energy is the capacity to do work. The various forms of energy include light energy, chemical energy, heat energy, and electrical energy.

■ Energy is often expressed in calories (English system) or joules (metric system); 1 calorie equals 4.186 joules.

■ Efficiency describes the effective work performed after muscle contraction and is usually expressed as the percentage of total work. Humans are approximately 20% efficient.

■ Gross efficiency (GE) is the ratio of the total work accomplished to the energy expended. Because resting metabolism is not accounted for, corrections have been made by subtracting baseline energy expenditure from total energy expenditure. Net efficiency, work efficiency, and delta efficiency each take resting energy expenditure into account.

- The energy content of 1 g of carbohydrate is 17.6 kJ (4.2 kcal). Fat contains between 36.0 kJ/g (8.6 kcal/g) and 40.2 kJ/g (9.6 kcal/g) (on average, about 39.3 kJ/g [9.4 kcal/g]), and protein contains about 23.7 kJ/g (5.65 kcal/g). The coefficient of digestibility represents the proportion of consumed food actually digested and absorbed by the body.

- Coefficients of digestibility average about 97% for carbohydrates, 95% for lipids, and 92% for proteins. The net energy values of carbohydrate, fat, and protein are therefore 16 kJ (4 kcal), 36 kJ (9 kcal), and 16 kJ (4 kcal), respectively, and these are referred to as the Atwater energy values or Atwater factors.

- Ways to measure (or estimate) human energy expenditure include direct but complex measurements of heat production (direct calorimetry), relatively simple indirect metabolic measurements (indirect calorimetry), expensive tracer methods (doubly labeled water), and relatively inexpensive and convenient rough estimations of energy expenditure (heart rate monitoring and accelerometry).

- Human energy expenditure can be divided into several components: resting metabolic rate, thermic effect of food, and exercise-related energy expenditure. RMR is the largest component (60% to 75%) of the daily energy expenditure in relatively sedentary people, and the thermic effect of food represents about 10%, leaving 15% to 30% for exercise-related energy expenditure.

- Respiratory exchange measurements can be used to calculate energy expenditure, as well as the contributions of carbohydrate and fat to energy expenditure.

- The energy balance is usually calculated over longer periods (days or weeks) and represents the difference between energy intake and energy expenditure. When energy intake exceeds energy expenditure, a positive energy balance occurs, which results in weight gain. When energy intake is below energy expenditure, a negative energy balance occurs, which results in weight loss.

- Female gymnasts, ballet dancers, and ice dancers often have energy intakes between 4 MJ (1,000 kcal) and 8 MJ (2,000 kcal). In some cases this intake is only 1.2 to 1.4 times the resting metabolic rate. Such low energy intakes can result in nutritional deficiency.

- Cycling, triathlon, and ultraendurance running are sports that may require energy expenditures as high as 36 MJ/day (8,600 kcal/day).

RECOMMENDED READINGS

Burke, L.M. 2001. Energy needs of athletes. *Canadian Journal of Applied Physiology* 26 (suppl): S202–S219.

Burke, L.M., A.B. Loucks, and N. Broad. 2006. Energy and carbohydrate for training and recovery. *Journal of Sports Sciences* 24 (7): 675–685.

King, N.A., P. Caudwell, M. Hopkins, N.M. Byrne, R. Colley, A.P. Hills et al. 2007. Metabolic and behavioral compensatory responses to exercise interventions: Barriers to weight loss. *Obesity (Silver Spring)* 15 (6): 1373–1383.

Loucks, A.B. 2004. Energy balance and body composition in sports and exercise. *Journal of Sports Sciences* 22 (1): 1–14.

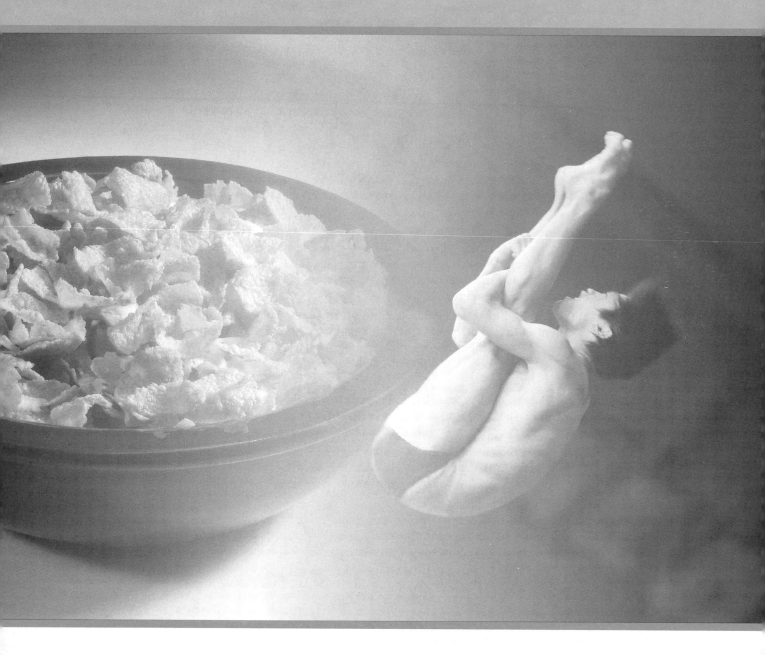

OBJECTIVES

After studying this chapter, you should be able to do the following:

- Describe the functions of the gastrointestinal system and list its anatomical components and structures

- Describe the digestion processes of carbohydrate, fat, and protein

- Describe the absorption processes of carbohydrate, fat, and protein

- Describe the absorption process of water

- Describe the absorption processes of vitamins and minerals

- Describe the factors that regulate gastric emptying

- State the approximate transit times within each compartment of the gastrointestinal tract

- Describe the effects of exercise on gastric emptying and absorption

- Describe the gastrointestinal problems that may occur during exercise and know which factors may augment or reduce these problems

5

Gastric Emptying, Digestion, and Absorption

Key Terms

The primary function of the gastrointestinal (or alimentary) tract is to provide the body with nutrients, water, and electrolytes from ingested foodstuffs. When food moves through the gastrointestinal tract (see highlight box), it is broken down into small units that can be absorbed in a process called digestion. Absorption (i.e., the transport of nutrients from the intestine into the blood or lymph system) takes place in various parts of the gastrointestinal tract for different nutrients. Here, we give an overview of the anatomy and physiology of the gastrointestinal tract, the various digestion and absorption processes that take place within it, and the changes that occur during exercise.

Anatomy of the Gastrointestinal Tract

The gastrointestinal tract is a long tubular structure that reaches from the mouth to the anus and includes the esophagus, stomach, small intestine, large intestine, rectum, anus, and several accessory digestive glands including the salivary glands, gallbladder, liver, and pancreas (see figure 5.1). In this 6 to 8 m tube, digestion of food and absorption of nutrients take place. The mouth, stomach, pancreas, and gallbladder have a predominantly digestive function, and most of the absorption occurs in the small and large intestine. After absorption,

most nutrients are transported to the liver, and from there they enter the main circulation.

Mouth

Chewing (or masticating) of food is the first step of digestion. It is often referred to as mechanical digestion. The anterior teeth or incisors provide strong cutting action, and the posterior teeth (molars) are used for grinding. The forces applied to cut and grind the food can be as much as 25 kg on the incisors and 90 kg on the molars. Chewing of food serves three major purposes: (1) It mechanically reduces the size of the food particles, which increases the rate of gastric emptying. (2) It increases the surface area of the food, which in turn increases the contact area for digestive enzymes that are released from the salivary glands and stomach (enzymatic digestion). Increasing the total surface area of the food increases the rate of digestion. (3) It mixes the food particles with saliva and digestive enzymes. The mouth has three pairs of salivary glands: the parotid glands, the sublingual glands, and the submandibular glands (see figure 5.2). Chewing is especially important for

Major Functions of Different Parts of the Gastrointestinal Tract

Organ		Function
Mouth	→	Mechanical digestion
Salivary glands	→	Secretion of fluid and digestive enzymes
Stomach	→	Secretion of HCl and protein-digesting enzymes (proteases)
Pancreas	→	Secretion of $NaHCO_3$ and digestive enzymes
Liver	→	Secretion of bile acids
Gallbladder	→	Temporary storage and concentration of bile
Small intestine	→	Digestion of food, absorption of water, nutrients, and electrolytes
Large intestine	→	Absorption of electrolytes

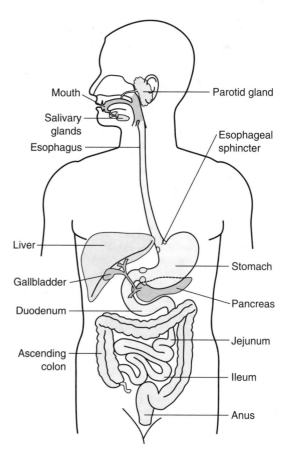

Figure 5.1 The gastrointestinal tract.

plant material (fruits and raw vegetables) because indigestible cellulose cell walls must be mechanically destroyed to release the nutrients.

Esophagus

When the food is small and soft enough to swallow, it moves past the pharynx at the back of the mouth into the esophagus. The esophagus moves the food particles to the stomach. This transport process is caused by rhythmic contractions and relaxations of the esophagus. The esophagus contains an inner layer of smooth muscle consisting of circular bands and an outer layer of smooth muscle that runs longitudinally. Contraction of these muscles causes peristalsis, a squeezing action involving progressive and recurring contractions, which mixes and moves the food to the stomach. This mechanism makes swallowing possible even when a person is hanging upside down or in space with zero gravity.

At the end of the esophagus, a valve of smooth muscle called the esophageal sphincter relaxes to allow food into the stomach. After some food particles have passed the esophageal sphincter, it contracts, preventing reflux of food or fluids from the stomach into the esophagus. People in whom this sphincter does not function properly may experience some acid leaking from the stomach, or heartburn. This gastrointestinal problem is common among runners and cyclists.

Stomach

The stomach, which is about 20 to 25 cm long, is divided in three parts (see figure 5.3): the corpus, or body; the antrum; and the fundus. The corpus and the antrum have different physiological functions. Although the fundus is a different part of the stomach from an anatomical point of view, from a functional point of view it is considered part of the corpus. The end of the stomach is a circular valve called the pyloric sphincter (pylorus), which controls the emptying of food from the stomach into the small intestine. When this muscle relaxes, food leaves the stomach; when it contracts, food stays in the stomach. The functions of the stomach include

- storage of large quantities of food until it can be accommodated in the intestine,
- mixing of this food with gastric secretions to form a homogeneous, acidic, souplike liquid or paste called chyme, and
- regulation of the emptying of the chyme into the duodenum (upper part of the small intestine) at a rate suitable for proper digestion and absorption.

Normally, food that enters the stomach forms concentric circles in the corpus and fundus so that the latest food is closest to the esophagus and the oldest food is nearest to the wall of the corpus. The stomach volume is normally around 1.5 L, but this volume can change from almost nothing when the stomach is empty to about 6 L when the stomach is full. The muscular tone of the stomach wall decreases as soon as food enters the stomach, which allows the stomach wall to stretch outward to accommodate more food.

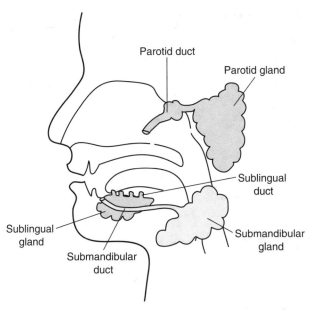

Figure 5.2   The mouth and its three pairs of salivary glands.

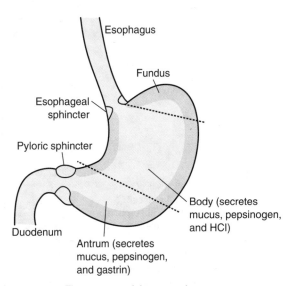

Figure 5.3   The anatomy of the stomach.

The wall of the corpus contains gastric glands that secrete digestive juices. These secretions come in contact with the food portions nearest to the stomach wall. The stomach can also contract and relax, which mixes the food into chyme. Chyme can be a fluid or a paste, depending on the relative amounts of food and secretions and the degree of digestion. The chyme is passed down to the small intestine by a strictly controlled process of gastric emptying. Little absorption takes place in the stomach (with the exception of some water and alcohol).

Small Intestine

The small intestine is approximately 2 to 3 m in length and 3 to 5 cm in diameter, and it can be divided into the duodenum (about 30 cm), the jejunum (next 1 to 2 m), and the ileum (last 1 m). About 95% of all absorption takes place in the duodenum and jejunum. The intestinal mucosa of the duodenum and jejunum contains many folds called the folds of Kerkring (see figure 5.4).

These folds increase the surface area of the intestine about three times that of a similarly sized flat internal lining. These folds are covered by millions of small fingerlike structures called villi, which project about 1 mm from the surface of the mucosa (see figure 5.5). The villi increase the total surface area of the small intestine another 10-fold. The intestinal cells that form the border of the villi are covered by a brush border consisting of about 600 microvilli approximately 1 μm long. These microvilli increase the total surface area a further 20-fold. The highly specialized construction of the small intestine, including the folds of Kerkring, the villi, and the microvilli, increases the absorption about 600-fold compared with a simple tube with a flat internal surface. The total surface area of the small intestine may be as large as 250 m², an area larger than a tennis court, which has a surface area of about 195 m².

Villi

Villi are finger-shaped and highly vascularized (see figure 5.5). The wall of a villus consists of a layer of epithelial cells, each with its own brush border (brush border is the name for the microvilli-covered surface of the intestine). Water, water-soluble particles, and electrolytes require transport or diffusion across the luminal and contraluminal membranes of the epithelial cell into the blood vessels. These nutrients are then transported to the liver through the hepatic portal vein. Each villus also contains a lacteal, which is located in the central part of a villus. The lacteal transports

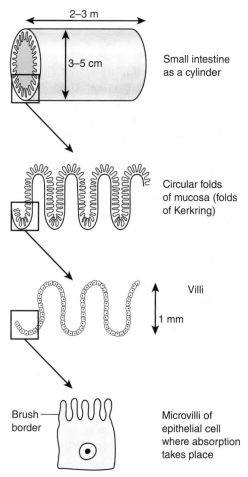

Figure 5.4 The organization of the small intestine increases the surface area about 600-fold over a simple tube with a flat internal surface.

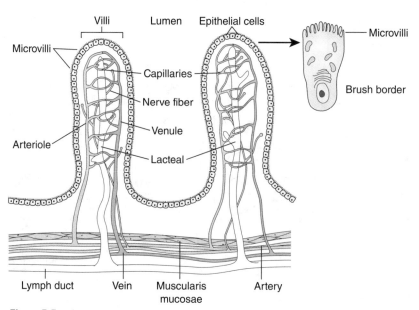

Figure 5.5 Functional organization of the villis.

particles that are not readily water soluble (e.g., long-chain FAs) via the lymphatic vessels. These vessels drain into large veins near the heart.

Motility and Transit Time

Food spends 1 to 3 days in the gastrointestinal tract before it is eliminated. The time spent in a section of the gastrointestinal tract is the transit time. For instance, the transit time in the small intestine is approximately 3 to 10 hours, depending on the composition of the food and the motility (movement of food) of the gastrointestinal tract. The small-intestine wall contains two layers of smooth muscle with longitudinal and circular muscle fibers that allow peristalsis and mixing contractions that push the chyme in the distal direction toward the large intestine (like squeezing toothpaste out of a tube). These contractions occur at a rate of 0.5 to 2.0 cm/s, with the fastest movement in the proximal intestine and the slowest movement in the distal intestine. The average speed of chyme along the small intestine is approximately 1 cm/s.

Peristalsis increases after a meal and can increase greatly after intense irritation of the intestinal mucosa, such as during infectious diarrhea. Mixing, or segmentation, contractions differ from peristalsis. The circular muscles contract, giving the small intestine the look of linked sausages. These intermittent contractions (8/min to 12/min) cause the chyme to move both forward and backward. The chyme moves backward before it advances. The function of these circular contractions is to mix the chyme with bile from the gallbladder, pancreatic juices, and intestinal juices. The juices get extra time to digest the food, and the contact time and area are increased.

Gallbladder

The gallbladder stores, concentrates, and releases bile. Bile, which is produced by liver cells, consists of water, electrolytes, bile salts, cholesterol, lecithin, and bilirubin. The gallbladder can store approximately 30 to 60 ml, but it secretes as much as 1,200 ml into the duodenum every day. The gall bladder stores up to 12 hours of bile secretion by concentrating the bile constituents. Bile facilitates the digestion and absorption of fat and is released through the hepatic duct, which joins the pancreatic duct just before entering the duodenum (see figure 5.6). Bile secretion increases after a meal, especially when the meal contains a large amount of fat.

Pancreas

The pancreas is a large gland situated parallel to and just beneath the stomach (see figures 5.1 and 5.6). It secretes sodium bicarbonate to buffer the hydrochloric acid of the stomach and digestive enzymes to break down carbohydrate, protein, and fat. Pancreatic juice is mainly secreted in response to chyme in the upper portions of the small intestine. The regulatory mechanisms for sodium bicarbonate secretion and digestive enzyme secretion are different, and the secretion rates are highly dependent on the type and amount of food ingested. The concentration of various enzymes in pancreatic juice also depends to some extent on the type of food ingested.

Ileocecal Valve

From the small intestine, the chyme moves into the large intestine through the ileocecal valve (see figure 5.7). This valve prevents backflow of indigestible fecal material into the small intestine. The valve can resist pressure equal to about 50 to 60 cm of water. The distal end of the small intestine, or ileum, has a thicker muscular coat that controls the emptying from the ileum. Contraction of the ileocecal sphincter is regulated by a variety of factors, including (1) distension of the cecum (a blind pouch, open only at one end, at the beginning of the large intestine), (2) irritating substances in the cecum, and (3) fluidity of the chyme. An inflamed appendix (a nonfunctional part of the intestine that is short, thin, and outpouching from

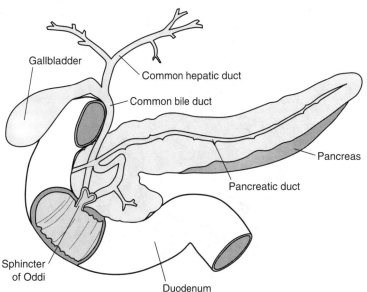

Figure 5.6 Duodenum, pancreas, and gallbladder.

the cecum) restricts the emptying of the ileum. Increased fluidity of chyme, on the other hand, increases emptying from the ileum.

Large Intestine

In the large intestine, the chyme is called feces. The large intestine consists of the colon, the rectum, and the anal canal. The colon is usually divided into the ascending colon, the transverse colon, the descending colon, and the sigmoid colon (see figure 5.7). The functions of the colon are (1) absorption of water and electrolytes from the chyme and (2) storage of feces until they can be expelled. Absorption takes place mainly in the first part of the colon, and storage mainly occurs in the distal parts. The peristaltic movements of the colon are slower than those of the small intestine. The colon also has circular and longitudinal smooth muscle layers and moves the feces toward the distal parts of the colon by rhythmic contractions. The fecal material is slowly rolled over and mixed so that contact with the surface of the large intestine increases and as much water as possible is absorbed. Normally only 80 to 150 ml of water are present in approximately 300 ml of feces.

Regulation of the Gastrointestinal Tract

The gastrointestinal tract is innervated by both the sympathetic and the parasympathetic components of the autonomic nervous system. Parasympa-

thetic stimulation in general stimulates motility. The vagus nerve is the source of parasympathetic activity in the esophagus, stomach, pancreas, gallbladder, small intestine, and upper section of the large intestine. The lower portion of the large intestine receives parasympathetic innervation from spinal nerves in the sacral region (the lower end of the spine). Autonomic regulation, which is "extrinsic" to the gastrointestinal tract, is over-ruled by "intrinsic" modes of regulation. Sensory neurons in various parts of the gastrointestinal tract have their cell bodies in the gut wall but are not part of the autonomic nervous system. In addition, hormonal regulation plays an important role. Endocrine glands secrete hormones into the circulation, whereas paracrine glands or cells secrete products that influence the secretion of another product secreted by a local gland or cell. For example, gastrin is a hormone secreted by the stomach that increases hydrochloric acid and pepsinogen secretion in the stomach. Another example is secretin, a hormone produced by the small intestine that increases water and bicarbonate secretion by the pancreas.

Substances within the tissues of the gastrointestinal tract and hormones released by organs in the gastrointestinal tract affect secretion and motility. An overview of the effects of gastrointestinal hormones and their functions is given in table 5.1.

Digestion

Digestion starts the moment food is ingested and may take 4 to 6 hours to complete. Specific enzymes are responsible for the digestion of different macronutrients.

Carbohydrate Digestion

The digestion of carbohydrates starts in the mouth as saliva is added to the food. Saliva is secreted from the parotid glands, the sublingual glands, and the submandibular glands (see figure 5.2). The daily secretion of saliva normally ranges between 800 and 1,500 ml (see table 5.2). In the unstimulated state, saliva secretion rate is about 0.5 ml/min, but this rate can increase by up to 10-fold during the chewing of food. Saliva consists primarily of water (99.5%) derived from extracellular fluid. In addition, it contains α-amylase (also referred to as ptyalin), an enzyme responsible for the breakdown of starch into smaller units; mucoid proteins; bicarbonate; electrolytes; lysozymes, enzymes that break down proteins and attack bacteria; lingual lipase; and protein antibodies (the major secre-

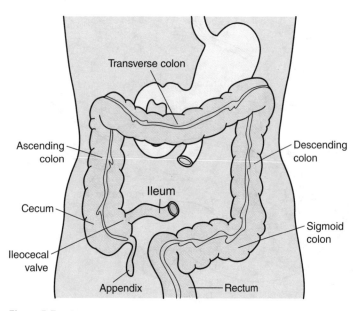

Figure 5.7 The ileocecal valve and large intestine.

■ **TABLE 5.1** ■

Effects of Gastrointestinal Hormones

Hormone	Secreted by	Effect
Gastrin	Stomach	Stimulates HCl production in the stomach; stimulates secretion of pepsinogen in the stomach
Secretin	Small intestine	Stimulates water and bicarbonate secretion in pancreatic juice
Cholecystokinin (CCK)	Small intestine	Stimulates secretion of enzymes in pancreatic juice; stimulates gallbladder contractions; inhibits gastric motility and secretion
Gastric inhibitory peptide (GIP)	Small intestine	Inhibits gastric motility and secretion
Glucagonlike peptide I (GLP-I)	Ileum and colon	Inhibits gastric motility and secretion
Guanylin	Ileum and colon	Causes removal of NaCl and water from feces

■ **TABLE 5.2** ■

Daily Secretion of Intestinal Juices

Intestinal juices	Daily volume (ml)
Saliva	1,000
Gastric secretions	1,500
Pancreatic secretion	1,000
Bile	1,000
Small intestine	2,000
Large intestine	200
Total	6,700

tory antibody being immunoglobulin A [IgA]) that can help to destroy oral bacteria. Thus, besides a digestive function, saliva has a protective function against invading bacteria (see chapter 16). An overview of digestive enzymes is given in table 5.3.

The mucoid proteins give saliva its viscous quality, which helps lubricate food and makes it easier to swallow. Chewing food mixes saliva with the food and increases the contact area so that amylase can start breaking down the glucose chain in starches. Prolonged chewing of a cracker will cause it to taste sweeter because some starch breaks down to disaccharide sugars such as maltose, which tastes much sweeter than starch.

When food is swallowed and arrives in the acid environment of the stomach, the amylase activity decreases. Carbohydrate digestion still takes place but at a much slower rate. In the mouth and stomach, before the stomach content is completely mixed with gastric secretions, approximately 30% to 40% of the carbohydrate may be digested, predominantly to maltose, maltotrioses, and small oligosaccharides (see figure 5.8).

When the carbohydrates are emptied from the stomach into the duodenum and the acid is neutralized by sodium bicarbonate from the pancreas, digestion again proceeds at a high rate. In the duodenum, additional α-amylase will be secreted in the pancreatic juice. This α-amylase, like salivary amylase, hydrolyzes the starches into small glucose polymers (dextrins) and maltose (see figure 5.8). Almost complete hydrolysis of all starches to maltose has taken place when the chyme enters the ileum. The disaccharides and small polysaccharides are further digested by specific enzymes located in the brush borders of intestinal epithelial cells. As soon as disaccharides come in contact with the brush border, they are digested by the enzymes lactase, sucrase, and maltase (see figure 5.8). Lactase breaks lactose down into glucose and galactose, sucrase breaks sucrose down into glucose and fructose, and maltase breaks maltose down into two glucose molecules.

Problems with the digestive process can result when a deficiency of one or more of these enzymes exists. Lactose intolerance is caused by an absence or deficiency of the intestinal enzyme lactase. When lactose, the main carbohydrate component of milk, is not digested, diarrhea and fluid loss result. In addition, bacteria in the large intestine metabolizes the lactose to produce large quantities of gas, which causes bloating and pain.

■ **TABLE 5.3** ■
Digestive Enzymes and Their Functions

Enzyme	Site of action	Source	Substrate	Product	Optimum pH
CARBOHYDRATES					
Salivary amylase	Mouth	Salivary glands	Starch	Maltose	6.7
Pancreatic amylase	Duodenum	Pancreatic juice	Starch	Maltose, maltotriose, and oligosaccharides	6.7–7.0
Maltase	Small intestine	Brush border	Maltose	Glucose	5.0–7.0
Sucrase	Small intestine	Brush border	Sucrose	Glucose and fructose	5.0–7.0
Lactase	Small intestine	Brush border	Lactose	Glucose and galactose	5.8–6.2
LIPIDS					
Lingual lipase	Mouth	Lingual salivary glands	Starch	Maltose	3.5–6.0
Pancreatic lipase	Small intestine	Pancreatic juice	Triacylglycerols	Fatty acids and monoacylglycerols	8.0
PROTEINS					
Pepsin	Stomach	Gastric glands	Protein	Polypeptides	1.6–2.4
Trypsin	Small intestine	Pancreatic juice	Polypeptides	Amino acids, dipeptides, and tripeptides	8.0
Chymotrypsin	Small intestine	Pancreatic juice	Polypeptides	Amino acids, dipeptides, and tripeptides	8.0
Carboxypeptidase	Small intestine	Pancreatic juice	Polypeptides	Amino acids, dipeptides, and tripeptides	8.0
Elastase	Small intestine	Pancreatic juice	Polypeptides	Amino acids, dipeptides, and tripeptides	8.5

Fiber, a form of dietary carbohydrate, contains cellulose, which is a structural component of plant cells and is resistant to human digestive enzymes. Cellulose can be excreted in the feces. Some of it, however, is fermented by the bacteria present in the large intestine. Similar to the way in which yeast ferments the sugars in grape juice to produce wine, the bacteria in the large intestine ferment cellulose to produce hydrogen and carbon dioxide gases, volatile FAs, and in many instances methane gas (which has an unpleasant odor). Changes in the diet or in the type of microorganisms can influence the amount of gas produced.

Peristaltic movements push undigested carbohydrates, including fibrous substances, to the colon, where more digestion occurs. Indigestible carbohydrates (predominantly cellulose) move to the rectum for expulsion though the anus.

Lipid Digestion

Digestion of lipids begins in the mouth because saliva contains small amounts of lingual lipase, the enzyme that splits triacylglycerols (triglycerides) into FAs and glycerol. In the stomach, this acid-stable lipase continues to hydrolyze the triacylglycerols (see figure 5.9). Hydrolysis, however, is slow because triacylglycerols are not soluble in water and therefore do not mix well with the water fraction in which lipase is found. The lingual and gastric lipases act together but mainly on the short-chain (C4 to C6) and medium-chain (C8 to C10) triacylglycerols, whereas the majority of the fat (long-chain triacylglycerols; C12 to C24) is digested in the small intestine. Lingual lipase is responsible for 10% to 30% of the triacylglycerol digestion. When the chyme enters the duodenum,

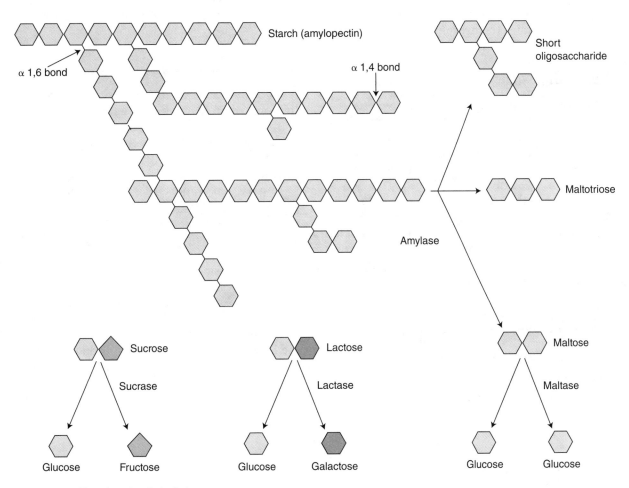

Figure 5.8   Digestion of carbohydrates.

bile is added and acts on the triacylglycerols, which by this time are organized into large lipid globules. Pancreatic lipase is secreted into the duodenum and further hydrolyzes the triacylglycerols.

After initial hydrolysis starts and the triglycerides are converted into FAs, monoglycerides and diglycerides organize themselves into small emulsion droplets. The fat-soluble part of the FA faces inward, and the water-soluble part forms the core of these droplets. When bile salts (bile acids), stored in the gallbladder, are secreted into the duodenum, micelles are formed (see figure 5.9). Micelles are well-defined structures with a disklike shape, on which phospholipids and FAs form a bilayer. The bile salts occupy the edge positions, rendering the edge of the disk hydrophilic (i.e., more attractive to water). The bile salts emulsify the lipids into small

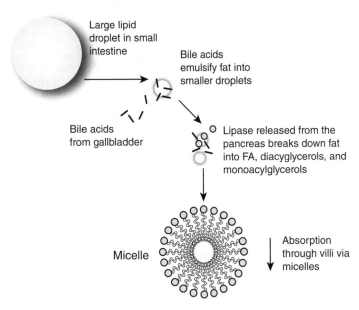

Figure 5.9   Digestion of fat.

droplets, which increases the total surface area and thus facilitates the hydrolysis (breakdown) of triacylglycerols by pancreatic lipase.

Protein Digestion

Protein digestion breaks down the ingested proteins into simple amino acids, dipeptides, and tripeptides for absorption across the intestinal mucosa (see figure 5.10). This process (protein hydrolysis) takes place within the stomach and small intestine and depends on specific protein-digesting enzymes (proteases) and the acidity of the stomach. Specific cells produce and secrete hydrochloric acid (HCl), a strong acid, into the stomach. These parietal cells secrete an isotonic 160 mM HCl solution with a pH of about 0.8, illustrating its extreme acidity. The pH within the stomach and of the gastric contents is typically around 2.0.

HCl, and thereby the acidic ingested food, has various functions; among other things it

■ activates the protease enzyme pepsin,

■ kills many pathogenic organisms,

■ increases the absorption of iron and calcium,

■ inactivates hormones of plant and animal origin, and

■ denatures (breaks down) food proteins, making them more vulnerable to enzyme action.

Proteases (see table 5.3) are often stored in the form of an inactive precursor, but as soon as it is released into the stomach or small intestine it becomes active. This mechanism prevents the digesting of the cells in which the proteases are produced and stored.

Pepsin (an important group of proteases), secreted as its precursor pepsinogen from the cells of the stomach wall, is initially inactive. As soon as pepsinogen comes in contact with the HCl of the stomach, it is automatically converted into the active pepsin that breaks down protein. Pepsin degrades the collagenous connective tissue fibers of meat. After dismantling these fibers, other proteases can effectively digest the remaining animal protein. Stomach enzymes and acids attack the long, complex protein strands and hydrolyze approximately 10% to 20% of the ingested proteins. The low pH causes denaturation of the protein, meaning that the three-dimensional

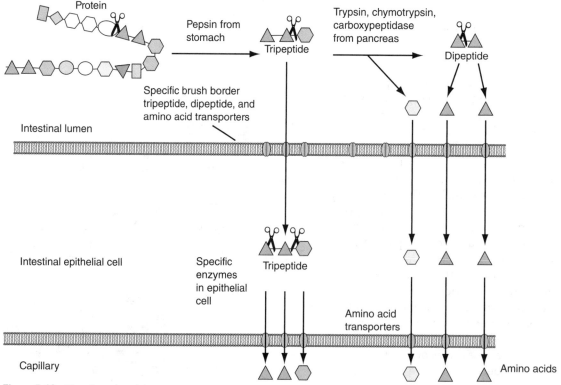

Figure 5.10 Digestion of protein.

structure of protein is uncoiled and breaks into smaller polypeptide and peptide units. When the chyme passes into the small intestine, pepsin becomes inactivated by the relatively high pH in the duodenum.

Other proteases (alkaline enzymes), including trypsin, are released and become active to digest the remaining proteins and polypeptides. The pancreatic juice is rich in precursors of endo-peptidases, carboxypeptidases, enteropeptidases, trypsinogen, and trypsin (see figure 5.10). These proteases digest the polypeptides into tripeptides, dipeptides, and single amino acids. Amino acids, dipeptides, and tripeptides can be transported across the enterocyte.

Absorption

Absorption of nutrients across the intestinal walls occurs either by active transport or by simple diffusion. Active transport requires energy and usually takes place against a concentration gradient or an electrical potential. Active transport often requires specialized carrier proteins. Diffusion is the movement of substances across a membrane along, rather than against, an electrochemical gradient. Simple diffusion does not require transport proteins or energy in the form of ATP, but many nutrients are transported by facilitated diffusion, which requires a protein transporter or channel.

Absorption of Carbohydrates

The major monosaccharides that result from digestion of polysaccharides and disaccharides are glucose, fructose, and galactose. These monosaccharides are absorbed by carrier-mediated transport processes. The transporters that mediate the uptake of monosaccharides in the epithelial cell (see figure 5.11) are (1) a sodium monosaccharide cotransporter (most commonly the sodium dependent glucose transporter [SGLT1]) and (2) a sodium-independent facilitated-diffusion transporter with specificity for fructose (GLUT5). For each molecule of glucose, two sodium ions will be transported into the epithelial cell. The sodium is then actively transported back into the gut lumen through a Na^+-K^+-ATPase pump. Galactose also uses SGLT1.

A separate monosaccharide transporter on the contraluminal side of the epithelial cell accepts all three monosaccharides (GLUT 2). The monosaccharides then enter the circulation in the hepatic portal vein, which will transport them to the liver.

Absorption of Fats

The monoacylglycerols and FAs incorporated into micelles are transported to the villi and move into the spaces between the microvilli. Here FAs diffuse across the membrane of the epithelium and enter the epithelial cell. The micelles then move away from the villi, incorporate new FAs, and transport them to the villi.

Micelles formed within the intestinal lumen, therefore, perform an important ferrying function. In the presence of **bile salts** (and, thus, micelles), fat absorption is almost complete (97%), whereas in the absence of bile, only about 50% of the FAs are absorbed.

The absorption of FAs through the epithelial membranes is by diffusion (because they are highly soluble in the lipid membranes) (see figure 5.12). In the epithelial cell, FAs are reesterified to triacylglycerols in the endoplasmic reticulum. Once formed, triacylglycerols combine with cholesterol and phospholipids to form chylomicrons (see also figure 1.5, p. 13). In this chylomicron, the fatty sides of the phospholipids face toward the center, and the polar parts form the surface. Chylomicrons make possible

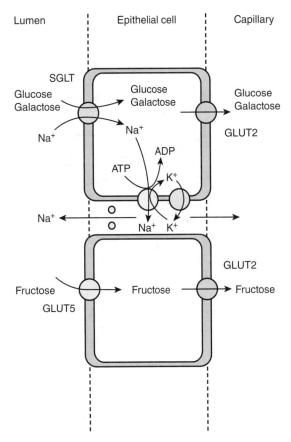

Figure 5.11 Absorption of carbohydrate.

the transport of fat in the aqueous environment of the lymph and blood plasma. These large molecules move toward the central lacteal of the villi and are slowly transported through the lymphatic system, reaching the circulation in the subclavian veins.

Short-chain and medium-chain FAs are more water soluble than long-chain FAs and therefore follow a slightly different route of absorption. They enter the epithelial cell, and, without being reesterified to triacylglycerols, they directly diffuse through the contraluminal membrane into the portal blood, where they are bound to the plasma protein albumin and passed to the liver via the hepatic portal vein. The bile salts are reabsorbed again in the intestinal mucosa of the distal ileum. They enter the portal blood and pass to the liver. In the liver, they are resecreted into the bile. In this way, 94% of the bile salts are reutilized. The recirculation of bile salts is called the enterohepatic circulation.

Absorption of Amino Acids

Amino acids, dipeptides, and tripeptides are absorbed by active transport (coupled to the trans-port of sodium) in the small intestine and delivered to the liver via the hepatic portal vein. Dipeptides and tripeptides that have been transported across the epithelial membrane are broken down inside the cell into their amino acid constituents by specific dipeptidases and tripeptidases (see figure 5.10).

Most amino acids are transported across the epithelium against a concentration gradient, and, therefore, carrier-mediated transport is needed (see figure 5.13). At least seven brush border–specific transport proteins have been identified. The luminal membrane usually contains sodium-dependent transport systems, whereas the contraluminal membrane transport does not require sodium. The small intestine has a large and effective capacity to absorb amino acids and small peptides. Most amino acids can use more than one transporter for absorption. Less than 1% of the ingested protein is usually found in feces. After amino acids have passed the epithelium, they are transported to the liver where they can be converted to glucose, fat, or protein, or they can be released into the bloodstream as free amino acids.

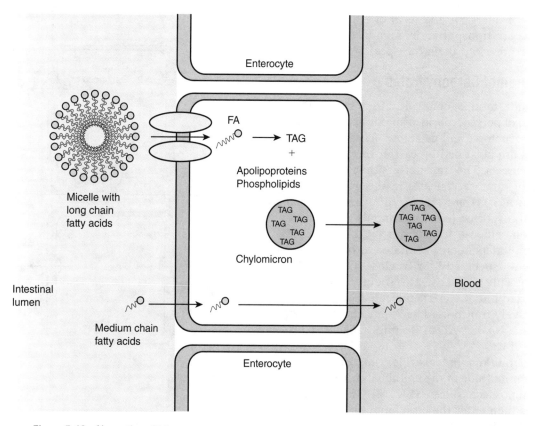

Figure 5.12 Absorption of fat.

Absorption of Water

Most water absorption (99%) takes place in the small intestine, mainly in the duodenum (72%), entirely by simple diffusion. This absorption obeys the laws of osmosis (see figure 5.14). A membrane that is impermeable to solutes but permeable to water separates two compartments with the same amount of fluid but different numbers of solute particles.

Water diffuses across this membrane in both directions, but relatively more water flows toward the compartment with the lower water concentration (higher solute concentration). This net movement of water eventually results in a similar solute concentration on both sides of the membrane. But the amount of water in the compartment with the lower water concentration increases.

The term *osmole* describes the number of solute particles, and the solute particle density is usually expressed as milliosmoles (mOsm) per unit mass (kg) or volume (L): mOsm/kg (osmolality) or mOsm/L (osmolarity), respectively. The osmolarity of most body fluids is around 290 mOsm/L (see table 5.4). Therefore, when the osmolarity of the chyme is low (<280 mOsm/L), water moves toward the epithelial cell and the blood plasma in which the osmolarity is higher. If the osmolarity of the chyme is high (>300 mOsm/L, as, for example, in a concentrated glucose solution), water moves into the gut lumen. With the absorption of solutes (e.g., glucose and sodium), the osmotic gradient changes and pulls water into the epithelium (a process known as solvent drag).

The secretions into the intestine can amount up to 7 L/day in a sedentary adult (see table 5.2). Those 7 L of water are produced by the combined secretions of the salivary glands, stomach

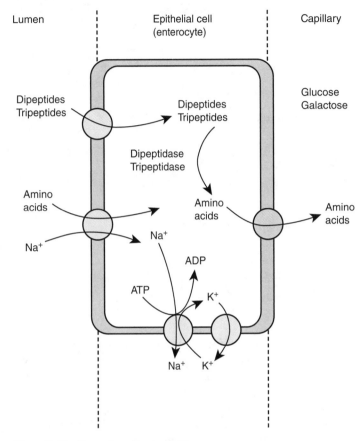

Figure 5.13 Absorption of amino acids.

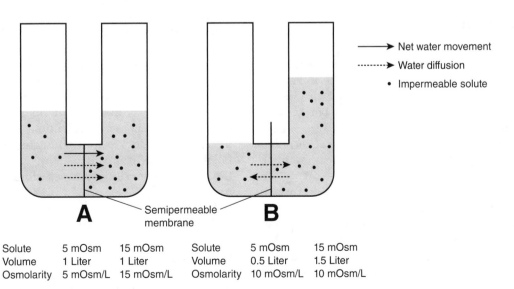

Figure 5.14 The process of osmosis.

■ **TABLE 5.4** ■

Osmolarity of Body Fluids and Commercially Available Drinks

Solution	Osmolarity (mOsm/L)
Water	10–20
Sweat	170–220
Gastric fluids	280–303
Blood serum	300
Lucozade Sport	280
Isostar	296
Gatorade	349
Powerade (UK)	285
Powerade (U.S.)	381
Allsport	516
Pepsi-Cola	568
Coca-Cola	650
Fruit juice	450–690

wall, gallbladder, pancreas, and intestine. Daily water intake may average 2 L, and the total daily water absorption may therefore be as high as 9 L. During exercise, especially in hot conditions when fluid losses and intakes are high, daily water absorption can easily exceed 10 L. With diarrhea, absorption of water is minimal, and the losses of fluid from the body can be high and, in some cases, life threatening.

Absorption of Vitamins

Most of the vitamin absorption takes place in the jejunum and ileum and is usually a passive process (diffusion). Fat-soluble vitamins (A, D, E, and K) are absorbed along with FAs. They are also incorporated into chylomicrons and transported through the lymph system into the systemic circulation to liver and other tissues. Most of the absorption of fat-soluble vitamins takes place in the small intestine.

Water-soluble vitamins are also mostly absorbed in the small intestine, by diffusion. The water-soluble vitamins are not retained to any great extent by different tissues, and when large amounts are ingested, they are mostly excreted in urine. Most vitamin C is absorbed in the distal portion of the small intestine. Excess intake of vitamin C (above approximately 1,200 mg/day) decreases the efficiency of renal reabsorption of vitamin C, and much of the excess intake appears in the urine. B vitamins are often ingested as part of coenzymes in food; digestion liberates the vitamins. For example, pantothenic acid is usually present in food as part of coenzyme A. Digestion releases the vitamin from its coenzyme, and absorption takes place. Thiamin and vitamin B_6 are mainly absorbed in the jejunum. Biotin and riboflavin are mainly absorbed in the proximal part of the small intestine. Niacin is partly absorbed in the stomach but mostly in the small intestine. Vitamin B_{12} is mainly absorbed in the ileum. Its absorption is more complex, involving binding to a specific protein (called intrinsic factor, which is secreted by the parietal cells of the gastric mucosa). Absorption of folic acid depends on the presence of the intestinal enzyme conjugase, which facilitates the absorption of folic acid in the small intestine. An overview of various vitamins and their absorption is given in table 5.5.

Absorption of Minerals

Minerals are not well absorbed in the human intestine. The intake in food is therefore usually far in excess of the actual requirements. Mineral absorption often depends on its chemical form. The best-known example of this requirement is probably the difference in absorption between nonheme and heme iron. (Heme iron is found in meat; nonheme iron is obtained from plants.) About 15% of all ingested heme iron is absorbed in the small intestine, whereas only 2% to 10% of nonheme iron is absorbed. Absorption of other minerals is also relatively poor. A maximum of only 35% of ingested calcium is absorbed, 20% to 30% of ingested magnesium is absorbed, 14% to 41% of ingested zinc is absorbed, and less than 2% of ingested chromium is absorbed. Besides poor absorption, excretion rates by urine are also high. About 65% of absorbed phosphorus and 50% of absorbed calcium is excreted by urine. When daily mineral intake is insufficient, increased intake may result in increased retention. For example, many women in Western countries have insufficient intake of iron and calcium, and increasing the intake generally increases storage of these minerals.

Sodium is actively transported out of the epithelial cell into the portal circulation, a process requiring ATPase carrier enzymes and energy (in the form of ATP). The transport of sodium out of the epithelial cell creates a low sodium concentration in the cell, which increases diffusion of sodium from the gut lumen into the epithelial cell. About

30 g of sodium is secreted in intestinal secretions every day. Daily sodium ingestion is about 5 to 8 g. Thus, about 25 to 35 g of sodium must be reabsorbed each day, representing a large percentage of the body sodium stores. This requirement explains why extreme diarrhea results in large sodium losses, which can be dangerous and even life threatening.

Function of Bacteria in the Colon

The adult human gut contains about 1 kg of various bacteria (colon bacilli). The gastrointestinal tract contains an immensely complex ecology of microorganisms. A typical person harbors more than 500 distinct species of bacteria. The composition and distribution of these microorganisms vary with age, state of health, and diet.

The number and type of bacteria in the gastrointestinal tract vary dramatically by region. In healthy people the stomach and proximal small intestine contain few microorganisms, largely a result of the bacteriocidal activity of gastric acid. One interesting testimony to the ability of gastric acid to suppress bacterial populations is seen in patients with achlorhydria, a genetic condition that prevents secretion of gastric acid. Patients with achlorhydria who are otherwise healthy may have as many as 10,000 to 100,000,000 microorganisms per milliliter of stomach contents.

In sharp contrast to the stomach and small intestine, the colon literally teems with bacteria, predominantly strict anaerobes (bacteria that survive only in environments virtually devoid of oxygen) (see table 5.6). Between these two extremes is a transitional zone, usually in the ileum, where moderate numbers of both aerobic and anaerobic bacteria are found. The gastrointestinal tract is sterile at birth, but colonization typically begins within a few hours of birth, starting in the small intestine and progressing caudally over a period of several days. In most circumstances, a mature microbial flora is established by 3 to 4 weeks of age.

■ TABLE 5.5 ■
Absorption of Vitamins

Vitamin	Absorption mechanism
Vitamin C	Almost all absorption (90%) takes place in the distal portion of the small intestine.
Thiamine	Absorption occurs predominantly in the jejunum.
Riboflavin	Absorption occurs in the proximal part of the small intestine.
Niacin	Some absorption occurs in the stomach, but most occurs in the small intestine.
Pantothenic acid	This vitamin exists as part of coenzyme A, but absorption occurs readily throughout the small intestine when the vitamin is released from CoA.
Biotin	Absorption occurs in upper one-third to one-half of the small intestine.
Folic acid	Absorption occurs in small intestine with the help of a specialized intestinal enzyme system called conjugase.
Vitamin B_6	Absorption occurs in the jejunum.
Vitamin B_{12}	Absorption occurs mainly in the ileum and requires an intrinsic factor secreted from parietal cells of the stomach.

■ TABLE 5.6 ■
Microbial Populations in the Digestive Tract of Normal Humans

	Stomach	Jejunum	Ileum	Colon
Viable bacteria per gram	$0-10^3$	$0-10^4$	10^5-10^8	$10^{10}-10^{12}$
pH	3.0	6.0–7.0	7.5	6.8–7.3

Probiotics and Prebiotics

Probiotics are potentially beneficial bacteria or yeasts. They can be found in certain foods or can be bought as a supplement. The most common probiotics are the lactic acid bacteria (LAB). These microbes have been used in the food industry for many years. LAB are able to convert sugars (including lactose) and other carbohydrates into lactic acid. This conversion not only provides the characteristic sour taste of fermented dairy foods such as yogurt but also by lowering the pH may create fewer opportunities for "bad bacteria" to grow, hence creating possible health benefits by preventing gastrointestinal infections. Strains of the *Lactobacillus* and *Bifidobacterium* are the most widely used probiotic bacteria. Probiotic bacterial cultures are intended to help the body's naturally occurring gut flora, an ecology of microbes (the "good bacteria"), to reestablish themselves. They are sometimes recommended after a course of antibiotics. Claims are made that probiotics strengthen the immune system and gastrointestinal barrier function to help combat infections, allergies, excessive alcohol intake, stress, exposure to toxic substances, and other diseases.

Instead of consuming probiotics, people can eat foods for the "good" bacteria to feed on. These foods, known as prebiotics, consist of indigestible food fibers and complex carbohydrates that specifically stimulate the growth of good bacteria in the bowel. It has been argued that it may be more effective to take prebiotics that boost growth of the good bacteria already present in the gut rather than take supplements of live bacteria that may be destroyed by the acidity of the stomach as soon as they are swallowed. Prebiotics are found naturally in small amounts in foods such as wheat, oats, bananas, asparagus, leeks, garlic, and onions. But to get an adequate daily dose, people may want to look for foods in the supermarket that have been enriched with prebiotics or even consider prebiotic supplements.

The latest research shows that both probiotics and prebiotics may have widespread health benefits including the treatment and prevention of acute diarrhea and antibiotic-induced diarrhea. Likely mediated through immune influences, the effects of prebiotics and probiotics may reach beyond the gastrointestinal tract and include systemic effects such as reduced severity of colds or other respiratory conditions (see chapter 16), lower incidence and reduced symptoms of allergy, and fewer absences from work or daycare.

Bacterial populations in the large intestine digest carbohydrates, proteins, and lipids that escape digestion and absorption in the small intestine. The bacteria are responsible for the fermentation of small amounts of cellulose. More important, however, is the production of vitamin K, vitamin B_{12}, thiamine, riboflavin, and other substances. Vitamin K is especially important because the daily vitamin K intake in foodstuffs is normally insufficient.

Regulation of Gastric Emptying

After the ingestion, food usually takes 1 to 4 hours to leave the stomach, depending on the content of the meal. Gastric motility and secretion are to some extent automatic. Contraction of the stomach increases the intragastric pressure to push chyme through the pyloric sphincter. Such contractions are initiated by pacemaker cells in the stomach wall. Gastric emptying is further controlled by a variety of signals directly from the stomach or the duodenum (see figure 5.15). The signals are either nervous or hormonal signals.

The stomach signals include (1) nervous signals caused by stretching and extension of the stomach wall and (2) the release of the hormone gastrin by the antral mucosa. Gastrin is released in response to both internal (thought of food and extension of the stomach) and external (sight and smell of food) stimuli. These signals from the stomach are always positive feedback signals. The increased amount of food relaxes the pyloric sphincter and increases gastric emptying. Signals from the duodenum usually provide negative feedback (i.e., inhibit gastric emptying). The duodenum contains receptors that can detect acidity, distension of the duodenum, osmolarity, and possibly carbohydrate, fat, and protein. When these receptors are stimulated, the enterogastric reflex is initiated, which increases the contraction of the pylorus. This mechanism prevents dumping of an excessive amount of chyme into the small intestine. Too rapid delivery of the chyme into the intestine could mean insufficient time for digestion and absorption to take place, and

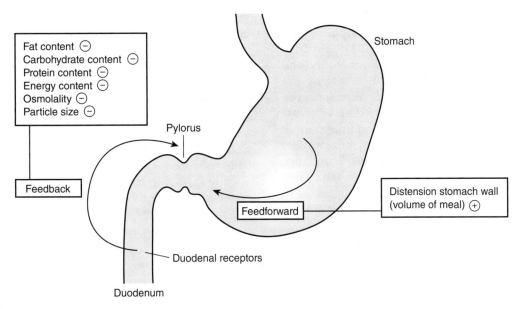

Figure 5.15 Regulation of gastric emptying by feedforward and feedback mechanisms.

some nutrients would be lost in the feces. Factors that have been suggested to affect gastric emptying include

- smell and sight of food,
- thought of food,
- volume of a drink,
- energy density of a drink,
- temperature of a drink,
- osmolarity of a drink,
- body temperature and dehydration,
- type of exercise,
- exercise intensity,
- gender, and
- psychological stress and anxiety.

These factors operate in the following ways:

- *Volume of the food ingested.* The stomach walls can extend to accommodate larger volumes, and as a result the volume of the stomach increases without a change in pressure. When maximal distension is reached, pressure will increase. The rate of gastric emptying of a fluid is highly dependent on the volume of the fluid in the stomach (Hunt and Donald 1954). Therefore, the rate of gastric emptying from a fluid bolus is exponential (see figure 5.16). The gastric-emptying phase is initially rapid, and when the volume is reduced, the rate of gastric emptying is reduced accordingly. The rate of gastric emptying is regulated

through positive-feedback signals to the pyloric sphincter.

- *Exercise intensity.* The rate of gastric emptying is not affected by exercise intensity, up to an intensity of 80% of $\dot{V}O_2$max. Above this intensity a reduction may occur in fluid and nutrient delivery to the small intestine (Sole and Noakes 1989; Costill and Saltin 1974). From a practical point of view, however, this reduction may not be important because exercise intensities of greater than 80% of $\dot{V}O_2$max generally cannot be sustained long enough to cause a limitation in fluid or carbohydrate delivery. Eating and drinking at these high intensities are problematic anyway because of exercise-induced hyperventilation. Gastric emptying of liquids is slowed during brief intermittent high-intensity exercise compared with rest or steady-state moderate exercise (Leiper et al. 2001a). Gastric emptying measured after a five-a-side indoor soccer match decreased even though the average intensity of the activity was only 54% to 63% of $\dot{V}O_2$max (Leiper et al. 2001b). The relatively short bouts of very high-intensity exercise were clearly enough to reduce gastric emptying.

- *Osmolarity.* Osmolarity has always been considered an important factor in controlling the rate of gastric emptying. Increased beverage osmolarity not only increases gastric secretions but also increases intestinal secretions. Osmolarity is therefore an important factor to consider when selecting a beverage for ingestion during exercise. Higher osmolarity may reduce gastric emptying and decrease water absorption. But osmolarity and the concentration of simple carbohydrates are related. A high-energy or high-carbohydrate content is usually related to high osmolarity, and the effects of concentration and osmolarity are therefore difficult to distinguish. Studies, however, suggest that although osmolarity reduces the rate of gastric emptying, this factor is not important in beverages with osmolarities in the range of 200 to 400 mOsm/L (Brouns et al. 1995). This range is typical for most sports drinks (see table 5.4). Osmolarity possibly becomes more important in beverages with extremely high osmolarities (>500 mOsm/L).

■ *Energy density.* Energy density has a strong effect on the rate of gastric emptying. Whether this effect is an effect of energy density per se or of specific nutrients is not clear. Several nutrients exert a strong inhibitory effect on gastric emptying. For example, fat is a strong inhibitor of gastric emptying. Increasing the carbohydrate or protein content of a beverage, however, also slows gastric emptying. Carbohydrate–electrolyte solutions with 2% carbohydrate already show a tendency to empty slower than water does (Vist and Maughan 1994), but solutions of 8% or more significantly inhibit gastric emptying. The energy content of the solution is a more important factor than the osmolarity (Vist and Maughan 1995).

■ *Meal or beverage temperature.* The effect of meal or beverage temperature is probably not important physiologically. Lambert et al. 1999 showed that after ingestion of a ^2H_2O-containing beverage, deuterium (^2H) accumulation in plasma was similar in drinks at varying temperatures. Gastric emptying was not different despite the differences in beverage temperature. This study reflects the findings in the literature that, generally, no effects of meal

temperature have been found on the rate of gastric emptying. Some studies, however, have found a reduction in the rate of gastric emptying with very cold or very hot drinks, and gastric emptying may be influenced by beverage temperature when the intragastric temperature is much higher or lower than body temperature.

■ *Psychological stress.* Stress affects gastrointestinal motility and the rate of gastric emptying. This reduction in the rate of gastric emptying is usually related to changes in circulating hormone concentrations because of stress. Some of these hormones (e.g., epinephrine) reduce blood flow to the gastrointestinal tract.

■ *Other factors.* Besides the factors mentioned earlier, other factors may affect gastric emptying. Studies in hot conditions have shown that dehydration and hyperthermia can cause a slowing of gastric emptying (Rehrer et al. 1990; Neufer et al. 1989). Because subjects in these studies became dehydrated and hyperthermic at the same time, determining what the mechanisms were and whether dehydration, hyperthermia, or a combination of the two was responsible for the reduced gastric-emptying rate is not possible.

Women have slower gastric-emptying rates than men (Notivol et al. 1984), although gastric-emptying rates seemed to increase somewhat during ovulation. Women are reported to be more prone to gastrointestinal complaints after prolonged endurance exercise. This finding could be related to a slower rate of gastric emptying.

Considerable differences exist in the rate of gastric emptying between individuals. Some people may empty 70% to 80% of a solution in 15 minutes, whereas others empty only 20% to 30% of that same solution in 15 minutes. The reasons for these individual differences are not known, but diet has been suggested as an important factor. The gastrointestinal tract possibly adapts to the intake of certain nutrients, and a high habitual fat intake may result in a high gastric-emptying rate of fat. Whatever the mechanisms, they highlight the importance of individual fluid intake recommendations.

Gastrointestinal Problems During and After Exercise

Gastrointestinal complaints are common among endurance athletes. An estimated 30 to 50% of distance runners experience intestinal problems

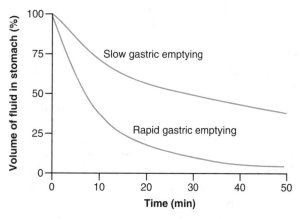

Figure 5.16 An example of a gastric-emptying curve.

related to exercise. Bill Rodgers, the marathon legend who won both the Boston Marathon and New York City Marathon four times between 1975 and 1980 said, "More marathons are won or lost in the porta-toilets than at the dinner table." This comment illustrates the magnitude of the problem for endurance athletes, in particular long-distance runners.

The most common complaints include nausea, gastroesophageal reflux (or heartburn), abdominal pains, loose stool, diarrhea or even bloody diarrhea, and vomiting. The complaints are normally divided into two categories: symptoms of the upper intestinal tract and symptoms of the lower intestinal tract (see the highlight box). Several symptoms are not classified as either upper or lower gastrointestinal problems but might be related to the gastrointestinal tract (for example, stitch).

The vast majority (83%) of 471 marathoners who completed a survey reported suffering from gastrointestinal (GI) problems occasionally or frequently during or after running; 53% experienced the urge to defecate, and 38% reported diarrhea. Women were more likely than men to experience these problems. Among 155 mountain marathoners, 24% had intestinal symptoms and 2 dropped out because of GI troubles.

A study by Keeffe et al. (1984) surveyed 1,700 participants after a marathon race. Lower gastrointestinal symptoms, such as diarrhea, abdominal cramps, urge to defecate, flatulence, and gastrointestinal bleeding were found to be more common than upper gastrointestinal symptoms such as nausea, vomiting, heartburn, bloating, and side ache (stitch).

The most common symptom experienced was the urge to defecate (36% to 39% of the participants), both during and immediately after running. Bowel movements (35%) and diarrhea (19%) were reported frequently and immediately after running. During the race, some runners (16% to 18%) had to stop to defecate, and some runners (8% to 10%) had to stop because of diarrhea. Bloody bowel movements were reported by 1% to 2% of the participants. Similar results were obtained by Jeukendrup et al. (2000), who found that 93% of the participants of a long-distance triathlon reported at least one symptom of gastrointestinal discomfort; 29% of these symptoms were rated as serious (complaints about symptoms that affect exercise performance).

Lower gastrointestinal symptoms are more often observed in women than in men, and some symptoms are more frequently reported by younger than older participants. Problems seem to occur more frequently during running than during activities such as cycling or swimming, possibly because of the vertical (i.e., up and down) movements of the gut during running. People with preexisting GI issues (such as reflux, lactose intolerance, or irritable bowel syndrome) are more likely to get GI symptoms during competition.

Causes of Gastrointestinal Problems

The causes of gastrointestinal symptoms are not completely understood. The symptoms are difficult to investigate because they are often specific to race situations and cannot be simulated in a laboratory. Nevertheless, some laboratory studies have been performed, and field studies have correlated the symptoms with nutritional intake and other factors. From these studies a number of potential causes and contributors have been identified. They can be divided into three categories: (1) physiological, (2) mechanical, and (3) nutritional.

Physiological Causes Physiological causes of GI symptoms include reduced blood flow and increased anxiety (especially before competition). With exercise, blood flow is preferentially redirected to the working muscles and blood flow

---

Frequently Reported Gastrointestinal and Related Problems

Upper gastrointestinal symptoms

- Heartburn
- Bloating
- Vomiting

Lower gastrointestinal symptoms

- Urge to defecate
- Loose stool
- Diarrhea
- Bleeding

Related symptoms

- Nausea
- Dizziness
- Side ache (stitch)
- Urge to urinate

to the gut can be reduced by as much as 80%. The low blood supply can compromise gut function and result in commonly experienced GI symptoms such as cramping. In severe cases it can even result in ischemic colitis (injury of the large intestine as a result of inadequate blood supply). Although, with training, this decrease in blood flow becomes less pronounced, no clear evidence shows that less fit people are more prone to symptomatic ischemia. Anxiety has an effect on hormone secretion, which in turn can affect gut motility, resulting in incomplete absorption and loose stool.

Mechanical Causes The mechanical causes of GI problems are related to either impact or posture. Gastrointestinal bleeding is common among runners. This condition is thought to be a result of the repetitive high-impact mechanics of running and subsequent damage to the intestinal lining. This repetitive gastric jostling is also thought to contribute to lower GI symptoms such as flatulence, diarrhea, and urgency. Estimates of the incidence of occult blood (blood in feces) after a race range from 8% to 85% mostly because of the wide range of race distances in various studies. The longer the distance, the greater the incidence. As many as 16% of runners in one study report having bloody diarrhea on at least one occasion after a race or hard run. The mechanical trauma suffered by the gut from the repetitive impact of running in combination with gut ischemia is probably the cause of the bleeding. Presence of bloody bowel movements after an endurance event raise the possibility of ischemic colitis and hemorrhagic gastritis. Posture can also have an effect on GI symptoms. For example, in a cyclist upper GI symptoms are more prevalent possibly because of increased pressure on the abdomen because of the cycling position, specifically when in the aero position. "Swallowing" air as a result of increased respiration and drinking from water bottles can result in mild to moderate stomach distress.

Nutritional Causes Finally, nutrition can have a strong influence on gastrointestinal distress. Fiber, fat, protein, and fructose have all been associated with a greater risk of developing GI symptoms. Dehydration, possibly because of inadequate fluid intake, may also exacerbate the symptoms. A study by Rehrer et al. (1992) demonstrated a link between nutritional practices and gastrointestinal complaints during a half-Ironman triathlon. Gastrointestinal problems were more likely to occur with the ingestion of fiber, fat, protein, and

concentrated carbohydrate solutions during the triathlon. Beverages with high osmolarities (>500 mOsm/L) seemed especially to be responsible for some of the reported complaints. The intake of dairy products may also be linked to the occurrence of gastrointestinal distress. Mild lactose intolerance is common and could result in increased bowel activity and mild diarrhea (Noakes 1986). Although some risk factors have been identified it is still unclear why some people seem to be more prone to develop GI problems than others. To minimize gastrointestinal distress, all these risk factors must be taken into account. Milk products, fiber, high-fat, and high-protein intake must be avoided 24 hours before competition and during exercise. A detailed discussion of preventative measures follows.

Prevention of Gastrointestinal Problems

To help prevent gastrointestinal distress, a few guidelines should be considered. Although these suggestions are based on limited research, anecdotally they seem to be effective:

■ *Avoid milk products that contain lactose because even mild lactose intolerance can cause problems during exercise.* For instance, people can avoid milk completely or drink lactose-free milk. Soy, rice, and almond milks generally do not contain lactose.

■ *Avoid high-fiber foods in the day or even days before competition.* For the athlete in training, a diet with adequate fiber will help keep the bowel regular. Fiber before race day is different. By definition, fiber is not digestible, so any fiber that is eaten essentially passes through the intestinal tract. Increased bowel movements during exercise are not desirable, will accelerate fluid loss, and may result in unnecessary gas production that might cause gastrointestinal discomfort (e.g., cramping). Especially for those who are prone to develop GI symptoms, a low-fiber diet the day before (or even a couple of days before) is recommended. People should choose processed white foods like regular pasta, white rice, and plain bagels instead of whole-grain bread, high-fiber cereals, and brown rice. Athletes can check food labels for fiber content. Most fruits and vegetables are high in fiber, but some are not; zucchini, tomatoes, olives, grapes, and grapefruit all have less than 1 g of fiber per serving.

■ *Avoid aspirin and nonsteroidal anti-inflammatory drugs (NSAIDs) such as ibuprofen.* Athletes commonly use both aspirin and NSAIDs, but they have been shown to increase intestinal permeability and may increase the incidence of GI complaints. The use of NSAIDs in the prerace period should be discouraged.

■ *Avoid high-fructose foods (in particular drinks that contain exclusively fructose as the carbohydrate component).* Fructose is found not only in fruit but also in most processed sweets (candy, cookies, and so forth) in the form of high-fructose corn syrup. Some fruit juices are almost exclusively fructose. Fructose is absorbed by the intestines more slowly, and fructose is much less tolerated than glucose (and may lead to cramping, loose stool, and diarrhea). Having said that, in chapter 6 we will describe that fructose in combination with glucose may not cause problems and may even be better tolerated.

■ *Avoid dehydration.* Because dehydration can exacerbate GI symptoms, avoiding dehydration is important. Competitors should start races well hydrated (see chapter 9 for further details).

■ *Practice new nutrition strategies.* Competitors should experiment with their prerace and race-day nutrition plans many times before race day to figure out what does and does not work for them and to reduce the chances that GI issues will ruin their race.

KEY POINTS

■ The primary function of the gastrointestinal (or alimentary) tract, a 6 to 8 m long tubular structure that reaches from the mouth to the anus, is to provide the body with nutrients.

■ Chewing food makes the food particles smaller and increases the surface area of the food. This increases the contact area for digestive enzymes. Chewing also mixes the food particles with saliva and digestive enzymes.

■ In the stomach, food is mixed with gastric secretions (hydrochloric acid and digestive enzymes).

■ Gastric emptying is influenced by volume of food, energy density, osmolarity, dehydration, psychological stress and anxiety, and to a lesser degree by exercise intensity, meal temperature, and gender.

■ Pancreatic juices and bile are added to the chyme in the duodenum to digest the carbohydrate, fat, and protein. Specialized enzymes split these macronutrients into the smallest subunits for absorption. Bile is added to emulsify lipid droplets and facilitate digestion and absorption.

■ About 90% to 95% of all absorption takes place in the duodenum and jejunum (first parts of the small intestine).

■ The large intestine is a storage place for undigested food residues, and the final water and electrolyte absorption occurs there.

■ Gastrointestinal problems are a common phenomenon, mainly among endurance athletes, and the incidence is increased by physiological factors, mechanical factors, and nutrition.

RECOMMENDED READINGS

Brouns, F., and E. Beckers. 1993. Is the gut an athletic organ? Digestion, absorption and exercise. *Sports Medicine* 15:242–257.

Guyton, A.C., and J.E. Hall. 2005. *Textbook of medical physiology.* Philadelphia: Saunders.

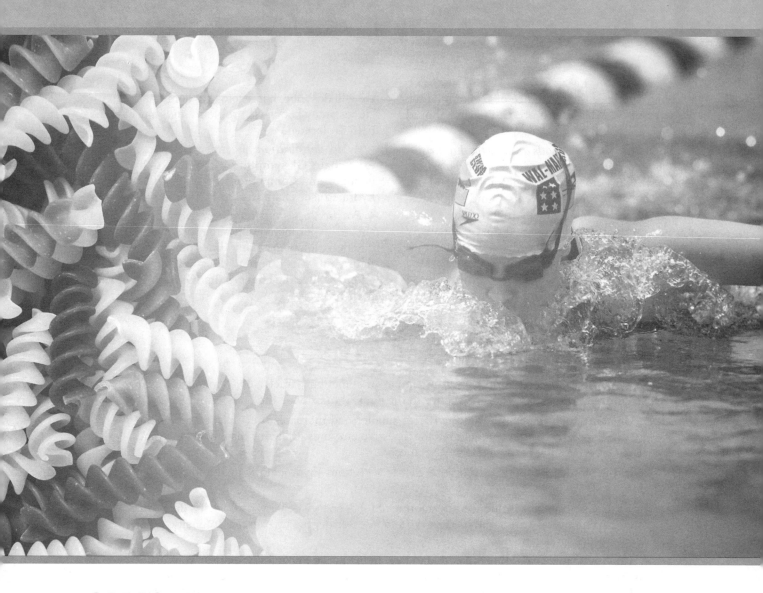

OBJECTIVES

After studying this chapter, you should be able to do the following:

- Describe the main biochemical pathways involved in carbohydrate metabolism
- Describe the changes that occur in carbohydrate metabolism at different intensities of exercise
- Describe how blood glucose concentrations are maintained and regulated
- Describe the metabolic and performance effects of carbohydrate ingestion 3 to 4 hours before exercise
- Describe the metabolic and performance effects of carbohydrate ingestion 1 hour before exercise
- Describe the metabolic and performance effects of carbohydrate ingestion during exercise
- Describe the mechanisms involved in glycogen synthesis
- Give generally accepted guidelines for carbohydrate intake before and during exercise
- Give generally accepted guidelines for carbohydrate intake to improve recovery in the short term and long term
- Describe the dietary requirements for carbohydrate in a variety of sports

6

Carbohydrate

Key Terms

One hundred years ago beef was believed to be the most important component of an athlete's diet, but nowadays pasta, bread, and rice seem to form the central part of the same diet. Athletes are often advised to eat a high-carbohydrate diet, consume carbohydrate before exercise, ensure adequate carbohydrate intake during exercise, and replenish carbohydrate stores as soon as possible after exercise.

Since the beginning of the 20th century, carbohydrate intake has been known to be related to exercise performance. The availability of carbohydrate as a substrate for skeletal muscle contraction and the central nervous system (e.g., the brain) is important for endurance exercise performance. But carbohydrate availability may influence not only the performance of prolonged exercise but also the performance of intermittent-intensity and high-intensity exercise. Because carbohydrate is the most important fuel for the central nervous system, various cognitive tasks and motor skills that play a crucial role in skill sports may also be affected by carbohydrate availability.

Carbohydrate is, therefore, an important component of the athlete's diet, and various strategies have been developed over the past 30 years to optimize carbohydrate availability and hence performance. Generally, these goals can be achieved by (1) carbohydrate feedings before exercise to replenish muscle and liver glycogen stores and (2) carbohydrate feeding during exercise to maintain blood glucose levels and hence high rates of glucose oxidation derived from the plasma. In this chapter the effects of carbohydrate on exercise metabolism and performance are explained. The results of some classic experimental studies are discussed, along with practical implications arising from this work. This chapter is subdivided into four distinct sections:

- Carbohydrate intake in the days before competition (or training)
- Carbohydrate intake in the hours before competition
- Carbohydrate intake during competition or training
- Carbohydrate intake after training or competition

First, however, we start with a short historical tour, beginning with the first studies that investigated the role of carbohydrate in the body as well as the effects of carbohydrate on exercise performance.

History

Krogh and Lindhardt (1920) were probably the first investigators to recognize the importance of carbohydrate as a fuel during exercise. In their study, subjects consumed a high-fat diet for 3 days (bacon, butter, cream, eggs, and cabbage) and then ate a high-carbohydrate diet (potatoes, flour, bread, cake, marmalade, and sugar) for 3 days. The subjects performed a 2-hour exercise test and reported various symptoms of fatigue when they consumed the high-fat diet. But when they consumed the high-carbohydrate diet, the exercise was reported as easy. The investigators also demonstrated that after several days of a low-carbohydrate, high-fat diet, the average respiratory exchange ratio (RER) during 2 hours of cycling declined to 0.80 as compared with 0.85 to 0.90 when a mixed diet was consumed. Conversely, when subjects ate a high-carbohydrate, low-fat diet, RER increased to 0.95.

Important observations were also made by Levine, Gordon, and Derick (Levine et al. 1924). They measured blood glucose in some of the participants of the 1923 Boston Marathon and observed that in most runners, glucose concentrations declined markedly after the race. These investigators suggested that low blood glucose levels were a cause of fatigue. To test that hypothesis,

---

Carbohydrate Intake and Dental Health

Much has been written in the popular press about the potential of sports drinks to have a negative effect on dental health. The frequent intake of acidic drinks (pH ~3–4) during training and competition could lead to dental erosion, which is characterized by painless chemical dissolution of the dental hard tissue not involving bacterial action. Although numerous factors can cause enamel erosion, the acidic properties of soft drinks such as pH, type of acid, and buffering capacity are among the principal factors in the etiology of enamel erosion. Manufacturers are looking into ways around this by increasing the pH of beverages or adding calcium. These steps can dramatically reduce enamel erosion. A study showed that a sports drink was as erosive as orange juice but that a modified drink with higher pH and calcium had an erosive effect equal to that of water (Venables et al. 2005).

they encouraged several participants of the same marathon 1 year later to consume carbohydrate during the race. This practice, in combination with consuming a high-carbohydrate diet before the race, prevented hypoglycemia (low blood glucose) and significantly improved running performance (i.e., time to complete the race).

The importance of carbohydrate for improving exercise capacity was further demonstrated by Dill, Edwards, and Talbott (1932). These investigators let their dogs, Joe and Sally, run without feeding them carbohydrate. The dogs became hypoglycemic and fatigued after 4 to 6 hours. When the test was repeated with the only difference being that the dogs were fed carbohydrate during exercise, the dogs ran for 17 to 23 hours.

Christensen (1932) showed that with increasing exercise intensity, the proportion of carbohydrate utilized increased. A group of Scandinavian scientists (Bergstrom et al. 1966, 1967a) expanded this work in the late 1960s by reintroducing the muscle biopsy technique. These studies indicated the critical role of muscle glycogen. The improved performance after a high-carbohydrate diet was linked with the higher muscle glycogen concentrations observed after such a diet. A high-carbohydrate diet (approximately 70% of dietary energy from carbohydrate) elevated muscle glycogen stores and seemed to enhance endurance capacity compared with a normal-carbohydrate (~50%) and a low-carbohydrate (~10%) diet. These observations have led to the recommendations to carbohydrate-load (i.e., eat a high-carbohydrate diet) before competition (Costill et al. 1980; Sherman et al. 1984).

In the 1980s the effects of carbohydrate feeding during exercise on exercise performance and metabolism were further investigated (Coyle et al. 1984, 1986). Costill et al. (1973) were the first to study the contribution of ingested carbohydrate to total energy expenditure, and in the following years, studies were conducted using isotopic tracers (i.e., ^{14}C-glucose or ^{13}C-glucose) to investigate differences in oxidation rates and metabolism of different types of carbohydrate, different amounts of carbohydrate, different feeding schedules, and various other factors that influence the efficacy of carbohydrate ingestion. Although Costill et al. (1973) concluded

that ingested carbohydrates were not oxidized to any major extent, later studies have convincingly shown that ingested carbohydrates are an important energy source during prolonged exercise.

Role of Carbohydrate

As discussed in chapter 1, carbohydrate plays many roles in the human body, but one of its main functions is to provide energy for the contracting muscle. Glycogen, the storage form of carbohydrate, is found mainly in muscle and the liver.

Muscle Glycogen

Muscle glycogen is a readily available energy source for the working muscle. The glycogen content of skeletal muscle at rest is approximately 12 to 16 g/kg w.w. (65 mmol to 90 mmol glucosyl units/kg w.w. [see the highlight box]), equating to a total of 300 to 400 g of carbohydrate (see chapter

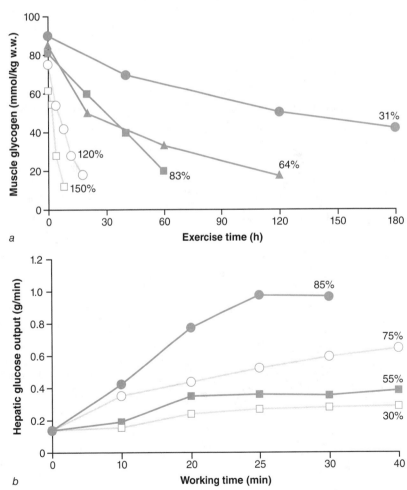

Figure 6.1 The effects of exercise intensity (shown as a percentage of V̇O$_2$max) on (a) muscle glycogen breakdown and (b) liver glucose output.

Data from P.D. Gollick, K. Peel, and B. Salting, 1974, "Selective glycogen depletion pattern in human muscle fibers after exercise of varying intensity and at varying pedaling rates," *Journal of Physiology* 214(1): 45-57.

Muscle Glycogen Units

In the literature, muscle glycogen is expressed in various ways, making possible comparison of results of different studies. The units used most frequently are millimole glycosyl (glucose) units per kilogram of dry mass or per kilogram of wet mass. To express the results per kilogram of dry mass, the muscle biopsy sample must be freeze dried. All the water is removed by placing the frozen biopsy sample in a freeze dryer. Muscle contains approximately 75% to 80% water, and to convert values from wet mass to dry mass the concentration is usually multiplied by 4.5.

2). The rate at which muscle glycogen is oxidized depends largely on exercise intensity. At low to moderate exercise intensity, most of the energy can be obtained from oxidative phosphorylation of acetyl-CoA derived from both carbohydrate and fat. As the exercise intensity increases to high levels, the oxidation of carbohydrate and fat cannot by itself meet the energy requirements. Muscle glycogen becomes the most important substrate, because anaerobic energy delivery (ATP resynthesis from glycolysis) is mostly derived from the

breakdown of muscle glycogen. Figure 6.1 shows the effects of exercise intensity on muscle glycogen breakdown and liver glucose output. At very high exercise intensity, muscle glycogen is broken down very rapidly and becomes nearly depleted in a relatively short time when this type of exercise is performed intermittently.

Liver Glycogen

The main role of glycogen in the liver is to maintain a constant blood glucose level. Glucose is the main, and in normal circumstances the only, fuel used by the brain. The liver is often referred to as the glucoregulator or glucostat—the organ responsible for the regulation of the blood glucose concentration. An average liver weighs approximately 1.5 kg, and approximately 80 to 110 g of glycogen is stored in the liver of an adult human in the postabsorptive state. Glycogen is broken down in the liver to glucose and then released into the circulatory system. The kidneys also store some glycogen and release glucose into the blood, but from a quantitative point of view the kidneys are far less important than the liver. In this book, the terms liver glucose output or hepatic glucose output includes the release of glucose from the liver and kidneys. This release is also often called endogenous glucose production. Glycogen that is broken down in the muscle is not released as glucose into the circulation, because muscle lacks the enzyme glucose-6-phosphatase (the enzyme that removes a phosphate group from glucose-6-phosphate) (figure 6.2). After glucose has been phosphorylated in the muscle cell by the enzyme hexokinase (the enzyme that attaches a phosphate group to glucose), it cannot be dephosphorylated (see chapter 3). Because a phosphorylated glucose molecule cannot be transported out of the cell, glucose-6-phosphate is trapped within the muscle cell.

The liver has a much higher concentration of glycogen (per kilogram of tissue) than does muscle. Only because of the much larger mass of muscle does muscle contain more glycogen than the liver does (in absolute terms, 300 to 600 g versus 80 to 110 g). After an overnight fast, the liver glycogen content can be reduced to low levels (< 20 g) because tissues such as the brain use glucose at a rate of about 0.1 g/min in resting conditions. During exercise, the rate

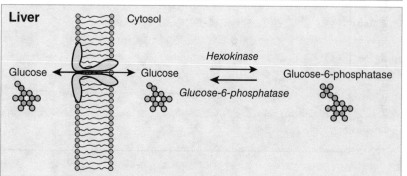

Figure 6.2 Glucose enters the cytosol of the cell by facilitated transport. In the cell it is phosphorylated by hexokinase, and after it is phosphorylated, glucose cannot leave the cell. The exceptions are liver and kidney cells. Liver and kidney cells have an enzyme called glucose-6-phosphatase that reverses the glucokinase reaction.

of glucose utilization by tissues other than muscle does not change much (~0.1 g/min).

Circulation (of blood) can be regarded as a sink (see figure 6.3) from which various tissues, especially exercising muscle, can tap glucose. An extremely precise mechanism, however, regulates

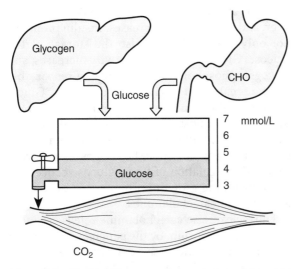

Figure 6.3   The bloodstream can be regarded as a sink in which the blood glucose concentration is accurately controlled. During exercise, muscle glucose uptake increases dramatically, and to prevent the blood glucose concentration from dropping, the liver must produce glucose at an equally high rate.

the blood glucose concentration in this sink at 4.0 to 4.5 mmol/L. (This is equivalent to a plasma glucose concentration of 5 to 6 mmol/L because the concentration of free glucose inside the red blood cells is somewhat less than that in the plasma; see the sidebar.) Note that 5.55 mmol/L equates to 1 g of glucose per liter. When the blood glucose concentration drops, the liver releases glucose. If the demand for glucose is less, the liver produces less glucose or even takes up glucose from the bloodstream to synthesize glycogen. After a meal, for instance, when a large amount of glucose enters the liver through the hepatic portal vein, the liver uses this glucose to synthesize glycogen. Despite the changes in glucose flux, both after feeding and during exercise (or fasting), normoglycemia is usually nicely maintained.

Liver glycogen plays an important role in regulating the blood glucose concentration both at rest and during exercise. Although this has been known for many years, the exact role of the liver during exercise is still incompletely understood. The main reason for this puzzlement is that liver glycogen is notoriously difficult to measure. Although some studies using liver biopsies were performed in the 1960s, limited information is available about liver glycogen synthesis after exercise and its potential effect on performance. A noninvasive technique

Differences Between Whole Blood, Plasma, and Serum

Blood refers to the red liquid in our arteries and veins. It is composed of cells (red blood cells, or erythrocytes; white blood cells, or leukocytes; and cell fragments called platelets, or thrombocytes) that are suspended in a fluid called plasma. The plasma contains proteins, lipoproteins, electrolytes, and small organic molecules such as glucose, fatty acids, glycerol, lactate, and amino acids, but by weight it is about 93% water. After taking a blood sample from a person, plasma can be separated from the cellular components by centrifugation if an anticoagulant (a substance that prevents the activation of clot formation) is added to the blood sample soon after it is collected.

Typical anticoagulants that can be used include heparin, oxalate, citrate, and ethylene-diamine-tetraacetate (EDTA). If an anticoagulant is not added, the blood will clot within a matter of minutes. Centrifuging the clotted blood will separate the cellular elements and the insoluble clotting protein fibrin from the fluid; this fluid is called serum.

Hence, the difference between plasma and serum is that plasma has an anticoagulant in it and still contains soluble fibrinogen, whereas serum does not. Substances such as glucose can be measured in whole blood (after lysing all the blood cells), plasma, or serum. But the glucose concentrations measured in each of these fluids will be a little different because the concentration of free glucose inside the red blood cells is somewhat less than that in the plasma. This means that whole blood will have a lower glucose concentration than plasma or serum. The concentration of most substances in plasma is pretty much the same as in serum, providing that the blood is not left too long to clot before centrifugation takes place. If left at room temperature, blood cell metabolism will use up glucose at a rate of about 0.5 $mmol \cdot L^{-1} \cdot h^{-1}$. In this situation, the serum glucose concentration will be less than that in plasma if the latter was obtained by centrifugation immediately after blood sampling.

that has been used to address this problem is nuclear magnetic resonance (NMR) imaging. Using ^{13}C-NMR, Casey et al. (2000) measured liver glycogen concentrations after exercise and during 4 hours of recovery. They observed that liver glycogen resynthesis was evident after glucose and sucrose ingestion but not with water. Relatively small amounts of carbohydrate were ingested (1 g/kg b.w.), and these amounts were sufficient to initiate postexercise liver glycogen resynthesis.

Early studies in Scandinavia with liver biopsies showed that liver glycogen is decreased by about 50% after 1 hour of exercise at 75% of $\dot{V}O_2$max. Later studies have used stable isotopes to measure the oxidation of liver glucose indirectly. These studies clearly show that liver glycogen is a significant substrate during exercise, and its importance (in absolute terms) increases when exercise intensity increases (Romijn et al. 1993; van Loon et al. 2001).

The liver can also produce glucose through newly formed glucose (gluconeogenesis). Substrates such as lactate, glycerol, pyruvate, alanine, glutamine, and some other amino acids can be used for the synthesis of glucose. These substrates are usually formed in other organs of the body and transported to the liver. For example, during exercise most of the lactate is formed in skeletal muscle, and most of the glycerol is from adipose tissue.

In resting conditions, the glucose output by the liver is approximately 150 mg/min (0.8 mmol/min). About 60% of this output (90 mg/min) is derived from liver glycogenolysis (the breakdown of liver glycogen), and about 40% (60 mg/min) is gluconeogenesis (Hultman et al. 1971; Nilsson et al. 1973). During exercise, the liver glucose output increases dramatically. During high-intensity exercise (>75% of $\dot{V}O_2$max), liver glucose output increases to about 1 g/min, and the majority (>90%) of this glucose is derived from the breakdown of liver glycogen. The rate of gluconeogenesis increases only marginally during exercise compared with resting conditions. Gluconeogenesis increases in the presence of high plasma concentrations of cortisol, epinephrine (adrenaline), and glucagon, whereas insulin has the opposite effect. The longer the exercise is, the greater the relative contribution of gluconeogenesis is to liver glucose production and output. During periods of starvation gluconeogenesis increases, whereas after carbohydrate consumption gluconeogenesis decreases.

Regulation of Glucose Concentration

Blood glucose concentrations are normally maintained within a narrow range (a normal resting blood glucose concentration is usually between 4.0 and 4.5 mmol/L; plasma glucose concentrations are between 5 and 6 mmol/L). Hormones play a key role in this regulation. In resting conditions, insulin is the most important glucoregulatory hormone. It increases the uptake of glucose into various tissues. After a meal, plasma insulin concentrations increase, and as a result glucose uptake by muscle, liver, and other tissues increases. Insulin promotes not only the uptake but also the storage of the glucose. Glycogen synthase activity increases, and glycogen phosphorylase (the enzyme responsible for the breakdown of glycogen) decreases. Glucagon is the most important counteractive hormone. Secretion of glucagon causes the breakdown of liver glycogen and the release of glucose into the circulation. Several other hormones may have a role in the regulation of blood glucose concentrations, including growth hormone, cortisol, somatostatin, and catecholamines.

During exercise catecholamine release reduces the secretion of insulin by the pancreas, and plasma insulin concentrations can decrease to extremely low levels. Muscle glucose uptake is enhanced by contraction-stimulated glucose transport. As mentioned previously, however, despite dramatically increased glucose uptake by the muscle during exercise, blood glucose levels are well maintained in most conditions.

But a mismatch between glucose uptake and glucose production by the liver occurs during high-intensity exercise. At an intensity of approximately 80% of $\dot{V}O_2$max or more, the liver produces glucose at a higher rate than it is taken up by the muscle. This increased hepatic glucose release is most likely caused by neural feedforward mechanisms and results in slightly elevated blood glucose concentration compared with rest. Another situation in which a mismatch occurs is during the later stages of prolonged exercise. As liver glycogen becomes depleted, the rate of glucose production may become insufficient to compensate for the glucose uptake by the muscle and other tissues. As a result hypoglycemia develops, and blood glucose levels sometimes drop below 3 mmol/L.

Hypoglycemia

If blood glucose concentrations drop below a critical level (often 3 mmol/L), the rate of glucose uptake by the brain is insufficient to meet its metabolic requirements, and symptoms of hypoglycemia result. Hypoglycemia is characterized by a variety of symptoms, including dizziness, nausea, cold sweat, reduced mental alertness and ability to concentrate, loss of motor skill, increased heart rate, excessive hunger, and disorientation. Hypoglycemia is a common problem in exercise and sport and can be treated simply by carbohydrate consumption. Hypoglycemia has received considerable attention because preexercise carbohydrate feeding seemed to induce reactive hypoglycemia (also referred to as **rebound hypoglycemia).** Note that although the symptoms of hypoglycemia that may occur during prolonged exercise are identical to those resulting from rebound hypoglycemia, the cause is very different. This topic is discussed in more detail in the section "Carbohydrate Intake 30 Minutes to 60 Minutes Before Exercise."

Athletes often train (or compete) on consecutive days, in which case rapid replenishment of muscle glycogen can be crucial. Costill et al. (1971) reported that in subjects running 16.1 km on 3 consecutive days, a diet containing only moderate amounts of carbohydrate (40% to 50%) may not be enough to restore muscle glycogen fully (see figure 6.4). A marked decrease in muscle glycogen occurred immediately after the run, and although some glycogen was synthesized before the run the next day, the starting muscle glycogen concentrations were lower. After 3 days of running, the muscle glycogen concentration had dropped considerably.

Sherman et al. (1993) fed subjects a diet containing either 5 or 10 g of carbohydrate · kg b.w.$^{-1}$ · day^{-1} during 7 days of training. The diet containing 5 g of carbohydrate · kg b.w.$^{-1}$ · day^{-1} resulted in a decline in muscle glycogen concentration in the first 5 days, which was then maintained for the remainder of the study. With the high-carbohydrate diet (10 g · kg b.w.$^{-1}$ · day^{-1}), muscle glycogen concentrations were maintained despite daily training.

In another study, well-trained cyclists exercised 2 hours per day at 65% of $\dot{V}O_2$max (Coyle et al. 2001). They ingested a diet containing 581 g, 718 g, or 901 g of carbohydrate. These high carbohydrate intakes made maintaining high muscle glycogen concentrations possible (120 mmol/kg w.w., 155 mmol/kg w.w., and 185 mmol/kg w.w., respectively). The muscle glycogen concentrations were even higher than the values reported after the classical supercompensation diet. The amount of carbohydrate ingested between two exercise bouts on consecutive days is, therefore, extremely important in determining the total amount of muscle glycogen stored. A higher carbo-

hydrate intake can also reduce some symptoms of overreaching (an early stage of overtraining) such as changes in mood state and feelings of fatigue, although it cannot completely prevent them. Achten et al. (2003) observed such an effect in runners who increased their training volume and intensity and controlled their carbohydrate intake at either 5.4 or 8.5 g · kg b.w.$^{-1}$ · day^{-1}.

Unless large amounts of carbohydrate are ingested, muscle glycogen does not normalize on a day-to-day basis (Costill et al. 1971). But just how much carbohydrate must we eat to replenish our glycogen stores within 24 hours? Costill et al. (1981) suggested that increasing carbohydrate intake from 150 to 650 g results in a proportional increase in muscle glycogen. Intakes greater than 600 g/24 h, however, do not result in a further increase in glycogen resynthesis. Studies that are more recent seem to suggest that with daily exercise, an almost linear increase in glycogen storage occurs in relation to carbohydrate intake (Coyle et al. 2001). These findings and others have led sport nutrition experts to recommend increasing carbohydrate intake to 10 to 13 g · kg b.w.$^{-1}$ · day^{-1} when exercising for 3 hours or more on a daily basis.

What does a high-carbohydrate diet look like? Is a carbohydrate intake of 70% of total energy intake high? That depends; guidelines expressed in percentages have muddled the advice given to athletes. For example, a 50% carbohydrate diet may contain a large amount of carbohydrate for a triathlete or cyclist who expends 6,000 kcal/day (25 MJ/day) but contain only a small amount of carbohydrate for a distance runner who has an intake of 2,000 kcal/day (8.4 MJ/day). A more sensible expression of carbohydrate intake is grams per kilogram of bodyweight per day (g · kg b.w.$^{-1}$ · day^{-1}).

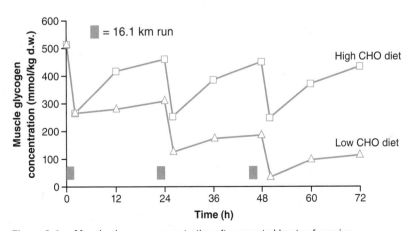

Figure 6.4 Muscle glycogen concentration after repeated bouts of running.
Data from Costill et al. 1971.

Carbohydrate Type

To stimulate glycogen resynthesis after exercise, the amount of carbohydrate ingested may be the most important factor, but the type of carbohydrate may also play a role. One study investigated the effects of the GI on muscle glycogen resynthesis. Subjects performed a bout of exercise that depleted their glycogen stores on two occasions and received a diet of high-GI carbohydrate on one occasion and a diet of low-GI carbohydrate on the other (Coyle et al. 2001). The total carbohydrate intake over 24 hours was 10 g/kg b.w. The increase in muscle glycogen was more than 50% greater when the high-GI carbohydrate was consumed. Therefore, high-GI foods are important for complete muscle glycogen resynthesis within 24 hours. The higher insulin responses of the high-GI meals are likely responsible for the increased glycogen synthesis. Jozsi et al (1996) compared two forms of starch (100% amylose and 100% amylopectin) with maltodextrins and glucose and reported slower glycogen resynthesis with the amylose starch compared with the other carbohydrate types.

Recommendations for Carbohydrate Intake

The following are some recommendations based on the International Olympic Committee's consensus on sport nutrition (Burke et al. 2004). These recommendations are general and should be tailored to specific individual needs with consideration of total energy needs, specific training needs, and feedback from training performance. These rec-

Postexercise Carbohydrate Intake Recommendations

Immediately after exercise (0–4 hours)	1.0–1.2 g · kg b.w.$^{-1}$ · h^{-1} carbohydrate, ingested at frequent intervals
Daily recovery from moderate duration, low-intensity training	5–7 g · kg b.w.$^{-1}$ · day^{-1}
Daily recovery from moderate to heavy endurance training	7–12 g · kg b.w.$^{-1}$ · day^{-1}
Daily recovery from an extreme exercise program (4–6 h training per day)	10–12+ g · kg b.w.$^{-1}$ · day^{-1}

ommendations should enable athletes to restore muscle glycogen on a 24-hour basis, although they may become depleted in a training session.

- Depending on the exercise intensity and duration, consume 5-12 g · kg b.w.$^{-1}$ · day^{-1} (see highlight box).
- Choose high-GI carbohydrates (see table 6.1).
- Consume a sports drink to provide a convenient source of carbohydrate in the first hour after exercise when appetite is suppressed. Carbohydrate solutions have the advantage of providing fluid that helps to restore fluid balance (see chapter 9).
- Choose nutrient-rich carbohydrate foods and add other foods to recovery meals and snacks to provide a good source of protein and other nutrients. These nutrients may assist in other recovery processes and, in the case of protein, may promote additional glycogen recovery when carbohydrate intake is suboptimal or when frequent snacking is not possible.
- When the period between exercise sessions is less than 8 hours, the athlete should begin carbohydrate intake as soon as practical after the first workout to maximize the effective recovery time between sessions. Meeting carbohydrate intake targets as a series of snacks during the early recovery phase may offer some advantages.
- During longer recovery periods (24 hours), the athlete should organize the pattern and timing of carbohydrate-rich meals and snacks according to what is practical and comfortable for his or her individual situation. Glycogen synthesis is the same whether liquid or solid forms of carbohydrate are consumed.
- Carbohydrate-rich foods with a moderate to high glycemic index provide a readily available source of carbohydrate for muscle glycogen synthesis and should be the major carbohydrate choices in recovery meals.
- Adequate energy intake is important for optimal glycogen recovery; the restrained eating practices of some athletes, particularly females, make it difficult to meet carbohydrate intake targets and to optimize glycogen storage from that intake.

Carbohydrate Intake Days Before Competition

Carbohydrate can play an important role in preparation for competition. Carbohydrate intake in the days before competition mainly replenishes muscle glycogen stores, whereas carbohydrate intake in the hours before competition optimizes liver glycogen stores.

Glycemic Index (GI) and Glycemic Load (GL)

Food	GI	Serving size (g)	Available carbohydrate (g)	GL (per serving)
HIGH GI (>70)				
Boiled potato	101	150	17	17
Glucose	99	10	10	10
Baked potato	85	150	30	26
Lucozade, original	95	250 (ml)	42	40
Pancakes, buckwheat	102	77	22	22
Pretzels	83	30	20	16
Scones	92	25	9	7
Gatorade	78	250 (ml)	15	12
Isostar	70	250 (ml)	18	13
Bagel	72	70	35	25
Baguette, white, plain	95	70	37	27
Cheerios cereal	74	30	20	15
Corn flakes	81	30	26	21
Shredded wheat	75	30	20	15
K-time strawberry crunch bar	77	30	25	19
Puffed rice cakes	78	25	21	17
Watermelon	72	120	6	4
Popcorn	72	20	11	8
Stir fried vegetables	73	360	75	55
MODERATE GI (56–70)				
Doughnut	67	47	23	17
Croissant	67	57	26	17
Blueberry muffin	60	57	29	17
Coca-Cola	58	250 (ml)	26	16
French baguette with butter and strawberry jam	62	70	41	26
Porridge	58	250 (ml)	22	13
Rice, white, boiled	64	150	36	23
Long-grain rice, boiled	56	150	41	23
Digestives (cookies)	59	25	16	10
Oreo cookies	64	40	32	20
Ice cream, regular	61	50	13	8
Fruit cocktail, canned	55	120	16	9
Mars bar	65	60	40	26
Snickers bar	55	60	35	19
Power bar, chocolate	56	65	42	24
Ironman PR bar	39	65	26	10

(continued) ▶

Food	GI	Serving size (g)	Available carbohydrate (g)	GL (per serving)
LOW GI (<55)				
Honey	55	25	18	10
Potato crisps/chips	54	50	21	11
Sweet corn	54	80	17	9
Pizza, Super Supreme (Pizza Hut)	36	100	24	9
Wheat bread	53	30	20	11
Carrots	47	80	6	3
Orange juice	50	250 (ml)	26	13
Apple juice	40	250 (ml)	29	12
Rye bread	41	30	12	5
All-Bran cereal	42	30	23	9
Baked beans	48	150	15	7
Kidney beans	28	150	25	7
Lentils	30	150	17	5
Smoothie, raspberry	33	250 (ml)	41	14
M&Ms (peanut)	33	30	17	6
Muesli	49	30	20	10
Prince Fourre chocolate cookies	52	45	30	16
Ice cream, low-fat, vanilla	50	50	6	3
Spaghetti, boiled	38	180	48	18
Chocolate milk, plain	43	50	28	12
Skim milk	32	250 (ml)	13	4
Milk, full-fat	27	250 (ml)	12	3
Yogurt	36	200	9	3
Low-fat yogurt	24	200	14	3
Apple	38	120	15	6
Banana	52	120	24	12
Orange	42	120	11	5
Grapes	46	120	18	8
Peach	42	120	11	5
Peanuts	14	50	6	1
Fructose	19	10	10	2

Reprinted with permission from *American Journal of Clinical Nutrition,* "International table of glycolic index and glycolic load values: 2002," K. Foster-Powell and J.C. Brand-Miller, 76(1): 556, 2002; permission conveyed through Copyright Clearance Center, Inc.

Because carbohydrate intake in the days before competition has distinctly different effects than carbohydrate intake immediately before competition, these issues will be discussed separately.

Scandinavian researchers discovered that muscle glycogen could be supercompensated by changes in diet and exercise (Bergstrom et al. 1967b). In a series of studies, they developed a so-called **supercompensation** protocol, which resulted in extremely high muscle glycogen concentrations. This diet and exercise regimen started with a glycogen-depleting exercise bout (see figure 6.5). The exercise was then followed by 3 days of a high-protein, high-fat diet. Another exhausting exercise bout was performed on day 4, after which the subjects were placed on a high-carbohydrate diet for 3 days. Another group of subjects followed the same exercise protocol, but their diets were in reverse order. This study revealed that the subjects who received the high-protein, high-fat, low-carbohydrate diet first followed by the high-carbohydrate diet had higher rates of muscle glycogen resynthesis. The authors therefore concluded that a period of carbohydrate deprivation further stimulated glycogen resynthesis when carbohydrates were given after exercise.

The regimen that was proposed is generally referred to as the classical supercompensation protocol (see figure 6.5). Several top athletes have used it successfully, including the legendary British runner Ron Hill. In fact, nowadays many marathon runners use this method to optimize their performance. Although the supercompensation protocol has been effective in increasing muscle glycogen to very high concentrations, it also has several important (potential) disadvantages of which athletes should be aware:

- Hypoglycemia during the low-carbohydrate period
- Practical problems (difficulty in preparing extreme diets)
- Gastrointestinal problems (especially on the low-carbohydrate diet)
- Poor recovery when no carbohydrate is ingested
- Tenseness during a week without training
- Increased risk of injury
- Mood disturbances (lethargy and irritability) during the low-carbohydrate period

The main problem may be the incidence of gastrointestinal problems when using this regimen. Diarrhea has often been reported on the days when the high-protein, high-fat diet is consumed. During the first 3 days, athletes may also experience hypoglycemia, and they may not recover well from the exhausting exercise bout when no carbohydrate is ingested. Also, the fact that athletes cannot train in the week before an event is not ideal, because the worst punishment for most athletes seems to be asking them to avoid training. These factors may also have an effect on mental preparation for an event.

Because of the numerous disadvantages of the classical supercompensation protocol, studies have focused on a more moderate supercompensation protocol that would achieve similar results. Sherman et al. (1981) studied three types of muscle glycogen supercompensation regimens in runners. The subjects slowly reduced their training over a 6-day period from 90 minutes of running at 75% of $\dot{V}O_2max$ to complete rest on the last day. During each taper, they ingested one of the following three diets:

- A mixed diet with 50% carbohydrate
- A low-carbohydrate diet (25% carbohydrate) for the first 3 days followed by 3 days of a high-carbohydrate diet (70%) (classical supercompensation protocol)
- A mixed diet for the first 3 days (50% carbohydrate) followed by 3 days of a high-carbohydrate diet (70%) (moderate supercompensation protocol)

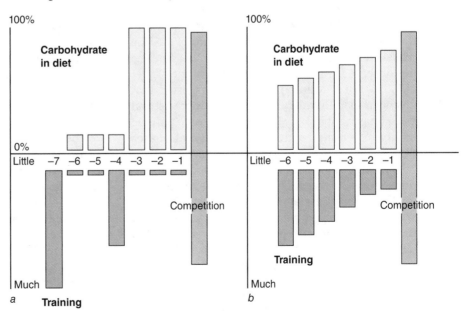

Figure 6.5 *(a)* The classical supercompensation protocols consisting of a glycogen-depleting exercise bout followed by 3 days of a high-protein, high-fat diet, another exhausting exercise bout on day 4, followed by a 3-day high-carbohydrate diet. *(b)* A more moderate protocol was later suggested to be almost as effective.

The classical protocol resulted in very high muscle glycogen stores (211 mmol/kg w.w.), confirming the results of earlier studies. But the moderate approach produced similar muscle glycogen levels (204 mmol/kg w.w.). Therefore, a normal training taper in conjunction with a moderate-carbohydrate to high-carbohydrate diet proved just as effective as the classical supercompensation protocol. A slightly modified and commonly applied strategy of the moderate supercompensation protocol is depicted in figure 6.5b. Because it does not have the disadvantages of the classical protocol, the moderate supercompensation protocol is the preferred regimen.

More recently, various glycogen-loading protocols have been used successfully. In one study endurance-trained athletes performed very high-intensity exercise for only 2 min (cycling for 150 s at 130% of $\dot{V}O_2$max followed by 30 s of all-out cycling) and then consumed a very high-carbohydrate diet (Fairchild et al. 2002). This protocol resulted in very high muscle glycogen concentrations 24 hours later (198 mmol/kg w.w.). Clearly, an exhausting bout of exercise is not necessary to achieve very high (supercompensated) glycogen stores (Bussau et al. 2002). Finally, note that after glycogen stores are high they will stay high for several days if limited exercise is performed.

Early reports suggested that women have reduced ability to synthesize glycogen (Tarnopolsky et al. 1995), but this view has changed because the research findings may have been a result of the smaller amount of carbohydrate that the female subjects ingested in that study. When men and women consume a comparable amount of carbohydrate (expressed in grams per kilogram of fat-free mass, FFM), no differences in glycogen loading are observed (McLay et al. 2007; Tarnopolsky et al. 1997). In addition, it has been suggested that glycogen loading might be affected by menstrual cycle phase, but a study found no differences in the ability to synthesize glycogen in different phases of the menstrual cycle (McLay et al. 2007).

Carbohydrate loading, or increased carbohydrate stores, increases time to exhaustion (endurance capacity) on average by about 20% and reduces the time required to complete a set task (time trial, endurance performance) by 2% to 3% (Hawley et al. 1997). But the available studies seem to suggest that the duration of exercise has to be at least 90 minutes before performance benefits occur. Carbohydrate loading seems to have no effect on sprint performance and high-intensity exercise up to about 30 minutes compared with normal diets (~50% carbohydrate). This finding is

expected, because at these high intensities glycogen depletion is probably not the performance-limiting factor. But several days on a very low-carbohydrate diet (< 10%) after a prolonged cycle ride to exhaustion has been shown to impair endurance capacity at 100% of $\dot{V}O_2$max (Maughan et al. 1997).

Carbohydrate loading has also been reported to improve performance in team sports involving high-intensity intermittent exercise and skills, such as soccer and hockey (Balsom et al. 1999), although this result has not always been confirmed. A study was performed in elite Swedish soccer players who played two matches separated by 3 days (Saltin 1973). One group consumed a high-carbohydrate diet, and the other group consumed a normal diet between the matches. Before the second match, muscle glycogen concentrations were 50% lower in the group that consumed the control diet. At halftime (after 45 minutes), muscle glycogen was virtually depleted in this group, whereas the high-carbohydrate group still had some glycogen left (see table 6.2). This glycogen status was related to the distance covered during the match, which was significantly lower with the control diet and low muscle glycogen concentrations. The players also spent less time sprinting and thus were believed to have impaired running performance.

So several strategies can optimize muscle glycogen, and these do not necessarily involve a complicated approach. The approach is similar for men and women. In essence, carbohydrate intake should be very high in the days before the event and muscle activity should be limited.

Supercompensation in Practice

Although muscle glycogen is important in most endurance sports, supercompensation strategies are not always applicable. In some sports supercompensation strategies are impractical or even impossible given the time frame and the rules of the sport. For instance in cycling, stage races consist of several days of consecutive competition. Although a supercompensation regimen can theoretically be followed before the first stage, the nature of the sport does not allow the athletes to prepare for a week or more of daily hard exercise. Similar problems occur in sports in which consecutive competitions follow each other within 1 to 5 days. This supercompensation protocol, however, seems suitable for marathon running and triathlon competing.

Muscle glycogen supercompensation is not of great importance to athletes involved in events that are short and explosive. Muscle glycogen avail-

■ TABLE 6.2 ■
Diet and Performance in Soccer

MUSCLE GLYCOGEN CONCENTRATION (g/kg w.w.)			
	Before	Halftime	End
High-carbohydrate diet	15	4	1
Normal diet	7	1	0
DISTANCE COVERED			
	First half (m)	Second half (m)	Walk (%)	Sprint (%)
High-carbohydrate diet	6,100	5,900	27	24
Normal diet	5,600	4,100	50	15

Adapted from Salting 1973.

ability per se is not usually responsible for fatigue during high-intensity exercise (> 95% of $\dot{V}O_2$max), if the preexercise glycogen store is not depleted below 25 mmol/kg w.w. (4 g/kg w.w.). Even so, athletes involved in high-intensity training do need to consume sufficient carbohydrate in their diet. Diets very low in carbohydrate content can compromise exercise performance at intensities around 95% to 100% of maximum oxygen uptake (Maughan et al. 1997).

Note that every gram of carbohydrate is stored with approximately 3 g of water, which means that storage of 500 g (8,000 kJ or 2,000 kcal) of carbohydrate is accompanied by an increase in body mass of approximately 2 kg. In some sports or disciplines (especially weight-bearing activities) this increase in body mass may not be desirable.

Carbohydrate Intake in Practice

Although the recommendations are generally to consume fairly large amounts of carbohydrate, what do athletes actually do? Discussing in depth the many reports of dietary intake among athletes would be beyond the scope of this book. Here we will only summarize the findings. The interested reader is referred to an excellent publication (Burke 2001) in which this topic is discussed in detail. In the publication it was concluded that most male athletes achieve a dietary intake of 5 to 7 g · kg b.w.$^{-1}$ · day^{-1} for regular training needs and 7 to 10 g · kg b.w.$^{-1}$ · day^{-1} during periods of increased training or competition. Female athletes, in particular endurance runners, are less likely to achieve their specific carbohydrate intake targets because they sometimes try to reduce their energy intake to achieve or maintain low levels of body fat, without paying enough attention to carbohydrate intake.

Carbohydrate Intake Hours Before Exercise

Athletes should have the last fairly large meal 3 to 5 hours before competition. This meal (usually breakfast) can be important after an overnight fast when the liver is almost depleted of glycogen. The advantages of a meal in the hours before exercise are related to the increased carbohydrate availability in muscle and the liver. In the 3 to 5 hours before exercise, some carbohydrate is incorporated into muscle glycogen. Carbohydrate intake in the last hour before competition will not affect muscle glycogen but still has an effect on liver glycogen and increases the delivery of carbohydrate to the muscle during exercise.

Ingestion of a carbohydrate-rich meal (containing 140 to approximately 330 g of carbohydrate) 3 to 5 hours before exercise increases muscle glycogen levels and improves exercise performance (Hargreaves et al. 2004). Such a meal could include carbohydrate sources such as bread and jam or honey, cereals, porridge, bananas, canned fruit, and fruit juice. Following is an example of a daily diet containing 150 g of carbohydrate representing at least 80% of the energy intake:

■ Meal 1: one large bowl of porridge with skim milk, one banana, one glass (250 ml) of sweetened orange juice

■ Meal 2: four slices of bread with jam or honey, one can of a soft drink

■ Meal 3: 3 cups of rice made into a light stir fry with small amounts of lean ham or chicken, peas, corn, mushrooms and onion, and one glass (250 ml) of fruit juice

The enhanced performance observed in research studies is likely related to small increases in pre-exercise muscle glycogen. But replenishing liver glycogen levels may be even more important. Liver glycogen concentrations are substantially reduced after an overnight fast. Ingestion of carbohydrate increases these reserves and contributes, together with any ongoing absorption of the ingested carbohydrate, to the maintenance of blood glucose concentrations during the subsequent exercise bout. Plasma glucose and insulin concentrations return to basal levels within 30 to 60 minutes after ingestion. But ingestion of carbohydrate in the hours before exercise has three important effects:

■ Transient fall in plasma glucose with the onset of exercise

■ Increased carbohydrate oxidation and accelerated glycogen breakdown

■ Blunting of FA mobilization and fat oxidation

The effects on FA mobilization can persist for a long time after carbohydrate ingestion. Montain et al. (1991) showed a blunting of FA mobilization 6 hours after ingestion of a carbohydrate meal.

These metabolic changes, however, do not appear to be detrimental to exercise performance because increased carbohydrate availability compensates for the greater carbohydrate utilization. No differences in exercise performance were observed after ingestion of meals that produced marked differences in plasma glucose and insulin levels (Wee et al. 1999). From a practical perspective, if access to carbohydrate during exercise is limited or nonexistent, ingestion of 200 to 300 g of carbohydrate 3 to 4 hours before exercise may be an effective strategy for enhancing carbohydrate availability during the subsequent exercise period.

Carbohydrate Intake 30 to 60 Minutes Before Exercise

The ingestion of carbohydrate in the hour before exercise results in a large rise in plasma glucose and insulin. With the onset of exercise, however, a rapid fall in blood glucose occurs. This phenomenon is called rebound or reactive hypoglycemia. Up to only a few years ago, athletes were often advised not to consume carbohydrate in the hour

before exercise because this was thought to induce hypoglycemia and negatively affect performance. This view has gradually changed as will be discussed here.

A combination of several metabolic events causes the fall in blood glucose. First, hyperinsulinemia stimulates glucose uptake, and in addition, contractile activity further stimulates muscle glucose uptake. The exercise-induced increase in the normal liver glucose output is inhibited by carbohydrate ingestion (Marmy-Conus et al. 1996), despite ongoing absorption of the ingested carbohydrate. Enhanced uptake and oxidation of blood glucose by skeletal muscle may account for the increased carbohydrate oxidation after preexercise carbohydrate ingestion. In addition, in some studies, an increase in muscle glycogen degradation has been observed.

The increase in plasma FA with exercise is attenuated after preexercise carbohydrate ingestion because of insulin-mediated inhibition of lipolysis (Horowitz et al. 1997). Even small increases in plasma insulin (e.g., after fructose ingestion) can result in a marked reduction of lipolysis. Fat oxidation is reduced not only because of the lower plasma FA availability (Horowitz et al. 1997) but also because of inhibition of fat oxidation in skeletal muscle. Artificially increased plasma FA availability did not completely return fat oxidation to levels seen during exercise in the fasted state (Horowitz et al. 1997). Some evidence indicates that the hyperinsulinemia and hyperglycemia reduce the uptake of FA into the mitochondria (Coyle et al. 1997).

Factors that determine the glycemic response during exercise include

■ the combined stimulatory effects of insulin and contractile activity on muscle glucose uptake,

■ the balance of inhibitory and stimulatory effects of insulin and catecholamines on liver glucose output, and

■ the magnitude of ongoing intestinal absorption of glucose from the ingested carbohydrate.

Because the metabolic effects of preexercise carbohydrate ingestion are a consequence of hyperglycemia and hyperinsulinemia, interest has developed in strategies that minimize the changes in plasma glucose and insulin before exercise. These strategies include the ingestion of fructose or carbohydrate types other than glucose that have a lower **glycemic index** (see the side bar for an explanation of glycemic index), varying the carbohydrate load or the ingestion schedule, the addition of fat, and the inclusion of warm-up exercise in the preexercise period. In general, although these various interventions do modify the metabolic response to exercise, blunting the preexercise glycemic and insulinemic responses appear to offer no advantage for exercise performance.

The metabolic alterations associated with ingestion of carbohydrate in the 30 to 60 minutes before exercise have the potential to influence exercise performance. The increase in muscle glycogenolysis and suppression of fat metabolism could possibly result in earlier onset of fatigue during exercise as suggested in a study by Foster, Costill, and Fink (Foster et al. 1979). Indeed, this early study reported a reduction in exercise performance. Since

then, however, the overwhelming majority of more than 100 studies have shown either unchanged or even enhanced endurance exercise performance after ingestion of carbohydrate in the hour before exercise.

Interestingly in a series of studies (Jentjens et al. 2003a; Moseley et al. 2003) it was demonstrated that certain individuals may develop hypoglycemia when carbohydrate is ingested in the hour before exercise, although this was not a predictor of performance. Note that the causes of hypoglycemia in this situation are different from the causes of hypoglycemia that occurs after prolonged exercise when endogenous carbohydrate stores become depleted. Hypoglycemia seemed to be more prevalent when the carbohydrate was ingested 75

Glycemic Index

The glycemic index (GI) refers to the increase in blood glucose and insulin in response to a standard amount of food and is determined by measuring the area under the glucose curve. The GI measurements are usually based on the ingestion of 50 g of carbohydrate and measurements of blood glucose over a 2-hour period. The greater the glucose response is and the greater the area under the curve is, the greater the GI of a food is. A greater GI indicates rapid absorption and delivery of the carbohydrate into the circulation. The GI is calculated using the following formula:

GI = area under the glucose curve of test food / area under the glucose curve of reference food × 100

The reference food, usually glucose or white bread, has a glycemic index of 100. Foods are generally divided into low-GI foods, moderate-GI foods, and high-GI foods. Low-GI foods have a GI of 55 or less, moderate-GI foods have a GI between 56 and 70, and high-GI foods have a GI of 71 or higher. Apples or lentils, for example, result in a slow and small rise of blood glucose concentration, whereas white bread or potatoes result in a rapid rise in blood glucose concentration. The apples and the lentils, therefore, are classified as low-GI foods, and bread and potatoes are classified as high-GI foods. A list of high-GI, moderate-GI, and low-GI foods is given in table 6.1.

The use of the GI as a tool is controversial, mainly because the GI for any given food might vary considerably between individuals. The tables usually provide an average value that is not necessarily useful in controlling a person's blood glucose concentration. The GI of foods is also sometimes confusing. In general, foods with large amounts of refined sugar (simple carbohydrates) have a high GI, and sugars with high fiber content and complex carbohydrates have a lower GI. Some complex carbohydrates (starches), however, can have a high GI. On the other hand, adding relatively small amounts of fat to a high-GI carbohydrate can lower the GI of the food substantially. Therefore, the GI must be interpreted and used with caution. It can probably be a useful tool if its limitations and pitfalls are well understood.

The glycemic load (GL) is a relatively new way to assess the effect of carbohydrate consumption that takes the GI into account but gives a fuller picture than GI does alone. A GI value indicates only how rapidly a particular carbohydrate appears as glucose in the circulation but does not take into account the amount of the food that is normally consumed. For example, the carbohydrate in watermelon has a high GI, but there is not a lot of it, so the GL of watermelon is relatively low. The GL is calculated by multiplying the GI by the amount of carbohydrate (g) in one serving and dividing by 100. For example, a carrot weighing 60 g contains only 4 g of carbohydrate. To get 50 g, a person would have to eat about 750 g of carrots. GL takes the GI value and multiplies it by the actual amount of carbohydrate in a serving. A GL is low if it is between 1 and 10, medium if it is between 11 and 19, and high if it is 20 or higher. Foods that have a low GL almost always have a low GI. Foods with an intermediate or high GL range from a very low to a very high GI.

minutes before exercise compared with 45 minutes, and when it was ingested 15 minutes before exercise few people developed hypoglycemia (Moseley et al. 2003). Other studies have demonstrated that hypoglycemia can be completely prevented when carbohydrate is taken 5 minutes before exercise or during a warm-up.

In conclusion, despite the well-documented metabolic effects of preexercise carbohydrate ingestion, little evidence appears to support the practice of avoiding carbohydrate ingestion in the hour before exercise, if sufficient carbohydrate is ingested. Some people, however, may be more prone to develop hypoglycemia; therefore, it is recommended to determine individual practice based on experience with various preexercise carbohydrate ingestion protocols.

Finally, when carbohydrate is ingested during prolonged exercise, the potential negative effects of the preexercise carbohydrate feedings are reduced. When a high-GI food is ingested before exercise, it has little or no effect on metabolism and performance if carbohydrate is ingested during exercise (Burke et al. 1998).

Carbohydrate Intake During Exercise

Convincing evidence from numerous studies indicates that carbohydrate feeding during exercise of about 45 minutes or longer (Jeukendrup 2004, 2008; Jeukendrup et al. 1997) can improve endurance capacity and performance. Studies have also addressed questions of which carbohydrates are most effective, what feeding schedule is the most effective, and what amount of carbohydrate to consume is optimal. Other studies have looked at factors that could possibly influence the oxidation of ingested carbohydrate, such as muscle glycogen levels, diet, and exercise intensity. Mechanisms by which carbohydrate feeding during exercise may improve endurance performance include the following.

■ *Maintaining blood glucose and high levels of carbohydrate oxidation.* Coyle et al. (1986) demonstrated that carbohydrate feeding during exercise at 70% of $\dot{V}O_2$max prevents the drop in blood glucose that was observed when water (placebo) was ingested. In the placebo trials, the glucose concentration started to drop after 1 hour of exercise and reached extremely low concentrations (2.5 mmol/L) at exhaustion after 3 hours. With carbohydrate feeding, glucose concentrations were maintained above 3 mmol/L, and subjects continued to exercise for

4 hours at the same intensity. Total-carbohydrate oxidation rates followed a similar pattern. A drop in carbohydrate oxidation occurred after about 1.5 hours of exercise with placebo, and high rates of carbohydrate oxidation were maintained with carbohydrate feeding. When subjects ingested only water and exercised to exhaustion, they were able to continue again when glucose was ingested or infused intravenously. These studies showed the importance of plasma glucose as a substrate during exercise.

■ *Glycogen sparing in the liver and possibly muscle.* Carbohydrate feedings during exercise "spare" liver glycogen (Jeukendrup et al. 1999), and Tsintzas and Williams (Tsintzas et al. 1998) discussed a potential muscle glycogen sparing effect. Generally, muscle glycogen sparing is not found during cycling (Jeukendrup et al. 1999), but it may be important during running (Tsintzas et al. 1995).

■ *Promoting glycogen synthesis during exercise.* After intermittent exercise, muscle glycogen concentrations were higher when carbohydrate was ingested than when water was ingested (Yaspelkis et al. 1993). This finding could indicate reduced muscle glycogen breakdown. But the ingested carbohydrate was possibly used to synthesize muscle glycogen during the low-intensity exercise periods (Keizer et al. 1987a).

■ *Affecting motor skills.* Few studies have attempted to study the effect of carbohydrate drinks on motor skills. One such study investigated 13 trained tennis players and observed that when players ingested carbohydrate during a 2-hour training session (Vergauwen et al. 1998), stroke quality improved during the final stages of prolonged play. This effect was most noticeable when the situations required fast running speed, rapid movement, and explosiveness.

■ *Affecting the central nervous system.* Carbohydrate may also have central nervous system effects. Although direct evidence for such an effect is lacking, the brain can sense changes in the composition of the mouth and stomach contents. Evidence, for instance, suggests that taste influences mood and may influence perception of effort. An interesting observation provides support for a central nervous system effect. When a hypoglycemic person bites a candy bar, that person's symptoms almost immediately decrease, and the person feels better again long before the carbohydrate reaches the systemic circulation and the brain. The central nervous system effect may also explain why some studies report positive effects of carbohydrate during exercise on performance lasting approximately 1 hour (Jeukendrup et al. 1997). During exercise of such short duration, only a small amount of the carbohydrate becomes available as a substrate. Most of the ingested carbohydrate is still in the stomach or intestine. Studies in which athletes rinsed their mouths with carbohydrate (but did not ingest any) during 1-hour time trials showed performance improvements similar to those that occurred when the athletes ingested the carbohydrate (Carter et al. 2004). Others (Pottier et al. 2008) recently confirmed these findings.

Whether the central nervous system effects of glucose feeding are mediated by sensory detection of glucose or perception of sweetness is not known, although studies with placebo solutions with identical taste to glucose solutions suggest that sweetness is not the key factor. Brain imaging studies also show that increased brain activity is specific to carbohydrates.

Feeding Strategies and Exogenous Carbohydrate Oxidation

A greater contribution of exogenous (external) fuel sources (carbohydrate) spares endogenous (internal) sources, and the notion that a greater contribution from exogenous sources increases endurance capacity is enticing. The contribution of exogenous substrates can be measured using stable (or radioactive) isotopic tracers. The principle of this technique is simple: The ingested substrate (e.g., glucose) is labeled, and the label can be measured in expired gas after the substrate has been oxidized. The more the ingested substrate has been oxidized, the more of the label (tracer) will be recovered in the expired gas. Knowing the amount of tracer ingested, the amount of tracer in the expired gas, and the total CO_2 production enables us to calculate exogenous substrate oxidation rates.

The typical pattern of exogenous glucose oxidation rates is shown in figure 6.6. The labeled CO_2 starts to appear 5 minutes after ingestion of the labeled carbohydrate. During the first 75 to 90 minutes of exercise, exogenous carbohydrate oxidation continues to rise as more and more carbohydrate is emptied from the stomach and absorbed in the intestine. After 75 to 90 minutes a leveling off occurs, and the exogenous

carbohydrate oxidation rate reaches its maximum value and does not increase further. Several factors have been suggested to influence exogenous carbohydrate oxidation including feeding schedule, type and amount of carbohydrate ingested, and exercise intensity.

Timing of Intake The timing of carbohydrate feedings seems to have relatively little effect on exogenous carbohydrate oxidation rates. Studies in which a large bolus (100 g) of a carbohydrate in solution was given produced exogenous carbohydrate oxidation rates similar to those in studies in which 100 g carbohydrate was ingested at regular intervals.

Amount of Carbohydrate From a practical point of view, the amount of carbohydrate that needs to be ingested to attain optimal performance is important. The optimal amount is likely to be the amount that results in maximal exogenous oxidation rates without causing gastrointestinal problems. Rehrer, Wagenmakers, et al. (1992) studied the oxidation of different amounts of carbohydrate ingested during 80 minutes of cycling exercise at 70% of $\dot{V}O_2$max. Subjects received either a 4.5% glucose solution (a total of 58 g glucose during 80 minutes of exercise) or a 17% glucose solution (220 g during 80 minutes of exercise). Total exogenous carbohydrate oxidation was measured and found to be slightly higher with the larger carbohydrate dose (42 g versus 32 g in 80 minutes). So, even though the amount of carbohydrate ingested was increased almost fourfold, the oxidation rate was barely affected.

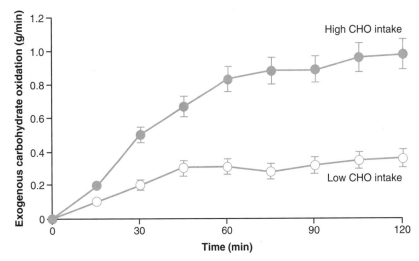

Figure 6.6 Exogenous carbohydrate oxidation during exercise. The curve shows the typical pattern of the oxidation of carbohydrate ingested at regular intervals.

Reprinted, by permission, from A.E. Jeukendrup and R. Jentjens, 2000, "Oxidation of carbohydrate feedings during prolonged exercise: Current thoughts, guidelines, and directions for future research," *Sports Medicine* 29(6): 407-424. Reproduced with permission from Adis, A Wolters Kluwer business (Copyright Adis Data Information BV 1994. All rights reserved.)

Jeukendrup et al. (1999) investigated the oxidation rates of carbohydrate intakes up to 3.00 g/min and found oxidation rates of up to 0.94 g/min at the end of 120 minutes of cycling exercise.

The results from a large number of studies were used to construct figure 6.7 (Jeukendrup and Jentjens 2000). The peak exogenous carbohydrate oxidation rates are plotted against the rate of ingestion. The maximal rate at which a single ingested carbohydrate can be oxidized is about 1.0 g/min. The horizontal line depicts the absolute maximum just below 1.1 g/min. The dotted line represents the line of identity where the rate of carbohydrate ingestion equals the rate of exogenous carbohydrate oxidation. This graph suggests that oxidation of orally ingested carbohydrate may already be optimal at ingestion rates around 1.2 g/min. Thus, athletes should ensure a carbohydrate intake of about 70 g/h for optimal carbohydrate delivery. Adopting an ingestion rate of 70 g/h optimizes exogenous carbohydrate oxidation. Ingesting more than this amount of a single carbohydrate does not result in higher carbohydrate oxidation rates and is more likely to cause gastrointestinal discomfort. This amount of carbohydrate can be found in the following sources:

■ 1 L sports drink (Gatorade, Powerade, Isostar, Lucozade Sport)

■ 600 ml cola drink

■ 1 1/2 Power bars

■ 1 1/2 Gatorade energy bars

■ Three medium bananas

■ 120 to 150 g wine gums

Type of Carbohydrate Studies have compared the oxidation rates of various types of carbohydrate to the oxidation of ingested glucose during exercise (Jeukendrup 2004, 2008; Jeukendrup et al. 2000). Glucose is oxidized at relatively high rates (up to about 1 g/min). The other two monosaccharides, fructose and galactose, are oxidized at much lower rates because they have to be converted into glucose in the liver before they can be metabolized. They are, therefore, a relatively slow energy source.

The oxidation rates of maltose, sucrose, and glucose polymers (maltodextrins) are comparable to those of glucose. Starches with a relatively large amount of amylopectin are rapidly digested and absorbed, whereas those with high amylose content have a relatively slow rate of hydrolysis. Ingested amylopectin is oxidized at very high rates (similar to glucose), whereas amylose is oxidized at very low rates. Carbohydrates are divided into two categories according to the rate at which they are oxidized: a higher rate group (~1 g/min) and a lower rate group (~0.6 g/min). These two categories of carbohydrates are listed in the highlight box that follows.

Shi et al. (1995) suggest that the inclusion of two or three different carbohydrates (glucose, fructose, and sucrose) in a drink may increase water and carbohydrate absorption despite the increased osmolality. This effect is attributed to the separate transport mechanisms across the intestinal wall for glucose, fructose, and sucrose. The monosaccharides glucose and galactose are transported across the luminal membrane by a glucose transporter called SGLT1 (see chapter 3) and fructose is transported by GLUT5. Interestingly, fructose absorption from a certain amount of the disaccharide sucrose is more rapid than the absorption of the same amount of fructose. If a combination of glucose and fructose is ingested, more carbohydrate will be absorbed and made available for oxidation. Ingestion of relatively large amounts of glucose and fructose can result in exogenous carbohydrate oxidation rates well over 1 g/min (Jeukendrup 2004, 2008) (see figure 6.8).

Drinks, Gels, or Energy Bars To ingest 50 g of carbohydrate, a person can take two bottles (1 L) of a sports drink, two carbohydrate gels (typically 25 g each), or one energy bar. The solid and semi-solid food is more energy dense and

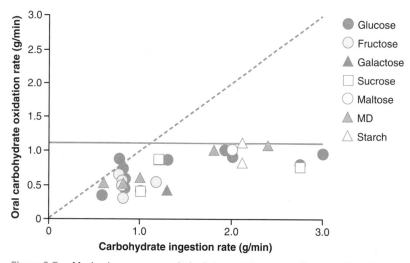

Figure 6.7 Maximal exogenous carbohydrate oxidation versus the rate of ingestion.

easier to carry during sporting events, but solid food may have a slowing effect on gastric emptying, especially when the food contains fiber and fat. Few studies have compared the efficacy of drinks versus gels and energy bars. Personal preference

and tolerance are probably the main factors when choosing between these carbohydrate sources.

Exercise Intensity With increasing exercise intensity, the active muscle mass becomes more dependent on carbohydrate as a source of energy. Both increased muscle glycogenolysis and increased plasma glucose oxidation contribute to the increased energy demands (Romijn et al. 1993). Therefore, exogenous carbohydrate oxidation increases with increasing exercise intensity. Indeed, Pirnay et al. (1982) reported lower exogenous carbohydrate oxidation rates at low exercise intensity compared with moderate intensity, but exogenous carbohydrate oxidation tended to level off between 51% and 64% of $\dot{V}O_2max$. But when exercise intensity increased from 60% to 75% of $\dot{V}O_2max$, exogenous carbohydrate oxidation rates leveled off or even decreased (Pirnay et al. 1995).

Lower exogenous carbohydrate oxidation rates are possibly observed only at very low exercise intensities when the reliance on carbohydrate as an energy source is minimal. In this situation, part of the ingested carbohydrate may be directed toward nonoxidative glucose disposal (storage in the liver or muscle) rather than toward oxidation. Studies with carbohydrate ingestion during intermittent exercise have suggested that during low-intensity exercise, glycogen can be resynthesized (Kuipers et al. 1989).

Thus, at exercise intensities below 50% of $\dot{V}O_2max$, exogenous carbohydrate oxidation increases with increasing total carbohydrate oxidation rates. Usually, above approximately 60% of $\dot{V}O_2max$, oxidation rates will not increase further.

Oxidation Rates of Ingested Carbohydrate During Exercise

Rapidly Oxidized Carbohydrates (~1 g/min)

- Glucose (a sugar formed by the breakdown of starch)
- Sucrose (table sugar—glucose plus fructose)
- Maltose (two glucose molecules)
- Maltodextrins (from starch breakdown)
- Amylopectin (from starch breakdown)

Slowly Oxidized Carbohydrates (~0.6 g/min)

- Fructose (a sugar found in honey, fruits, and so on)
- Galactose (a sugar found in sugar beets)
- Isomaltulose (a sugar found in honey and sugarcane)
- Trehalose (a sugar found in fungi, some plants, and invertebrate animals)
- Amylose (from starch breakdown)

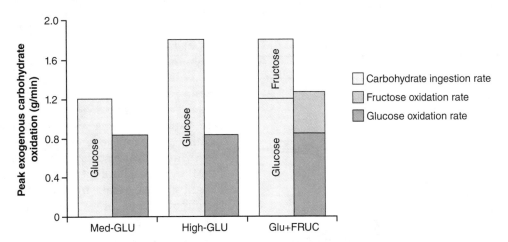

Figure 6.8 The oxidation rate of glucose plus fructose in a combined drink is higher than the oxidation rate of similar amounts of either glucose or fructose alone.

Limitations to Exogenous Carbohydrate Oxidation

As discussed earlier, exogenous carbohydrate oxidation seems to be limited to rates of 1.0 g/min to 1.1 g/min (see figure 6.7). This finding is supported by most of the studies using either radioactive or stable isotopes to quantify exogenous carbohydrate oxidation during exercise. Understanding the causes of this limitation is important so that strategies can be developed to make the exogenous supply of fuel more effective.

A number of factors could possibly limit the oxidation of ingested carbohydrate:

- Gastric emptying
- Digestion of the carbohydrate
- Intestinal carbohydrate absorption
- Retention of carbohydrate by the liver
- Glucose uptake by the muscle
- Metabolism in the muscle (glycolysis, TCA cycle, and oxidative phosphorylation)

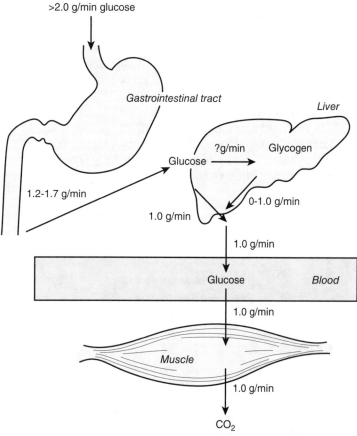

Figure 6.9 Gastric emptying of glucose, absorption, and uptake in skeletal muscle. Glucose travels from the gut after ingestion to the muscle. The suggested maximal flux at each of the stages is indicated.

One of the possible limiting factors could be the rate of gastric emptying (see figure 6.9). Some studies, however, indicate that gastric emptying is unlikely to affect exogenous carbohydrate oxidation rates (Rehrer et al. 1992b; Saris et al. 1993). Because in these studies only a small percentage (32%–48%) of the carbohydrate delivered to the intestine was oxidized, gastric emptying was determined not to be limiting exogenous carbohydrate oxidation.

Another potential limiting factor is the rate of absorption of carbohydrate into the systemic circulation from the small intestine. Studies using a triple-lumen technique have measured glucose absorption and estimated whole-body intestinal absorption rates of a 6% glucose–electrolyte solution (Duchman et al. 1997). The estimated maximal absorption rate of the intestine ranged from 1.2 to 1.7 g/min. Studies using stable isotopes have observed a reduction in the glucose output by the liver when carbohydrate is ingested. When very large amounts of glucose are ingested, hepatic glucose output can be blocked completely (Jeukendrup et al. 1999). At low to moderate ingestion rates, no net storage of glucose occurs in the liver. Instead, all ingested glucose appears in the bloodstream. The glucose output from the liver can vary from nothing to approximately 1 g/min when no carbohydrate is ingested, the intensity of exercise is high enough ($>60\%$ of $\dot{V}O_2max$), and the duration is long enough (>1 hour).

Glucose appearing in the bloodstream was taken up at rates similar to its rate of appearance (Ra), and 90% to 95% of this glucose was oxidized during exercise. When a larger dose of carbohydrate was ingested (3 g/min), the rate of appearance of glucose from the intestine was one-third the rate of carbohydrate ingestion (0.96 g/min to 1.04 g/min). Thus, only part of the ingested carbohydrate entered the systemic circulation. A large proportion of the glucose appearing in the blood, however, was taken up by tissues (presumably mainly by the muscle) and 90% to 95% was oxidized. Therefore, entrance into the systemic circulation is a limiting factor for exogenous glucose oxidation, rather than intramuscular factors. Hawley et al. (1994) bypassed both intestinal absorption and hepatic glucose uptake by infusing glucose into the circulation of subjects exercising at 70% of $\dot{V}O_2max$. When large amounts of glucose were infused and subjects were hyperglycemic (10 mmol/L), blood glucose oxidation rate increased substantially above 1 g/min.

Exogenous carbohydrate oxidation is limited by the rate of digestion, absorption, and subsequent release of glucose into the systemic circulation. During high-intensity exercise (e.g., >80% of $\dot{V}O_2max$), reduced blood flow to the gut may result in decreased absorption of glucose and water (Brouns et al. 1993) and hence a low rate of absorption relative to the rate of ingestion. Taken together, this information suggests that intestinal absorption is a contributing factor in limiting the oxidation of ingested carbohydrate at rates higher than 1.1 g/min, but it may not be the sole factor. The liver may also play an additional important role. Hepatic glucose output is highly regulated, and the glucose output derived from the intestine and from hepatic glycogenolysis and gluconeogenesis possibly does not exceed 1.1 g/min, even though the maximal rate of glucose absorption is slightly in excess of this rate. If supply from the intestine is too large (>1.0 g/min), glycogen synthesis may be stimulated in the liver.

Multiple Transportable Carbohydrates

It has been suggested that by feeding a single carbohydrate source (e.g., glucose, fructose, or maltodextrins) at high rates, the specific transporter proteins that aid in absorbing that carbohydrate from the intestine become saturated. After these transporters are saturated, feeding more of that carbohydrate will not result in greater intestinal absorption and increased oxidation rates. In 1995 Shi et al. suggested that the ingestion of carbohydrates that use different transporters might increase total carbohydrate absorption. Subsequently, a series of studies was conducted at the University of Birmingham in the United Kingdom using different combinations of carbohydrates to determine their effects on exogenous carbohydrate oxidation during exercise. In the first study subjects ingested a drink containing glucose and fructose (Jentjens et al. 2004a). Glucose was ingested at a rate of 1.2 g/min and fructose at a rate of 0.6 g/min. In the control trials, the subjects ingested glucose at a rate of 1.2 g/min and 1.8 g/min (matching glucose intake or energy intake). It was found that the ingestion of glucose at a rate of 1.2 g/min resulted in oxidation rates of about 0.8 g/min. Ingesting glucose at 1.8 g/min did not increase the oxidation rate. But after ingesting glucose plus fructose, the rate of total exogenous carbohydrate oxidation increased to 1.23 g/min, an increase in oxidation of 45% compared with a similar amount of glucose. In subsequent studies different combinations and amounts of carbohydrates were evaluated in an attempt to determine the maximal rate of oxidation of mixtures of exogenous carbohydrates (Jentjens et al. 2005a, 2004a, 2005b, 2006, 2004b;

Jeukendrup et al. 2005; Wallis et al. 2005). Very high oxidation rates were observed with combinations of glucose plus fructose, with maltodextrins plus fructose, and with glucose plus sucrose plus fructose. The highest rates were observed with a mixture of glucose and fructose ingested at a rate of 2.4 g/min. With this feeding regimen, exogenous carbohydrate oxidation peaked at 1.75 g/min, a rate 75% greater than what was previously thought to be the absolute maximum.

In subsequent studies, subjects ingested more practical but still quite large amounts of carbohydrate (1.5 g/min). It was observed that the subjects' ratings of perceived exertion (RPE) tended to be lower with the mixture of glucose and fructose compared with glucose alone (Jeukendrup et al. 2006). More recently it was demonstrated that a glucose and fructose blend of carbohydrate can improve performance significantly more than a glucose-only drink can (Currell et al. 2008).

The term oxidation efficiency was introduced to describe the percentage of the ingested carbohydrate that is oxidized (Jeukendrup et al. 2000). High oxidation efficiency means that smaller amounts of carbohydrate remain in the gastrointestinal tract, reducing the risk of causing gastrointestinal discomfort that is frequently reported during prolonged exercise. Therefore, compared with a single source of carbohydrate, ingesting multiple carbohydrate sources results in a smaller amount of carbohydrate remaining in the intestine, and osmotic shifts and malabsorption may be reduced. This probably means that drinks with multiple transportable carbohydrates are less likely to cause gastrointestinal discomfort. This finding has occurred consistently in studies that have attempted to evaluate gastrointestinal discomfort during exercise (Jeukendrup 2008). Subjects tended to feel less bloated with the glucose plus fructose drinks compared with drinking glucose-only solutions. A further advantage of the carbohydrate blend (glucose plus fructose) is that fluid delivery seems to be improved compared with glucose-only drinks.

Metabolic Effects of Carbohydrate Intake

The metabolic effects of carbohydrate intake during exercise depend on various factors, including the amount ingested, the timing of the intake, and the intensity and duration of exercise. Generally, carbohydrate ingestion early in exercise has large effects on insulin response, fat mobilization, and substrate utilization, whereas ingestion late in exercise has relatively little effect. If carbohydrate is ingested at the onset of exercise, plasma

Caffeine

The main factor that limits the oxidation of carbohydrate from a drink seems to be absorption. In a study it was suggested that caffeine might increase glucose absorption. This notion led to the idea that caffeine added to a carbohydrate drink may not only increase absorption but also result in greater delivery of carbohydrate to the muscle and higher exogenous carbohydrate oxidation rates. Yeo et al. (2005) tested this hypothesis and found that exogenous carbohydrate oxidation increased by 17% when relatively large amounts of caffeine were added. So caffeine may not only have a direct effect on exercise performance (see chapter 11) but also may aid the absorption and oxidation of carbohydrates. The exact dose of carbohydrate and caffeine required is still unclear because a follow-up study with a lower dose of caffeine did not find a significant increase in exogenous carbohydrate oxidation rate, although time-trial performance was improved compared with carbohydrate alone or a placebo (Hulston and Jeukendrup 2008). More on caffeine can be found in chapter 11.

insulin concentrations rise in the first minutes of exercise and lipolysis is suppressed. FA availability is lowered, and this condition may partly explain the lower fat oxidation rates observed in this situation. But carbohydrate intake during exercise also inhibits fat oxidation by hindering the transport of FA into the mitochondria.

When carbohydrate is ingested later in exercise, the already raised catecholamine levels blunt the insulin response, and hence fat oxidation is less affected. Similarly, when a small amount of carbohydrate is ingested during exercise, the effect on the plasma insulin concentration is also small, whereas larger intakes result in an increased insulin response. Exercise intensity may be important as well. Studies suggest that the suppressive effect of carbohydrate feeding on fat metabolism is greater at low exercise intensity than at high exercise intensity.

Carbohydrate Intake After Exercise

The main purpose of carbohydrate intake after physical activity is to replenish depleted stores of liver and muscle glycogen. The replenishment of muscle glycogen is directly related to recovery of endurance capacity, and glycogen loading, or carboloading, between training sessions has become common practice among endurance athletes.

Regulation of Glucose Uptake and Glycogen Synthesis

Glucose uptake in the muscle is through facilitated diffusion by the glucose transporter GLUT4, which is largely responsible for transporting glucose across the sarcolemma. GLUT4 is normally stored in intracellular vesicles but can translocate to the cell membrane, merge with the cell membrane, and allow increased transport of glucose into the cell (see figure 6.10). Both muscle contraction (through Ca^{2+} ions) and insulin secretion will stimulate the translocation of GLUT4 and hence glucose transport into the cell.

After its transport across the sarcolemma, glucose is phosphorylated to glucose-6-phosphate (G6P) by the enzyme hexokinase (see figure 6.10). G6P is next converted to glucose-1-phosphate (G1P) by the enzyme phosphoglucomutase, and G1P is combined with uridine triphosphate to form uridine diphosphate (UDP)–glucose and pyrophosphate (PPi) in a reaction catalyzed by 1-phosphate uridyltransferase. UDP is a carrier of glucose units and takes the glucose molecule to the terminal glucose residue of a preexisting glycogen molecule. UDP-glucose can be considered an activated glucose molecule. The UDP-glucose then forms an α-1,4 glycosidic bond, a reaction catalyzed by glycogen synthase, resulting in one long straight chain of glucose molecules. Branch points (α-1,6 glycosidic bond), however, are introduced into the glycogen structure by a branching enzyme. When the length of a chain is about 12 glucose residues long, the branching enzyme detaches a chain about 7 residues long and reattaches it to a neighboring chain by an α-1,6 glycosidic bond. Branching results in the formation of a large but compact glycogen molecule.

The rate of glycogen synthesis depends on several factors:

1. the availability of glucose;
2. the transport of glucose into the cell, which in turn depends on
   a. prior exercise (exercise stimulates glucose uptake for 1–2 hours postexercise and increases insulin sensitivity),
   b. insulin concentration (high insulin stimulates glucose uptake), and
   c. muscle glycogen content (low muscle glycogen stimulates glucose uptake); and
3. the activity of enzymes (in particular glycogen synthase), which also depends on insulin concentration (high insulin stimulates glycogen synthesis).

As a result of the changing activity of these enzymes and the effectiveness of these transport mechanisms, two phases can be distinguished in the process of glycogen synthesis after exercise. These phases are the initial insulin-independent, or rapid, phase and the insulin-dependent, or slow, phase.

Rapid Phase of Glycogen Synthesis After Exercise

The rate-limiting enzyme for glycogen resynthesis after exercise, glycogen synthase, exists in an inactive D-form and an active I-form. More glycogen synthase is present in the active I-form when muscle glycogen concentrations are low. As glycogen stores are replenished, more glycogen synthase is transformed back into the D-form. Exercise activates glycogen synthase (immediately

after exercise, as much as 80% of all glycogen synthase may be in the active I-form), but glycogen can be formed only if the substrate (UDP-glucose) is available. Another important factor in glycogen resynthesis, therefore, is the availability of glucose, which is mainly dependent on glucose transport across the sarcolemma. During exercise and in the first hour after exercise, an abundance of GLUT4 is available at the cell membrane, and glucose uptake into the muscle is facilitated. This exercise-induced effect on glucose transport, however, lasts only a few hours in the absence of insulin. The increase in the permeability of the sarcolemma for glucose after exercise seems to be directly related to the amount of glycogen in the muscle. When muscle glycogen concentrations are very low, the enhanced glucose uptake may last longer. With high muscle glycogen concentrations, the effect is rapidly reversed.

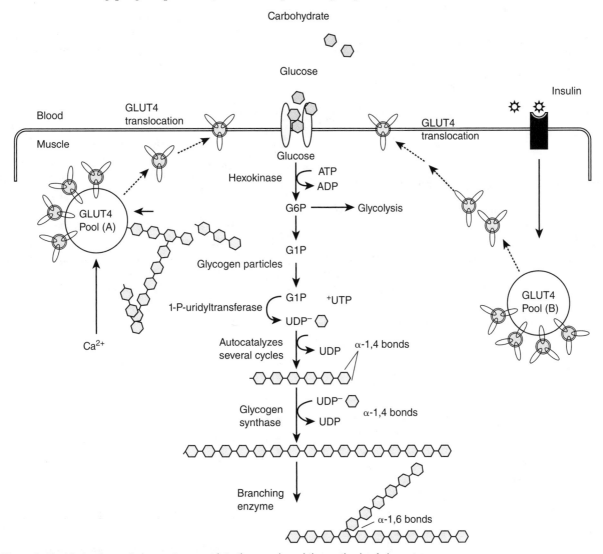

Figure 6.10 Mechanisms of glucose transport into the muscle and the synthesis of glycogen.

Reprinted, by permission, from L.P.G. Jentjens and A.E. Jeukendrup, 2003, "Glycogen resynthesis after exercise," *Sports Medicine* 33(2): 117-144. Reproduced with permission from Adis, A Wolters Kluwer business (Copyright Adis Data Information BV 2003. All rights reserved.)

Slow Phase of Glycogen Synthesis After Exercise

When the effect of the exercise-induced increase in glucose transport wears off, glycogen resynthesis occurs at a much slower rate. The rate at which glycogen synthesis occurs during the slow phase depends largely on the circulating insulin concentration, which increases GLUT4 translocation to the cell membrane and increases glucose transport into the muscle cell.

In addition, muscle contraction increases insulin sensitivity, and this effect may last for several hours. This increased insulin sensitivity after exercise is thought to be an important component of the slow phase of glycogen synthesis. The glycogen synthase activity decreases during this phase as muscle glycogen is restored.

After it is inside, the muscle cell glucose is directed toward muscle glycogen rather than oxidation. This effect is mediated by an increased glycogen synthase activity. An increase in the amount of GLUT4 present in the cell may also contribute to higher glycogen synthesis rates (Ren et al. 1994). After exercise, a rapid increase in GLUT4 expression may occur, resulting in increased synthesis of this protein, which in turn results in a proportional increase in insulin-stimulated glucose uptake and glycogen synthesis.

Postexercise Feeding and Rapid Recovery

A high rate of glycogen synthesis in the hours after exercise depends on the availability of substrate. In the absence of carbohydrate ingestion, glycogen resynthesis rates are extremely low, despite increased insulin sensitivity, increased glycogen synthase activity, and increased permeability of the sarcolemma to glucose (Ivy et al. 1988b). Often, the time available to recover between successive athletic competitions or training sessions is short. In such cases, rapid glycogen synthesis is even more important. Although muscle glycogen concentrations are unlikely to be completely restored to preexercise levels, all methods of carbohydrate supplementation that maximize glycogen restoration may benefit performance. Five factors have been recognized as potentially important in promoting restoration of muscle glycogen stores: (1) timing of carbohydrate intake, (2) rate of carbohydrate ingestion, (3) the type of carbohydrate ingested, (4) the ingestion of protein and carbohydrate after exercise, and (5) the intake of caffeine.

Timing of Carbohydrate Intake The timing of carbohydrate intake can have an important effect on the rate of muscle glycogen synthesis after exercise (Ivy et al. 1988a). When carbohydrate intake is delayed until 2 hours after exercise, muscle glycogen concentration after 4 hours is 45% lower compared with ingestion of the same amount of carbohydrate immediately after exercise. Average glycogen resynthesis rates in the 2 hours after ingestion are 3 to 4 mmol · kg w.w.$^{-1}$ · h^{-1} when carbohydrate is ingested after 2 hours and 5 to 6 mmol · kg w.w.$^{-1}$ · h^{-1} when it is ingested immediately after exercise (see figure 6.11). When carbohydrate intake is delayed until after the rapid phase, less glucose is taken up and stored as glycogen, primarily because of decreasing insulin sensitivity after the first few hours after exercise. A substantial intake of carbohydrate immediately after exercise seems to prevent this developing insulin resistance quite effectively.

Rate of Carbohydrate Ingestion When no carbohydrate is ingested after exercise, the rate of muscle glycogen synthesis is extremely low (1 to 2 mmol · kg w.w.$^{-1}$ · h^{-1}) (Ivy et al. 1988a). The ingestion of carbohydrate, especially in the first hours after exercise, results in enhanced muscle glycogen restoration, and glycogen is generally synthesized at a rate between 4.5 and 11 mmol · kg w.w.$^{-1}$ · h^{-1}. In figure 6.12 the results of a large number of studies performed in various laboratories have been compiled. The rate of muscle glycogen synthesis plotted against the ingestion rate shows that, with an increase in intake, an increase in synthesis also occurs in the first 3 to 5 hours after exercise. This graph shows a trend toward a higher glycogen synthesis rate when more carbohydrate is ingested, up to intakes of about 1.4 g/min, which is higher than previously suggested (Blom et al. 1987). At a given rate of carbohydrate intake, large variability exists in the rate of glycogen synthesis, probably

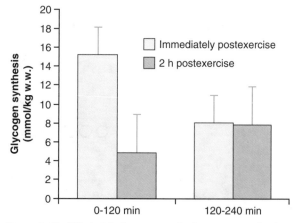

Figure 6.11 Effect of timing on muscle glycogen resynthesis.

Adapted from J.L. Ivy et al., 1998, "Muscle glycogen synthesis after exercise: Effect of time of carbohydrate ingestion," *Journal of Applied Physiology* 64: 1480-1485. Used with permission.

indicating that other factors such as timing, type of carbohydrate ingested, and training are also important.

Type of Carbohydrate Ingested Ingestion of different types of carbohydrate has different effects on glycogen synthesis. Blom et al. (1987) demonstrated that fructose ingestion resulted in lower rates of muscle glycogen synthesis after exercise compared with glucose or sucrose ingestion. Fructose must be converted to glucose in the liver before it can be used for glycogen synthesis in the muscle. Because this process takes time, glycogen synthesis occurs at a lower rate compared with a directly available carbohydrate source such as glucose. Other studies confirmed that glycogen synthesis from fructose occurs at only 50% of the rate of glycogen synthesis from glucose. In the study by Blom et al. (1987), sucrose intake resulted in muscle glycogen levels 4 hours after exercise similar to those that occurred after glucose intake.

Glycogen synthesis depends on the GI of the meal consumed after exercise. After 6 hours of recovery, muscle glycogen is more restored with a high-GI meal compared with a low-GI meal. Thus, the absorption rate and the availability of glucose seem to be important factors for glycogen synthesis. Low-GI foods result in lower glycogen resynthesis in the first hours after exercise.

Because the delivery of carbohydrate seems to be a factor and because combinations of multiple transportable carbohydrates such as glucose and fructose have been shown to increase absorption and delivery to the muscle during exercise, it is possible that these carbohydrate mixtures can also increase muscle glycogen synthesis after exercise. But it was recently observed that a combination

of glucose and fructose ingested at relatively high rates did not improve glycogen synthesis compared with the ingestion of glucose only. It is possible that the fructose is preferentially stored in the liver postexercise and therefore does not reach the muscle. Note, however, that the glucose–fructose mix did not result in less glycogen synthesis either.

Protein and Carbohydrate Ingestion After Exercise Certain amino acids have a potent effect on the secretion of insulin. The effects of adding amino acids and proteins to a carbohydrate solution have been investigated to optimize glycogen synthesis. Zawadzki et al. (1992) compared glycogen resynthesis rates after ingestion of carbohydrate, protein, or carbohydrate plus protein. As expected, little glycogen was stored when protein alone was ingested. Glycogen storage increased when carbohydrate was ingested. But most interestingly, glycogen storage increased further when carbohydrate was ingested together with protein.

The increased glycogen synthesis also coincided with higher insulin levels. Van Loon et al. (2000) used a protein hydrolysate and amino acid mixture ($0.8 \text{ g} \cdot \text{kg}^{-1} \cdot \text{h}^{-1}$ of carbohydrate and $0.4 \text{ g} \cdot \text{kg}^{-1} \cdot \text{h}^{-1}$ of protein–amino acid) that had previously been shown to result in a marked insulin response in combination with carbohydrate. When subjects ingested carbohydrate and this protein–amino acid mixture, they had higher glycogen resynthesis rates than when they ingested only carbohydrate. In this study, subjects also ingested an isoenergetic carbohydrate solution. Despite a larger insulin response with the added protein, glycogen resynthesis was highest with the isoenergetic amount of carbohydrate (see figure 6.13). These results suggest that insulin is an important factor, but the main limiting factor is the availability of carbohydrate. When a protein–amino acid mixture ($0.4 \text{ g} \cdot \text{kg}^{-1} \cdot \text{h}^{-1}$) was added to a large amount of carbohydrate ($1.2 \text{ g} \cdot \text{kg}^{-1} \cdot \text{h}^{-1}$), insulin concentrations increased, but the increase did not further increase glycogen resynthesis (Jentjens et al. 2001). These studies are summarized in figure 6.13. The maximal capacity to store muscle glycogen is likely reached, and, therefore, no additional effect of elevated insulin concentration is found. Thus, to achieve rapid muscle glycogen replenishment, ingesting an adequate amount of carbohydrate is more important than adding protein or amino acid mixtures to a recovery meal or drink.

Solid Versus Liquid

Few studies have investigated the effect of solid versus liquid carbohydrate foods on glycogen

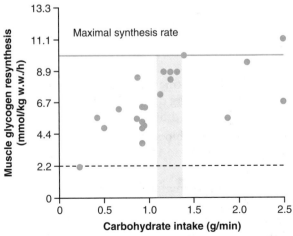

Figure 6.12 Muscle glycogen resynthesis after exercise as a function of carbohydrate intake.

Adapted from J.L. Ivy et al., 1998, "Muscle glycogen synthesis after exercise: Effect of time of carbohydrate ingestion," *Journal of Applied Physiology* 64: 1480-1485. Used with permission.

synthesis in the early hours after exercise. Keizer et al. (1987b) demonstrated that glycogen synthesis rates were similar after consumption of either a liquid or a solid carbohydrate meal. But the solid meal in that study contained slightly more carbohydrate than the liquid meal did, and differences in fat and protein content between the two meals were substantial.

Other investigators also found no difference in the rate of muscle glycogen storage between liquid and solid carbohydrate feedings. Therefore, no difference in glycogen synthesis with solid or liquid feedings is believed to exist. In the studies mentioned previously the investigators used a high-GI carbohydrate, probably resulting in rapid delivery of glucose. Low-GI solid meals are likely to result in lower rates of glycogen synthesis compared with carbohydrate solutions. For further reading about glycogen synthesis after exercise, see reviews by Jentjens and Jeukendrup (Jentjens et al. 2003b), Ivy (1998), and Ivy and Kuo (Ivy et al. 1998).

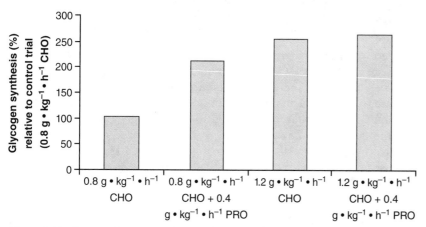

Figure 6.13 The rate of muscle glycogen synthesis after ingestion of various carbohydrate and carbohydrate–protein beverages. The synthesis rate for a drink containing 0.8 g · kg^{-1} · h^{-1} of carbohydrate is set at 100%, and all other synthesis rates are expressed relative to this baseline.

Caffeine and Glycogen Restoration

Caffeine has been shown to reduce insulin-stimulated glucose uptake and as such has been claimed to impair glucose metabolism. Caffeine ingestion before either an oral glucose tolerance test or a hyperinsulinemic euglycemic clamp results in significant impairment in insulin-mediated glucose disposal and carbohydrate storage. Although caffeine ingestion exerts a negative effect on skeletal muscle glucose disposal in resting humans, exercise appears to diminish such effects. As discussed earlier the coingestion of caffeine with carbohydrate during exercise increased glucose delivery to the muscle and oxidation (Yeo et al. 2005). If caffeine can increase the delivery of glucose during exercise, it might do the same following exercise, potentially increasing muscle glycogen synthesis. In a study by Pedersen et al. (2008), caffeine was added to a carbohydrate drink and given to subjects during a 4-hour recovery period from exhaustive glycogen-depleting exercise. Glycogen restoration was greatest with caffeine. Although evidence is thin, these initial results seem promising.

KEY POINTS

■ Muscle glycogen is a readily available energy source for the working muscle. The glycogen content of skeletal muscle at rest is approximately 54 to 72 g/kg d.m. (65 to 90 mmol glucosyl units/kg w.w.), equating to about 300 to 600 g of carbohydrate.

■ The main role of glycogen in the liver is to maintain a constant blood glucose level. An average liver weighs approximately 1.5 kg, and approximately 80 to 110 g of glycogen is stored in the liver of an adult human in the postabsorptive state.

■ In resting conditions the glucose output of the liver is approximately 150 mg/min, of which 60% is derived from the breakdown of liver glycogen and 40% from gluconeogenesis. During exercise, the liver glucose output increases dramatically, up to about 1 g/min, and most of this glucose (>90%) is derived from the breakdown of liver glycogen.

■ The classical supercompensation protocol results in very high muscle glycogen stores. But a moderate approach results in similar muscle glycogen levels without the disadvantages of the classical protocol and is therefore the preferred regimen.

- The brain is highly dependent on glucose as a fuel. As blood glucose concentrations drop, hypoglycemia may develop, resulting in dizziness, nausea, cold sweat, reduced mental alertness and ability to concentrate, loss of motor skill, increased heart rate, excessive hunger, and disorientation.

- The primary role of carbohydrate in the days leading up to competition is to replenish muscle glycogen stores fully.

- Carbohydrate loading, or increased carbohydrate stores, increases time to exhaustion (endurance capacity) on average by about 20% and reduces time taken to complete a set task (time trial, endurance performance) by 2% to 3%.

- In the 3 to 5 hours before exercise, some carbohydrate may be incorporated into muscle glycogen, but most will be stored as liver glycogen.

- Carbohydrate intake in the hours before exercise results in a transient fall in plasma glucose with the onset of exercise, increases carbohydrate oxidation and accelerates glycogen breakdown, and results in a blunting of fatty acid mobilization and fat oxidation.

- Carbohydrate feeding during exercise of about 45 minutes or longer is believed to improve endurance capacity and performance. The mechanisms may be the maintenance of blood glucose levels and high carbohydrate oxidation rates, glycogen sparing, or central nervous system effects.

- Oxidation of ingested carbohydrate during exercise depends on the type of carbohydrate, the amount ingested, and the exercise intensity, but the maximum oxidation rate seems to be about 1 g/min.

- Ingestion of 70 g of carbohydrate per hour (1.2 g/min) is recommended during prolonged exercise.

- Multiple transportable carbohydrates (e.g., glucose and fructose) in a beverage can increase oxidation rates during exercise.

- Two phases can be distinguished in the process of glycogen synthesis after exercise, which have often been referred to as the initial insulin-independent, or rapid phase, and the insulin-dependent, or slow, phase.

- Restoration of muscle glycogen stores after exercise may depend on the timing of carbohydrate intake, the rate of carbohydrate ingestion, the type of carbohydrate consumed, and the addition of other macronutrients (e.g., protein).

- As a general guideline, the recommended carbohydrate ingestion during periods of moderate training intensity is 5 to 7 g $\cdot$ kg^{-1} $\cdot$ day^{-1} and 7 to 10 g $\cdot$ kg^{-1} $\cdot$ day^{-1} when training is increased. For endurance athletes who are involved in extreme training programs, increasing carbohydrate intake to 10 to 13 g $\cdot$ kg^{-1} $\cdot$ day^{-1} when exercising daily is generally recommended.

RECOMMENDED READINGS

Hargreaves, M., J.A. Hawley, and A.E. Jeukendrup. 2004. Pre-exercise carbohydrate and fat ingestion: Effects on metabolism and performance. *Journal of Sports Sciences* 22:31-38.

Hawley, J.A., E.J. Schabort, T.D. Noakes, and S.C. Dennis. 1997. Carbohydrate loading and exercise performance: An update. *Sports Medicine* 24:73-81.

Ivy, J. 1998. Glycogen resynthesis after exercise: Effect of carbohydrate intake. *International Journal of Sports Medicine* 19:S142-S145.

Ivy, J.L., and C.-H. Kuo. 1998. Regulation of GLUT4 protein and glycogen synthase during muscle glycogen synthesis after exercise. *Acta Physiologica Scandinavica* 162: 295-304.

Jentjens, L.P.G., and A.E. Jeukendrup. 2003. Glycogen resynthesis after exercise. *Sports Medicine* 33 (2): 117-144.

Jeukendrup, A.E., and R. Jentjens. 2000. Oxidation of carbohydrate feedings during prolonged exercise: Current thoughts, guidelines and directions for future research. *Sports Medicine* 29 (6): 407-424.

Jeukendrup, AE. 2008. Carbohydrate feeding during exercise. *European Journal of Sport Science* 8:77-86.

Jeukendrup, A.E. 2004. Carbohydrate intake during exercise and performance. *Nutrition* 20:669-677.

Maughan, R.J., and M. Gleeson. 2004. *The biochemical basis of sports performance.* Oxford: Oxford University Press.

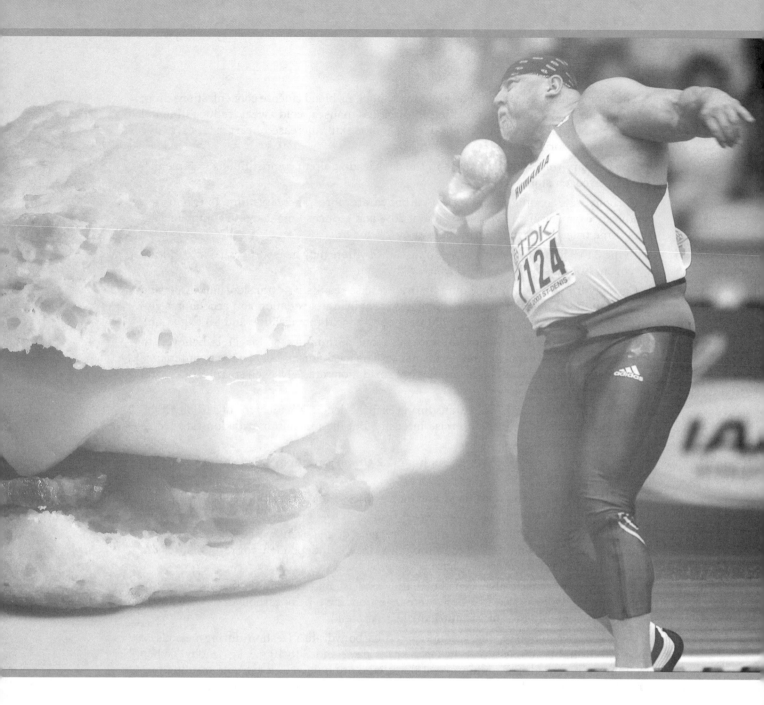

OBJECTIVES

After studying this chapter, you should be able to do the following:

- Describe the main biochemical pathways in fat metabolism
- Describe the changes that occur in fat metabolism at different intensities of exercise
- Discuss the factors that limit fat oxidation
- Describe the interactions between carbohydrate and fat metabolism at rest and in response to exercise
- Describe the metabolic and performance effects of fat intake 3 to 4 hours before exercise
- Describe the metabolic and performance effects of short-term high-fat diets
- Describe the metabolic and performance effects of long-term high-fat diets

7

Fat

ietary fat is frequently undervalued as a contributor to health and performance of athletes. Fat is an extremely important fuel for endurance exercise, along with carbohydrate, and some fat intake is required for optimal health. Dietary fat provides the essential fatty acids (EFA) that cannot be synthesized in the body.

The fat stores of the body are very large in comparison with carbohydrate stores. In some forms of exercise (e.g., prolonged cycling or running), carbohydrate depletion is possibly a cause of fatigue and depletion and can occur within 1 to 2 hours of strenuous exercise (see chapter 6). The total amount of energy stored as glycogen in the muscles and liver has been estimated to be 8,000 kJ (2,000 kcal). Fat stores can contain more than 50 times the amount of energy contained in carbohydrate stores. A person with a body mass of 80 kg and 15% body fat has 12 kg of fat (see table 7.1).

Most of this fat is stored in subcutaneous adipose tissue, but some fat can also be found in muscle as intramuscular triacylglycerol (IMTG). In theory, fat stores could provide sufficient energy for a runner to run at least 1,300 km.

Ideally, athletes would like to tap into their fat stores as much as possible and save the carbohydrate for later in a competition. Researchers, coaches, and athletes have therefore tried to devise nutritional strategies to enhance fat metabolism, spare carbohydrate stores, and thereby improve endurance performance. Understanding the effects of various nutritional strategies requires an understanding of fat metabolism and the factors that regulate fat oxidation during exercise. This chapter therefore describes fat metabolism in detail and discusses various ways in which researchers and athletes have tried to enhance fat metabolism by nutritional manipulation. Finally, the effects of both low-fat and high-fat diets on metabolism, exercise performance, and health are discussed.

■ TABLE 7.1 ■
Availability of Substrates in the Human Body

Substrate	Weight (kg)	Energy kJ (kcal)
CARBOHYDRATES		
Plasma glucose	0.01	160 (40)
Liver glycogen	0.1	1,600 (400)
Muscle glycogen	0.4	6,400 (1,600)
Total (approximately)	0.51	8,000 (2,000)
FAT		
Plasma fatty acid	0.0004	16 (4)
Plasma triacylglycerols	0.004	160 (40)
Adipose tissue	12.0	430,000 (108,000)
Intramuscular triacylglycerols	0.3	11,000 (2,700)
Total (approximately)	12.3	442,000 (111,000)

Values given are estimates for a "normal" man of 80 kg (176 lb) and 15% body fat, not an athlete, who might be leaner and have more stored glycogen. The amount of protein in the body is not mentioned, but it would be about 10 kg (22 lb [40,000 kcal or 167,440 kJ]), mainly located in the muscles.

Fat Metabolism During Exercise

FAs that are oxidized in the mitochondria of skeletal muscle during exercise are derived from various sources. The main two sources are adipose tissue and muscle triacylglycerols. A third fuel, plasma triacylglycerol may also be utilized, but the importance of this fuel is subject to debate. Figure 7.1 gives an overview of the fat substrates and their journey to the muscle. Triacylglycerols in adipose tissue are split into FAs and glycerol. The glycerol is released into the circulation, along with some of the FAs. A small percentage of FAs is not released into the circulation but is used to form new triacylglycerols within the adipose tissue, a process called reesterification. The other FAs are transported to the other tissues and taken up by skeletal muscle during exercise. Glycerol is transported to the liver, where it serves as a gluconeogenic substrate to form new glucose.

Besides the FAs in plasma, two other sources of FAs for oxidation in skeletal muscle are available. Circulating triacylglycerols (for example in a very low-density lipoprotein [VLDL]) can temporarily bind to lipoprotein lipase (LPL), which splits off FAs that can then be taken up by the muscle. A source of fat exists inside the muscle in the form of intramuscular triacylglycerol. These triacylglycerols are split by a hormone-sensitive lipase (HSL), and FAs are transported into the mitochondria for

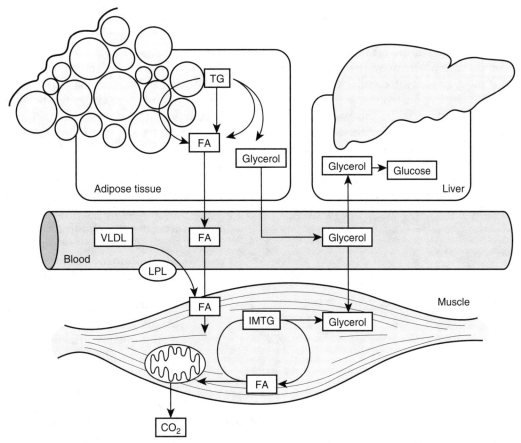

Figure 7.1 Overview of fat metabolism and the main organs involved. TG = triacylglycerol; FA = fatty acid; IMTG = intramuscular triacylglycerol; LPL = lipoprotein lipase; VLDL = very low-density lipoprotein.

oxidation in the same way that FAs from plasma and plasma triacylglycerol are utilized.

Limits to Fat Oxidation

Despite the fact that humans have large fat stores, in many situations using these large amounts of fat as a fuel seems impossible. Why can fat not be oxidized at higher rates in some conditions? Is it because the FAs cannot be mobilized? To find the factor that causes this limitation, we examine all the steps that are important in the process of fat oxidation—from the mobilization of FAs to the transport and oxidation of FAs in the mitochondrion itself.

The steps that could potentially limit fat oxidation are

- **lipolysis,** the breakdown of triacylglycerols to FAs and glycerol;
- removal of FAs from the fat cell;
- transport of fat by the bloodstream;
- transport of FAs into the muscle cell;

- transport of FAs into the mitochondria; and
- oxidation of FAs in the β-oxidation pathway and TCA cycle.

Lipolysis in Adipocytes

Most FAs are stored in the form of triacylglycerols in subcutaneous adipose tissue. Before these FAs are oxidized, they must be mobilized and transported to the site of oxidation. The **adipocyte** contains lipases that break down triacylglycerols. Hormone-sensitive lipase (HSL) splits triacylglycerols into FAs and glycerol and, as its name implies, is regulated by hormones (see figure 7.2). Adipocytes also contain triacylglycerol lipase and enzymes that split off the first FAs resulting in the formation of a diacylglycerol (DAG). HSL may be translocated to the triacylglycerol in the cell and subsequently activated. Conversion of the inactive form of HSL into the active form mainly depends on the sympathetic nervous system and circulating epinephrine. Norepinephrine is released from nerve endings of the sympathetic nervous system, whereas epinephrine is produced in the adrenal medulla, especially during high-intensity exercise. The effects are mediated through adrenergic receptors found on the adipocyte membrane. Insulin is probably the most important counter-regulatory hormone, and its secretion from the pancreatic islets is usually suppressed in the presence of elevated concentrations of epinephrine.

When lipolysis is stimulated, the glycerol released by this reaction diffuses freely into the blood. The adipocyte cannot reuse it, because the enzyme glycerokinase, which is required to phosphorylate the glycerol before

reesterification with FAs, is only present in extremely low concentrations. Therefore, almost all the glycerol produced by lipolysis is released into the plasma, and the measurement of glycerol in the blood is often used as a measure of lipolysis. FAs released by lipolysis are either reesterified within the adipocyte or transported into the bloodstream for use in other tissues (see figure 7.3).

At rest, approximately 70% of all FAs released during lipolysis are reesterified (Wolfe et al. 1990). During exercise, reesterification is suppressed, which results in increased availability of FAs in the adipocyte. The availability of FAs increases even more because lipolysis is stimulated by β-adrenoreceptors during exercise. Catecholamines released from the adrenal gland stimulate lipolysis during exercise.

Lipolysis is usually in excess of the demand for FAs both at rest and during exercise. Reesterification is therefore believed to play an important role in regulating FA mobilization. Reesterification depends on the rate at which FAs are removed from the adipocyte by the blood, the rate of glycerol-3-phosphate production, and the activity of triacylglycerol synthesizing enzymes. Because glycerol cannot be recycled to any major extent in human adipocytes (or myocytes), the backbone for a triacylglycerol molecule is derived from glycerol-3-phosphate, an intermediate of the glycolytic pathway.

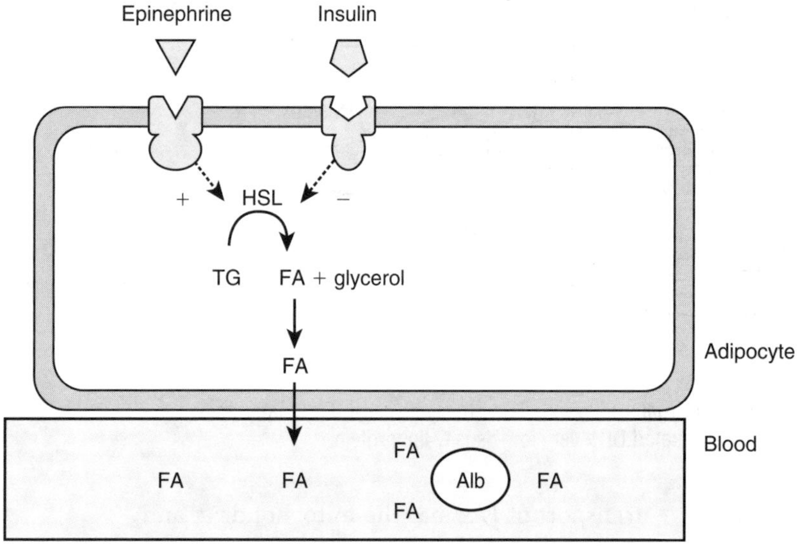

Figure 7.2 Mobilization of FAs from adipose tissue. TG = triacylglycerol; HSL = hormone-sensitive lipase; Alb = albumin.

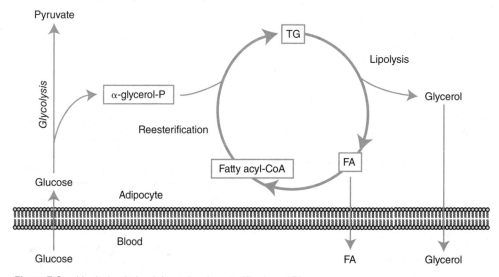

Figure 7.3 Lipolysis of triacylglycerol and reesterification of FAs.

International Journal of Sports Medicine: From A.E. Jeukendrup et al., 1998, "Fat metabolism during exercise. Part I. Fatty acid mobilization and muscle metabolism," 19(4): 231-244. Adapted by permission.

FAs are not soluble in the aqueous environment of the adipocyte cytoplasm. They are therefore bound to so-called FA-binding proteins (FABPs) that transport the FAs to the cell membrane. At least during low-intensity to moderate-intensity exercise, the increase in lipolysis and the reduction in esterification of FAs result in a substantially increased level of FAs in the blood (Romijn et al. 1993; Wolfe et al. 1990).

Removal of FAs and Transport in the Blood

The removal of FAs from the adipocyte into the bloodstream depends on several factors, the most important being blood flow to the adipose tissue, the albumin concentration in the blood, and the number of free binding sites for FAs on the albumin molecule. Albumin is the most abundant protein in plasma, and one of its functions is as a carrier protein that transports FAs. When it arrives at the target tissue (for example, muscle) it binds to specific albumin-binding proteins (ABP). Binding to this protein then aids the release of FAs from albumin and their uptake.

A typical plasma albumin concentration is around 0.7 mmol/L (45 g/L), and albumin has at least three high-affinity binding sites for FAs, which provide a large capacity to bind FAs. Therefore, most FAs in the blood are bound to albumin (>99.9%), and only a small fraction (<0.1%), dissolved in the plasma water, circulates freely. Under most conditions, only a fraction of the total number of binding sites of albumin are occupied. At rest, in the postabsorptive state, the plasma FA concentration is about 0.2 to 0.4 mmol/L. However, during prolonged exercise, the FA concentration in the blood can rise to about 2 mmol/L. At this concentration the maximum capacity of albumin to bind FAs may be reached. When the FA concentration rises further, the percentage of unbound FAs increases, which is believed to be toxic for cells because of detergent-like properties of unbound FAs. These extremely high FA levels, however, are unusual, and the body seems to have protective mechanisms to prevent rises much above 2 mmol/L. One of these mechanisms could be increased incorporation of FAs into plasma triacylglycerol. During every pass through the liver, a fraction of the FAs is extracted from the circulation and incorporated into VLDL particles.

Plasma Lipoproteins

Triacylglycerols bound to lipoproteins (VLDLs and chylomicrons) are another potential source of FAs (Havel et al. 1967). The enzyme lipoprotein lipase (LPL) in the vascular wall hydrolyzes some of the triacylglycerols in circulating lipoproteins passing through the capillary bed. As a result FAs are released, and the muscle takes them up to use for oxidation. But the FA uptake from plasma lipoprotein triacylglycerols occurs slowly and accounts for fewer than 3% of the energy expenditure during prolonged exercise (Havel et al. 1967). Therefore, it is generally believed that plasma triacylglycerols contribute only minimally to energy production during exercise. Some interesting observations need further investigation. For instance, LPL activity increases significantly after training and after consumption of a high-fat diet; in both situations, fat oxidation increases markedly. In addition, acute exercise also stimulates LPL activity.

Transport of FAs Into the Muscle Cell

For a long time, the transport of FAs into the muscle cell was believed to be a passive process. This belief was based on early observations that FA uptake increased linearly with FA concentration. Recently, however, specific carrier proteins have been identified (see figure 7.4). In the sarcolemma, at least two proteins are involved in the transport of FAs across the membrane—a specific plasma membrane FA-binding protein (FABPpm) and a FA transporter (FAT/CD36) protein. These proteins are likely to be responsible for the transport of most FAs across the sarcolemma. Animal studies indicate that the transporters become saturated at plasma FA concentrations around 1.5 mmol/L. FAT/CD36 can translocate from intracellular vesicles to the cell membrane in a similar manner as the GLUT4 protein, indicating that FA transport can also be regulated acutely (Bonen et al. 1999; van Oort et al. 2008). Muscle contraction increases plasma membrane FAT/CD36 and decreases the concentration of FAT/CD36 in the sarcoplasm (cytoplasm of muscle cells). Along with a higher density of FAT/CD36 at the cell membrane, increased FA transport into the cell was observed. What triggers the translocation of the FAT/CD36 to the cell membrane is currently not known. Similar factors that result in GLUT4 translocation might also be responsible for the translocation of FAT/CD36.

In the sarcoplasm the FAs are bound to another specific cytoplasmic FA-binding protein (FABPc). FABPc is thought to be responsible for the transport of FAs from the sarcolemma to the mitochondria. At present, little is known about the roles of these FA-binding proteins and transporters, and whether they are a limiting factor for fat oxidation is unknown.

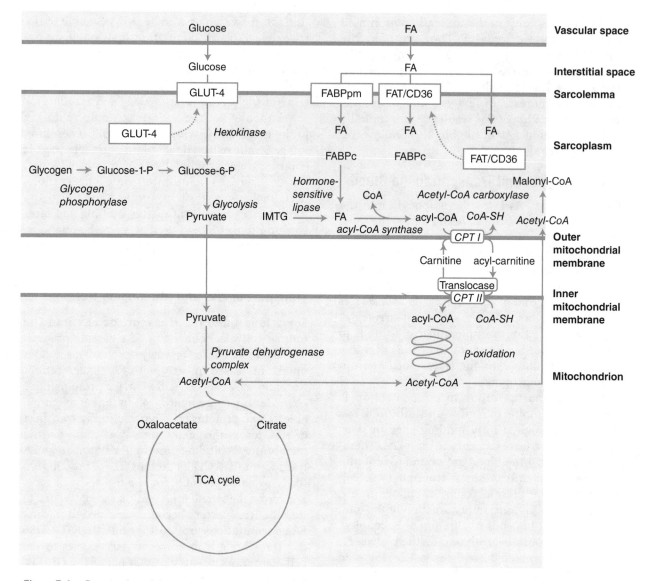

Figure 7.4   Presentation of the transport of glucose and FAs from the blood into the mitochondria. CoASH = free coenzyme A; CPT I = carnitine palmitoyl transferase I; CPT II = carnitine palmitoyl transferase II; FABP = fatty acid binding protein; IMTG = intramuscular triacylglycerol.

Reprinted, by permission, from A.E. Jeukendrup, 2002, "Regulation of skeletal muscle fat metabolism," *New York Academy of Sciences* 967: 1-19.

Intramuscular Triacylglycerols

Another source of FAs are the IMTG stores in the muscle itself. Type I muscle fibers have a higher content of IMTG than type II muscle fibers. IMTG stores, usually located adjacent to the mitochondria as lipid droplets (see figure 7.5), have been recognized as an important energy source during exercise. Studies in which muscle samples were investigated under a microscope revealed that the size of these lipid droplets decreases during exercise. Also, indirect measures of IMTG breakdown provide evidence for its use during exercise. The location of the droplets seems to be important as well. In trained muscle, the lipid droplets are believed to be located next to the mitochondria, whereas in untrained muscle, the lipid droplets may not be so intricately linked with the mitochondria and may be dispersed throughout the cytoplasm. It has been shown that exercise training increases the number of intramuscular triacylglycerols next to the mitochondria (Devries et al. 2007). Like adipose tissue, muscle contains a HSL that is activated by β-adrenergic stimulation and inhibited by insulin. FAs liberated from IMTGs may be released into the blood, reesterified, or oxidized within the muscle. Because the lipid droplets are located close to the mitochondria, at least in trained muscle, most of the FAs released after lipolysis are assumed to be oxidized. The FAs released are bound to FABPc until they are transported into the mitochondria.

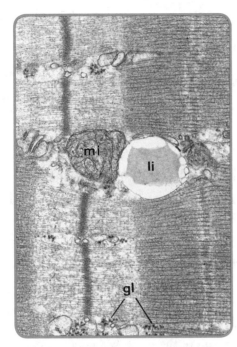

Figure 7.5 An electromyograph of skeletal muscle showing intramuscular triacylglycerols. A large lipid droplit (li) is located adjacent to the mitochondria (mi). Compare the enormous stores of lipid with the small stores of glycogen (gl) in this muscle.

International Journal of Sports Medicine: From A.E. Jeukendrup et al., Fat metabolism during exercise Part I. Fatty acid mobilization and muscle metabolism, 1998, 19(4): 231-244. Adapted by permission.

Transport of FAs into the Mitochondria

FAs in the cytoplasm may be activated by the enzyme acyl-CoA synthetase or thiokinase to form an acyl-CoA complex (often referred to as an activated FA) (see figure 7.6). This acyl-CoA complex is used for the synthesis of IMTGs, or it is bound to carnitine under the influence of the enzyme carnitine palmitoyl transferase I (CPT I, which is also known as carnitine acyl transferase I or CAT-I), which is located at the outside of the outer mitochondrial membrane.

The bonding between carnitine and the activated FA is the first step in the transport of the FA into the mitochondria. As carnitine binds to the FA, free CoA is released. The fatty acyl-carnitine complex is transported with a translocase and reconverted into fatty acyl-CoA at the matrix side of the inner mitochondrial membrane by the enzyme carnitine palmitoyl transferase II (CPT II). The carnitine that is released diffuses back across the mitochondrial membrane into the cytoplasm and thus becomes available again for the transport of other FAs. Fatty acyl-carnitine crosses the inner membrane in a 1:1 exchange with a molecule of free carnitine. Although short-chain FAs (SCFAs) and medium-chain FAs (MCFAs) are believed to diffuse freely into the mitochondrial matrix, car-

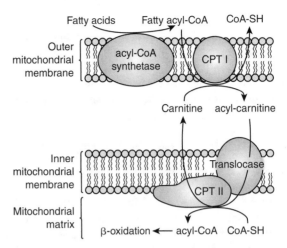

Figure 7.6 Transport of FAs into the mitochondria.

rier proteins with a specific maximum affinity for short-chain or medium-chain acyl-CoA transport at least some of these FAs. In addition, it has recently been discovered that another protein (FAT/CD36) is involved in the transport of fatty acids across the mitochondria. FAT/CD36 is translocated to the mitochondrial membrane before it can transport FA across.

β-Oxidation

After it is in the mitochondrial matrix, the fatty acyl-CoA is subjected to β-oxidation, a series of reactions that splits a two-carbon acetyl-CoA molecule of the multiple-carbon FA chain (see figure 7.7). The β-oxidation pathway uses oxygen and generates some ATP through substrate-level phosphorylation. The

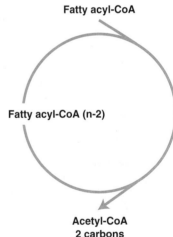

Figure 7.7 The β-oxidation process.

acetyl-CoA is then oxidized in the tricarboxylic acid (TCA) cycle. The complete oxidation of FAs in the mitochondria depends on several factors, including the activity of enzymes of the β-oxidation pathway, the concentration of TCA-cycle intermediates and activity of enzymes in the TCA cycle (these factors determine the total TCA-cycle activity), and the presence of oxygen.

Fat as a Fuel During Exercise

Carbohydrate and fat are always oxidized as a mixture, and whether carbohydrate or fat is the predominant fuel depends on a variety of factors, including the intensity and duration of exercise, the level of aerobic fitness, diet, and carbohydrate intake before or during exercise.

The changes in fat metabolism that occur in the transition from rest to exercise as well as the various factors that influence fat mobilization and oxidation are discussed in the following sections.

Fat Utilization at Rest and During Exercise

After an overnight fast, most of the energy requirement is covered by the oxidation of FAs derived from adipose tissue. The rate of lipolysis in adipose tissue depends mostly on the circulating concentrations of hormones (epinephrine stimulates lipolysis, and insulin inhibits lipolysis). Most of the FAs liberated after lipolysis seem to be reesterified within the adipocyte. Some FAs enter the bloodstream, but only about half of them are oxidized. Resting plasma FA concentrations are typically between 0.2 and 0.4 mmol/L.

When exercise is initiated, the rate of lipolysis and the rate of FA release from adipose tissue increase. During moderate-intensity exercise, lipolysis increases approximately threefold, mainly because of an increased β-adrenergic stimulation (by catecholamines). In addition, during moderate-intensity exercise, blood flow to adipose tissue is doubled and the rate of reesterification is halved. Blood flow in skeletal muscle increases dramatically, and, therefore, the delivery of FAs to the muscle increases.

During the first 15 minutes of exercise, plasma FA concentrations usually decrease because the rate of FA uptake by the muscle exceeds the rate of FA appearance from lipolysis. Thereafter, the rate of appearance is in excess of the utilization by muscle, and plasma FA concentrations increase. The rise in FA depends on the exercise intensity. During moderate-intensity exercise, FA concentrations may reach 1 mmol/L within 60 minutes of exercise, but at higher exercise intensities, the rise in plasma FAs is small or may even be absent.

Fat Oxidation and Exercise Duration

Fat oxidation increases as exercise duration increases. Edwards et al. (1934) reported fat oxidation rates of over 1.0 g/min after 6 hours of

running. Christensen and Hansen (Christensen et al. 1939) observed that the contribution of fat could even increase to levels as high as 90% of energy expenditure when a fatty meal was consumed, leading to fat oxidation rates of 1.5 g/min. The mechanism of this increased fat oxidation as exercise duration increases is not entirely clear but seems to be linked to the decrease in muscle glycogen stores.

Fat Oxidation and Exercise Intensity

Fat oxidation is usually the predominant fuel at low exercise intensities, whereas during high exercise intensities, carbohydrates are the major fuel. In absolute terms, fat oxidation increases as the exercise intensity increases from low to moderate intensities, although the percentage contribution of fat may actually decrease (see figure 7.8). For the transition from low-intensity to moderate-intensity exercise, the increased fat oxidation is a direct result of the increased energy expenditure. At higher intensities of exercise (>75% of $\dot{V}O_2max$) fat oxidation is inhibited and both the relative and absolute rates of fat oxidation decrease to negligible values. Achten et al. (2002, 2003) studied this relationship over a wide range of exercise intensities in a group of trained subjects and found that on average the maximal rates of fat oxidation were observed at 62 to 63% of $\dot{V}O_2max$.

During exercise at 25% of $\dot{V}O_2max$, most of the fat oxidized is derived from plasma FAs and only small amounts come from IMTGs (Romijn et al. 1993) (see figure 7.9). During moderate-intensity exercise (65% of $\dot{V}O_2max$), however, the contribution of plasma FAs declines whereas the contribu-

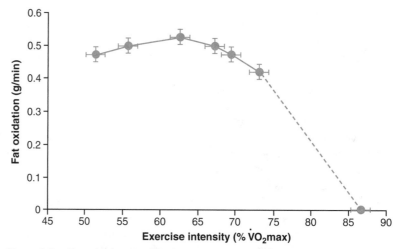

Figure 7.8 Fat oxidation as a function of exercise intensity.

International Journal of Sports Medicine: From J. Achten and A.G. Jeukendrup. Maximal fat oxidation during exercise in trained men, 2003, 24(8): 603-608. Reprinted by permission.

tion of IMTGs increases and provides about half of the FAs used for total fat oxidation (Romijn et al. 1993). Training also decreases the contribution of plasma FAs, despite a dramatic increase in total fat oxidation. This decrease in plasma FA oxidation is accounted for by a marked increase in the contribution of muscle triacylglycerols to energy expenditure.

When the exercise intensity is further increased, fat oxidation decreases, although the rate of

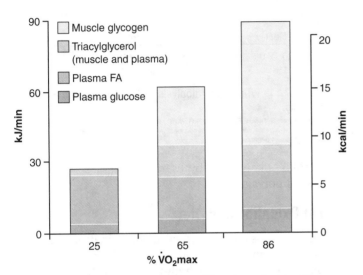

Figure 7.9 Substrate utilization at different exercise intensities.

Reprinted from J.A. Romijn et al., 1993, "Regulation of endogenous fat and carbohydrate metabolism in relation to exercise intensity and duration," *Journal of Applied Physiology* 265: E380-E391. Used with permission.

lipolysis is still high. The blood flow to the adipose tissue may decrease (because of sympathetic vasoconstriction), which may result in decreased removal of FAs from adipose tissue. During high-intensity exercise, lactate accumulation may also increase the rate of reesterification of FAs. As a result, plasma FA concentrations are usually low during intense exercise. But this decreased availability of FAs can only partially explain the reduced fat oxidation observed in these conditions. When Romijn et al. (1995) restored FA concentrations to levels observed at moderate exercise intensities by infusing triacylglycerols (Intralipid) and heparin, fat oxidation increased only slightly and was still lower than at moderate intensities (see the sidebar and figure 7.10). Therefore, an additional mechanism in the muscle must be responsible for the decreased fat oxidation observed during high-intensity exercise.

Sidossis et al. (1997) and Coyle et al. (1997) suggested that the decreased fat oxidation is related to the transport of FAs into the mitochondria. They observed that during high-intensity exercise, the oxidation of long-chain FAs (LCFA) is impaired, whereas the oxidation of medium chain FAs is unaffected. Because the medium-chain FAs are less dependent on transport mechanisms into the mitochondria, these data provide evidence that carnitine-dependent FA transport is a limiting factor.

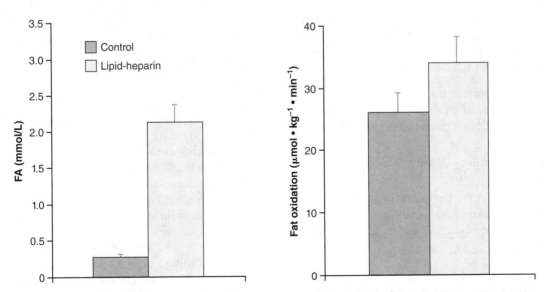

Figure 7.10 FA concentrations are usually low at high exercise intensities (>85% of V̇O₂max), which could explain the relatively low oxidation rates of fat compared with moderate exercise intensities (gray bars). When lipid and heparin are infused, high plasma FA concentrations are achieved but do not restore fat oxidation to the levels observed at moderate exercise intensities (65% of V̇O₂max).

Data from J.A. Romijn et al., 1995, "Relationship between fatty acid delivery and fatty acid oxidation during strenuous exercise," *Journal of Applied Physiology* 79(6): 1939-1945. Used with permission.

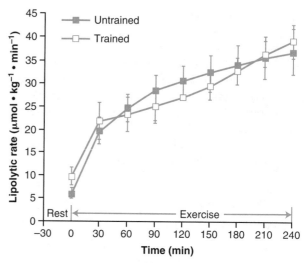

Figure 7.11 Whole-body lipolysis in trained and untrained subjects.

Reprinted from S. Klein, E.F. Coyle, and R.R. Wolfe, 1994, "Fat metabolism during low-intensity exercise in endurance trained and untrained men," *Journal of Applied Physiology* 267: E934-E940. Used with permission.

Triacylglycerol and Heparin Infusion

To increase plasma FA concentrations for experimental purposes, researchers have used the infusion of triacylglycerol and heparin. Because FAs are not soluble in water (plasma), they cannot be infused directly. Therefore, a lipid emulsion is used (often Intralipid) in combination with a heparin injection. Heparin releases lipoprotein lipase (LPL) from the capillaries. After LPL becomes freely available in the circulation, it starts to break down the plasma triacylglycerol, and FA concentrations rise rapidly.

Fat Oxidation and Aerobic Capacity

Endurance training affects both substrate utilization and exercise capacity. Studies involving both animals and humans have established a marked adaptive increase in oxidative potential in response to increased regular physical activity (Holloszy and Booth 1976; Holloszy and Coyle 1984). A consequence and probably contributing factor to the enhanced exercise capacity after endurance training is the metabolic shift to greater use of fat and a concomitant sparing of glycogen. The contribution of fat to total energy expenditure increases after training at both the relative and the absolute exercise intensities. The adaptations that contribute to stimulation of fat oxidation in trained subjects include

- increased mitochondrial density and an increase in the number of oxidative enzymes in trained muscle, which increases the capacity to oxidize fat;
- increased capillary density, which enhances FA delivery to the muscle;
- increased FABP concentrations, which may facilitate uptake of FAs across the sarcolemma;
- increased CPT concentration, which facilitates the transport of FAs into the mitochondria.

One factor that does not seem to be influenced by training is lipolysis in adipose tissue (Klein et al. 1994) (see figure 7.11). After training, the rate of lipolysis at the same absolute exercise intensity does not seem to be affected. At the same relative exercise intensity, the rate of lipolysis increases after training (Klein et al. 1996). Increased lipolysis

of IMTG likely contributes to this increased whole-body lipolysis.

Fat Oxidation and Diet

Diet also has marked effects on fat oxidation. Generally, a high-carbohydrate, low-fat diet reduces fat oxidation, whereas a high-fat, low-carbohydrate diet increases fat oxidation. Some scientists have argued that the results seen in most of these studies are the effects of the last meal, which is known to influence substrate utilization. But Burke et al. (1999) showed that a high-fat, low-carbohydrate diet had a similar effect on substrate utilization, even after a day on a high-carbohydrate diet. The results indicate that some chronic effects of diet cannot be directly explained by substrate availability. In the study by Burke et al. (1999), for example, subjects consumed a high-fat diet or a high-carbohydrate diet for 5 days followed by 1 day on a high-carbohydrate diet. The 1-day high-carbohydrate intake replenished glycogen stores in both conditions, and muscle glycogen concentrations were identical. Yet large differences existed in substrate utilization between the two diets.

The respiratory exchange ratio (RER) changed from 0.90 to 0.82 after 5 days on a high-fat diet. After consuming a high-carbohydrate diet for 1 day, RER was still lower compared with baseline values (0.87). Because these changes were not caused by alterations in muscle glycogen availability, they are likely to be related to metabolic adaptations in the muscle.

Chronic diets can have marked effects on metabolism. These effects seem only partly related to the effects of diets on substrate availability. Adaptations at the muscular level, which result in changes in substrate utilization in response to a diet, may occur within a period as short as 5 days.

Response to Carbohydrate Feeding

The fastest way to alter fat metabolism during exercise is probably by carbohydrate feeding. Carbohydrate increases the plasma insulin concentration, which reduces lipolysis and causes a marked reduction in FA availability. In a study by Horowitz et al. (1997), carbohydrate was ingested 1 hour before exercise. Both lipolysis and fat oxidation were reduced. Plasma FA concentrations decreased to extremely low levels during exercise. But when Intralipid was infused and heparin was injected to increase the plasma FA concentrations, fat oxidation was only partially restored. These findings indicate that reduced availability of FAs is indeed a factor that limits fat oxidation, but because increasing the plasma FA concentrations does not completely restore fat oxidation, other factors must play a role as well. These factors must be located inside the muscle itself.

When a large amount of glucose is ingested 1 hour before exercise, plasma insulin levels are very high at the start of exercise, whereas plasma FA and glycerol concentrations are very low (Coyle et al. 1997). This circumstance results in a 30% reduction in fat oxidation compared with no carbohydrate intake. In a study by Coyle et al. (1997), trace amounts of labeled medium-chain or long-chain FAs were infused, and the oxidation rates of these FAs were determined. The oxidation of long-chain FAs appeared to be reduced, whereas the oxidation of medium-chain FAs appeared to be unaffected (see figure 7.12). Because medium-chain FAs are not as dependent on transport mechanisms into the mitochondria, but the long-chain FAs are highly dependent on this mechanism, these results provide evidence that this transport is an important regulatory step. Although the exact mechanisms are still unclear, carbohydrate feeding before exercise reduces fat oxidation by reducing lipolysis and plasma FA availability and exerts an inhibitory effect on carnitine-dependent FA transport into the mitochondria.

Regulation of Carbohydrate and Fat Metabolism

In all situations, carbohydrate and fat together constitute most, if not all, of the energy provision. The percentage contribution of these two fuels, however, varies depending on the factors discussed previously. The rate of carbohydrate utilization during prolonged strenuous exercise is closely related to the energy needs of the working muscle. In contrast, fat utilization during exercise is not tightly regulated. No mechanisms closely match

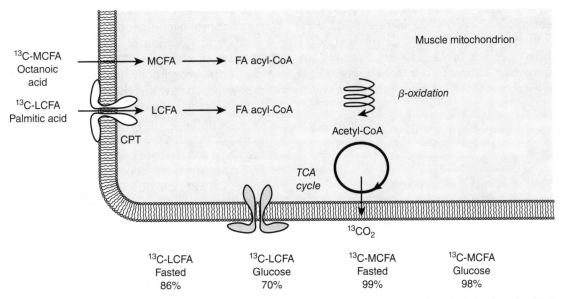

Figure 7.12 Oxidation of medium-chain FAs (MCFAs) and long-chain FAs (LCFAs) in the mitochondria during fasted and fed conditions (glucose). Glucose intake reduced the oxidation of LCFAs but not MCFAs. Because LCFAs use a transport protein to enter the mitochondria, and MCFAs are less dependent on this protein, glucose availability possibly regulates the entry of FA into the mitochondria.

Data from Coyle et al. 1997.

the metabolism of FAs to energy expenditure. Fat oxidation is therefore mainly influenced by fat availability and the rate of carbohydrate utilization.

Some evidence suggests that increases in plasma FA concentration can cause a decrease in the rate of muscle glycogen breakdown. This action could theoretically be beneficial, because muscle glycogen depletion is one of the prime causes of fatigue. Researchers have artificially elevated plasma FA concentrations by raising plasma triacylglycerol concentrations by means of a fat meal or intravenous infusion of triacylglycerol (Intralipid), followed by a heparin injection. Using this method, it has been repeatedly shown that an increase in FA concentration can reduce carbohydrate dependence.

In a study by Costill et al. (1977), Intralipid was infused and heparin was injected during exercise at 70% of V̇O₂max. After 60 minutes, a muscle biopsy was taken and muscle glycogen was measured before and after the exercise bout. Muscle glycogen breakdown decreased with the elevated plasma FA concentrations (see figure 7.13). Similar results were obtained when a fat feeding was given in combination with heparin infusion (Vukovich et al. 1993). Although elevating FA levels seems to reduce muscle glycogen breakdown during exercise, the mechanisms are still incompletely understood.

The classical glucose–FA cycle was originally thought to explain this interaction between carbohydrate and fat metabolism (see figure 7.14). This theory states that with an increase in plasma FA concentration, uptake of FAs increases and these FAs undergo β-oxidation in the mitochondria, in which they are broken down to acetyl-CoA. An increasing concentration of acetyl-CoA (or increased acetyl-CoA/CoA ratio) inhibits the pyruvate dehydrogenase complex that breaks down pyruvate to acetyl-CoA. In addition, increased formation of acetyl-CoA from FA oxidation in the mitochondria increases muscle citrate levels, and after diffusing into the sarcoplasm, citrate could inhibit phosphofructokinase, the rate-limiting enzyme in glycolysis. The effect of increased acetyl-CoA and citrate levels is, therefore, a reduction in the rate of glycolysis. This reduced rate of glycolysis, in turn, may cause accumulation of glucose-6-phosphate (G6P) in the muscle sarcoplasm, which inhibits hexokinase activity and thus reduces muscle glucose uptake.

With increased fat availability the disturbance in the cellular homeostasis declines. Increasing FA availability decreases intramuscular inorganic phosphate (Pi) and adenosine monophosphate (AMP) accumulation during exercise, possibly because of a greater accumulation of mitochondrial reduced nicotinamide adenine dinucleotide (NADH) (Dyck et al. 1996, 1993). Pi and AMP are indicators of the energy charge of the cell; high concentrations indicate low energy status, whereas low concentrations reflect ample energy availability. Because Pi and AMP are known to stimulate the enzyme glycogen phosphorylase, the reduction in Pi and AMP levels may be at least partially responsible for reduced muscle glycogen breakdown.

Some studies offer an alternative explanation for reduced muscle glycogen breakdown after elevation of plasma FA concentrations. When studied in more detail, the plasma FA concentrations appear significantly elevated (by infusion of TG and injection of heparin) compared with the control condition. The FA concentrations in the control condition, however, were below 0.2 mmol/L. Conceivably, these FA levels are too low to provide the muscle with sufficient fat substrate. As a result, muscle glycogen breakdown may have been increased in the control condition. Therefore, the observed "sparing" of glycogen with the high FA concentrations could have been caused by increased breakdown of glycogen in the control condition. Blocking lipolysis and reducing FA availability by giving nicotinic acid or a derivative increases muscle glycogen breakdown during exercise.

A more recent theory about the regulation of carbohydrate and fat metabolism proposes that fat does not regulate carbohydrate metabolism, but rather that carbohydrate regulates fat metabolism. An increase in the rate of glycolysis decreases fat oxidation. Figure 7.15 shows some of the factors that regulate carbohydrate and fat metabolism.

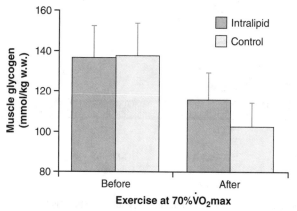

Figure 7.13 Glycogen "sparing" with increased FA availability. This increased availability of FAs was achieved by infusing a triacylglycerol emulsion with heparin.

Data from Costill et al. 1977.

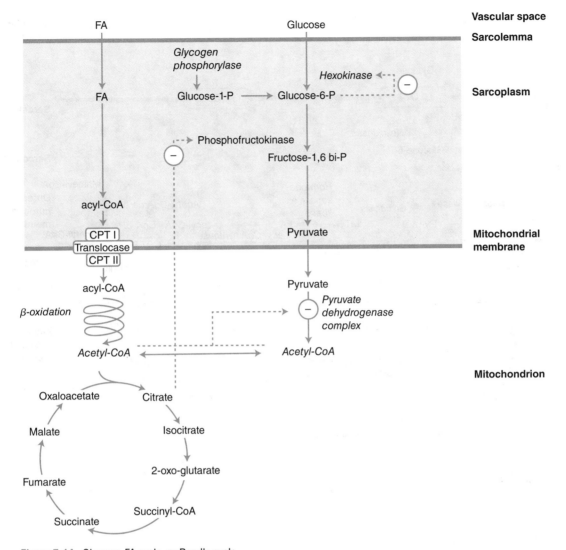

Figure 7.14 Glucose–FA cycle, or Randle cycle.

Reprinted, by permission, from A.E. Jeukendrup, 2002, "Regulation of fat metabolism in skeletal muscle," *New York Academy of Sciences* 967: 217-235.

Regulation of fat metabolism involves the transport of FAs into the mitochondria, which is controlled mainly by the activity of CPT I. CPT I is regulated by several factors, including the malonyl-CoA (a precursor of FA synthesis) concentration. The high rate of glycogenolysis during high-intensity exercise increases the amount of acetyl-CoA in the muscle cell, and some of this acetyl-CoA is converted to malonyl-CoA by the enzyme acetyl CoA carboxylase (ACC). Malonyl-CoA inhibits CPT I and could thus reduce the transport of FAs into the mitochondria. Although evidence suggests that malonyl-CoA may be an important regulator at rest, studies in exercising humans indicate no important role of malonyl-CoA (Odland et al. 1996, 1998). Reductions in intramuscular pH that may occur during high-intensity exercise may also inhibit CPT I and hence FA transport into the mitochondria (Starritt et al. 2000).

Another explanation is that reduced free carnitine concentration plays a role. When glycogenolysis accelerates, acetyl-CoA accumulates during intense exercise and some of this acetyl-CoA is bound to carnitine. As a result, the free carnitine concentration drops and less carnitine is available to transport FAs into the mitochondria (Greenhaff et al. 1998). Finally, it has been proposed that pyruvate-derived acetyl-CoA competes with the FA-derived acetyl-CoA for entrance into the TCA cycle.

The rate of carbohydrate utilization during prolonged strenuous exercise is closely related to the energy needs of the working muscle. In contrast, fat utilization during exercise is not tightly regulated. No mechanisms closely match the metabolism of FAs to energy expenditure. Fat oxidation is, therefore, mainly influenced by fat availability and the rate of carbohydrate utilization. The importance of each of these factors may

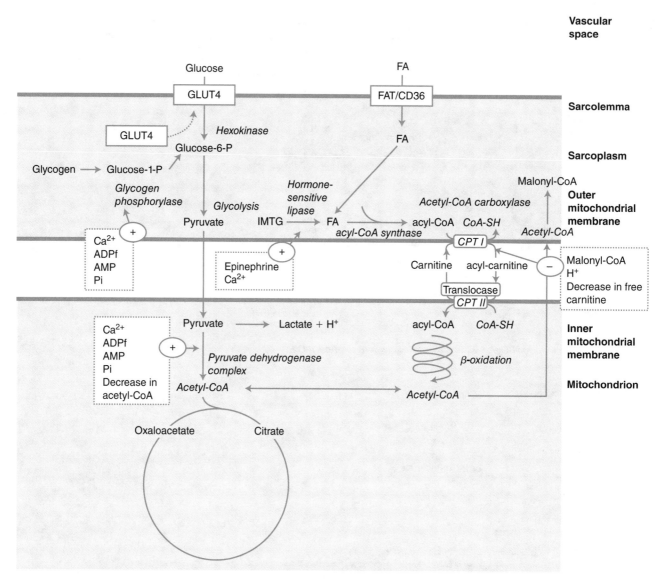

Figure 7.15 Glucose FA cycle reversed. An increase in glycolysis can reduce the FA transport into the mitochondria. CPT I = carnitine palmitoyl transferase I; CPT II = carnitine palmitoyl transferase II; ADPf = free ADP.

Reprinted, by permission, from A.E. Jeukendrup, 2002, "Regulation of metabolism in skeletal muscle," *New York Academy of Sciences* 967: 217-235.

depend on the situation. For example, carbohydrate utilization may be a more important factor during exercise, whereas the availability of FAs may be more important at rest.

Fat Supplementation and Exercise

The effects of eating fat before or during exercise have been studied as a method to increase FA availability and increase fat oxidation to reduce muscle glycogen breakdown. Initial studies looked at fatty meals consisting mainly of long-chain triacylglyerols (LCTs); later studies have also looked at alternative lipid fuels such as medium-chain triacylglycerols (MCTs).

Long-Chain Triacylglycerols

Nutritional fats include triacylglycerols (containing mostly C16 and C18 FAs), phospholipids, and cholesterol, of which only triacylglycerols can contribute to any extent to energy provision during exercise. In contrast to carbohydrates, nutritional fats reach the circulation slowly because they are potent inhibitors of gastric emptying. Furthermore, the digestion in the gut and absorption of fat are also rather slow processes compared with the digestion and absorption of carbohydrates.

Bile salts, produced by the liver, and lipase, secreted by the pancreas, are needed for lipolysis of the long-chain triacylglycerols (LCTs) into glycerol and three LCFAs or monoacylglycerol and two FAs.

The FAs diffuse into the intestinal mucosa cells and are reesterified in the cytoplasm to form LCTs. These LCTs are encapsulated by a coat of proteins, forming chylomicrons, to make them water soluble. These chylomicrons are then released in the lymphatic system, which ultimately drains in the systemic circulation. Exogenous LCTs enter the systemic circulation much more slowly than carbohydrates do, which are absorbed as glucose (or to minor extents, as fructose or galactose) and directly enter the main circulation through the portal vein. Long-chain dietary FAs typically enter the blood 3 to 4 hours after ingestion.

The fact that these LCFAs enter the circulation in chylomicrons is also important, and the rate of breakdown of chylomicron-bound triacylglycerols by muscle is generally believed to be relatively low. The primary role of these triacylglycerols in chylomicrons may be the replenishment of IMTG stores after exercise (Oscai et al. 1990). The intake of fat during exercise should therefore be avoided. Many so-called sports bars or energy bars, however, contain relatively large amounts of fat. Food labels of these products should be checked when choosing an energy bar.

Medium-Chain Triacylglycerols

Medium-chain triacylglycerols (MCTs) contain FAs with a chain length of C8 or C10. MCTs are normally present in our diet in extremely small quantities, and they have few natural sources. Intake from these sources is small, and, therefore, MCTs are often consumed as a supplement. MCTs are sold as a supplement to replace normal fat because MCTs are not stored in the body and could therefore help athletes lose body fat. MCT supplements are popular among bodybuilders and have been used as an alternative fuel source during exercise (see chapter 11).

Fish Oil

Fish oil is a natural source of long-chain omega-3 FAs. It contains both docosahexaenoic (DHA) and eicosapentaenoic acid (EPA). Fish oil is said to improve membrane characteristics and improve membrane function when more of these omega-3 FAs are incorporated into the lipid bilayer of the membrane (see chapter 11).

Effect of Diet on Fat Metabolism and Performance

Another strategy that has been used to increase fat oxidation and reduce reliance on carbohydrate stores has involved longer-term manipulations of the diet lasting days or weeks. These methods included fasting and high-fat, low-carbohydrate diets.

Fasting

Fasting has been proposed as a way to increase fat utilization, spare muscle glycogen, and improve exercise performance. In rats, short-term fasting increases plasma epinephrine and norepinephrine concentrations, stimulates lipolysis, and increases the concentration of circulating plasma FAs. These effects, in turn, increase fat oxidation and "spare" muscle glycogen, leading to a similar (Koubi et al. 1991) or even increased running time to exhaustion in rats (Dohm et al. 1983). In humans, fasting also results in increased concentration of circulating catecholamines, increased lipolysis, increased concentration of plasma FAs (Dohm et al. 1986), and decreased glucose turnover (Knapik et al. 1988). Muscle glycogen concentrations, however, are unaffected by fasting for 24 hours when no strenuous exercise is performed (Knapik et al. 1988; Loy et al. 1986). Although fasting has been reported to have no effect on endurance capacity at low exercise intensities (45% of $\dot{V}O_2max$), decreases in performance have been observed for exercise intensities between 50% and 100% of $\dot{V}O_2max$. The observed decreased performance was not reversible by carbohydrate ingestion during exercise (Riley et al. 1988).

Some investigators argued that the effects observed in most of these studies were seen because, in the control situation, the last meal was provided 3 hours before the exercise to exhaustion. The effects, therefore, result from the improvement in endurance capacity after feeding rather than from decreased performance after fasting. But the studies that compared a prolonged fast (>24 hours) to a 12-hour fast also reported decreased performance (Knapik et al. 1988; Maughan and Gleeson 1988; Zinker et al. 1990), and thus the conclusion that fasting decreases endurance capacity seems justified. The mechanism remains unclear, although certainly liver glycogen stores are substantially depleted after a 24-hour fast. Thus, euglycemia may not be as well maintained during exercise. Some degree of metabolic acidosis may also be observed after prolonged fasting. When hepatic glycogen stores are exhausted (e.g., after 12 to 24 hours of total fasting), the liver produces ketone bodies (acetoacetate, β-hydroxybutyrate, and acetone) to provide an energy substrate for peripheral tissues. These keto-acids lower blood pH, although the acidosis is usually only mild.

Short-Term High-Fat Diet

Christensen and Hansen (1939) showed that short-term exposure to a high-fat diet resulted in impaired fatigue resistance. After muscle biopsy techniques were redeveloped, a high-fat, low-carbohydrate diet was shown to result in decreased muscle glycogen levels, and this was the main factor causing lack of fatigue resistance during prolonged exercise (Bergstrom and Hultman 1967b; Hultman 1967). Plasma FA concentrations increase at rest and increase more rapidly when a low-carbohydrate diet is consumed (Conlee et al. 1990; Martin et al. 1978; Maughan et al. 1978). These changes in plasma FA concentrations are attributed to changes in the rate of lipolysis. After consumption of a low-carbohydrate diet, both plasma FAs and plasma glycerol concentrations increase.

Jansson and Kaijser (1982) reported that the uptake of FAs by the muscle during 25 minutes of cycling at 65% of $\dot{V}O_2$max was 82% higher in subjects receiving a low-carbohydrate diet (5%) for 5 days, compared with subjects receiving a high-carbohydrate diet (75%) for 5 days. Plasma FAs contributed 24% and 14%, respectively, to energy expenditure. Increased FA concentrations in the blood after a period of carbohydrate restriction leads to increased ketogenesis with elevated plasma levels of β-hydroxybutyrate and acetoacetate. After a few days of high-fat feeding, the ketone body production increases 5-fold (Fery and Balasse 1983) and the arterial concentration of ketone bodies may increase 10- to 20-fold (Fery and Balasse 1983). During the first phase of light to moderate exercise, ketone body concentrations usually decline, and after 30 to 90 minutes, they increase again (Fery and Balasse 1983; Knapik et al. 1988; Zinker et al. 1990). But the observed plasma concentrations under those conditions are still higher after a high-fat diet compared with those associated with a low-fat diet. Carbohydrate-restricted diets may also lead to increased breakdown of muscle triacylglycerols.

Long-Term High-Fat Diet

A 3- to 4-day alteration in dietary composition has been suggested to be an insufficient time to induce an adaptive response to the changed diet. A high-fat diet over a prolonged period, however, may result in decreased utilization of carbohydrates and increased contribution of fat to energy metabolism. In rats, adaptation to a high-fat diet leads to considerable improvements in

endurance capacity (Miller et al. 1984; Simi et al. 1991) (see figure 7.16). These adaptations can be attributed to the increased number of oxidative enzymes and decreased degradation of liver glycogen during exercise (Simi et al. 1991). The results suggest that after adaptation to a high-fat diet, the capacity to oxidize FAs instead of carbohydrates increases because of an adaptation of the oxidative enzymes in the muscle cell. These adaptations are much like the adaptations that occur after endurance training.

One of the first studies that investigated the effects of prolonged high-fat diets on humans was conducted by Phinney et al. (1980). They investigated exercise performance in obese subjects who followed a high-fat diet (90% of energy intake from fat) for 6 weeks. Before and after the diet, subjects exercised at 75% of $\dot{V}O_2$max until exhaustion. Subjects were able to exercise as long on the high-fat diet as they did on their normal diet, but after the high-fat diet, fat became the main substrate. Results of this study, however, may have been influenced by the fact that these subjects were not in energy balance and lost 11 kg of body weight. So, although no differences were seen in absolute $\dot{V}O_2$max before and after the dietary period, considerable differences were apparent in relative exercise intensity.

The observed improvement in performance may have been an artifact rather than a positive effect of the adaptation period. Therefore, Phinney and colleagues (Phinney, Bistrian, Evans, et al. 1983; Phinney, Bistrian, Wolfe, and Blackburn 1983) conducted a follow-up study in which trained subjects were studied before and after a 4-week high-fat diet (< 20 g/day of carbohydrates). The diet reduced the preexercise muscle glycogen concentration by 50%,

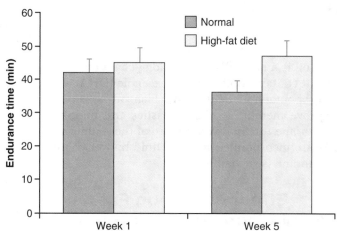

Figure 7.16 Running performance with high-fat diets in rats.
Data from Miller, Bryce, and Conlee 1984.

but no difference in the average time to exhaustion at 62% to 64% of V̇O₂max before and after the diet was found. The results are difficult to interpret, however, because of the large variability of the subjects' performance times (times to exhaustion). One subject exercised 57% longer, whereas other subjects showed no improvement or even had decreased times to exhaustion. In addition, exercise intensity was relatively low and subjects' reliance on carbohydrates during exercise at 62% to 64% of V̇O₂max was low. In such a situation, reduced carbohydrate stores may not be limiting. At higher exercise intensities, performance may have been impaired. Nevertheless, the fact that performance did not decline in all subjects, even though muscle glycogen levels measured before exercise decreased by almost 50% and fat oxidation during exercise increased markedly, is remarkable. These observations have been attributed to enzymatic adaptations (including a 44% increase in carnitine palmitoyl transferase activity and a 46% decrease in hexokinase activity) (Phinney, Bistrian, Evans, et al. 1983). In subsequent studies, maintained or improved performance was seen at relatively low exercise intensities (60% to 65% of V̇O₂max), which are far below the intensities observed during competition. How these results translate into practical applications in training and competition for most athletes is unclear.

Eating large amounts of fat has been associated with the development of obesity and cardiovascular disease. Whether this association is true for athletes is not known. Few studies have described the effects of high-fat diets on cardiovascular risk factors in athletes who train regularly. Pendergast et al. (1996) reported no changes in plasma LDL, HDL, or total cholesterol levels in male and female runners with diets in the range of 17% to 40% fat. Although the risk of obesity and cardiovascular disease increases with the consumption of high-fat diets in sedentary people, regular exercise or endurance training seems to attenuate these risks (Sarna and Kaprio 1994). Exposure to high-fat diets has also been associated with insulin resistance, which has traditionally been linked to an effect of the IMTG pools on glucose uptake (Pan et al. 1997). This observation was made in obese subjects, however, and whether these results can be extrapolated to athletes is not clear, especially because athletes seem to have larger IMTG stores and increased insulin sensitivity. Because little information is available about the negative effects of high-fat diets on athletes, and because the effects of these diets on performance are unclear, we

suggest caution when recommending high-fat diets to athletes.

Although chronic high-fat diets induce persistent enzymatic adaptations in skeletal muscle that favor fat oxidation, the effects on performance may not be visible because muscle glycogen levels are suboptimal. A period of adaptation to a high-fat diet, followed by acute carbohydrate feeding, might theoretically induce the enzymatic adaptations in the muscle while also allowing optimizing of preexercise glycogen stores. If the high glycogen levels are accompanied by a slightly lower rate of glycogenolysis, an improvement in exercise capacity is expected. Indeed, in rats after 3 to 8 weeks of adaptation to a high-fat diet (0% to 25% carbohydrate) followed by 3 days of carbohydrate feeding (70% carbohydrate), muscle and liver glycogen were restored to extremely high levels.

In humans, Helge et al. (1998) studied trained subjects who, after 7 weeks of adaptation to a high-fat diet (62% fat, 21% carbohydrate), changed to a high-carbohydrate diet (65% carbohydrate, 20% fat) for 1 week (see figure 7.17). A control group followed a high-carbohydrate diet for 8 weeks. Although exercise time to exhaustion increased from week 7 to week 8 in the subjects who received a high-fat diet followed by the high-carbohydrate diet, their performance was inferior to those in the group that received the high-carbohydrate diet for 8 weeks. Because switching to a high-carbohydrate diet after 7 weeks of a high-fat diet did not reverse the negative effects, these authors concluded that the negative effects of 7 weeks of a high-fat diet on performance are caused not simply by a lack of carbohydrate as a fuel but rather by suboptimal adaptations to the training (i.e., improvements in

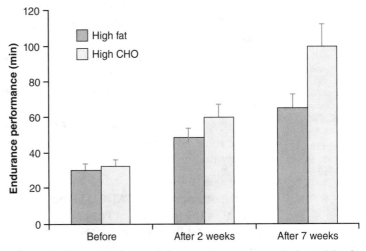

Figure 7.17 High-fat diets and performance improvements during training in humans.

Data from Helge et al. 1998 and Helge et al. 1996.

endurance capacity were smaller compared with the group that consumed the high-carbohydrate diet).

In another study by Burke et al. (1999), trained cyclists received a high-fat diet for a relatively short period (5 days), followed by a day of carbohydrate loading on day 6. On day 7 substrate oxidation during exercise was measured, and a performance ride followed. No significant performance improvement was observed. The potential benefits of an adaptation period to a high-fat diet followed by a period of carbohydrate loading are not clear. A fat-adaptation period beyond 4 weeks may decrease exercise performance, which cannot be reversed by a week on a high-carbohydrate diet.

Although the hypothesis that chronic high-fat diets may increase the capacity to oxidize fat and improve exercise performance during competition is attractive, little evidence indicates that it is true. The available studies that indicate a positive effect on performance were conducted at exercise intensities lower than typical intensities during competition.

Recently, another explanation for the apparent adaptations in fat metabolism was brought forward. Stellingwerff et al. (2006) found reduced pyruvate dehydrogenase activation after fat adaptation. This finding could indicate that the increase in fat oxidation is at least partly caused by a reduction in the ability to oxidize carbohydrate because pyruvate dehydrogenase is a key enzyme in carbohydrate metabolism catalyzing the conversion of pyruvate to acetyl-CoA in the mitochondrion, and thus controlling the entry of substrate into the TCA cycle.

Therefore, additional well-controlled studies are needed to clarify the importance of the effect of dietary carbohydrate and fat content on athletic performance. At this time, because little information is available about the negative effects of high-fat diets for athletes, caution should be exercised when recommending a high-fat diet to athletes.

Supplements That Increase Fat Oxidation

Several nutritional supplements on the market are claimed to increase fat oxidation, increase fat loss and lean body mass, and promote weight loss. Supplements that have been associated with fat oxidation are

- caffeine,
- pyruvate,
- carnitine,
- vanadium (vanadyl-sulphate),
- chromium,
- yohimbine, and
- dihydroxyacetone.

Caffeine is thought to stimulate lipolysis and the mobilization of FAs. Carnitine is believed to help transport FAs into the mitochondria. Pyruvate and dihydroxyacetone are often sold as supplements to increase fat oxidation. Similarly, the trace elements chromium and vanadium are claimed to promote fat oxidation and promote weight loss (see chapter 11 for further details).

KEY POINTS

- In contrast to carbohydrate stores, fat stores are large in humans and are regarded as practically unlimited. The stores of fat are located mainly in adipose tissue, but significant amounts also exist as IMTGs.

- The steps that could potentially limit fat oxidation are lipolysis, removal of FAs from the fat cell, transport of fat by the bloodstream, transport of FAs into the muscle cell, transport of FAs into the mitochondria, or oxidation of FAs in the β-oxidation pathway and TCA cycle.

- Most FAs are stored in the form of triacylglycerols in subcutaneous adipose tissue, and FAs are released along with glycerol after the breakdown of triacylglycerols (lipolysis) by the enzyme hormone-sensitive lipase.

- Most FAs in the blood (>99.9%) are bound to albumin.

- Transporter proteins (FAT/CD36) have been identified that are likely to be responsible for most of the transport of FAs across the sarcolemma. After they are in the muscle cell, FAs are bound to FA-binding proteins.

- In the muscle, FAs are stored as IMTG, which can provide an important fuel during exercise.

- The enzyme CPT I plays a crucial role in the transport of FAs into the mitochondria.

■ Carbohydrate and fat are always oxidized as a mixture, and the relative contribution of these two substrates depends on exercise intensity and duration, the level of aerobic fitness, diet, and carbohydrate intake before and during exercise.

■ In absolute terms, fat oxidation increases as exercise intensity increases from low to moderate levels, although the percentage contribution of fat may actually decrease. At higher intensities of exercise (>75% of $\dot{V}O_2$max), fat oxidation is inhibited and both the relative and absolute rates of fat oxidation decrease to negligible values. In trained people, the maximal rates of fat oxidation were observed at 63% of $\dot{V}O_2$max.

■ Diet also has marked effects on fat oxidation. Generally a high-carbohydrate, low-fat diet reduces fat oxidation, whereas a high-fat, low-carbohydrate diet increases fat oxidation.

■ Carbohydrate feeding before exercise reduces fat oxidation by reducing lipolysis and plasma FA availability and by inhibiting the carnitine-dependent FA transport into the mitochondria.

■ The rate of carbohydrate utilization during prolonged strenuous exercise is closely related to the energy needs of the working muscle. In contrast, fat utilization during exercise is not tightly regulated. No mechanisms exist that closely match the metabolism of FAs to energy expenditure. Fat oxidation is therefore mainly influenced by fat availability and the rate of carbohydrate utilization.

■ Long-chain triacylglycerol ingestion during exercise is not desirable because they slow gastric emptying, they appear only slowly in the systemic circulation, and they enter the systemic circulation in chylomicrons, which are believed to be an insignificant fuel source during exercise.

■ Medium-chain triacylglycerols (MCTs) are rapidly emptied from the stomach, absorbed, and oxidized, but the ingestion of larger amounts of MCTs resulted in gastrointestinal distress. When ingested in smaller amounts MCTs do not appear to have the positive effects on performance that are often claimed.

■ Fasting increases the availability of lipid substrates, resulting in increased oxidation of FAs at rest and during exercise. But because the liver glycogen stores are not maintained, fatigue resistance and exercise performance are impaired.

■ High-fat diets for 3 to 5 days increase the availability of lipid substrates but reduce the storage of glycogen. As a result, fat oxidation increases during exercise, but fatigue resistance and exercise performance are compromised.

■ Although the hypothesis that chronic high-fat diets may increase the capacity to oxidize fat and improve exercise performance during competition is attractive, little evidence indicates that the hypothesis is true.

RECOMMENDED READINGS

Hawley, J.A., F. Brouns, and A. Jeukendrup. 1998. Strategies to enhance fat utilization during exercise. *Sports Medicine* 26:241–257.

Jeukendrup, A.E. 1999. Dietary fat and physical performance. *Current Opinion in Clinical Nutrition Metabolic Care* 2:521–526.

Jeukendrup, A.E. 2002. Regulation of skeletal muscle fat metabolism. *Annals of the New York Academy of Science* 967:217–35.

Jeukendrup, A.E. 2003. Modulation of carbohydrate and fat utilization by diet, exercise and environment. *Biochemical Society Transactions* 31: 270–1273.

Jeukendrup, A.E., W.H.M. Saris, and A.J.M. Wagenmakers. 1998. Fat metabolism during exercise: A review. Part I: Fatty acid mobilization and muscle metabolism. *International Journal of Sports Medicine* 19:231–244.

Jeukendrup, A.E., W.H.M. Saris, and A.J.M. Wagenmakers. 1998. Fat metabolism during exercise: A review. Part II: Regulation of metabolism and the effects of training. *International Journal of Sports Medicine* 19:293–302.

Jeukendrup, A.E., W.H.M. Saris, and A.J.M. Wagenmakers. 1998. Fat metabolism during exercise: A review. Part III: Effects of nutritional interventions. *International Journal of Sports Medicine* 19:371–379.

Van der Vusse, G.J., and R.S. Reneman. 1996. Lipid metabolism in muscle. In *Handbook of physiology*, Section 12, eds. L.B. Rowell and J.T. Shephard. New York: Oxford University Press.

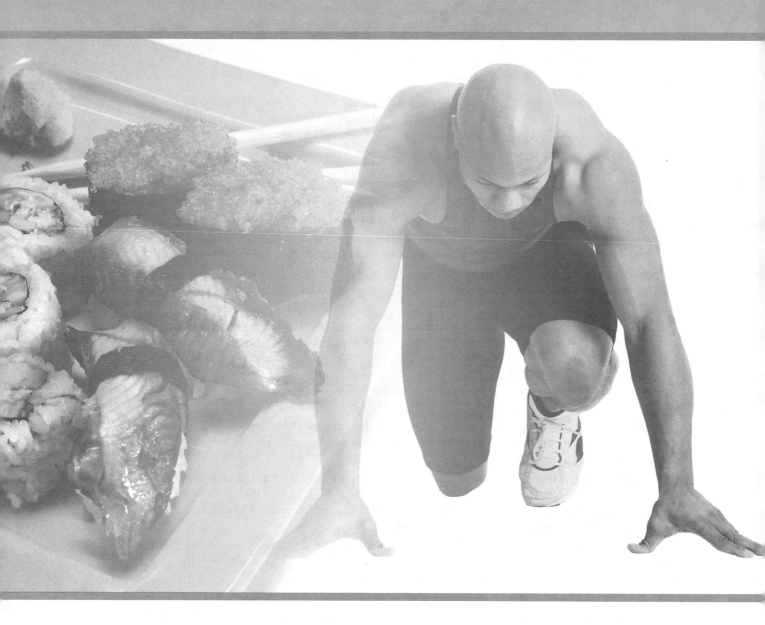

OBJECTIVES

After studying this chapter, you should be able to do the following:

- Give a general description of amino acids and name the most abundant amino acids

- Give a general description of protein and amino acid metabolism

- Describe the effects of training on body proteins

- List techniques available to study protein metabolism and to discuss the advantages and disadvantages of these techniques

- Discuss the contribution of protein to energy expenditure at rest and during exercise

- Discuss the effect of exercise and feeding on protein synthesis and breakdown

- Describe the recommendations for protein intake generally given for strength and endurance athletes

- Discuss the need for protein supplementation in athletes

- Describe the potential health hazards of excess intake of protein

- Discuss the effects of ingesting single amino acids

8

Protein
and Amino Acids

Key Terms

Debate has long raged over how much dietary protein is required for optimal athletic performance. Because muscle plays a crucial role in exercise performance and contains the largest proportion of the protein in a human body (about 40%), the presence of this controversy is not surprising. Body proteins are continually "turning over," that is, they are constantly being synthesized and degraded to maintain optimal function. Proteins turn over at different rates, ranging from minutes to days. Despite the mass of protein in muscle, however, its rate of protein turnover accounts for only 25% to 35% of total protein turnover in the body. Muscle proteins turn over quite slowly compared with, for example, blood proteins. The most abundant proteins in muscle are the contractile proteins actin and myosin. Together they account for approximately 80% to 90% of all muscle protein. Both the structural proteins that make up the myofibrils and the proteins that act as enzymes within a muscle cell change as an adaptation to exercise training. Indeed, muscle mass, muscle protein content, and muscle protein composition change in response to training (see chapter 12).

Interest in protein consumption is high among amateur and professional athletes. Therefore, the fact that meat, which contains high-quality protein (high biological value), is a popular protein source for athletes (especially strength athletes) is not surprising. This preference for meat probably dates back to ancient Greece, where athletes in preparation for Olympic Games consumed large quantities of meat.

A strong belief, especially among strength athletes, is that a large protein intake or the ingestion of certain protein or amino acid supplements increases muscle mass and strength. Despite the long history of protein use in sport, debate continues even over questions such as whether protein requirements are greater in athletes. Protein and amino acid metabolism is complex, and many organs and tissues are involved. Thus, no uniform opinion exists about what should be measured as an endpoint. For example, the effectiveness of protein intake or supplements could be assessed by measuring performance, muscle mass, or strength, or it could be measured by nitrogen balance (nitrogen balance is essentially the balance of protein because nitrogen in our diets comes exclusively from protein) over several days or by short-term methods involving the incorporation of labeled amino acids into muscle proteins.

The use of different techniques to estimate protein turnover may give different results. Therefore, the principles of the techniques and their limita-

tions must be understood. This chapter discusses the various techniques available to investigate protein metabolism. Then, a brief overview of protein and amino acid metabolism is given. Subsequently, protein metabolism during exercise and dietary protein needs for endurance and strength-training athletes are examined. Finally, the effects of supplementing the diet with various individual amino acids are discussed.

Amino Acids

Muscle contains all the naturally occurring amino acids, and thus both meat and dairy products are valuable foods (both have high biological value; dairy sources have higher values). The most abundant amino acids in muscle are the branched-chain amino acids (BCAAs) leucine, valine, and isoleucine, which together account for 20% of the total amino acids found in muscle protein. Both meat and dairy protein have high BCAA content.

Amino Acid Transport

The concentrations of amino acids in muscle and in blood differ, suggesting that maintaining these concentration gradients is important. Because concentration gradients of amino acids differ, different transporters move individual or groups of amino acids across membranes. Amino acid transporters are membrane-bound proteins that recognize specific amino acid shapes and chemical properties (e.g., neutral, basic, or anionic). The transporters are divided into sodium-dependent and sodium-independent carriers. Generally, the sodium-dependent transporters maintain a larger gradient than the sodium-independent transporters. Note that all these transporters are facilitative and usually coupled to cotransport with sodium and thus are not directly energy dependent. To date, some transporter proteins have been identified, but many more are yet to be discovered.

Amino Acid Metabolism

The metabolism of most amino acids is linked to the metabolism of other amino acids, and some amino acids can be synthesized from other amino acids. This feature is especially important in conditions of limited dietary protein intake or when metabolic requirements increase. Some amino acids are essential and are not synthesized in the body, whereas others can be synthesized in the body (nonessential amino acids) (see chapter 1, figure 1.6 [p. 16]).

Amino acids are involved in a variety of biochemical and physiological processes, some of which are common to all and some of which are highly specific to certain amino acids. Amino acids are constantly incorporated into proteins (protein synthesis), and proteins are constantly broken down (protein breakdown or degradation). This constant turnover of proteins is summarized in figure 8.1. The vast majority of the amino acids in the body are incorporated into tissue proteins, but a small pool of free amino acids also exists (about 120 g of free amino acids is present in the skeletal muscle of an adult). Amino acids are constantly extracted from the free amino acid pool for synthesis of various proteins, and breakdown of protein (protein degradation) makes amino acids available for the free amino acid pool.

Protein Breakdown

The breakdown of protein serves three main purposes:

1. It degrades potentially damaged proteins to prevent a decline in their function. Note that there is usually a net replacement of these degraded proteins (see figure 8.1).

2. It provides energy when some of its individual amino acids are converted into acetyl-CoA or TCA-cycle intermediates and are oxidized in the mitochondria.

3. Individual amino acids can be used for the synthesis of other compounds, including neurotransmitters (e.g., serotonin), hormones (e.g., epinephrine), and other peptides and proteins.

This breakdown of protein and incorporation of the amino acids into a new protein links protein degradation with protein synthesis. Amino acids can also be incorporated into compounds that are not proteins. In this case, the body loses protein. For example, some amino acids are converted into glucose (gluconeogenesis), ketones (ketogenesis), or fat (lipogenesis) and subsequently stored in adipose tissue.

Before amino acids can be oxidized, the amino group must be removed. Removal of the amino group can be achieved for some amino acids by transferring it to another molecule called a keto-acid, which results in the formation of a different amino acid. This process, called transamination, is catalyzed by enzymes called aminotransferases. A good example is the transfer of the amino group

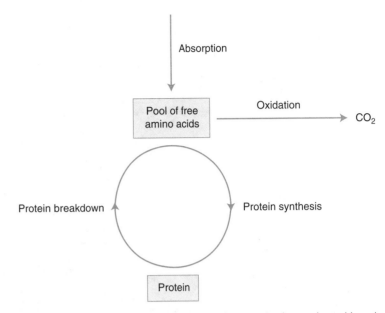

Figure 8.1 Protein metabolism. Amino acids enter the free amino acid pool from the diet (absorption) or from breakdown of protein. Amino acids leave the free amino acid pool for protein synthesis or oxidation to CO_2.

from the amino acid leucine to the keto-acid α-ketoglutarate forming α-ketoisocaproate (which can be further metabolized to form acetyl-CoA) and glutamate, respectively. Each amino acid has its own, unique corresponding keto-acid. Alternatively, the amino group can be removed from the amino acid to form free ammonia (NH_3), in a process called oxidative deamination. One example is the breakdown of asparagine to form aspartate and NH_3. Because free ammonia is a toxic substance, it is used either to form glutamine from glutamate within the muscle or is transported to the liver, where it is converted to urea and eventually excreted by the kidneys. Both ammonia and urea can be excreted in urine and sweat.

After the removal of the amino group from an amino acid, the remaining carbon skeleton (the keto-acid) is eventually oxidized to CO_2 in the TCA cycle. The carbon skeleton of amino acids can enter the TCA cycle in several ways. Some can be converted to acetyl-CoA and enter the TCA cycle just like acetyl-CoA from carbohydrate or fat. They can also enter the TCA cycle as α-ketoglutarate or **oxaloacetate** as metabolites of glutamate and aspartate, respectively (see figure 8.2).

Some amino acids can serve as glucogenic or lipogenic (ketogenic) precursors. The amino acids that can be converted into α-ketoglutarate, oxaloacetate, or pyruvate can also be used for the synthesis of glucose in the liver (gluconeogenesis). Amino acids or keto-acids that are eventually broken

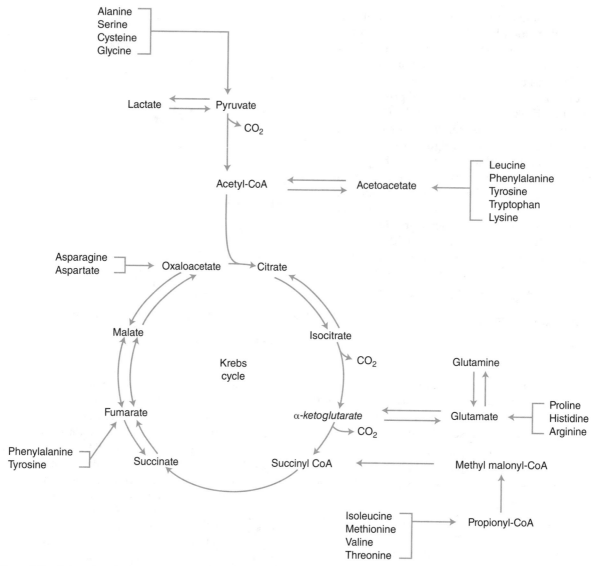

Figure 8.2 Interactions between amino acids and the TCA cycle.

down to acetyl-CoA can also be used in the synthesis of FAs. Acetyl-CoA units can be used in an elongation process to form "longer" FAs by adding on to the hydrocarbon chain of the 16-carbon FA, palmitate. The following are examples of some common aminotransferase reactions:

L-glutamate + oxaloacetate → α-ketoglutarate + L-aspartate

L-alanine + α-ketoglutarate → pyruvate + L-glutamate

Several amino acids undergo reversible transamination. These amino acids include alanine, aspartate, glutamate, and the BCAAs—leucine, isoleucine, and valine. The BCAAs are the only essential amino acids that can undergo transamination. Transamination is usually rapid, and the main limiting factor is the fact that these pro-

Amino Acids That Can Undergo Transamination With Glutamate

- Leucine
- Valine
- Isoleucine
- Alanine
- Aspartate
- Glutamine
- NH_3 + α-ketoglutarate

cesses sometimes take place in different tissues. Amino acids thus have to be transported by the circulation. Glutamate serves a central role in these transamination reactions because several amino acids can undergo transamination with glutamate (see highlight box on p. 172).

Most of the nitrogen from amino acid degradation is transferred to α-ketoglutarate to form glutamate and subsequently glutamine; these two amino acids (glutamate and glutamine) are the most abundant free amino acids in muscle. Although all carbon skeletons of amino acids can be used for oxidation, only 6 of the available 20 amino acids in protein are oxidized in significant amounts by muscle—asparagine, aspartate, glutamate, isoleucine, leucine, and valine. An outline of the pathways involved in degradation of the various amino acids is provided in table 8.1.

■ TABLE 8.1 ■
Pathways of Amino Acid Degradation

Metabolic pathway	Important enzymes	Nitrogen end product	Carbon end product
AMINO ACIDS CONVERTED TO OTHER AMINO ACIDS			
Asparagine	Asparaginase	Aspartate + NH_3	
Glutamine	Glutaminase	Glutamate + NH_3	
Arginine	Arginase	Ornithine + urea	
Phenylalanine	Phenylalanine hydroxylase	Tyrosine	
Proline		Glutamate	
Cysteine		Taurine	
TRANSAMINATION TO FORM GLUTAMATE			
Alanine		Glutamate	Pyruvate
Aspartate		Glutamate	Oxaloacetate
Leucine		Glutamate	Ketones
Isoleucine		Glutamate	Succinate
Valine		Glutamate	Succinate
Ornithine		Two glutamates	α-ketoglutarate
Tyrosine		Glutamate	Ketone + fumarate
Cysteine		Glutamate	Ketone + SO_4^{2-}
OTHER PATHWAYS			
Serine	Serine dehydratase	NH_3	Pyruvate
Threonine	Threonine dehydratase	NH_3	Ketobutyrate
Histidine	Histidase	NH_3	Urocanate
Tryptophan		NH_3	Kynurenine
Glycine		NH_3	CO_2
Methionine		NH_3	Ketobutyrate
Lysine		Two glutamates	Acetate

Adapted from Matthews 1999.

Amino Acid Synthesis

The discussion of synthesis of amino acids is by definition limited to the nonessential amino acids because the essential amino acids cannot be synthesized in the body. Figure 8.3 provides a summary of the synthetic pathways of nonessential amino acids. Again, glutamate plays a central role. Glutamate serves as the donor of nitrogen in the synthesis of many amino acids, which occurs by transferring NH_3 to a carbon skeleton precursor (keto-acid) from the TCA cycle, from another nonessential amino acid, or from an essential amino acid.

Synthesis of amino acids by the transfer of NH_3 to a carbon skeleton precursor from the TCA cycle is rarely limited because of the ample availability of the substrates (carbon skeleton precursors and NH_3). On the other hand, synthesis of amino acids from other amino acids can sometimes be limited because of limited dietary supply. Cysteine and tyrosine are special cases because they are synthe-

sized from essential amino acids and are therefore indirectly dependent on adequate protein (and thus amino acid) intake.

Incorporation of Amino Acids Into Protein

Different proteins are synthesized and degraded at different rates. Generally, the proteins that have a regulatory function (such as enzymes) or that act as signals (hormones) have a relatively rapid rate of turnover (minutes, hours, or days). The structural proteins, such as collagen and contractile proteins (actin and myosin), have a relatively slow turnover (days, weeks, or months). In humans who are weight stable, the overall synthesis and degradation of proteins must be in balance, which means that the amount of nitrogen consumed in the diet equals the amount of nitrogen excreted in urine, feces, and other routes.

Protein turnover is several times greater than protein intake, as is illustrated in figure 8.4 for a healthy 70 kg (154 lb) person. A normal daily protein intake is approximately 90 g. In this example, the intake of protein provides only about 25% of the amino acids that enter the free amino acid pool each day (340 g). Most of the amino acids that appear in and disappear from the free amino acid pool are derived from proteins in the gut, kidneys, and liver. Although this protein is a relatively small portion of the total mass of protein, it represents about two-thirds of the total protein turnover because of the rapid turnover in these tissues. Muscle has a relatively slow protein turnover and provides most of the remainder. Various techniques are used to study protein metabolism, including nitrogen balance. These techniques are reviewed later in this chapter.

Incorporation of Amino Acids Into Other Compounds

Amino acids are used for the synthesis of amino acid–like compounds. A list of the most important products is provided in table 8.2. Amino acids glutamate, tyrosine, and tryptophan, for example, are precursors of neurotransmitters. Glutamate is a special amino acid in this respect because it is not only a precursor of neurotransmitters but also a neurotransmitter. Tyrosine is the precursor of catecholamines (dopamine, ephinephrine, and norepinephrine) and tryptophan is the precursor of serotonin (5-hydroxytryptamine). The roles of amino acids as precursors of creatine and carnitine synthesis are discussed in detail in chapter 11.

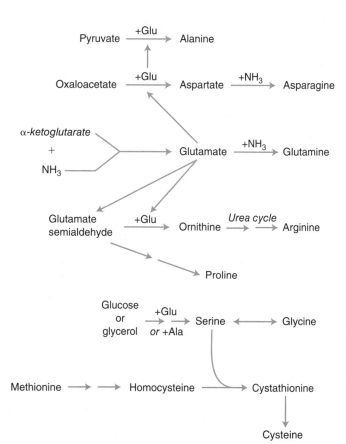

Figure 8.3 Synthetic pathways of the nonessential amino acids. Glu = glutamate; Ala = alanine.

Adapted from Matthews 1998.

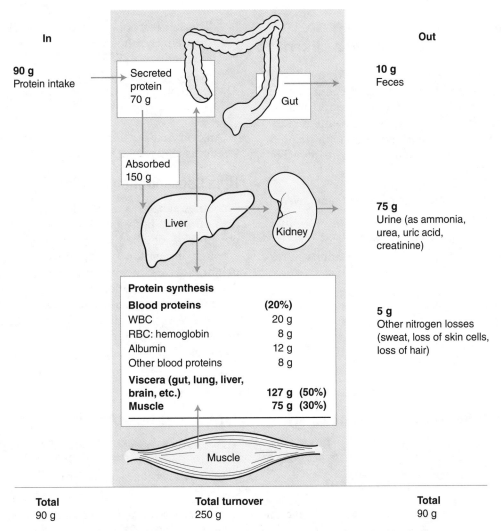

In
90 g
Protein intake

Out
10 g
Feces

Secreted protein 70 g

Gut

Absorbed 150 g

Liver

Kidney

75 g
Urine (as ammonia, urea, uric acid, creatinine)

Protein synthesis

Blood proteins	**(20%)**
WBC	20 g
RBC: hemoglobin	8 g
Albumin	12 g
Other blood proteins	8 g
Viscera (gut, lung, liver, brain, etc.)	**127 g (50%)**
Muscle	**75 g (30%)**

5 g
Other nitrogen losses (sweat, loss of skin cells, loss of hair)

Muscle

Total
90 g

Total turnover
250 g

Total
90 g

Figure 8.4   Daily protein balance in humans. RBC = red blood cells, WBC = white blood cells.
Adapted from Matthews 1998.

■ TABLE 8.2 ■

Products Synthesized From Amino Acids

Product	Synthesized from	Product	Synthesized from
Creatine	Arginine Glycine Methionine	Pyrimidines	Aspartate Glutamine
Glutathione	Cysteine Taurine Glutamine	Histamine	Histidine
		Carnitine	Lysine
Neurotransmitters	Glutamate Tyrosine Tryptophan	Choline Serine	Methionine
Purines	Aspartate Glutamine Glycine	T3, T4 Epinephrine	Tyrosine

Techniques to Study Protein and Amino Acid Metabolism

The following is a list of currently available techniques to study protein metabolism. These techniques range from simple techniques such as the measurement of urea in urine to complex techniques that involve expensive and sophisticated equipment in combination with more invasive techniques.

- Urea concentration in urine, blood, and sweat
- 3-methylhistidine in urine and blood (indication of myofibrillar protein breakdown)
- Nitrogen balance (nitrogen intake minus nitrogen excretion in sweat, feces, and urine)
- Arteriovenous measurements of amino acids across a tissue bed
- Radiolabeled isotopes
- Stable isotopes, including the following:

– Tracer incorporation into a specific protein (protein synthesis), often called fractional synthetic rate (FSR)

– Tracer release from a specific protein (protein breakdown), often called fractional breakdown rate (FBR)

An overview of these techniques, including their strengths and weaknesses, is given in table 8.3.

Urea Concentration in Urine

The amount of urea excreted in urine is an indication of whole-body protein breakdown but does not provide detailed information and gives only a rough indication of protein breakdown. The urinary urea concentration depends on many disturbing factors, such as the level of hydration and the diet (e.g., increasing or decreasing protein intake will result in increased or decreased urea production independent of changes in tissue protein breakdown). When urine is collected over 24

▪ **TABLE 8.3** ▪

Methods for Estimating Protein Metabolism

Method	Advantages	Disadvantages and limitations
Urea concentration in urine and sweat	Easy; relatively cheap	Only rough estimate; heavily affected by diet (protein intake)
3-methylhistidine in urine	Simple measure of myofibrillar protein breakdown	Only rough estimate of myofibrillar protein breakdown; requires strict control of meat intake; does not provide information about actual changes in muscle mass
Nitrogen balance (nitrogen intake minus nitrogen excretion in sweat and urine)	Accurate method when used over relatively long periods	Difficult and time consuming; tends to overestimate nitrogen retention; usually ignores nitrogen loss in sweat; highly dependent on subject compliance; gives no insight into metabolic pathways
Arteriovenous measurements of amino acids across a tissue bed	Gives information about net exchange of amino acids across a tissue; net uptake of essential amino acids related to rate of protein synthesis	Invasive; can have high variability, depending on blood flow measurement
Radiolabeled isotopes	Relatively cheap; relatively easy to measure; small amounts of tracer needed	Potential health risk
Stable isotopes	No health risk	Relatively expensive; sophisticated equipment needed for analyses
Tracer incorporation into a specific protein (protein synthesis)	Gives direct information about protein synthesis in a tissue	Invasive (tissue biopsies needed); relatively expensive; sophisticated equipment needed for analyses
Fractional synthetic rate (FSR) and fractional breakdown rate (FBR)	Uses stable isotopes so no health risk	Short-term measurement; does not provide information about actual changes in muscle mass; relatively expensive; sophisticated equipment needed for analyses

hours, the results become slightly more meaningful because total daily urea excretion can be determined, but the results are still highly dependent on protein intake.

Nitrogen Balance

Most experts in various countries have used nitrogen balance studies to determine the recommended dietary intakes for protein. Subjects are fed a diet with a certain level of protein intake, and for a time (3 to 14 days), urine and feces are collected over 24-hour periods. The nitrogen intake (protein intake) and nitrogen excretion are measured as accurately as possible. A week or more may be required before collection reflects the adaptations to a particular diet.

Nitrogen excretion can be measured from urine, feces, and sweat. Nitrogen is detectable in feces because not all protein is completely absorbed, and some of the nitrogen secreted (often in the form of cells from the GI tract itself) into the gastrointestinal tract is not reabsorbed. When nitrogen balance is measured in exercising subjects, nitrogen excretion in sweat is substantial and must be included in the measurements. Nitrogen is excreted mainly in the form of urea (about 90%) but also in creatinine, ammonia, uric acid, and other nitrogen-containing compounds. Urinary nitrogen is often the only measure taken and assumptions are made for the excretion in sweat and feces, but nitrogen excretion may be underestimated when using this measure alone.

When nitrogen intake exceeds excretion, a person is in positive nitrogen balance and so must be retaining nitrogen (i.e., protein). When nitrogen excretion exceeds nitrogen intake, a person is in negative nitrogen balance and thus nitrogen or protein loss is occurring. The latter situation cannot continue for a long time. The body uses protein, and because it does not contain large stores of protein, the breakdown and atrophy of tissues and organs will occur. Only when nitrogen intake matches nitrogen excretion is a person in nitrogen balance.

Although the estimation of nitrogen balance is an often-used technique, it is not easy to apply, and it has been criticized for numerous reasons. The technique is time consuming and involves several 24-hour periods of urine collection. It is labor intensive for the investigators. Its success is highly dependent on subject compliance. This technique also tends to underestimate nitrogen excretion and thus overestimate nitrogen retention, and it gives only a measure of the net nitrogen balance. Because of its "black box" nature, the technique does not provide any insight into the metabolic pathways involved in changes in protein metabolism. Furthermore, nitrogen balance measurements, especially at high protein intakes, often result in physiologically impossible estimates of positive nitrogen balance. For example, in some studies weightlifters who ate approximately 2.5 g protein/kg of body weight per day had positive nitrogen balances of about 17 g/day. That number would represent about 110 kg of lean tissue gained in 1 year! Clearly, this number cannot possibly be correct, and the methodology must be in error. Nevertheless, done properly and with the appropriate understanding of the limitations, important information may be gleaned from nitrogen balance studies.

3-Methylhistidine Excretion

Another method of estimating protein metabolism is the measurement of 3-methylhistidine or N-methylhistidine excretion in the urine. When proteins are degraded, 3-methylhistidine cannot be recycled within the muscle and is excreted in the urine. The amount of 3-methylhistidine in urine is, therefore, a measure of contractile protein breakdown. Diet can confound the results of this relatively simple technique. Meat and fish contain a relatively large amount of 3-methylhistidine and could cause erroneous results. The measurement of 3-methylhistidine is, therefore, meaningful only when the diet is strictly controlled, usually with a meat-free diet. The urinary 3-methylhistidine is also highly dependent on the renal clearance rate. Thus, 3-methylhistidine excretion is often expressed relative to creatinine excretion to allow corrections for renal clearance and individual differences in muscle mass. The technique has several limitations but is regarded as a relatively easy and noninvasive way to get an idea of muscle protein breakdown.

Arteriovenous Differences

Nitrogen balance can also be determined across a specific organ. When arterial and venous blood across a certain tissue is sampled, the difference in the amino acid concentration gives information about the net exchange of specific amino acids. The arterial blood delivers amino acids to a tissue, and some of these amino acids are taken up and used for protein synthesis. The venous blood contains amino acids from protein breakdown. Depending on the tissue of interest, measuring arteriovenous differences (AV-differences) can be more or less invasive. For example, AV-differences from tissues like the gut, liver, and brain are difficult to obtain in humans. On the other hand, AV-differences across an arm or leg muscle are relatively easy to obtain. Recently, techniques have been developed to sample across adipose tissue. Independent of the tissue sampled, measurements of AV-differences always require a medically qualified person with good skills.

The AV-difference provides a measure of net uptake and release of amino acids by a tissue. The most valuable information is obtained from amino acids that are not metabolized. For example, the AV-difference of phenylalanine, tyrosine, and lysine (which are not metabolized in the muscle) is assumed to reflect the difference between net amino acid uptake from protein synthesis and the release of amino acids from muscle protein breakdown. The most often used amino acid is phenylalanine because it may give the best representation of overall amino acid metabolism. The assumption is that the amino acid measured reflects overall amino acid metabolism, but this may not always be the case because different amino acids may behave differently. Furthermore, the AV-difference measurement reflects the balance across the leg (or arm) and would thus represent metabolism not only in skeletal muscle but also in bone, skin, and adipose tissue. This method measures the uptake of amino acids into tissues but does not measure incorporation into a protein, and the method does not provide information about specific metabolic pathways in that tissue. Adding a tracer improves the value of the measurement and allows for firmer conclusions about metabolic pathways that play a role in the tissue. AV-differences of 3-methylhistidine across a muscle may be used as a specific marker of contractile protein breakdown.

Tracer Methods

Labeled tracers are used to follow amino acids in the body. These tracers have properties identical to the amino acid or metabolite they are meant to trace. They are, however, distinguishable because they either emit radiation (radioactive isotopes) or are slightly heavier (stable isotopes). Radioactively labeled tracers such as ^{3}H (hydrogen) and ^{14}C (carbon) have been used most often in the past, but many laboratories now use stable isotopic tracers because, unlike radioisotopes, they do not pose a health risk. Stable isotopes have a different number of neutrons and, therefore, a different molecular mass. The difference in mass can be detected with mass spectrometry.

Stable isotopes occur naturally, and most elements have one abundant mass and up to three less abundant masses. For example, the abundant mass for hydrogen is ^{1}H, and the less abundant mass is ^{2}H. For carbon the abundant and less-abundant isotopes are ^{12}C and ^{13}C, respectively. The highlight box lists some common stable isotopes and their abundance.

Most tracer techniques are based on the principle of dilution. A tracer is infused at a constant rate, and after an isotopic steady state is achieved (the appearance of tracer is equal to its disappearance), the dilution of the tracer gives information about release of the amino acid of interest. This principle can be illustrated by a simple analogy. If you want to know the amount of water in a bucket, you can add a known amount of dye. After mixing the dye with the water, a sample of the mixture can be taken and the concentration of the dye can be determined. From the dilution of the dye, the amount of water in the bucket can be calculated. This calculation is accurate, of course, only if the exact amount of dye is known, mixing with the water is complete, and the concentration of the dye can be determined after mixing. Similar measurements can be made in a dynamic system if the dye is infused at a known constant rate. For example, a dye could be used to calculate the flow of water through a stream. The same principle can be applied by infusing a tracer into the human circulation. Several variations to this technique exist to study whole-body protein metabolism or the metabolism of specific amino acids. Here we discuss only the principles. The interested reader should refer to other literature to learn more about stable and radioactive tracers (Matthews 1999; Wolfe 1992).

Commonly Used Stable and Radiolabeled Isotopes in Metabolic Research

Common stable	Rare stable	Radioactive
^{1}H	^{2}H (0.02%)	^{3}H
^{12}C	^{13}C (1.1%)	^{14}C
^{14}N	^{15}N (0.37%)	^{13}N*
^{16}O	^{18}O (0.04%)	^{17}O*

The asterisk (*) indicates no long-lived radioisotopes for these elements.

Methods have been developed to calculate the fractional synthetic rate (FSR) and fractional breakdown rate (FBR). These techniques, which use isotopic tracers, calculate the relative rate of protein breakdown and synthesis. By studying the incorporation of a labeled amino acid into a tissue, information can be obtained about the rates of protein synthesis. It is possible to get a measure of protein synthesis for that tissue (for example, mixed muscle protein synthesis), or if different protein fractions are extracted, it is possible to look at protein synthesis in those specific fractions (for example, myofibrillar proteins or mitochondrial proteins). Modern techniques even make it possible to study protein synthesis of specific proteins. Although the techniques to study protein metabolism in humans are constantly being improved, all methods have their limitations and no agreement has been reached on which method is best. Nevertheless, the available information allows us to draw some conclusions about exercise and protein requirements.

Protein Requirements for Exercise

The protein requirements and the recommendations for protein intake for athletes have not been without controversy. Generally, scientists seem to be divided into two camps—those who believe that participation in exercise and sport increases the nutritional requirement for protein and those who believe that protein requirements for athletes and exercising people are no different from the requirements for sedentary people. Evidence has been found for both arguments. Although this issue may be scientifically relevant, from a practical perspective, the requirement for protein—as most often defined—may not be relevant to most athletes. The scientists who believe that protein requirements are greater for athletes and exercising people offer two explanations:

1. Amino acids may be oxidized during exercise.
2. Increased protein synthesis is necessary to repair damage and forms the basis of training adaptations.

Let us look at the evidence. Acute endurance exercise results in increased oxidation of the BCAAs leucine, isoleucine, and valine. Because these are all essential amino acids and cannot be synthesized within the body, the implication is that they come from increased breakdown of proteins. Dietary protein requirements thus increase. Several studies using the nitrogen balance technique confirm that the dietary protein requirements for athletes involved in prolonged endurance training are higher than those for sedentary individuals. Based on nitrogen balance it can be estimated that protein contributes about 5% to 15% to energy expenditure at rest. During exercise, in relative terms more amino acids may be oxidized. In relative terms, however, protein as a fuel is not important because of the much greater increase of carbohydrate and fat oxidation. Therefore, during prolonged exercise the relative contribution of protein to energy expenditure is usually much lower than it is at rest, usually well below 5%. Only in extreme conditions, when carbohydrate availability is limited, can the contribution of protein increase up to about 10% of total energy expenditure. Nevertheless, it could be argued that leucine oxidation is increased and, therefore, the requirements are increased. The counterarguments are that leucine oxidation does not represent protein oxidation and grossly overestimates protein oxidation. For example, one study by Koopman and colleagues (Koopman et al. 2004) found an increase in leucine oxidation during prolonged endurance exercise but no change in phenylalanine oxidation, confirming that not all amino acids are oxidized to the same degree and suggesting that leucine oxidation overestimates protein oxidation. Furthermore, the oxidized amino acids do not appear to be derived from degradation of myofibrillar proteins (Kasperek et al. 1989). Finally, several nitrogen balance studies have not found differences or even improved nitrogen and leucine balance in active people.

After resistance exercise, muscle protein turnover increases because of an acceleration of both protein synthesis and degradation. Muscle protein breakdown increases after resistance exercise but to a smaller degree than muscle protein synthesis. The elevations in protein degradation and synthesis are transient but are still present at 3 and 24 hours after exercise, although protein turnover returns to baseline levels after 48 hours. These results seem to apply to resistance exercise or dynamic exercise at a relatively high intensity. Low-intensity to moderate-intensity dynamic endurance exercise does not seem to have the same effects on muscle protein turnover, although studies have shown that endurance exercise may result in increased protein oxidation, especially during the later stages of very prolonged exercise and in conditions of glycogen depletion.

Some studies have shown that the body adapts to training by becoming more efficient with protein

(Butterfield et al. 1984; Phillips et al. 1999). Protein turnover decreases after training, and less net protein degradation occurs. In other words, after training, athletes become more efficient and "waste" less protein (Butterfield et al. 1984). Another study has demonstrated that BCAA oxidation at the same relative workload is the same in untrained and trained individuals (Lamont et al. 1999). So although the protein requirement may increase initially, after adaptation to the training this increase seems to disappear. This finding has been used as an argument that protein requirements are not greater in athletes.

Recommendations for Endurance Athletes

Although most researchers agree that exercise increases protein oxidation to some extent and this increased oxidation is accompanied by increased nitrogen losses, controversy persists over whether athletes have to eat more protein than less active people do. Furthermore, nitrogen balance studies show that endurance athletes need to eat about 1.2 to 1.4 g/kg to maintain nitrogen balance. Several research groups claim that evidence supports the contention that athletes should eat more protein, whereas others believe that the evidence is insufficient to make such a statement. One interesting observation is that training seems to have a protein-sparing effect. The better trained a person is, the lower the protein breakdown and oxidation are during exercise. The research groups that advocate increased protein intake for endurance athletes usually recommend an intake of 1.2 to 1.8 g/kg b.w. of protein (as opposed to the recommended intake of 0.8 g/kg b.w. of protein for the average person).

Even if protein requirements are increased, in practice athletes have no problem meeting these needs. As an extreme example, we can look at the Tour de France. Cyclists in this event compete for 3 to 7 hours a day, and maintaining energy balance is often problematic (Jeukendrup et al. 2000). Nevertheless, in this situation, they seem to have no problems maintaining nitrogen balance (Brouns et al. 1989). With greater food intake, the intake of protein automatically increases because many food products contain at least some protein. A study by van Erp-Baart et al. (1989a) showed a linear relationship between energy intake and protein intake. Tour de France cyclists consumed 12% of their daily energy intake (26 MJ, or 6,500 kcal) in the form of protein, and they easily met the suggested increased requirements ($\sim$2.5 g · kg b.w.$^{-1}$ · day^{-1}). These results demonstrate that

if energy intake matches energy expenditure on a daily basis, endurance athletes do not need to supplement their diets with protein.

Recommendations for Strength Athletes

Unlike endurance exercise, resistance exercise does not increase the rate of leucine oxidation to any major degree. The suggested increased dietary protein requirements are related to increased need for amino acids as precursors for proteins being synthesized, resulting in increased muscle bulk (hypertrophy).

As with endurance exercise, the question of whether strength athletes have increased protein requirements is controversial. Nitrogen balance studies suggest that resistance athletes need about 1.5 g · kg b.w.$^{-1}$ · day^{-1}. But these nitrogen balance studies have been criticized because they generally have been of short duration and a steady-state situation may not be established in such circumstances (Rennie et al. 2000). Gontzea, Sutzeescu, and Dumitrache (1975) showed that the negative nitrogen balance used by many to indicate increased protein needs disappears after approximately 12 days of training (see figure 8.5). Note, however, that this study examined cycling exercise training, not resistance training. The protein requirements may therefore be only temporarily elevated. But with a further increase in training load, the protein requirement is likely to increase again. The recommendation for protein intake for strength athletes is often 1.6 to 1.7 g · kg b.w.$^{-1}$ · day^{-1}. Again, people seem to be able to meet this requirement easily with a normal diet, so they do not need extra protein intake. Protein supplements are often used, but they are not necessary to meet the recommended protein intake.

Reported Protein Intake by Athletes

The literature contains several reports of protein intake by athletes in a variety of sports. These intakes are usually self-reported but generally give a good indication of nutritional habits and can reveal whether the athlete is achieving the recommended protein intake. In the van Erp-Baart et al. study (1989b), protein intake in a variety of elite athletes was investigated. In this study the lowest recorded intake was in a group of field hockey players, but their intake was still over 1.0 g · kg b.w.$^{-1}$ · day^{-1}. The highest intakes were recorded for endurance cyclists who consumed almost 3 g · kg b.w.$^{-1}$ · day^{-1} and bodybuilders who consumed 2.5 g · kg b.w.$^{-1}$ · day^{-1}. Most athletes therefore consume far more than the RDA for protein (0.8 g · kg b.w.$^{-1}$ · day^{-1}). Some reports in the literature, however, describe intakes below 0.8 g · kg b.w.$^{-1}$ · day^{-1} in gymnasts and runners and well above 3.0 g · kg b.w.$^{-1}$ · day^{-1} in weightlifters and bodybuilders.

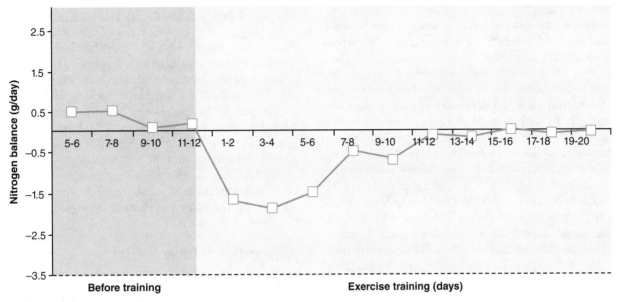

Figure 8.5 Nitrogen balance in response to exercise training.

Adapted from I. Gontzea, R. Sutzeescu, and S. Dumitrache, 1975, "The influence of adaptation to physical effort on nitrogen balance in man," *Nutrition Report International* 11(3): 231-236.

Carbohydrate and Protein During Exercise

The excitement about adding protein to carbohydrate drinks stems from a small number of studies that suggested that adding a small amount of protein (about 2% whey protein or about 20 g/L) to a carbohydrate drink produced improvements in endurance capacity compared with a carbohydrate drink alone (Ivy et al. 2003; Saunders et al. 2004, 2007). It has been speculated that increased endurance capacity with CHO + protein may be due to increased protein oxidation when muscle glycogen is depleted (Koopman et al. 2005) or because of attenuations in central fatigue (Blomstrand et al. 1991). None of these explanations seems plausible, and evidence is lacking. The few studies that reported positive effects have been criticized, and others have not been able to show any performance effects. In a study by van Essen et al. (2006) athletes performed an 80 km cycling time trial on three occasions and drank either a 6% carbohydrate blend, a 6% carbohydrate + 2% whey-protein blend, or a sweetened placebo. All the subjects consumed the solutions at a rate of 1 L/h. The average performance time was identical for the CHO and CHO + protein trials (roughly 135 min) and both were significantly faster (by approximately 4%) than the placebo trial (141 min). This study demonstrated that when athletes ingested a carbohydrate during exercise at a rate considered optimal for CHO delivery, protein provided no additional performance benefit during an event that simulated real-life competition. Therefore, there is now no reason to advise athletes to ingest protein during endurance exercise.

Protein (and in particular BCAA) is often associated with faster recovery and reductions in muscle damage and soreness, especially after eccentric exercise. Most studies have provided carbohydrate postexercise in combination with protein. Some of these studies have demonstrated that CHO + protein coingestion can reduce postexercise plasma CK and attenuate muscle soreness. It has also been suggested that greater reductions in postexercise CK found for CHO + protein beverages may help prolong endurance capacity during a second exercise test. Although evidence is accumulating that protein somehow affects muscle soreness postexercise, mechanisms are unclear and more research is needed to study the effects of carbohydrate and protein intake on recovery from exercise.

Recommendations for Athletes at Risk

People with extremely low protein intake may suffer from protein deficiency, which can compromise function and ultimately lead to loss of body protein (atrophy). Certain groups of athletes are primarily recognized as being at risk from protein and energy deficiency: female runners, male wrestlers, boxers and other athletes in weight category sports, ski jumpers, male and female gymnasts, and female dancers. Although protein intake for these groups may be adequate on average, certain individuals within these groups may have protein intakes well below the RDA. Energy intake can be very low for many individuals in these groups, and as a result protein intake may be low as well.

Another group that has been suggested to be at risk is vegetarian athletes. Plant food sources typically contain lower-quality proteins, which often contain low levels of one or more essential amino acids (for a definition of high- and low-quality proteins see chapter 1). In addition, the digestibility of plant protein can be low compared with animal protein. Although some concern exists that vegetarian athletes may struggle to meet the protein requirements, the evidence for this is lacking, and adequate protein intake seems possible through a balanced vegetarian diet.

Training and Protein Metabolism

Training can have profound effects on muscle morphology and function. Different types of training have distinct effects. For example, strength training results in muscle hypertrophy, increased muscle mass, and likely maintained, or slightly increased, mitochondrial mass (Tang et al. 2006). Endurance training has no effect on muscle mass, but the mitochondrial density inside the muscle fibers increases dramatically. Exercise training is often a combination of strength and endurance, and the improvements in either strength or endurance depend on the relative intensity and the strength required to complete the training sessions. Whatever the adaptation, protein synthesis is required and must occur in the recovery phase between training sessions. Both forms of exercise have recently been shown to stimulate exercise-specific rises in protein synthesis. That is, endurance training stimulates a rise in mitochondrial protein synthesis, whereas resistance exercise stimulates a rise in myofibrillar protein synthesis (Wilkinson et al. 2006). In chapter 12 the underlying mechanisms that explain the specific training adaptations will be explained in detail.

Effect of Protein Intake on Protein Synthesis

Nutrition always plays an important role in the establishment of training adaptations. In the hours after exercise, protein synthesis may exceed protein degradation but only after feeding. If feeding is delayed by several hours, net protein balance remains negative and no muscle hypertrophy occurs (Rennie et al. 2000). Therefore, the suggestion is often made that the timing of protein intake is crucial. Key factors affecting protein synthesis are the coingestion of other nutrients, the amount of protein, the timing of protein intake, and lastly the type of protein.

Coingestion of Other Nutrients

Feeding a mixed diet not only provides substrates but also results in a favorable hormonal milieu for protein synthesis. Increased availability of glucose and amino acids also results in increased plasma insulin concentrations, which, in turn, may cause a reduction of protein breakdown and a small increase in protein synthesis (Bennet et al. 1991; Biolo et al. 1999).

Carbohydrate ingestion per se may not have an effect on protein synthesis after exercise. But carbohydrate ingestion elevates plasma insulin concentrations and thereby may reduce the breakdown of protein that normally occurs with resistance exercise. The combined ingestion of protein and carbohydrate seems to be preferred after exercise. The protein delivers the substrate (amino acids), and carbohydrate further increases the anabolic hormonal milieu required for net protein synthesis.

In a study by Miller et al. (2003) volunteers performed leg resistance exercise and then ingested one of three drinks (amino acids [AA], carbohydrate [CHO], or AA + CHO) at 1 and 2 hours postexercise. Total net uptake of phenylalanine across the leg over 3 hours was greatest in response to AA + CHO and least in CHO. Stimulation of net uptake in AA + CHO was due to increased muscle protein synthesis (figure 8.6). In the control condition, a net protein breakdown was observed. These results suggest that the ingestion of a relatively small amount of amino acids with a larger amount of carbohydrate can increase net muscle protein synthesis in the hours after resistance exercise. Similar data is available for endurance exercise.

Fat also seems to have an effect on protein synthesis because whole milk seemed to give responses different from those of fat-free milk (Elliot et al. 2006). This was discovered in a study that was probably the first to investigate protein synthesis in response to an intact food. After a bout of resistance exercise, subjects consumed either fat-free milk or whole milk. Both milk drinks stimulated protein synthesis, but the greatest effect was seen with whole milk. The explanation for this is not immediately clear, but it was suggested that the fat in the whole milk would delay the delivery of the amino acids and provide a more sustained supply of amino acids for protein synthesis. More research is needed to look into the effects of added fat to protein synthesis.

Amount of Protein

In resting conditions, higher amino acid concentrations in plasma have a stimulatory effect on protein synthesis (Bennet et al. 1990, 1991). Immediately after exercise this effect of increased availability of amino acids on protein synthesis is exaggerated compared with the resting condition (Biolo et al. 1997). Amino acids and exercise thus seem to have an additive effect on net protein synthesis. Note, however, that in these studies, amino acids were infused and plasma amino acid concentrations were elevated to extremely high levels (much higher than those observed after oral ingestion of amino acid mixtures or protein). Intravenous infusion is not a practical method for athletes, and infused amino acids bypass the liver. The liver normally extracts over 20% and up to 90% of all amino acids after absorption from the gut (first-pass splanchnic extraction). Therefore, whether similar effects are to be expected after oral ingestion of amino acids is not clear. A follow-up study investigated this question (Tipton et al. 1999). In this study, a relatively large amount of amino acids was ingested after resistance exercise. Following exercise, muscle protein balance was negative after placebo ingestion, but when amino acids were ingested, the net balance was positive mainly because of increased muscle protein synthesis. From this study and a limited number of other studies, one can conclude that ingestion of amino acids or protein after exercise enhances net protein synthesis. The question remains: How much protein do we need to get optimal effects on

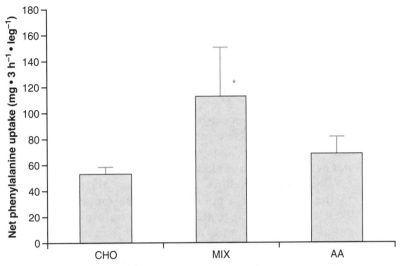

Figure 8.6 Protein synthesis over 3 hours after a bout of resistance exercise as measured by the area under the curve for net uptake of phenylalanine. Protein synthesis seems the lowest with CHO, followed by amino acids only. The combined effect of carbohydrate and amino acids, however, is significantly greater than the individual effects of carbohydrate or protein.

Reprinted, by permission, from S.L. Miller, 2003, "Independent and combined effects of amino acids and glucose after resistance exercise," *Medicine and Science in Sport and Exercise* 35(3): 449-455.

net protein balance? A study by Bohe et al. (2003) may have provided some initial information to answer this question. In this study it was observed that extracellular, and not intracellular, amino acids concentrations determined the rate of protein synthesis. The results showed that there appears to be a plateau above which protein synthesis is not further stimulated. Although it is difficult to determine exactly what amino acid intake is required to achieve this plateau, the amounts appear to be relatively small. A recent study suggests that 20 to 25 g of protein would be required, or 8 to 10 g of essential amino acids (Moore et al. 2009).

Timing of Protein Intake

The timing of food intake after exercise is important to the balance between protein synthesis and protein degradation. Studies have investigated protein ingestion immediately after exercise, delayed by 1 to 3 hours, or ingested before the exercise bout. In one study by Tipton et al. (2001) volunteers ingested 6 g of essential amino acids plus 35 g of carbohydrate immediately before initiation and immediately after completion of an intense, leg resistance exercise bout. Amino acid uptake also seemed to be greater when the nutrients were ingested before the exercise bout than immediately afterward, whereas the anabolic response was similar when the carbohydrate and amino acids were ingested at 1 or 3 h postexercise. Thus, it seems reasonable to assume that the anabolic response to exercise and amino acid and carbohydrate ingestion is greater with preexercise ingestion versus immediately postexercise, 1 h postexercise, and 3 h postexercise. Note that the studies were all performed with essential amino acids. When some of these studies were repeated with whey protein (and no carbohydrate), the difference between feeding before a bout of resistance exercise and after was not evident (Tipton et al. 2007).

These observed differences are likely related to the delivery of amino acids to the muscle. Free amino acids ingested before exercise may result in increased amino acid delivery (because of increased blood flow to active muscles during the exercise session) and lead to superior amino acid uptake compared with amino acids ingested after exercise. Apart from the delivery of amino acids, another factor may determine the anabolic response. Some amino acids, in particular leucine, can serve as signaling molecules and stimulate translation–initiation pathways, resulting in increased protein synthesis (Tipton et al. 1999). These effects will be discussed in detail in chapter 12, because they may form an essential role in the underlying mechanisms of training adaptations.

Type of Protein

Because the delivery of amino acids is important, digestive properties of proteins influence the anabolic response at rest and after exercise. Proteins are often classified as fast or slow (in regard to the speed at which they can be absorbed following ingestion). The increase in arterial amino acid concentrations during exercise was about threefold greater for essential amino acids than for whey proteins when ingested immediately before exercise. The interest in fast and slow proteins started with a series of studies by Boirie and colleagues (Boirie et al. 1997). Their comparison of fast and slow proteins involved comparing protein supplements containing whey with those containing casein (pronounced "kay-seen"). Both casein and whey are derived from whole milk. About 80% of milk protein is casein. The remaining 20% is composed of whey. Whey is considered a fast protein because the body absorbs it rapidly. Casein, on the other hand, is a slow protein that takes the body longer to break down and absorb. Casein seems to clot in the stomach, slowing gastric emptying. Casein intake also results in the release of peptides from the stomach during digestion that slows gastric emptying. Whey and casein vary in their effect on the rate at which proteins are synthesized and broken down. Similar to the concept of glycemic index, whereby foods differ in their effect on blood glucose concentrations over a 2- to 3-hour period, different sources of protein may be digested and absorbed at different rates.

In a series of studies from the lab of Dr. Phillips, it was found that milk protein results in greater rates of protein synthesis and a greater increase in muscle mass in weightlifters compared with soy protein (Hartman et al. 2007; Wilkinson et al. 2007). Although milk protein seems to be preferred to soy protein, it is difficult to recommend which source of protein would be optimal for protein accretion. The anabolic response postexercise depends not only on the type of protein but also on the timing of intake and the ingestion of other nutrients. A protein that is optimal in one condition is not necessarily optimal in all conditions. As research continues it is likely that we will be able to make clearer recommendations in the years to come.

Amino Acids as Ergogenic Aids

In the past, the amino acid needs of the body were primarily met by ingestion of whole proteins in the diet. But over the past few years, the supplementation of individual amino acids has become increasingly popular. Technological advances have made it possible to manufacture food-grade ultrapure amino acids. The individual amino acids, called free-form amino acids, are mostly produced by bacterial fermentation. Scientific studies are focusing on the pharmacologic and metabolic interactions of free-form amino acids. Considerable progress has been made in the area of clinical nutrition, where individual amino acids are used to reduce nitrogen losses and improve organ functions in traumatized and critically ill patients. Individual amino acids also are marketed as supplements for athletes and healthy people. Intake of separate amino acids is often claimed to improve exercise performance, stimulate hormone release, and improve immune function, among a variety of other positive effects. The following section reviews the facts and fallacies of these claims, which are summarized in table 8.4.

Arginine

Infusion of some amino acids into the blood can stimulate the release of growth hormone from the pituitary gland. Arginine is not the only amino acid

■ **TABLE 8.4** ■

Manufacturers' Claims for Amino Acids

Amino acid	Claim
Arginine	Improves immune function, increases tissue creatine levels, increases release of insulin and growth hormone, leads to fewer gastrointestinal problems, improves performance
Aspartate	Improves energy metabolism in muscle, reduces amount of fatigue-causing metabolites, improves endurance performance
Glutamine	Improves immune function (fewer colds), hastens recovery after exercise, improves performance, leads to fewer gastrointestinal problems
Ornithine	Increases growth hormone and insulin release, stimulates protein synthesis, reduces protein breakdown, improves performance
BCAAs	Provide fuel for working muscle, reduce fatigue, improve endurance, reduce muscle protein breakdown
Tyrosine	Increases blood concentration of catecholamines, improves fuel mobilization and metabolism during exercise
Tryptophan	Increases the release of growth hormone, improves sleep, decreases sensations of pain, improves performance
Taurine	Delays fatigue, improves performance, facilitates faster recovery, leads to less muscle damage and pain, leads to fewer gastrointestinal problems, scavenges free radicals
Glycine	Increases phosphocreatine synthesis, improves sprint performance, increases strength

that can have such an effect. Other amino acids that may stimulate the release of hormones from endocrine glands include lysine and ornithine. The intravenous administration of arginine to adults in a dose of 30 g in 30 minutes caused a marked increase in the secretion of human pituitary growth hormone (Knopf et al. 1966). Intravenous and oral arginine administration also resulted in a marked insulin release from the β-cells of the pancreas (Dupre et al. 1968). The finding that arginine increases the secretion of anabolic hormones such as human growth hormone and insulin has made it a popular supplement among bodybuilders and strength athletes. But the amount of arginine present in sport nutritional supplements is often rather small (between 1 and 2 g/day) in comparison with the intravenous doses that have been shown to have potent secretagogue actions (30 g/30 min). Well-controlled studies (double-blind, crossover) (Fogelholm et al. 1993; Lambert et al. 1993) failed to show an effect of oral L-arginine supplementation taken in low quantities on the plasma concentrations of growth hormone and insulin (measured over a 24-hour period) in male competitive weightlifters and bodybuilders. Note also that the growth hormone responses can be obtained simply by exercise. The response that can be obtained by

ingesting relatively large amounts of arginine are still smaller than those that can be obtained by 60 minutes of moderate-intensity exercise. Finally, the oral ingestion of large doses of arginine can cause severe gastrointestinal discomfort and is therefore not practical.

In summary, although arginine infused in large quantities can have anabolic properties, oral ingestion of tolerable doses (i.e., amounts that do not cause gastrointestinal problems) do not result in increased secretion of human growth hormone and insulin. Large increases in insulin secretion can be obtained by ingestion of carbohydrate, and much larger increases in plasma growth hormone are observed during exercise than with even large doses of arginine and other individual amino acids.

Aspartate

Aspartate is often claimed to improve aerobic exercise performance. Aspartate, a precursor for TCA-cycle intermediates, reduces plasma ammonia accumulation during exercise. Because ammonia formation is associated with fatigue, aspartate supplementation could theoretically be ergogenic.

In a study by Maughan and Sadler (Maughan et al. 1983), eight subjects cycled to exhaustion at 75% to 80% of $\dot{V}O_2max$ after ingestion of 6 g of aspartate (as magnesium and potassium salts) or placebo over 24 hours. No effect of aspartate supplementation was observed on plasma ammonia concentration or exercise time to exhaustion.

Branched-Chain Amino Acids

The three BCAAs—leucine, isoleucine, and valine—are not synthesized in the body. Yet they are oxidized during exercise, and they must therefore be replenished by the diet. In the late 1970s, BCAAs were suggested to be the third fuel for skeletal muscle after carbohydrate and fat (Goldberg et al. 1978). BCAAs are sometimes supplied to athletes in energy drinks to provide extra fuel. Many claims have been made about BCAAs:

- BCAAs are a fuel during exercise.
- BCAAs spare glycogen.
- BCAA supplementation can increase protein synthesis following exercise.
- BCAAs can reduce net protein breakdown in muscle during exercise.
- BCAAs reduce muscle damage.
- BCAAs reduce muscle soreness.
- BCAAs reduce fatigue.
- BCAAs enhance performance.
- BCAAs improve immune function (prevent immunodepression).

Despite the lack of strong evidence for the efficacy of BCAA supplements, athletes continue to use them. Normal food alternatives are available, however, and are almost certainly cheaper. For example, a typical BCAA supplement sold in tablet form contains 100 mg of valine, 50 mg of isoleucine, and 100 mg of leucine. A chicken breast (100 g) contains approximately 470 mg of valine, 375 mg of isoleucine, and 656 mg of leucine, or the equivalent of about 7 BCAA tablets. One quarter of a cup of peanuts (60 g) contains even more BCAAs and is equivalent to 11 tablets.

Fuel Source and Glycogen Sparing As mentioned earlier, a study by Goldberg and Chang (Goldberg et al. 1978) suggested that BCAAs can act as a fuel during exercise, in addition to carbohydrate and fat. More recently, however, the activities of the enzymes involved in the oxidation of BCAAs were shown to be too low to allow a major contribution of BCAAs to energy expenditure (Wagenmakers et al. 1989). Detailed studies with a ^{13}C-labeled BCAA (^{13}C-leucine) showed that the oxidation of BCAAs

increases only 2-fold to 3-fold during exercise, whereas the oxidation of carbohydrate and fat increases 10-fold to 20-fold (Knapik et al. 1991). Also, carbohydrate ingestion during exercise can prevent the increase in BCAA oxidation. A related claim is that BCAAs can spare glycogen because they are used as a fuel instead of muscle glycogen. Studies, however, have clearly demonstrated no glycogen sparing during exercise with BCAA ingestion. BCAAs therefore do not seem to play an important role as a fuel during exercise, and, from this point of view, the supplementation of BCAAs during exercise is unnecessary.

Protein Breakdown The claims that BCAAs reduce protein breakdown are mainly based on early in vitro studies, which showed that adding BCAAs to an incubation or perfusion medium stimulated tissue protein synthesis and inhibited protein degradation. Several in vivo studies in healthy individuals (Frexes-Steed et al. 1992; Nair et al. 1992) failed to confirm the positive effect on protein balance that had been observed in vitro. No BCAA supplementation studies to date have demonstrated improved nitrogen balance during or after exercise, although one study found that BCAA supplementation during exercise decreased negative net balance across the leg during exercise (MacLean et al. 1994).

Thus, limited scientific evidence supports the commercial claims that orally ingested BCAAs have an anticatabolic effect during and after exercise or that BCAA supplements may accelerate the repair of muscle damage after exercise.

Protein Synthesis It is claimed that BCAAs increase muscle mass. Resistance exercise increases muscle protein synthesis by stimulation of signaling pathways inside the muscle cells that have been contracted. But without increased availability of amino acids, from ingestion of protein or amino acids in food or in supplements, positive protein balance will not occur. Therefore, increased amino acid intake is necessary for two reasons—to stimulate the signaling pathways and to provide building blocks. BCAAs, in particular leucine, are able to stimulate the signaling pathways and protein synthesis. To date, however, no studies have examined the effects of leucine or BCAA ingestion on protein synthesis following exercise. It is likely, however, that BCAAs stimulate the signals in muscle, but this increased signaling would result in increased synthesis only if sufficient building blocks (other amino acids) are provided. One study demonstrated that the addition of protein to carbohydrates following resistance exercise increases muscle protein synthesis (Koopman et al. 2005). When extra leucine was added to the carbohydrate–protein mixture, however, protein did not increase further. Muscle protein synthesis was likely already fully stimulated by the combination of exercise and protein, so extra leucine could not increase it any further. So in summary, although BCAAs can theoretically help signaling and protein synthesis, in reality it is unlikely that BCAA ingestion will be effective when given in isolation (without other amino acids).

Central Fatigue Hypothesis The central fatigue hypothesis, illustrated in figure 8.7, was proposed in 1987 as a mechanism that contributed significantly to the development of fatigue during prolonged exercise (Newsholme et al. 1987). This hypothesis predicts that, during exercise, FAs are mobilized from adipose tissue and are transported by the blood to the muscles to serve as fuel. Because the rate of mobilization is greater than the rate of uptake by the muscle, the blood FA

concentration increases. Both FAs and the amino acid tryptophan bind to albumin and compete for the same binding sites. Tryptophan is prevented from binding to albumin by the increasing FA concentration, and, therefore, the free tryptophan (fTRP) concentration and the fTRP:BCAA ratio in the blood rise. Experimental studies in humans have confirmed that these events occur. The central fatigue hypothesis predicts that the increase in the fTRP:BCAA ratio results in increased fTRP transport across the blood–brain barrier, because BCAA and fTRP compete for carrier-mediated entry into the central nervous system by the large neutral amino acid (LNAA) transporter (Chaouloff et al. 1986; Hargreaves et al. 1988). After it is taken up, tryptophan is converted to serotonin, leading to a local increase of this neurotransmitter (Hargreaves et al. 1988).

Serotonin plays a role in the onset of sleep and is a determinant of mood and aggression. Therefore, the increase in serotoninergic activity might subsequently lead to central fatigue, forcing athletes to stop exercise or reduce exercise intensity. Of course, the assumption that increased fTRP uptake leads to increased serotonin synthesis and activity of serotoninergic pathways (i.e., increased synaptic serotonin release) is a large leap of faith.

The central fatigue hypothesis also predicts that ingestion of BCAA will raise the plasma BCAA concentration and hence reduce transport of fTRP into the brain. Subsequent reduced formation of serotonin may alleviate sensations of fatigue and in turn improve endurance exercise performance. If the central fatigue hypothesis is correct and the ingestion of BCAAs reduces the exercise-induced increase of brain fTRP uptake and thereby delays fatigue, the opposite must also be true; that is, ingestion of tryptophan before exercise should reduce the time to exhaustion. A few studies have included supplemental tryptophan in human subjects before or during exercise, and from these studies the conclusion must be drawn that tryptophan has no effects on exercise performance.

The effect of BCAA ingestion on physical performance was investigated for the first time in a field test by Blomstrand et al. (1991). One hundred and ninety-three male subjects were studied during a marathon in Stockholm. The subjects were randomly divided into an experimental group receiving BCAA in plain water and a placebo group receiving flavored water. The subjects also had free access to carbohydrate-containing drinks. No difference was observed in the marathon time of the

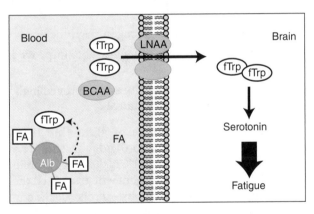

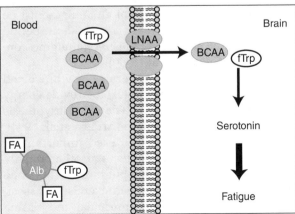

Figure 8.7 Central fatigue hypothesis.

two groups. When the original subject group was divided into fast and slower runners, however, a small significant reduction in marathon time was observed in the slower runners given BCAAs. This study has since been criticized for its design and statistical analysis. Later studies, with various exercise and treatment designs and several forms of administration of BCAA (infusion, oral, and with and without carbohydrates), failed to find a performance effect (Blomstrand et al. 1995, 1997; Madsen et al. 1996; Van Hall et al. 1995; Varnier et al. 1994). Van Hall et al. (1995) studied time-trial performance in trained cyclists who consumed carbohydrate during exercise with and without BCAAs. A high and a low dose of BCAA were given, but no differences were seen in time-trial performance (see figure 8.8).

Muscle Damage and Soreness BCAAs are often associated with reductions in muscle damage and soreness after eccentric exercise. Indeed, studies have shown some effect of acute or chronic BCAA supplementation on markers of muscle damage in the blood after endurance cycling exercise. Studies have consistently found reductions in muscle soreness, but no studies have found any differences in muscle function. Note that all these studies were performed in untrained, unaccustomed subjects. This finding suggests that the importance of BCAA supplementation may be limited to decreasing muscle soreness in untrained individuals.

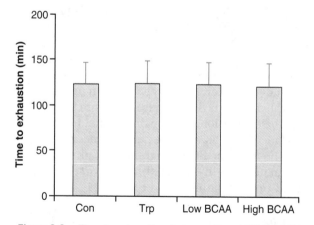

Figure 8.8 Time to exhaustion during cycling at 75% to 80% of V̇O₂max. No effect is seen with tryptophan, a small dose of branched-chain amino acids (BCAAs), or a large dose of BCAAs.

Reprinted from G. Van Hall et al., 1995, "Ingestion of branched-chain amino acids and tryptophan during sustained exercise in man: Failure to affect performance," *Journal of Physiology* 486: 789-794.

Glutamine

Glutamine is a naturally occurring nonessential amino acid; that is, it can be synthesized in the body. Glutamine is important as a constituent of proteins and as a means of nitrogen transport between tissues. It is also important in acid–base regulation and as a precursor of the antioxidant glutathione. Glutamine is the most abundant free amino acid in human muscle and plasma. Its alleged effects can be classified as anabolic and immunostimulatory. Relying somewhat on an uncritical evaluation of the scientific literature, various manufacturers and suppliers claim that glutamine supplements have the following beneficial effects:

- More rapid water absorption from the gut
- Improved intracellular fluid retention (i.e., a "volumizing" effect)
- Improved gut barrier function and reduced risk of endotoxemia
- Nutritional support for immune system and prevention of infection
- Stimulation of muscle protein synthesis and muscle tissue growth
- Stimulation of muscle glycogen resynthesis
- Reduction in muscle soreness and improved muscle tissue repair
- Enhanced buffering capacity and improved high-intensity exercise performance

The normal daily intake of glutamine from dietary protein is about 3 to 6 g/day (assuming a daily protein intake of 0.8 to 1.6 g/kg b.w. of protein for a 70 kg person). Researchers who examined the effects of glutamine on the postexercise decline in plasma glutamine concentration reported that a dose of about 0.1 g/kg b.w. of glutamine must be given every 30 minutes over a 2- to 3-hour period to prevent the fall in the plasma glutamine concentration (Nieman et al. 2000).

Glutamine is used at high rates by white blood cells (particularly lymphocytes) to provide energy and optimal conditions for nucleotide biosynthesis and, hence, cell proliferation (Ardawi et al. 1994). Indeed, glutamine is considered important, if not essential, to lymphocytes and other rapidly dividing cells, including the gut mucosa and bone marrow stem cells. Prolonged exercise is associated with a fall in the intramuscular and plasma concentration of glutamine, and this decrease in glutamine availability has been hypothesized to impair immune function (Parry-Billings et al. 1992). Periods of heavy training are associated with a chronic reduction in plasma glutamine levels, and this reduction may be partly responsible for the immunodepression apparent in many endurance athletes (Parry-Billings et al. 1992). The intramuscular concentration of glutamine is related to the rate of net protein synthesis (Rennie et al. 1989), and some evidence also indicates a role for glutamine in promoting glycogen synthesis (Bowtell et al. 1999). But the mechanisms underlying these alleged anabolic effects of glutamine remain to be elucidated.

Fluid Absorption Water transport from the gut into the circulation is promoted by the presence of glucose and sodium in drinks. Water movement is determined by osmotic gradients, and the cotransport of sodium and glucose into the gut epithelial cells is accompanied by the osmotic movement of water molecules in the same direction. Glutamine is transported into gut epithelial cells by both sodium-dependent and sodium-independent mechanisms, and the addition of glutamine to oral rehydration solutions increases the rate of fluid absorption above that of ingested water alone (Silva et al. 1998). The potential benefits of adding glutamine to commercially available sports drinks have not be adequately tested, however, and any additional benefit in terms of increased rate of fluid absorption and retention is likely to be small. Placebo-controlled studies that have investigated the effects of glutamine supplementation on extracellular buffering capacity and high-intensity exercise performance have not found any beneficial effect. Glutamine is not included in commercial sports drinks, mainly because of its relative instability in solution.

Muscle Protein Balance Research indicates that resistance exercise reduces the extent of protein catabolism, but an anabolic (muscle growth) response requires an intake of essential amino acids (dietary protein) in the recovery period after exercise (Borsheim et al. 2002). In one study, glutamine ingested in addition to carbohydrate and essential amino acids appeared to suppress a rise in whole-body proteolysis during the later stages of recovery (Wilkinson et al. 2006). The functional significance of this is yet to be elucidated. In general, if ingested protein contains all eight essential amino acids, taking supplements of individual nonessential amino acids is unlikely to provide any additional benefit. There is no evidence that glutamine alone will stimulate protein synthesis or reduce protein breakdown.

Muscle Glycogen Synthesis Some evidence exists for an effect of glutamine supplements in promoting glycogen synthesis in the first few hours of recovery after exercise (Bowtell et al. 1999). More recent work, however, suggests that the addition of glutamine to a beverage containing carbohydrate and essential amino acids has no effect on postexercise muscle glycogen resynthesis (Wilkinson et al. 2006). Therefore, at present limited evidence is available to substantiate claims that glutamine accelerates muscle glycogen synthesis.

Muscle Damage and Soreness Several scientists have suggested that exogenous provision of glutamine supplements may prevent muscle damage, muscle soreness, and the impairment of immune function after endurance exercise. Eccentric exercise-induced muscle damage, however, does not affect the plasma glutamine concentration (Walsh et al. 1998), and no scientific evidence supports a beneficial effect of oral glutamine supplementation on muscle repair after exercise-induced damage. No evidence supports reduced muscle soreness when glutamine is consumed compared with a placebo.

Immune System Prolonged exercise at 50% to 70% of $\dot{V}O_2$max causes a 10% to 30% fall in plasma glutamine concentration that may last for several hours during recovery (Castell et al. 1997; Parry-Billings et al. 1992; Walsh et al. 1998). This fall in plasma glutamine coincides with the theory of a "window of opportunity for infection" after prolonged exercise when an athlete is more susceptible to infections (Walsh et al. 1998).

One study showed that an oral glutamine supplement (5 g in 330 ml water) consumed immediately after and 2 hours after a marathon reduced the incidence of upper respiratory tract infection in the 7 days after the race (Castell et al. 1996). But in this study, plasma glutamine concentrations were not measured, and the amount of glutamine ingested was unlikely to have avoided a reduction in plasma glutamine concentrations. A number of review articles (Gleeson 2008; Gleeson et al. 2000; Nieman et al. 2000) concluded, however, that glutamine supplementation during exercise has no effect on various indices of immune function and studies failed to find any beneficial effects.

A larger dose of glutamine (0.1 g/kg b.w.) than that given by Castell et al. (1996) ingested at 0, 30, 60, and 90 minutes after a marathon race prevented the fall in the plasma glutamine concentration but did not prevent the fall in a number of markers of immune function (Gleeson 2008; Gleeson et al. 2000; Nieman et al. 2000). Similarly, maintaining the plasma glutamine concentration by consuming glutamine in drinks taken both during and after a prolonged bout of cycling did not affect a number of important indicators of immune function (Gleeson 2008; Gleeson et al. 2000; Nieman et al. 2000). Unlike the feeding of carbohydrate during exercise, glutamine supplements seem not to affect the immune function perturbations that have been examined to date (see chapter 16 for further details).

Glutamine is thought to be relatively safe and well tolerated by most people, although administration to people with kidney disorders is not recommended. No adverse reactions to short-term glutamine supplementation have been reported, and no information is available on long-term use exceeding 1 g/day. Excessive doses may cause gastrointestinal problems.

Glycine

Glycine is a nonessential amino acid that is involved in the synthesis of phosphocreatine. Therefore, it has been theorized to have ergogenic properties. Early studies indicated improvements in strength after glycine (or gelatin that contains about 25% glycine) supplementation, but these studies were poorly designed. Thus, the effects of glycine remain unconfirmed.

Ornithine

Ornithine is a **nonprotein amino acid** that has been suggested to stimulate growth hormone release from the pituitary gland (Evain-Brion et al. 1982) and insulin release from the pancreas. Growth hormone release after infusion of ornithine was even higher than that observed after arginine infusion. Most ornithine supplements, however, contain 1 to 2 g of ornithine, and this dosage does not affect the 24-hour hormone profile (Fogelholm et al. 1993). Therefore, ornithine supplementation does not seem to increase growth hormone release or increase muscle mass or strength. Although ornithine is often claimed to increase the secretion of insulin from the pancreas, a study in bodybuilders in which the effects of ornithine supplementation

on insulin release were investigated failed to show any effect (Bucci et al. 1992).

Taurine

Taurine is a nonprotein amino acid and a derivative of cysteine. Taurine has recently become a popular ingredient of many sports drinks. The concentrations of taurine in the brain, heart, and muscle are high, but its role is poorly understood. It has been suggested to act as a membrane stabilizer, an antioxidant, and a neuromodulator. Taurine plays an undefined role in calcium currents in cells, influences ionic conductance in excitable membranes, and plays a role in the regulation of cell volume. Many of the proposed effects remain largely unexplored, particularly in humans. The potential role for taurine within human skeletal muscle has yet to be identified, despite a high intramuscular content (50–60 mmol/kg of dry muscle) in relation to plasma (30–60 μmol/L in plasma) and an absence of incorporation of taurine into protein within skeletal muscle. A recent study found that 7 days of taurine supplementation did not alter skeletal muscle taurine content or carbohydrate and fat oxidation during exercise. Its value as a nutrition supplement is still unclear.

Tyrosine

Oral doses of tyrosine (5 to 10 g) result in increases in circulating concentrations of epinephrine, norepinephrine, and dopamine—hormones that are heavily involved in the regulation of body function during physical stress and exercise. Strength athletes, especially, use tyrosine supplements because of their supposed effect of activating metabolic pathways. But no controlled studies show an effect of tyrosine supplementation on exercise performance. Most tyrosine supplements use an extremely low dosage (less than 100 mg), whereas much larger doses are probably required to alter hormone levels. Tyrosine has been examined in animal models and human studies (mostly in military settings) and appears to prevent the substantial decline in various aspects of cognitive performance and mood associated with many kinds of acute stress (Lieberman 2003). For example, Banderet and Lieberman (Banderet et al. 1989) found that vigilance, choice reaction time, pattern recognition, coding, and complex behaviors, such as map and compass reading, were all improved by tyrosine administration when volunteers were exposed to the combination of cold and high altitude (hypoxia). It has been suggested that regular supplementation of large amounts (5 g to 10 g) may have adverse health effects in the long term because it affects sympathetic nervous system activity.

Tryptophan

Tryptophan has been suggested as a way to stimulate the release of growth hormone. The most common proposed ergogenic effect, however, is based on another function. Tryptophan is the precursor of serotonin, a neurotransmitter in the brain that may induce sleepiness, decrease aggression, and elicit a mellow mood. Serotonin has also been suggested to decrease the perception of pain. Segura and Ventura (Segura et al. 1988) hypothesized that tryptophan supplementation increases serotonin levels and the tolerance of pain and thereby improves exercise performance. They studied 12 subjects during running to exhaustion at 80% of $\dot{V}O_2$max with ingestion of tryptophan or placebo. Tryptophan was supplemented in four doses of 300 mg in the 24 hours before the endurance test, and the last doses were ingested 1 hour before the test (total tryptophan ingestion was 1,200 mg). The investigators observed a 49% improvement in endurance capacity and decreased ratings of perceived exertion after tryptophan ingestion. Because a 49% performance improvement seemed somewhat unrealistic, several other investigators have challenged the results of this study (Stensrud et al. 1992; Van Hall et al. 1995).

In a study by Stensrud et al. (1992), 49 well-trained male runners were exercised to exhaustion at 100% of $\dot{V}O_2$max, and no significant effect of tryptophan supplementation on endurance time was found. A very well-controlled study by Van Hall et al. (1995) of eight cyclists who were given tryptophan supplements found no effect on time to exhaustion at 70% of $\dot{V}O_2$max (see figure 8.8).

Both tryptophan and BCAAs have been suggested as supplements to reduce central fatigue. Yet the BCAAs and tryptophan have opposite effects. Whereas some claim that tryptophan reduces central fatigue (Segura et al. 1988), others have associated it with the development of central fatigue (Newsholme et al. 1992). Tryptophan could also exert some negative effects, including a blocking of gluconeogenesis and decreased mental alertness. Based on these studies, tryptophan does not seem to be ergogenic and may even be ergolytic in prolonged exercise.

Protein Intake and Health Risks

Excessive protein intake (more than 3 g · kg b.w.$^{-1}$ · day^{-1}) has been claimed to have various negative effects, including kidney damage, increased blood lipoprotein levels (which has been associated with arteriosclerosis), and dehydration. The latter may occur because of increased nitrogen excretion in urine, which results in increased urinary volume and dehydration. Athletes consuming a high-protein diet should therefore increase their fluid intake to prevent dehydration. The recommended protein intakes for athletes (1.2 to 1.8 g · kg b.w.$^{-1}$ · day^{-1}) and up to approximately 2 g · kg b.w.$^{-1}$ · day^{-1} are not harmful. Perhaps the main risk of increased protein intakes for athletes is the necessary reduction of carbohydrate (or fat) intake if energy levels are maintained. It is not possible to keep energy intake constant while increasing protein intake without lowering carbohydrate or fat intake. This risk is probably more important for endurance athletes, but it may also be a consideration for strength athletes who fancy extremely high protein intakes. Clear evidence shows that low glycogen levels before a training session impair intracellular signaling that leads to increased muscle protein synthesis.

No evidence demonstrates that intake of individual amino acids has any added nutritional value compared with the intake of proteins containing those amino acids. A possible advantage of the intake of individual amino acids is that larger amounts can be ingested. Purified amino acids were developed for clinical use in intravenous infusion of patients for adequate protein nutrition (particularly when oral consumption is compromised). Individual amino acids are also used as food additives to enhance the protein balance in case the diet is deficient in certain amino acids.

In 1989 an epidemic in the United States of the eosinophilia-myalgia syndrome (EMS), a neuromuscular disorder characterized by weakness, fever, edema, rashes, bone pain, and various other symptoms, was attributed to excessive intake of L-tryptophan. L-tryptophan has been classified as a neurotoxin and was banned for a while in the United States. It was later discovered that the EMS outbreak was caused by a contaminated batch of tryptophan, and in 2001 L-tryptophan was again sold in its original form.

KEY POINTS

■ Amino acids are constantly incorporated into proteins (protein synthesis), and proteins are constantly broken down (protein breakdown or degradation) to amino acids. This protein turnover is several times greater than our actual dietary requirement for protein. Some amino acids are essential and are not synthesized in the body, whereas others can be synthesized in the body (nonessential amino acids).

■ Muscle contains 40% of the total protein in a human body and accounts for 25% to 35% of all protein turnover in the body. The contractile proteins actin and myosin are the most abundant proteins in muscle, together accounting for 80% to 90% of all muscle protein.

■ Training has marked effects on body proteins. Both the structural proteins that make up the myofibrils and the proteins that act as enzymes within a muscle cell change as an adaptation to exercise training. Muscle mass, muscle protein composition, and muscle protein content all change in response to training.

■ Methods of studying protein metabolism include nitrogen excretion (urea and 3-methylhistidine), nitrogen balance, arteriovenous balance studies, and tracer methods. All methods available to measure protein turnover in humans have their limitations, and no method has been identified as the best one. Nonetheless, with consideration of their limitations, we can learn a great deal about protein metabolism and nutrition from studies that employ these methods.

■ Amino acids have many metabolic functions. They can be used to synthesize other amino acids, can be incorporated into proteins or other compounds (i.e., FAs and glucose), or can be oxidized in the TCA cycle.

■ The BCAAs are the most abundant amino acids in skeletal muscle, together accounting for 20% of all amino acids in muscle. Glutamine is the most abundant free amino acid in muscle and plasma.

■ Protein has been estimated to contribute up to only about 15% to energy expenditure in resting conditions. During exercise, this relative contribution likely decreases because of an increasing importance of carbohydrate and fat as fuels. During prolonged exercise, when carbohydrate availability becomes limited, amino acid oxidation may increase somewhat, but the contribution of protein to energy expenditure decreases to a maximum of about 10% of total energy expenditure.

■ In the hours after exercise, protein synthesis and breakdown increase. Protein synthesis increases more than breakdown does, but it will exceed protein degradation only after feeding of a source of amino acids.

■ The recommended protein intake for strength athletes is generally 1.6 to 1.7 g · kg b.w.$^{-1}$ · day^{-1}, about twice the value for the general population. The recommended protein intake for endurance athletes is usually 1.2 to 1.8 g · kg b.w.$^{-1}$ · day^{-1} of protein, although in extreme situations the amount may rise to as much as 2.5 g · kg b.w.$^{-1}$ · day^{-1}.

■ The vast majority of athletes consume ample protein to support their training needs, even if the higher recommended intakes are accepted. With increased food intake, the intake of protein automatically increases because many food products contain at least some protein. The relationship between energy intake and protein intake is linear.

■ In healthy people with no indication of kidney issues, there is no evidence that high protein intakes are dangerous. For most athletes the biggest danger of high protein intake is that it often comes at the cost of carbohydrate intake.

■ Arginine infused in large quantities can have anabolic properties in patients, but oral ingestion of tolerable amounts does not result in increased secretion of human growth hormone and insulin.

■ BCAAs are among the most popular nutrition supplements. The evidence for the manufacturers' claims, however, is not convincing.

RECOMMENDED READINGS

Phillips, S.M. 2004. Protein requirements and supplementation in strength sports. *Nutrition* 20:689–695.

Phillips, S.M. 2006. Dietary protein for athletes: from requirements to metabolic advantage. *Applied Physiology Nutrition and Metabolism* 31:647–654.

Rennie, M.J., and K.D. Tipton. 2000. Protein and amino acid metabolism during and after exercise and the effects of nutrition. *Annual Review of Nutrition* 20:457–483.

Tarnopolsky, M.A. 1999. Protein and physical performance. *Current Opinion in Clinical Nutrition Metabolic Care* 2:533-537.

Tipton, K.D., and A.A. Ferrando. 2008. Improving muscle mass: response of muscle metabolism to exercise, nutrition and anabolic agents. *Essays in Biochemistry* 44:85–98.

Tipton, K.D., and O.C. Witard. 2007. Protein requirements and recommendations for athletes: relevance of ivory tower arguments for practical recommendations. *Clinics in Sports Medicine* 26:17–36.

Tipton, K.D., and R.R.Wolfe. 2004. Protein and amino acids for athletes. *Journal of Sports Sciences* 22:65–79.

Wagenmakers, A.J. 1998. Protein and amino acid metabolism in human muscle. *Advances in Experimental Medicine and Biology* 441:307–319.

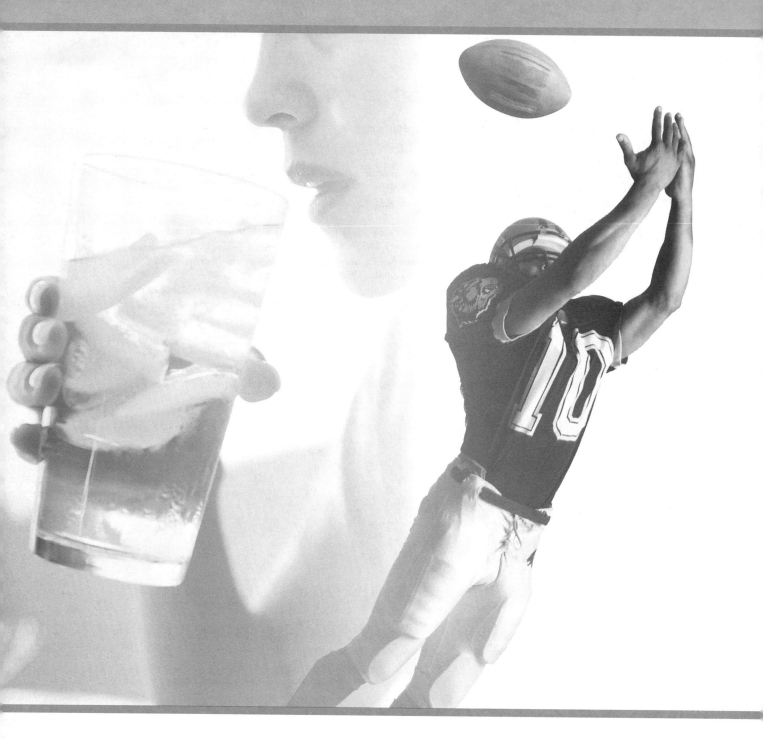

OBJECTIVES

After studying this chapter, you should be able to do the following:

- Describe how body temperature is regulated at rest and during exercise
- Describe the effect of dehydration on exercise performance
- Describe the effects of fluid intake before and during exercise on exercise performance
- Describe fluid intake strategies that help to ensure that the fluid requirements of athletes are met
- Describe the composition of drinks that are suitable for consumption by athletes during and after exercise

9

Water Requirements and Fluid Balance

Most athletes and coaches are aware that a reduction in the body's water content (dehydration) impairs exercise performance. Nevertheless, athletes do not always follow appropriate strategies to prevent or limit dehydration during training and competition. The hydration status of the body is determined by the balance between water intake and water loss. As with all the other nutrients, regular and sufficient water intake is required to maintain health and physical performance. Lack of water intake causes deficiency symptoms, and failure to drink water for more than a few days can result in death. Symptoms associated with overconsumption of water can also be observed.

In most people, water accounts for 50% to 60% of the body mass. Lean body tissues (e.g., muscle, heart, and liver) contain about 75% water by mass, whereas adipose tissue contains only about 5% water by mass, because the bulk of the adipocytes are filled with triacylglycerol fat. The fat content of the body, therefore, largely determines the normal body-water content. For a healthy, lean young male who weighs 70 kg (154 lb), body water amounts to about 42 L (i.e., 60% of body weight). A healthy, lean young female who weighs 70 kg has a total body-water volume of about 35 L, equivalent to 50% of her body weight (see table 9.1 and the illustration below it). The water content of the female body is less than that of the male because (1) the female body is lighter than that of the male and (2) the female body contains a higher proportion of fat (see table 9.1). Thus, for a typical female who weighs 60 kg (132 lb), body-water content is about 30 kg. The total body water is distributed among various body fluid compartments, as shown in table 9.2.

An important route of water (and electrolyte) loss from the body is through sweating, which is the body's principal means of preventing an excessive rise in body temperature (hyperthermia) during exercise in the heat. Some understanding of the regulation

of body temperature is, therefore, fundamental to the discussion of fluid balance in the body and the formulation of drinks intended for consumption both during and after exercise. Hence, this chapter begins with a brief overview of heat production and **thermoregulation** during exercise. The chapter then considers the effects of dehydration on exercise performance and discusses the need for water and electrolyte consumption by athletes.

■ **TABLE 9.1** ■

Fat Content and Volumes of Body Fluid Compartments in Adults and Infants

Body fluid	Infants*	Adult men*	Adult women*
Plasma	4	5	4
Interstitial fluid	26	15	11
Intracellular fluid	45	40	35
Total	75	60	50
Fat	5	18	25

*Values are expressed as a percentage of body mass.

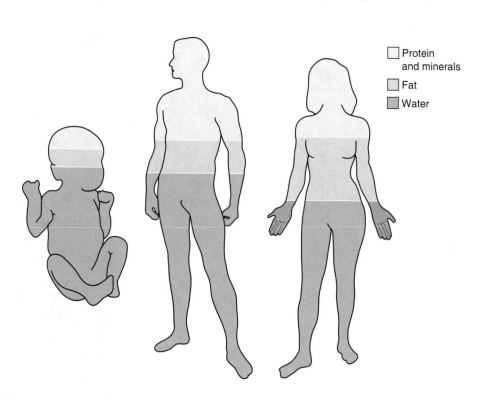

☐ Protein and minerals
☐ Fat
☐ Water

■ TABLE 9.2 ■
Distribution of Body Water* in a Young 70 kg (154 lb) Man

Volume (L)	Body mass (%)	Total-body water (%)
Intracellular fluid	28	40	62.5
Extracellular fluid	14	20	37.5
Interstitial fluid	10.5	15	30
Blood plasma	3.5	5	7.5

*Total body-water volume = 42 L, or 60% of body mass.

Thermoregulation and Exercise in the Heat

Increased muscular activity during exercise increases heat production in the body because of the inefficiency of the metabolic reactions that provide energy for muscle force development. Thermoregulation concerns the mechanisms that prevent excessive rises in body temperature.

Heat Production During Exercise

For every liter of oxygen consumed during exercise such as cycling or running, approximately 16 kJ (4 kcal) of heat is produced and only about 4 kJ (1 kcal) is used to perform mechanical work (to be precise, 1.0 kcal = 4.186 kJ; see chapter 4 for an explanation of this work efficiency). Thus, for an athlete consuming oxygen at a rate of 4 L/min during exercise, the rate of heat production in the body is about 16,000 × 4/60 = 800 J/s, or watts (W), or 16 × 4 × 60/1,000 = 3.84 MJ/h (917 kcal/h). Only a small proportion of the heat produced in active skeletal muscle is lost from the overlying skin. Rather, most of the heat is passed to the body core by the convective flow of venous blood returning to the heart. The rate of temperature increase in the belly of the quadriceps muscle group is close to 1 °C/min (1.8 °F/min) during the initial moments of high-intensity cycling (Saltin et al. 1968). This rate of heat storage cannot persist, because the muscle contractile proteins and enzymes would be inactivated by heat-induced denaturation within 10 minutes. Thus, most of the heat generated in the muscle is transferred to the body core. Increases in body core temperature are sensed by thermoreceptors located in the hypothalamus. This area of the brain also receives sensory input from skin thermoreceptors and integrates this information to produce appropriate reflex effector responses—increasing blood flow to the skin and initiating sweating—to increase heat loss and limit further rises in body temperature.

Heat Storage During Exercise

During exercise at a constant work rate, heat production increases in a square-wave fashion. The set point of the hypothalamic thermostat does not change during exercise, but some heat storage does occur. When heat loss from the body equals heat production, the rise in body temperature plateaus. During high-intensity exercise, however, particularly in an environment with a high ambient temperature and high humidity, core temperature continues to rise.

During exercise at an intensity equivalent to about 80% to 90% of $\dot{V}O_2$max, heat production in a fit person may exceed 1,000 W (resting heat production is about 70 W), which could potentially increase body temperature by 1 °C (1.8 °F) every 4 to 5 minutes if no changes occur in the body's heat-dissipating mechanisms. This estimate is based on the specific heat capacity of human tissues, which is 3.47 kJ · kg^{-1} · °C^{-1} (0.46 kcal · kg^{-1} · °F^{-1}) for lean tissue and 1.73 kJ · kg^{-1} · °C^{-1} (0.23 kcal · kg^{-1} · °F^{-1}) for fat. For a man weighing 70 kg (154 lb) with 15% body fat, the specific heat capacity of the body is (3.47 × 0.85) + (1.73 × 0.15) = 3.21 kJ · kg^{-1} · °C^{-1} (0.43 kcal · kg^{-1} · °F^{-1}). Using this value, we can calculate that at a rate of body heat production of 1,000 W, in 1 minute 1,000 J/s × 60 s = 60,000 J or 60 kJ (14.3 kcal) of heat energy is produced, which raises the body temperature of this 70 kg man by 60 kJ ÷ (70 kg × 3.21 kJ · kg^{-1} · °C^{-1}) = 0.27 °C (0.49 °F). Thus, within 12 to 15 minutes, core body temperature could approach dangerous levels or exercise will end because of the symptoms of fatigue that occur from this degree of hyperthermia.

Problems of hyperthermia and heat injury are not restricted to prolonged exercise in a hot environment. Heat production is directly proportional to exercise intensity, so extremely strenuous exercise, even in a cool environment, can cause a substantial rise in body temperature.

The absolute body temperature at the end of exercise depends on the starting body temperature. A vigorous warm-up causes a rise in body temperature and results in a higher final body temperature. When body temperature rises to about 39.5 °C (103 °F), central fatigue (i.e., fatigue in the brain rather than in the working muscles) ensues, so a high starting temperature is undesirable for athletes who are exercising in a hot environment. Such large increases in body temperature during exercise tend not to occur in individuals who run at a slower pace (e.g., those who run a marathon in 4 to 6 hours) but are common in the faster, highly motivated athletes.

A body temperature of 36 to 38 °C (96.8 to 100.4°F) is the normal range at rest and may rise to 38 to 40 °C (100.4 to 104 °F) during exercise. Further increases are commonly associated with heat exhaustion and occasionally with heatstroke, a life-threatening disorder characterized by lack of consciousness after exertion and by clinical symptoms of damage to the brain, liver, and kidneys (Gleeson 1998; Sutton and Bar-Or 1980). The elevated core temperature associated with exercise is not regulated at its elevated level (i.e., it is not caused by a resetting of the hypothalamic thermostat). Rather, the elevated temperature is caused by the temporary imbalance between the rates of heat production and dissipation during the early stages of exercise and the rapidity with which the heat-dissipating mechanisms respond to an increase in core temperature.

Environmental Heat Stress and Heat Loss by Evaporation of Sweat

Environmental heat stress is determined by the ambient temperature, relative humidity, wind velocity, and solar radiation (both directly from the sun and reflected from the ground) (see figure 9.1). During exercise, the working muscles produce heat at a high rate and body temperature rises. If the skin is hotter than the surroundings, heat is lost from the skin by physical transfer (evaporation of sweat, convection, and conduction) to the environment. If the environment is hotter than the skin, heat is gained by convection and conduction. If the environment is saturated with water vapor (i.e., relative humidity = 100%), evaporation of sweat does not occur and the body does not lose heat. Relative humidity is important because high humidity severely compromises the evaporative loss of sweat, and sweat must evaporate from the body surface to exert a cooling effect.

Evaporation of 1 L of water from the skin will remove 2.4 MJ (573 kcal) of heat from the body. The sweat rate during exercise must be at least 1.6 L/h if all the heat produced is to be dissipated by evaporative loss alone. In fact, the sweat rate probably has to be nearer 2 L/h, because at such high sweat rates, some of the sweat rolls off the skin, which has virtually no cooling effect. A reduction in skin blood flow and sweat rate as the body becomes progressively dehydrated or high humidity limits evaporative loss of sweat leads to further rises in core temperature, resulting in fatigue and possible heat injury to body tissues. The latter is potentially fatal.

A useful index of environmental heat stress is the wet bulb globe temperature (WBGT), which is calculated as follows:

$$WBGT = 0.7\ Twb + 0.2\ Tbg + 0.1\ Tdb$$

where Twb is the temperature (in °C) of a wet-bulb thermometer, Tbg is the temperature of a black-globe thermometer, and Tdb is the temperature of a dry-bulb thermometer. Note the 70% bias toward the Twb, which recognizes the greater relative importance of environmental humidity. Some typical environmental scenarios and physiological responses to exercise in various environmental conditions are illustrated in table 9.3.

Heat loss through the evaporation of sweat is largely determined by the water

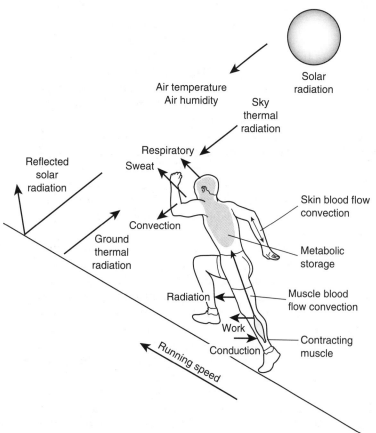

Figure 9.1 Sources of body heat-gain and heat-loss mechanisms.

■ **TABLE 9.3** ■
Sweat Loss and Heart Rates After 60 Minutes of Exercise

Ambient temperature	Humidity (%)	Sweat loss (L)	Core temperature	Heart rate (beats/min)
13 °C (55 °F)	7	0.8	38.0 °C (100.4 °F)	140
18 °C (64 °F)	50	1.2	38.3 °C (100.9 °F)	143
25 °C (77 °F)	50	1.4	38.7 °C (101.6 °F)	145
30 °C (86 °F)	30	2.1	39.3 °C (102.7 °F)	148
30 °C (86 °F)	90	2.8	39.5 °C (103.1 °F)	150
35 °C (95 °F)	30	3.0	39.9 °C (103.8 °F)	153

Exercise performed at about 60% to 70% of $\dot{V}O_2$max under various environmental conditions.

vapor pressure (humidity) of the air close to the body surface. The local humidity may be high if inappropriate, poorly ventilated clothing is worn because it reduces the convective flow of air over the skin surface. Sweat drips off the skin rather than evaporates, and heat loss by this route is severely restricted. If exercise continues at the same intensity, body core temperature rises further, a higher sweat rate is induced, and the athlete dehydrates more rapidly. This dehydration poses further problems for the athlete because progressive dehydration impairs the ability to sweat and, consequently, to thermoregulate. At any given exercise intensity, body temperature rises faster in the dehydrated state, and this condition is commonly accompanied by a higher heart rate during exercise, as shown in figure 9.2. Dehydration equivalent to the loss of only 2% of body mass (i.e., the loss of about 1.5 L of water for a typical 70 kg [154 lb] male athlete) is sufficient to cause significant impairment in exercise performance (Armstrong et al. 1985; Craig and Cummings 1966; Maughan 1991; Sawka and Pandolf 1990).

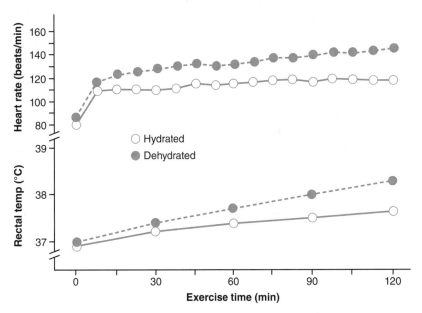

Figure 9.2 Effect of dehydration on heart rate and rectal temperature during 2 hours of cycling.

Heat Loss by Radiation and Convection

The other crucial effector mechanism in thermoregulation during exercise in the heat is increased blood flow through the skin capillaries. This mechanism allows increased heat loss from the body core to the environment by radiation and convection. Radiation is the transfer of energy waves by emission from one object and absorption by another. Convection is the exchange of heat between a solid medium (e.g., the human body) and one that moves (e.g., air or water). The rate of heat transfer away from the body core is the product of the skin blood flow and the temperature difference between the core and the skin.

High skin blood flow alone may not be sufficient to remove heat from the body core during exercise in hot, humid conditions when the skin temperature rises because of the inability to evaporate sweat. The effectiveness of this route of heat loss also depends largely on the amount of body surface available for heat exchange and the temperature gradient between the body surface and the surrounding atmosphere. When ambient temperature is close to body temperature, heat loss by the skin blood flow is minimal. The body then depends almost entirely on evaporative cooling. Inappropriate clothing impairs convection and radiation of heat from the body surface, so total heat dissipation will decrease to a critically low level.

Regulation of Body Temperature

Sensory information about body temperature is input to the central controller by nerves emanating from both deep-body and peripheral thermoreceptors. The latter, located in the skin, provide advance warning of environmental heat input. Central thermoreceptors, located in the hypothalamus, are sensitive to changes in internal core temperature and effectively monitor the temperature of blood flowing to the brain. Input from these receptors is more important than input from the peripheral receptors in eliciting appropriate effector responses designed to limit increases in body temperature. The central thermal controller, or "thermostat," located in the preoptic anterior hypothalamus also receives nonthermal sensory inputs that are capable of modulating the homeostatic regulation of body temperature.

These other inputs include nervous signals from osmoreceptors and pressure receptors, so changes in plasma osmolarity and blood volume are capable of affecting sweating and cutaneous vasodilation responses to rises in core temperature. These effects are summarized in figure 9.3. Some hormones (e.g., estrogen) and cytokines (e.g., interleukin-1 and interleukin-6) are also capable of influencing thermoregulatory responses. Interleukin-6, also known as endogenous pyrogen, is secreted from macrophages and is responsible for raising the set-point temperature of the hypothalamic "thermostat," causing a rise in core temperature during fever. The influence of other sensory inputs also appears to take place at the level of the hypothalamic neurons and is mediated by neurotransmitters, including dopamine, 5-hydroxytryptamine (5-HT or serotonin), norepinephrine (noradrenaline), and acetylcholine.

Exercise Training, Acclimatization, and Temperature Regulation

Exercise training improves temperature regulation during exercise at the same absolute work rate. To obtain thermoregulatory benefits from training, people must adequately stimulate thermoregulatory effector responses (i.e., sweating and increased skin blood flow). In other words, they must

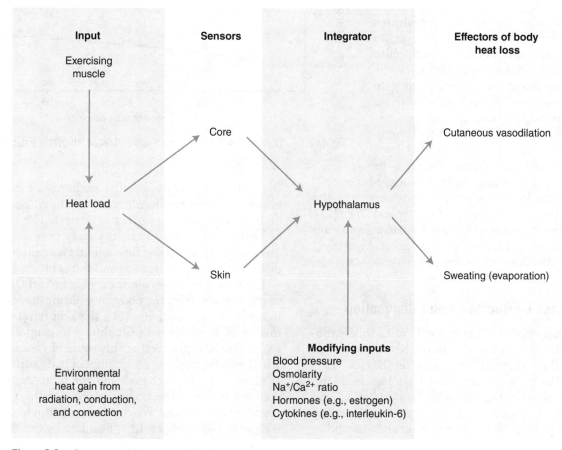

Figure 9.3 Summary of thermoregulation during exercise in the heat.

exercise at a sufficiently high intensity. Improvements in thermoregulatory responses to exercise have consistently been seen in studies in which subjects exercised at 70% to 100% of $\dot{V}O_2$max and increased their body temperature above 39 °C (102.2 °F). Studies in which subjects exercised at lower intensities (typically 35% to 60% of $\dot{V}O_2$max) have commonly shown little or no thermoregulatory benefit in response to training.

Most serious athletes regularly exercise at intensities above 70% of $\dot{V}O_2$max; such training allows them to achieve thermal equilibrium during exercise at 25% to 35% of $\dot{V}O_2$max in desert heat conditions, but, of course, this exercise intensity is not race pace. Appropriate training, however, increases tolerance of exercise in hot conditions, and acclimation to warm environments (achieved by exercising in a hot environment, not just resting in that environment) confers further benefits in terms of the ability to regulate body temperature during exercise in the heat at higher exercise intensities (Greenleaf 1979).

Marathon runners exhibit a lower resting body temperature and have a lower sweating (and shivering) threshold. Thus, the set-point temperature of endurance athletes seems to decrease as a result of training. Endurance athletes have also been reported to have a lower resting metabolic rate in thermoneutral conditions and a lower skin temperature. This effect appears to mimic the "insulative hypothermia" reported in Australian aborigines who sleep in the cold desert night; both skin and core temperature drop, reducing the temperature gradient between the body surface and the environment, which reduces heat loss and conserves energy. Heat and cold acclimatization are not mutually exclusive and can occur simultaneously in the same person.

Exercise training improves thermoregulation in the heat by earlier onset of sweat secretion and by increasing the total amount of sweat that can be produced. Thus, training increases the sensitivity of the relationship between sweat rate and core temperature as well as decreases the internal temperature threshold for sweating. Sweat rates can vary markedly between individuals (up to a maximum of about 3 L/h), even at the same relative exercise intensity (Maughan 1991), but evidence suggests that individuals characterized as heavy sweaters have larger sweat glands than light sweaters. Training appears to induce hypertrophy (enlarging) of existing sweat glands without increasing the total number.

Other adaptations to training include an increase in total blood volume and maximal cardiac output. As a result, blood flow in muscle and skin, with its heat flux, is better preserved during strenuous exercise in the heat. The body does not adapt to dehydration, so exercising in the heat without fluid intake does not confer additional adaptation in thermoregulation. In fact, progressive dehydration during exercise in the heat reduces the sensitivity of the relationship between sweat rate and core temperature as shown in figure 9.4 and thus results in relative hyperthermia and earlier onset of fatigue (Nadel et al. 1980; Sawka, Young, Francesconi et al. 1985). In practical terms, the athlete is less able to maintain training loads, so the physiological adaptation to training is not as great. Exercising for prolonged periods in the heat without fluid intake also increases the risk of cramps and heat illness. To summarize, aerobic exercise training improves the ability to maintain constant body temperature during exercise in the heat by the following means:

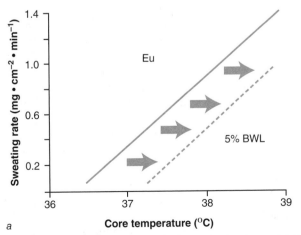

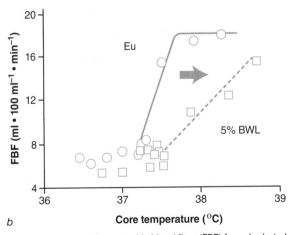

Figure 9.4 Relationship between body core temperature and (a) local sweating rate and (b) forearm skin blood flow (FBF) for euhydrated (normally hydrated) men (circles) and men dehydrated by 5% of body weight loss (BWL, squares) during exercise in the heat.

AMERICAN JOURNAL OF CLINICAL NUTRITION by M.N. Sawka and S.J. Montain. Copyright 2000 by American Society for Nutrition. Reproduced with permission of American Society for Nutrition in the format Textbook via Copyright Clearance Center.

- Increase in blood volume
- Increase in capacity for skin blood flow
- Increase in size of sweat glands
- Earlier onset of sweating (lower set-point core temperature for onset of sweating)
- Increase in sweat rate (increased sensitivity of the relationship between sweat rate and core temperature)

Effects of Dehydration on Exercise Performance

Fatigue toward the end of a prolonged sporting event may result as much from dehydration as from fuel substrate depletion. Exercise performance is impaired when a person is dehydrated by as little as 2% of body weight. Losses in excess of 5% of body weight can decrease the capacity for work by

about 30% (see figure 9.5) (Armstrong et al. 1985; Craig and Cummings 1966; Maughan 1991; Sawka and Pandolf 1990).

Sprint athletes are generally less concerned about the effects of dehydration than are endurance athletes. But the capacity to perform high-intensity exercise, which results in exhaustion within a few minutes, declines by as much as 45% by prior dehydration corresponding to a loss of only 2.5% of body weight (Sawka, Young, Cadarette, et al. 1985). Although sprint events offer little opportunity for sweat loss, athletes who travel to compete in hot climates are likely to experience acute dehydration, which persists for several days and may be serious enough to have a detrimental effect on performance in competition.

Even in cool laboratory conditions, maximal aerobic power ($\dot{V}O_2max$) decreases by about 5% when people experience fluid losses equivalent to 3% of body mass or more, as shown in figure 9.6 (Pinchan et al. 1988). In hot conditions, similar water deficits can cause a larger decrease in $\dot{V}O_2max$. Marginal dehydration (fluid loss of 1% to 2% of body weight) decreases endurance capacity during incremental exercise even if water deficits do not result in a decrease in $\dot{V}O_2max$. Endurance capacity is impaired much more in hot environments than in cool conditions, which implies that impaired thermoregulation is an important causal factor in reduced exercise performance associated with a body-water deficit. Dehydration also impairs endurance exercise performance. Fluid loss equivalent to 2% of body mass induced by a diuretic drug (furosemide) caused impairment of running performance at 1,500, 5,000, and 10,000 m distances (Armstrong et al. 1985). Running performance was impaired more at the longer distances (by approximately 5% at 5,000 and 10,000 m) compared with the shortest distance (approximately 3% at 1,500 m).

A study investigated the capacity of eight subjects to perform treadmill walking (at 25% of $\dot{V}O_2max$ and a target time of 140 minutes) in very hot, dry conditions (49 °C [120 °F], 20% relative humidity) when they were euhydrated and when they were dehydrated by a 3%, 5%, or 7% loss of body mass (Sawka,

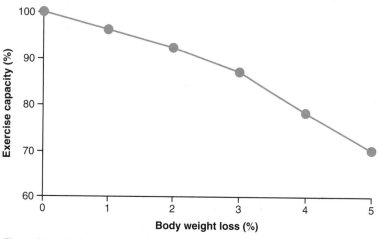

Figure 9.5 Reduction of work capacity with increasing degree of dehydration (body weight loss).

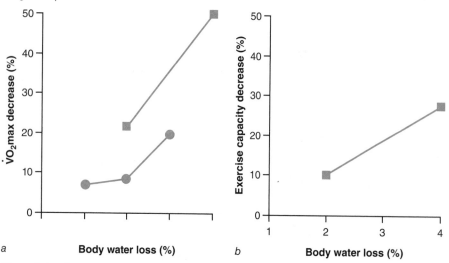

Figure 9.6 Effect of degree of dehydration (% loss of body water) on (a) decrement in maximal oxygen uptake ($\dot{V}O_2max$) and (b) reduction in physical work capacity during heat exposure.
Data from Craig and Cummings 1966; Pinchan et al. 1988.

Young, Francescone, et al. 1985). All eight subjects were able to complete 140 minutes walking when euhydrated and 3% dehydrated. Seven subjects completed the walk when 5% dehydrated, but when dehydrated by 7%, six subjects stopped walking after an average of only 64 minutes. Thus, even for relatively low-intensity exercise, dehydration clearly increases the incidence of exhaustion from heat strain. Sawka et al. (1992) had subjects walk to exhaustion at 47% of $\dot{V}O_2$max in the same environmental conditions as their previous study. Subjects were euhydrated and dehydrated to a loss of 8% of each individual's total body water. Dehydration reduced exercise endurance time from 121 minutes to 55 minutes. Dehydration also appeared to reduce the core temperature that a person could tolerate, because core temperature at exhaustion was about 0.4 °C (0.7 °F) lower in the dehydrated state. The main reasons dehydration has an adverse effect on exercise performance can be summarized as follows:

- Reduction in blood volume
- Decreased skin blood flow
- Decreased sweat rate
- Decreased heat dissipation
- Increased core temperature
- Increased rate of muscle glycogen use

Reduced maximal cardiac output (i.e., the highest pumping capacity of the heart that can be achieved during exercise) is the most likely physiological mechanism whereby dehydration decreases a person's $\dot{V}O_2$max and impairs work capacity in fatiguing exercise of an incremental nature. Dehydration causes a fall in plasma volume both at rest and during exercise, and decreased blood volume increases blood thickness (viscosity), lowers central venous pressure, and reduces venous return of blood to the heart. During maximal exercise, these changes can decrease the filling of the heart during diastole (the phase of the cardiac cycle when the heart is relaxed and is filling with blood before the next contraction), hence reducing stroke volume and cardiac output. Also, during exercise in the heat, the opening up of the skin blood vessels reduces the proportion of the cardiac output available to the working muscles.

Even for normally hydrated (euhydrated) people, climatic heat stress alone decreases $\dot{V}O_2$max by about 7%. Thus, both environmental heat stress and dehydration can act independently to limit cardiac output and blood delivery to the active muscles during high-intensity exercise. Dehydration also impairs the body's ability to lose heat. Both sweat rate and skin blood flow are lower at

the same core temperature for the dehydrated state compared with the euhydrated state (see figure 9.4) (Nadel et al. 1979, 1980; Sawka and Wenger 1988). Body temperature rises faster during exercise when the body is dehydrated. The reduced sweating response in the dehydrated state is probably mediated through the effects of both a fall in blood volume (hypovolemia) and elevated plasma osmolarity (i.e., dissolved salt concentration) (see figure 9.7) on hypothalamic neurons. As explained previously, as core temperature rises towards about 39.5 °C (103 °F), sensations of fatigue ensue. This critical temperature is reached more quickly in the dehydrated state.

Dehydration not only elevates core temperature responses but also negates the thermoregulatory advantages conferred by high aerobic fitness and heat acclimatization. The effects of dehydration (5% loss of body weight) on core temperature responses in the same people when unacclimated and when acclimated to heat are shown in figure 9.8. Heat acclimation lowered core temperature responses when subjects were euhydrated. When they were dehydrated, however, similar core temperature responses were observed in both unacclimated and acclimated states (Pinchan et al. 1988).

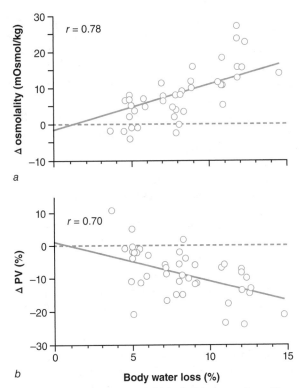

Figure 9.7 Effects of degree of dehydration (percentage of loss of body water) on *(a)* plasma osmolality and *(b)* plasma volume in heat-acclimated persons.

AMERICAN JOURNAL OF CLINICAL NUTRITION by M.N. Sawka and S.J. Montain. Copyright 2000 by American Society for Nutrition. Reproduced with permission of American Society for Nutrition in the format textbook via Copyright Clearance Center.

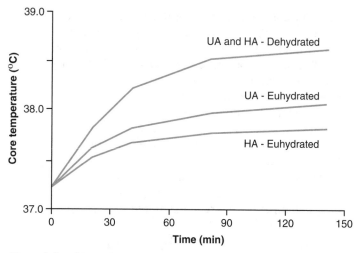

Figure 9.8 Core temperature responses during exercise in the heat in euhydrated or dehydrated (5% loss of body weight) persons both before (unacclimated, UA) and after becoming heat acclimated (HA).

AMERICAN JOURNAL OF CLINICAL NUTRITION by M.N. Sawka and S.J. Montain. Copyright 2000 by American Society for Nutrition. Reproduced with permission of American Society for Nutrition in the format textbook via Copyright Clearance Center.

A person's ability to tolerate heat strain appears to be impaired when dehydrated, so the critical temperature for experiencing central fatigue is likely to be near 39.0 °C (102.2 °F) when dehydrated by more than about 5% of body mass (Sawka et al. 1992). The larger rise in core temperature during exercise in the dehydrated state is associated with a bigger catecholamine response, and these effects may lead to increased rates of glycogen breakdown in the exercising muscle, which in turn may contribute to earlier onset of fatigue in prolonged exercise. Although it is well established that hypohydration (reduced total body water) impairs endurance exercise performance, the influence of hypohydration on muscular strength, power, and very high-intensity endurance (maximal activities lasting >30 seconds but <2 minutes) is poorly understood because of the inconsistent results reported in the literature. Several subtle methodological choices that exacerbate or attenuate the apparent effects of hypohydration explain much of this variability (Judelson et al. 2007). After accounting for these factors, hypohydration appears to attenuate strength, power, and high-intensity endurance by approximately 2%, 3%, and 10%, respectively, suggesting that alterations in total body water affect some aspect of force generation. Although the mechanisms are not well understood, the physiological demands of strength, power, and high-intensity endurance suggest alterations in cardiovascular, metabolic, or buffering function are responsible for the performance impairment associated with hypohydration. On the other hand, hypohydration might directly affect some component of the neuromuscular system, but this possibility awaits thorough evaluation. Hypohydration is, therefore, an important factor to consider when attempting to maximize intense muscular performance in athletic, military, and industrial settings.

Dehydration is associated with a reduced gastric emptying rate of ingested fluids during exercise in the heat. For example, one study reported a 20% to 25% reduction in gastric emptying when subjects were dehydrated by 5% of body mass (Neufer et al. 1989).

Fluid consumption should begin during the early stages of exercise in the heat, not only to minimize the degree of dehydration but also to maximize the bioavailability of ingested fluids. Dehydration poses a serious health risk in that it increases the risk of cramps, heat exhaustion, and life-threatening heatstroke (Sutton and Bar-Or 1980).

Mechanisms of Heat Illness

Heat injury is most common during exhaustive exercise in a hot, humid environment, particularly if the person is dehydrated. These problems affect not only highly trained athletes but also less well-trained sport participants. In fact, less well-trained individuals have less-effective thermoregulation during exercise, work less economically, use more carbohydrate for muscular work, and take longer to recover from exhausting exercise than do highly trained people.

During the initial stages of exercise in a hot environment, sweating begins and the skin blood vessels dilate, causing increased heat loss from the body. But as central blood volume and pressure fall, sympathetic nervous activity increases and the skin blood vessels constrict. A more powerful constriction of the blood vessels supplying the abdominal organs leads to cellular hypoxia in the region of the gastrointestinal tract, liver, and kidneys. Cellular hypoxia leads to the production of reactive oxygen species (ROS), including superoxide anion, hydrogen peroxide, hydroxyl radical, peroxynitrite, and nitric oxide (NO). The latter is a potent blood vessel dilator, and although its production can be viewed as protective (i.e., helping to conserve some blood flow through the capillary beds of the abdominal organs), ultimately the ROS may cause damage through their actions on membranes. The ROS cause peroxidation of lipids in cellular membranes, making them leaky. In the gastrointestinal tract, this action allows the passage of bacterial toxins (endotoxins) from the gut into the systemic circulation, leading to endotoxemia (blood poisoning) and a drastic fall in blood pressure (hypotension). Increased levels of NO probably contribute to the development of hypotension. The consequences for the athlete can be heat syncope (fainting) and organ injury (see figure 9.9).

Animal studies have shown a disappearance of manganese-superoxide dismutase (Mn-SOD), an important antioxidant enzyme that deactivates ROS, after 2 hours of heat exposure and a later induction of Mn-SOD in the liver cells of animals exposed to elevated core temperatures (41 °C [106 °F]) over a 24-hour period. Increased levels of hemoglobin-NO, semiquinone radical (a marker of mitochondrial oxidative stress), and ceruloplasmin (a copper-binding protein with antioxidant properties) have been found in the hepatic portal vein after exposure to heat stress.

A doubling of hepatic portal blood endotoxin levels has also been reported within 24 hours of the onset of heat exposure. Thus, ROS generation appears to increase within abdominal tissues during heat exposure. Antioxidant status is compromised within the first few hours but gradually recovers and is enhanced after 24 hours of heat exposure.

ROS generation probably increases most in areas of high metabolic activity and greatest potential for reduction in blood flow.

This ischemia–reperfusion mechanism involving the gastrointestinal tract may play a role in the vascular dysfunction and tissue injury associated with heat stress. Further studies are warranted about the possible benefits of antioxidant supplementation in people who regularly experience high body temperatures such as athletes who train and compete in hot, humid climates.

Although it is dramatically underreported, heat-related pathology contributes to significant morbidity as well as occasional mortality in athletic, elderly, children, and disabled populations. Among U.S. high school athletes, heat illness is the third-leading cause of death (Coris et al. 2004). Significant risk factors for heat illness include dehydration, hot and humid climate, obesity, low physical fitness, lack of acclimatization, previous history of heatstroke, sleep deprivation, medications (especially diuretics or antidepressants), sweat gland dysfunction, and upper respiratory or

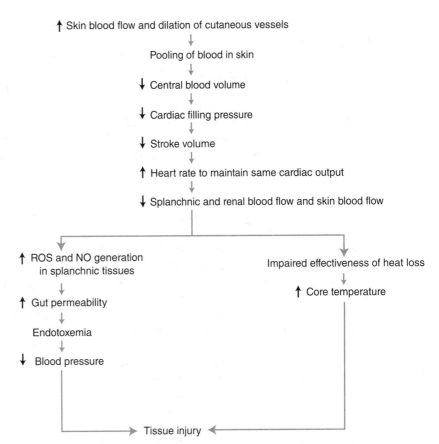

Figure 9.9 Potential mechanisms of heat-stress injury.

gastrointestinal illness. Many of these risk factors can be addressed with education and awareness of people at risk. Dehydration, with fluid loss occasionally as high as 6% to 10% of body weight, appears to be one of the most common risk factors for heat illness in people who exercise in the heat. Core body temperature has been shown to rise an additional 0.15 to 0.2 °C for every 1% of body weight lost during exercise. Identifying athletes at risk, limiting environmental exposure, and monitoring closely for signs and symptoms are all important components of preventing heat illness. But monitoring hydration status and promoting appropriate drinking strategies may be the most important factors in preventing severe heat illness.

Effects of Fluid Intake on Exercise Performance

Oral fluid ingestion during exercise helps restore plasma volume to near preexercise levels and prevents the adverse effects of dehydration on muscle strength, endurance, and coordination. Elevating blood volume just before exercise by various hyperhydration strategies has been suggested to be effective in enhancing exercise performance, but only a few studies have directly investigated this possibility.

Preexercise Hyperhydration

Because even mild dehydration has debilitating effects on exercise performance, hyperhydration (greater than normal body water content) has been hypothesized to improve thermoregulation by expanding blood volume and reducing plasma osmolarity, thereby improving heat dissipation and exercise performance. Although some studies report higher sweating rates, lower core temperatures, and lower heart rates during exercise after hyperhydration, several of these studies used control conditions that represented dehydration rather than euhydration, calling results into question. But the findings generally support the notion that hyperhydration reduces the thermal and cardiovascular strain of exercise. Relatively few studies have directly investigated the effects of hyperhydration on exercise performance, but one well-controlled study reported that expansion of blood volume by 450 to 500 ml improved cycling time-trial performance by 10% (81 minutes compared with 90 minutes).

Temporary hyperhydration is induced in test subjects by having them drink large volumes of water or water-electrolyte solutions for 1 to 3 hours before exercise. Much of the fluid overload is rapidly excreted, however, so expansion of body water and blood volume is only transient. Studies in which the blood volume was directly expanded by infusion reported decreased cardiovascular strain during exercise but yielded conflicting results on sweat loss, heat dissipation, and exercise performance. Some studies that limited the rise in plasma osmolarity during exercise reported improved heat dissipation but did not address the question of whether it affects exercise performance.

Greater fluid retention is achieved if glycerol is added to fluids consumed before exercise. When glycerol is consumed orally, it is rapidly absorbed primarily in the small intestine. It is reported to be evenly distributed among all fluid compartments, with the exception of the cerebrospinal fluid and aqueous humour, and promotes hyperhydration by inducing an osmotic gradient. Through an increase in the medullary concentration gradient of the kidney, water absorption in the kidney tubules (nephrons) is enhanced. When glycerol is consumed, the plasma glycerol concentration increases in proportion to the dose ingested, which easily exceeds the renal threshold for glycerol reabsorption resulting in urinary glycerol excretion.

Thus, without supplemental glycerol ingestion, a decrease in the osmotic gradient occurs, resulting in a loss of hyperhydration (Nelson and Rogbergs 2007).

One study has reported a higher sweating rate and lower core temperature when subjects exercised in the heat after hyperhydrating with glycerol (1 g/kg b.w.) and water (21.4 ml/kg b.w.) compared with an equal volume of water alone (Lyons et al. 1990). Other studies, however, report no thermoregulatory advantage during exercise after glycerol solution–induced hyperhydration (Inder et al. 1998; Latzka et al. 1997, 1998). In these studies, the volume of water consumed (500 ml) may have been too small. In a study by Murray et al. (1991), no indications of hyperhydration were found. Generally, however, the ingestion of 1 g/kg b.w. of glycerol with 1 to 2 L of water seems to protect against heat stress and thus may have some health benefits for people who exercise in hot conditions. A study examined the effect of ingestion of a large bolus of water (20 ml/kg b.w.) with or without added glycerol (1 g/kg b.w.) 2 hours before 90 minutes of submaximal cycling (98% of lactate threshold) in dry, hot conditions (35 °C [95 °F], relative humidity = 30%) followed by a 15-minute time trial (Anderson et al. 2001). Although preexercise glycerol ingestion did not affect skin temperature, muscle temperature, circulating catecholamine, or muscle metabolic responses to the steady state exercise, heart and core temperature were lower than with the ingestion of water alone. Furthermore, time-trial performance (total work performed) improved significantly, by 5%. In subsequent studies, this finding could not be confirmed, although those studies reported indications of improved thermoregulation. Why one study provides favorable results while another does not is unclear. Possible explanations may include subject characteristics; environmental factors; research design; whether fluids with or without glycerol were given during exercise; the rate at which fluids were initially given to induce hyperhydration; the time between peak hyperhydration and peak plasma glycerol concentration and the start of the exercise; the weight-specific glycerol dose (i.e., grams per kilogram of body mass) and the concentration of glycerol in the administered beverage (e.g., 5%, 10%, 20%); or perhaps the intensity, mode, and nature of the exercise test (time to exhaustion at a fixed work rate, time trial). What is clear is that glycerol has the capacity to enhance fluid retention. In so doing, glycerol hyperhydration may give a performance advantage by offsetting dehydration during subsequent exercise. Potential benefits of glycerol need to be explored further to identify the circumstances or factors that may contribute to an ergogenic effect. For more information on glycerol, see chapter 11.

Fluid Intake During Exercise

During exercise, especially in a hot environment, dehydration can be avoided only by matching fluid consumption with sweat loss. Achieving this goal, however, is difficult for a number of reasons:

■ Sweat rates during strenuous exercise in the heat can be around 2 to 3 L/h. A volume of ingested fluid in the stomach of more than about 1 L feels uncomfortable for most people when exercising, so achieving fluid intake that matches sweat loss during exercise is often not practical.

■ Sweat rates vary widely among individuals under the same ambient conditions. (Figure 9.10 shows the sweat rates of people competing in a marathon race in Scotland [Maughan 1985].) Hence, to prescribe the specific amount that a person should drink is difficult without knowing the person's sweat rate under the prevailing weather conditions.

■ Thirst is not a good indicator of body-water requirements or the degree of dehydration. In general, the sensation of thirst is not perceived until a person has lost at least 2% of body weight through sweating. As already mentioned, even this mild degree of dehydration is sufficient to impair exercise performance. Numerous studies show that ad libitum intake of water during exercise in the heat results in incomplete replacement of body-

water losses (observed values of fluid intakes and losses are shown in table 9.4).

■ The rules or practicalities of specific sports may limit the opportunities for drinking during competition.

Because even mild dehydration and small decreases in plasma volume impair endurance exercise capacity, athletes should try to minimize the extent of dehydration by ingesting fluids during exercise. Regular water intake during prolonged exercise is effective in improving both exercise capacity (time to exhaustion [see figures 9.11 and 9.12]) and exercise performance (time to complete a given amount of work [see figure 9.13]) in both thermoneutral and hot ambient conditions (Fallowfield et al. 1996; Maughan et al. 1987).

■ TABLE 9.4 ■
Fluid Losses and Intakes of Athletes

Sport	Ambient temperature	Sweat loss (ml/h)	Fluid intake (ml/h)
Marathon running	15–20 °C (59–68 °F)	800–1,200	500
Soccer	10 °C (50 °F) 25 °C (77 °F)	1,000 1,200	350 500
Basket-ball	20–25 °C (68–77 °F)	1,600	1,080
Rowing	10 °C (50 °F) 30 °C (86 °F)	1,165 1,980	580 960
Cycling	30 °C (86 °F)	2,000	800

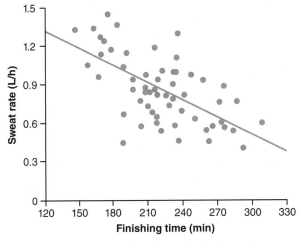

Figure 9.10 Sweat rates for subjects who competed in a marathon race held in cool (about 12 °C [54 °F]) conditions. The sweat rate was related to running speed, but a large variation existed between individuals, even those running at the same speed.

Data from Maughan 1985.

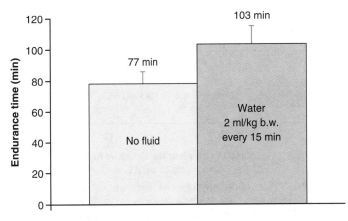

Figure 9.11 Effect of water intake on running endurance capacity in an ambient temperature of 20 °C.

Data from Fallowfield, Williams et al. 1996.

Fluid intake during prolonged exercise offers the opportunity to ingest some fuel as well. The addition of carbohydrate to some drinks consumed during exercise has an additional independent effect in improving exercise performance (see figures 9.12 and 9.13) (Below et al. 1995). Further details can found in chapter 6. Too much added

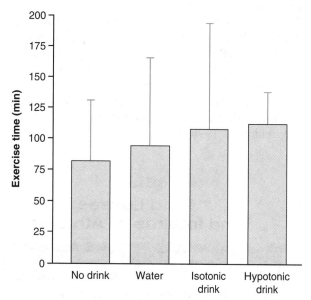

Figure 9.12 Effects of ingestion of different drinks on exercise capacity during a cycle ergometer test to exhaustion at 70% of V̇O₂max. Ingestion of water resulted in a longer time to exhaustion than in the no-drink trial, but ingestion of the two dilute carbohydrate–electrolyte drinks resulted in the longest endurance times.
Data from Maughan et al. 1987.

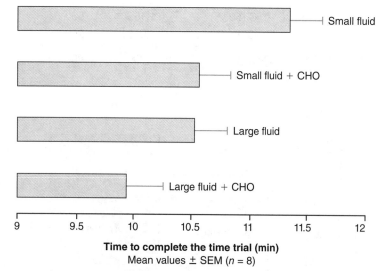

Time to complete the time trial (min)
Mean values ± SEM (*n* = 8)

Figure 9.13 Effect of carbohydrate and fluid ingestion on a cycling time trial performed at the end of a prolonged exercise test at 31 °C (88 °F) in which either a small (200 ml) or large (1,330 ml) fluid volume with either zero carbohydrate or a large amount (79 g) of carbohydrate was given. Ingestion of water and carbohydrate has independent and additive effects in improving exercise performance.
Data from Below et al. 1995.

carbohydrate in a sports drink, although providing more fuel for the working muscles, decreases the amount of water that can be absorbed. In this situation, water is drawn out of the interstitial fluid and plasma into the lumen of the small intestine by osmosis. This effect is demonstrated in figure 9.14, which shows that the ingestion of a concentrated (16.5% carbohydrate) glucose solution, hypertonic with respect to plasma, delays the restoration of plasma volume during exercise compared with the ingestion of a more dilute (3.6% carbohydrate) hypotonic glucose–electrolyte drink (Maughan et al. 1987).

As long as the fluid remains hypotonic with respect to plasma, the uptake of water from the small intestine is not adversely affected. In fact, the presence of small amounts of glucose and sodium tends to cause a slight increase in the rate of water absorption compared with pure water (Maughan and Murray 2000). Sodium and other electrolytes are added to sports drinks not to replace electrolytes lost through sweating but to provide the following benefits:

■ To increase palatability

■ To maintain thirst (and therefore promote drinking)

■ To prevent hyponatremia (low serum sodium concentration, which can occur when people ingest far more water than required)

■ To increase the rate of water uptake

■ To increase the retention of fluid

Replacement of the electrolytes lost in sweat can normally wait until the postexercise recovery period. Fluid intake during strenuous exercise of less than 30 minutes duration offers no advantage. Gastric emptying is inhibited at high work rates, and insignificant amounts of fluid are absorbed during exercise of such short duration. For exercise lasting more than 1 hour or exercise in hot or humid conditions, consumption of carbohydrate–electrolyte sports drink is warranted. These drinks supply fluid together with carbohydrate that helps maintain blood glucose and high levels of carbohydrate oxidation. The electrolyte (sodium) content partly offsets salt losses in sweat, but perhaps more important, it maintains the desire to drink.

Sweat-loss rates during exercise depend on exercise intensity, duration, and environmental conditions but vary considerably among individuals. Some people may lose up to 3 L/h of sweat during strenuous activity in a warm environment (see figure 9.15) (Sawka and Pandolf 1990), and even at low ambient temperatures of about 12 °C (54 °F), sweat loss can exceed 1 L/h (see figure 9.10) (Maughan 1985). Because the electrolyte composition of sweat is hypotonic to plasma (in other words, the total concentration of dissolved anions and cations is considerably lower in sweat than in plasma; see table 9.5), the replacement of water rather than electrolytes is the priority during exercise. Plasma volume falls by up to 20% during exercise, the magnitude of the fall being related to the relative exercise intensity. Typically, at work rates equivalent to 60% to 80% of the maximal oxygen uptake, plasma volume falls acutely by about 10% to 15% because of the increased capillary hydrostatic pressure and osmotic uptake of water into active skeletal muscle tissue. Without fluid intake, particularly in a warm, humid environment, further falls in plasma volume and increases in plasma osmolarity occur because of the loss of hypotonic sweat, as exercise proceeds.

As mentioned previously, the decrease in plasma volume that accompanies dehydration may be of particular importance in influencing work capacity. Blood flow to the muscles must be maintained at a high level to supply oxygen and fuel substrates (glucose and fatty acids), but high blood flow to the skin is also necessary to convect heat to the body surface, where it can be dissipated. When the ambient temperature is high and plasma volume decreases through sweat loss during prolonged exercise (as shown in figure 9.16), skin blood flow is likely to be compromised (Costill and Fink 1974), allowing central venous pressure and blood flow to the working muscle to be maintained but reducing heat loss and causing body temperature to rise to dangerous levels. To prevent dehydration, water must be replaced at a faster rate. Metabolic water production increases during exercise but not enough to compensate for water loss through sweating. Oral fluid ingestion during exercise helps restore plasma volume to near preexercise levels (see figure 9.16) and prevents the adverse effects of dehydration on

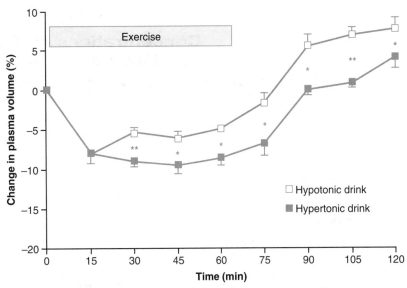

Figure 9.14 Plasma volume changes during exercise with consumption of a hypertonic (16.5% carbohydrate) or hypotonic (3.6% carbohydrate) glucose-containing beverage. Because of the faster gastric emptying and faster intestinal absorption of water, ingestion of the more dilute carbohydrate–electrolyte solution (open squares) is more effective in restoring plasma volume during exercise compared with ingestion of an equal volume of a concentrated glucose solution (closed squares).

European Journal of Applied Physiology, Vol. 45, 1988, pgs. 356-362, "Metabolic and circulatory responses to the ingestion of glucose polymer and glucose/electrolyte solutions during exercise in man," R.J. Maughan et al., © Springer Verlag. With kind permission of Springer Science+Business Media.

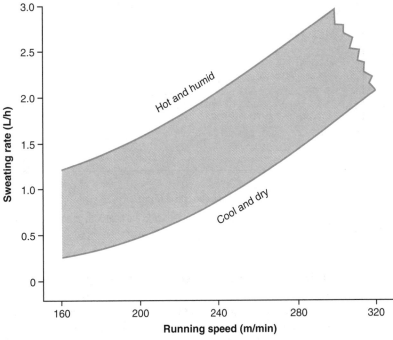

Figure 9.15 Approximate hourly sweating rates as a function of environmental conditions and running speed.

Reprinted, by permission, from M.N. Sawka and K.B. Pandolf, 1990, Effects of body water loss on physiological function and exercise performance. In *Perspectives in exercise science and sports medicine*, Vol. 3, edited by C.V. Gisolfi and D.R. Lamb (Traverse City, MI: Cooper Publishing), 1-38.

thermal and cardiovascular strain, muscle strength, endurance, and coordination.

A study compared time to exhaustion during cycling at 60% of $\dot{V}O_2max$ in warm ambient conditions

■ **TABLE 9.5** ■

Concentrations of Electrolytes in Sweat, Plasma, and Intracellular Water

Electrolyte	Sweat (mmol/L)	Plasma (mmol/L)	Intracellular water (mmol/L)
CATIONS			
Sodium	20–80	130–155	10
Potassium	4–8	3.2–5.5	150
Calcium	0.1–1.0	2.1–2.9	0.01
Magnesium	0.1–0.2	0.7–1.5	15
ANIONS			
Chloride	20–60	96–110	8
Bicarbonate	1–35	23–28	10
Phosphate	0.1–0.2	0.7–1.6	65
Sulphate	0.1–2.0	0.3–0.9	10

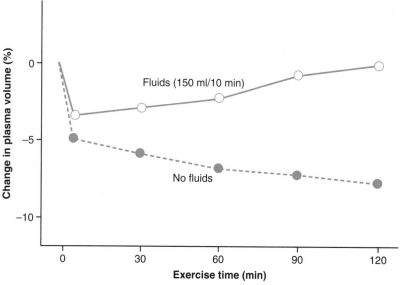

Figure 9.16 Changes in plasma volume during exercise in the heat with and without regular fluid ingestion.

Data from Costill and Fink 1974.

(30 °C [86 °F]) when six subjects were given (a) no drink, (b) 500 ml of a 15% carbohydrate–electrolyte drink immediately before exercise and 125 ml of the same drink every 10 minutes throughout exercise, or (c) 500 ml of a 2% carbohydrate–electrolyte drink immediately before exercise and 250 ml of the same drink every 10 minutes throughout exercise (Galloway and Maughan 2000). As shown in figure 9.17, with no drink, subjects fatigued after 71 minutes (median range 39 to 97 minutes). With the 15% carbohydrate–electrolyte drink, they could continue for longer times (median 84 minutes, range 63 to 145 minutes). But the best

performance was achieved with the 2% carbohydrate–electrolyte drink (median 118 minutes, range 83 minutes to 168 minutes). The median core temperature at exhaustion was the same in all three trials (39.5 °C [103 °F]). A significant fall in plasma volume occurred within the first 15 minutes of exercise on all trials. Subsequently, plasma volume remained below resting values on the no-drink and the 15% carbohydrate–electrolyte trials, but on the 2% carbohydrate–electrolyte trial, plasma volume was gradually restored during exercise.

Gonzalez-Alonso et al. (1998) showed that exercising-limb perfusion may decrease during prolonged exercise combined with heat stress and dehydration. The maintenance of plasma volume on the 2% carbohydrate–electrolyte trial may have resulted in better perfusion of active muscles during exercise and may have resulted in better maintenance of cellular hydration.

Ingestion of relatively cool fluid may have an additional small benefit during exercise in the heat because the additional volume of fluid in the body after drinking adds to the body's heat-storage capacity. The improvement in heat-storage capacity can be calculated based on the specific heat capacity of water, which is 4.184 kJ · kg⁻¹ · °C⁻¹ (0.555 kcal · kg⁻¹ · °F⁻¹). For example, the ingestion of 2 L of fluid at 10 °C (50 °F) increases heat-storage capacity by 4.184 × 2 × (37 − 10) kJ = 226 kJ (54 kcal).

In the study by Galloway and Maughan (2000), subjects ingested fluids cooled to 14 °C (57 °F). The investigators calculated that the extra fluid consumed on the 2% carbohydrate–electrolyte treatment (2.3 L) could have produced an 8-minute improvement in performance because of its effect in increasing body heat-storage capacity compared with the no-drink treatment.

Daily Water Balance

The typical daily water balance for a sedentary individual living in a cool or temperate climate (ambient temperature 10 to 20 °C [50 to 68 °F]) is shown in figure 9.18. Variable amounts of water are lost from the body through sweating in response to the requirement for thermoregulation, but for a sedentary person in cool conditions, evaporative loss of water through the skin amounts to only about 600 ml/day. Additional water is lost in the feces (about 100 ml/day) and urine. Normally, about 800 ml to 1,600 ml of urine is produced each day. The kidneys are able to regulate the amount of water lost in urine; although even in severe dehydration, some urine is still produced to maintain fluid flow through the kidney tubules (nephrons) and excrete toxic nitrogenous wastes such as ammonia and urea. Urinary water loss is not usually less than 800 ml/day.

Environmental conditions affect a person's water requirements by altering the losses that occur by the various routes. Water losses may be two to three times greater for a sedentary person living in a hot climate compared with a sedentary person living in a temperate climate. These higher rates of water loss are not caused exclusively by increased sweating; they may also be incurred by a marked increase in transcutaneous and respiratory water losses. These routes of water loss are heavily influenced by the humidity of the ambient air, which may be a more important factor than the ambient temperature. Respiratory water losses are greater when the relative humidity (RH) of the ambient air is low because air breathed out of the body is fully saturated with

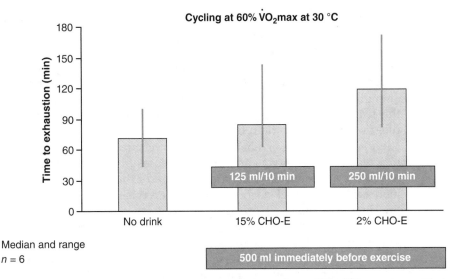

Median and range
$n = 6$

Figure 9.17 Time to exhaustion (median and range) during cycling at 60% of $\dot{V}O_2$max at an ambient temperature of 31°C (88 °F). Six subjects received *(a)* no drink, *(b)* 500 ml of a 15% carbohydrate–electrolyte drink (CHO–E) immediately preexercise and 125 ml of the same drink every 10 minutes throughout exercise, or *(c)* 500 ml of a 2% CHO–E drink immediately before exercise and 250 ml of the same drink every 10 minutes throughout exercise. The three treatments were significantly different from each other in terms of endurance performance.

JOURNAL OF SPORTS SCIENCES by Galloway and Maughan. Copyright 2000 by Taylor & Francis Informa UK Ltd - Journals. Reproduced with permission of Taylor & Francis Informa UK Ltd - Journals in the format Other book via Copyright Clearance Center.

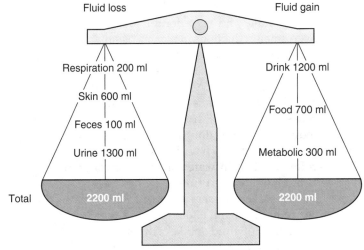

Figure 9.18 Daily water balance for a sedentary adult individual.

water vapor (RH = 100%). Although these losses are small for a sedentary individual in a moist, warm environment (about 200 ml/day), they may increase approximately twofold in low-humidity conditions (RH = 0% to 20%) and may rise up to 1,500 ml/day during periods of hard training in cold, dry air at altitude.

Water intake comes from drinks and food; some foods (especially plant material) have high water content. Water in food, in fact, makes a major contribution to total water intake. Water is also produced internally (metabolic water) from the catabolism of carbohydrate, fat, and protein. For example, in the complete oxidation of one molecule of glucose, six molecules of carbon dioxide and six molecules of water are produced. In a sedentary individual, metabolic water production amounts to about 300 ml/day, although most of this water is lost in expired gas, because oxidizing fuel in the body generates carbon dioxide, which stimulates breathing and hence increases respiratory water loss. Although an athlete increases his or her metabolic water production because of the increased rate of fuel catabolism during exercise, this increase, again, is offset by the obligatory increase in lung ventilation and respiratory evaporative water loss.

The body's water balance is under tight regulation involving nervous and hormonal factors that respond to a number of inputs. The osmolarity of the blood plasma is maintained within tight limits around 290 mOsmol/L. A rise or fall in the plasma osmolarity is sufficient to alter kidney function from maximum water conservation to maximum water excretion. Because sodium is the major electrolyte in the extracellular fluids (accounting for 50% of plasma osmolarity), the maintenance of osmotic balance is closely coupled to the intake and excretion of sodium and water. Even small reductions in plasma osmolarity invoke a marked increase in urine output (diuresis), and this increase is normally sufficient to prevent fluid overload when large volumes of water or low-electrolyte drinks such as beer are consumed. But some cases of hyponatremia (low plasma sodium concentration) have been reported, usually in people who have ingested excessively large volumes of plain water or low-electrolyte drinks in a relatively short time.

The subjective sensation of thirst initiates the desire to drink and is therefore a key factor in the regulation of fluid intake. Although the kidneys can effectively conserve water or electrolytes by reducing the rate of loss, they cannot restore a fluid deficit. Only consumption of fluid can correct this imbalance. The sensation of thirst is mainly evoked by the detection of elevated plasma osmolarity (and to a lesser extent, by reductions in blood volume and pressure) by osmoreceptors located in the hypothalamus of the brain. The thirst sensation results in a profound desire to drink and an increase in the secretion of antidiuretic hormone (ADH) from the posterior pituitary gland, which acts on the kidneys to reduce urine excretion. Other factors that promote thirst are learned responses such as dryness of the mouth or throat, salty tastes, and feeling hot. Thirst is quickly alle-

viated by drinking fluid, and alleviation can occur before a significant amount of the fluid is absorbed in the gut. This effect suggests a role for sensory receptors in the mouth and stomach. Distension of the stomach wall appears to reduce the perception of thirst and may result in premature cessation of fluid ingestion. Thus, the absence of the sensation of thirst cannot be used as an indicator that fluid balance (**euhydration**) is established; the perception of thirst is often not present until a significant degree of dehydration has occurred.

An electrolyte imbalance commonly called water intoxication, which results from hyponatremia (low plasma sodium) caused by excessive water consumption, is occasionally reported in endurance athletes. This condition appears to be most common among slow runners in marathon and ultramarathon races and probably arises because of the loss of sodium in sweat coupled with extremely high intakes (8 L to 10 L) of water (Noakes et al. 1985). The symptoms of hyponatremia are similar to those of dehydration and include mental confusion, weakness, and fainting. Therefore, this condition can be misdiagnosed when it occurs in people who participate in endurance races. The usual treatment for dehydration is administration of fluid intravenously and orally. If this treatment is given to a hyponatremic individual, the consequences can be fatal. The normal plasma sodium concentration is around 140 to 144 mmol/L. Symptomatic hyponatremia can occur when the plasma sodium concentration rapidly drops to 130 mmol/L or less. The longer that it remains low, the greater the risk is of developing swelling of the brain (the clinical term is dilutional encephalopathy) and accumulating extracellular fluid in the lungs (pulmonary edema). When plasma sodium falls well below 120 mmol/L, the risk of brain seizure, coma, and death increases. In long-distance events, symptomatic hyponatremia is more likely to occur in small, lean people who run slowly, sweat less, and ingest large volumes of water or hypotonic fluids before, during, and even after the event. People with genes for cystic fibrosis tend to be more prone to salt depletion and therefore may be at higher risk for developing exercise-associated hyponatremia. Women generally have lower sweating rates than men and are thus at higher risk for developing exercise-associated hyponatremia.

In a study the fluid requirements for American footballers performing two-a-day training sessions in a hot, humid environment were compared with cross country runners in the same conditions (Godek et al. 2005). Sweating rates during exercise were determined in both morning and afternoon practices or runs from the change in body weight adjusted for fluids consumed and urine produced. Overall sweat rate was higher in the footballers than in the cross country runners (2.14 vs. 1.77 L/h). Daily sweat losses were substantially higher in the footballers (9.4 vs. 3.5 L), but the footballers consumed much larger volumes of fluid during both morning and afternoon training sessions. For complete hydration, the necessary daily fluid consumption calculated as 130% of daily sweat loss in the footballers was 12.2 L compared with 4.6 L in the runners. Consuming such large volumes of hypotonic fluid may promote sodium dilution unless care is taken to ensure adequate electrolyte replacement. Thus, footballers and others (e.g., military personnel in hot conditions) whose fluid losses and replacement needs are high require careful guidance not only to avoid excessive dehydration but also to promote safe rehydration and avoid hyponatremia.

Fluid Requirements for Athletes

Athletes must be fully hydrated before they train or compete because the body cannot adapt to dehydration. Training quality will suffer if an athlete becomes dehydrated during training, as will performance quality if an athlete becomes dehydrated during competition.

Ensuring Adequate Hydration Before Exercise

An adequately hydrated state can be assured by high fluid intake in the last few days before competition. A useful check is to observe the color of the urine. It should be pale in color, although this simple test cannot be reliably used if the athlete is taking vitamin supplements, because some of the excreted water-soluble B vitamins add a yellowish hue to urine. A clearer indication of hydration status is obtained by measuring urine osmolality. (Note that the units of osmolality are Osmol/kg, whereas osmolarity is expressed as Osmol/L.) This measurement can be done quickly and simply using a portable osmometer. A urine osmolality of over 900 mOsmol/kg indicates that the athlete is relatively dehydrated; values of 100 to 300 mOsmol/kg indicate that the athlete is well hydrated. Measuring the athlete's body weight after rising and voiding

each morning may also prove useful. A sudden drop in body mass on any given day is likely to indicate dehydration. Approximate fluid intake requirements in liters per day in hot, dry conditions are shown in figure 9.19. The fluid intake requirement (to maintain water balance, or euhydration) increases as ambient temperature increases and as daily energy expenditure increases.

Ensuring Hydration During Exercise

Relying on feeling thirsty as the signal to drink is unreliable because a considerable degree of dehydration (certainly sufficient to impair athletic performance) can occur before the desire for fluid intake is evident. Ideally, athletes should consume enough fluids during activity to make body weight remain fairly constant before and after exercise. Guidelines for the amount of fluid to be consumed before, during, and after exercise can only be general because of the large variation in individual sweating responses. The American and Canadian Dietetic Associations recommend that approximately 500 ml of fluid be consumed 2 hours before exertion and another 500 ml be consumed about 15 minutes before prolonged exercise. In hot and humid environments, frequent consumption (every 15 to 20 minutes) of small volumes (120 to 180 ml) of fluid are recommended throughout exertion. Detailed recommendations on fluid replacement strategies during and following exercise have been given in the 2007 American College of Sports Medicine position stand on exercise and fluid replacement (available at www.acsm-msse.org). Athletes should become accustomed to consuming fluid at regular intervals (with or without thirst) during

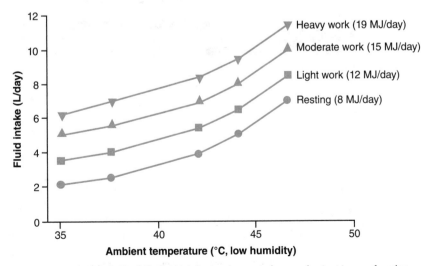

Figure 9.19 Approximate daily fluid intake requirements for people at rest or performing various amounts of physical work while living at different ambient temperatures.
Adapted from Sawka and Montain 2000.

training sessions so that they do not experience discomfort during competition. For most persons exercising for 30 to 60 minutes in moderate temperatures, an appropriate beverage is cool water.

Composition of Sport Drinks During Exercise

Fluid ingestion during exercise also supplies exogenous fuel substrate (usually carbohydrate) as well as helps maintain plasma volume and prevents dehydration. But the availability of ingested fluids may be limited by the rate of gastric emptying or intestinal absorption. Gastric emptying of fluids is slowed by the addition of carbohydrate or other macronutrients that increase the osmolarity of the solution ingested. Hence, with increasing glucose concentration in the fluid ingested, the rate of fluid volume delivery to the small intestine decreases, although the rate of glucose delivery increases.

Water absorption in the small intestine is by osmosis and is promoted by the coupled transport of glucose and sodium. Hence, the composition of fluids to be used during exercise depends on the relative needs to replace water and provide fuel substrate. Where rehydration is the main priority (e.g., for prolonged exercise in the heat), the solution should contain some carbohydrate as glucose or glucose polymers (20 to 60 g/L) and sodium (20 to 60 mmol/L) and should not exceed isotonicity (290 mOsmol/L). Most commercially available sports drinks contain 60 to 80 g/L of carbohydrate (predominantly as glucose, glucose polymers, or both, although some drinks may also contain fructose or sucrose) and 20 to 25 mmol/L of sodium. Table 9.6 compares the compositions of several commercially available drinks that athletes commonly consume during training or competition. In cool environments, where substrate provision to maintain endurance performance is more important, a concentrated solution incorporating large amounts of glucose polymers in concentrations of 550 to 800 mmol/L glucosyl units (100 to 150 g/L) is recommended. To minimize the limitation imposed by the rate of gastric emptying, the osmolarity of the beverage should be minimized by providing the glucose in the form of glucose polymers, and the volume of fluid in the stomach should be kept as high as is comfortable by frequent ingestion of small amounts of fluid.

The importance of practicing drinking during training is often neglected. This practice will accustom athletes to the feeling of exercising with fluid in the stomach. It also provides the opportunity to experiment with different volumes and flavorings to determine how much fluid intake they can tolerate and which formulations suit them best. Measuring fluid consumption and body mass changes before and after training gives an idea of the athlete's sweat rate under different environmental conditions. This information will help determine the athlete's requirements for fluid intake during competition.

The ideal drink for fluid replacement during exercise is one that tastes good to the athlete, does not cause gastrointestinal discomfort when

■ **TABLE 9.6** ■

Compositions of Commonly Consumed Sport Drinks

Drink	Carbohydrate (g/L)	Sodium (mmol/L)	Potassium (mmol/L)	Osmolality (mOsmol/kg)
Coca-Cola	105	3	0	650
Allsport	80	10	6	516
Gatorade	60	18	3	349
Isostar	65	24	4	296
Lucozade Sport	64	23	4	280
Lucozade	180	0	0	658
Powerade (UK)	60	24	4	285
Powerade (U.S.)	80	5	4	381

Note: Some drink bottles show carbohydrate content as % or % w/v (weight/volume), which is equivalent to g/100 ml; for example, in the table, Lucozade Sport carbohydrate content is 64 g/L, which is 6.4 g/100 ml or 6.4%. Sodium content may be given in milligrams (mg), which can be obtained from the table by multiplying the sodium concentration in mmol/L by 23 (the atomic mass of sodium). For example, Lucozade Sport sodium content is 23 mmol/L, which is 529 mg/L. Thus, a 500 ml bottle of Lucozade Sport contains 265 mg of sodium.

consumed in large volumes (this rules out all fizzy carbonated drinks), promotes rapid gastric emptying and fluid absorption to help maintain extracellular fluid volume, and provides some energy in the form of carbohydrate for the working muscles. Exercising subjects prefer cool, pleasantly flavored, sweetened beverages, and the presence of sodium in the drinks seems to promote their consumption, probably by maintaining thirst.

Rehydration After Exercise

Replacement of water and electrolytes in the postexercise recovery period may be of crucial importance when repeated bouts of exercise must be performed and rehydration must be maximized in the time available. As previously mentioned, dehydration is associated with impaired thermoregulation, increased cardiovascular strain, and the loss of the thermoregulatory advantages conferred by heat acclimation and high aerobic fitness. With progressive dehydration, loss of both intracellular and extracellular fluid volume occurs. Loss of intracellular volume may have important implications for recovery from exercise given the emerging evidence of a role for cell volume in the regulation of cell metabolism. Reduced intracellular volume reduces rates of glycogen and protein synthesis, whereas high cell volume stimulates these processes.

The main factors influencing the effectiveness of postexercise rehydration are the volume and composition of the fluid consumed. Plain water is not the ideal rehydration beverage when rapid and complete restoration of body fluid balance is necessary and when all intake is in liquid form. Ingestion of water alone causes a rapid fall in plasma sodium concentration and in plasma osmolarity. These changes reduce the stimulation to drink (thirst) and increase urine output, both of which delay the rehydration process. Plasma volume is more rapidly and completely restored if some sodium chloride (77 mmol/L, or 0.45 g/L) is added to the water consumed (Nose et al. 1988). This sodium concentration is similar to the upper limit of the sodium concentration found in sweat but is considerably higher than the sodium concentration of many commercially available sports drinks, which usually contain 10 to 25 mmol/L (see table 9.6). Optimal rehydration after exercise can be achieved only if the sodium lost in sweat is replaced along with the water.

Shirreffs et al. (1996) showed that if an adequate volume of fluid is consumed, euhydration is achieved when sodium intake is greater than sodium loss (see figure 9.20). Ingesting a beverage containing sodium not only promotes rapid fluid absorption in the small intestine but also allows the plasma sodium concentration to remain elevated during the rehydration period and helps maintain thirst while delaying stimulation of urine production. Sodium is the major cation in extracellular fluid. The inclusion of potassium in the beverage consumed after exercise would be expected to enhance the replacement of intracellular water and thus promote rehydration, but currently little experimental evidence supports this expectation. The rehydration drink should also contain carbohydrate (glucose or glucose polymers) because the presence of some glucose also stimulates fluid absorption in the gut and improves beverage taste. After exercise, the uptake of glucose into the muscle for glycogen resynthesis should also promote intracellular rehydration.

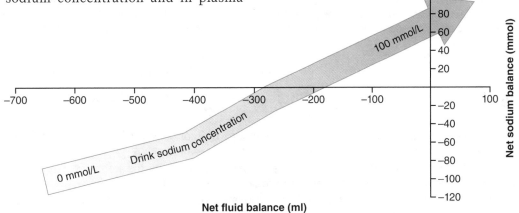

Figure 9.20 Net sodium balance plotted against net fluid balance 6 hours after the end of a rehydration period, during which subjects ingested various drinks in a volume equivalent to 150% of sweat loss. The drinks containing sodium at a concentration of 0, 25, 50, or 100 mmol/L (trials 0, 25, 50, and 100, respectively) were ingested after exercise. At the end of the 6-hour rehydration period, water balance was achieved only when the sodium intake was greater than the sodium sweat loss.

Reprinted, by permission, from S.M. Shirreffs and R.J. Maughan, 2000, "Rehydration and recovery of fluid balance after exercise," *Exercise and Sport Sciences Reviews* 28(1): 27-32.

Fluid Consumption After Exercise

For a person undertaking regular exercise, any fluid deficit incurred during one exercise session can potentially compromise the next exercise session if adequate fluid replacement does not occur. Fluid replacement after exercise can, therefore, frequently be thought of as hydration before the next exercise bout. Until recently, athletes were generally encouraged to consume a volume of fluid equivalent to their sweat loss incurred during exercise to rehydrate adequately in the postexercise recovery period. In other words, they were to consume about 1 L of fluid for every kilogram lost during an exercise session. This amount is insufficient because it does not take into account the obligatory urine losses that are incurred after beverage consumption over a period of hours. Existing data indicate that ingestion of 150% or

more of weight loss (i.e., 1.5 L of fluid consumed during recovery for every kilogram of weight lost during exercise) may be required to achieve normal hydration within 6 hours after exercise (Shirreffs et al. 1996; Shirreffs and Maughan 1998, 2000 [see figure 9.21]). Current (1996) American College of Sports Medicine (ACSM) guidelines on fluid ingestion before, during, and after exercise are shown in the highlight box.

Intake of caffeine and alcohol in the postexercise recovery period is generally discouraged because of their diuretic actions. The diuretic effect of alcohol appears to be blunted, however, when it is consumed by persons who are moderately dehydrated after exercise in a warm environment (Shirreffs and Maughan 1997). If shandy (a mixture of beer and lemonade) is consumed in the postexercise period, then (as expected) urinary output increases with increasing alcohol intake.

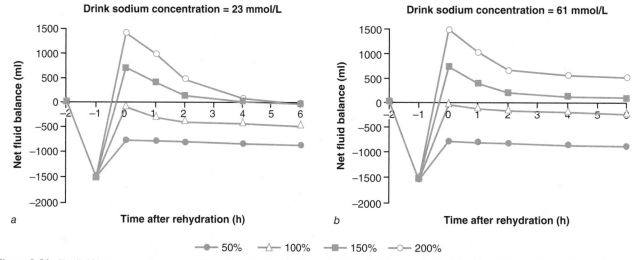

Figure 9.21 Net fluid balance plotted against time after dehydration (loss of 1,500 ml of body water) induced by mild exercise in a hot environment. Zero net fluid balance represents euhydration. Drink volume ingested was half of (50%), equal to (100%), one-and-a-half times (150%), and twice (200%) the sweat loss. The drink sodium concentration was either (a) 23 mmol/L or (b) 61 mmol/L. Mild dehydration was present 6 hours after rehydration when a large volume of the low-sodium drink (23 mmol/L) was consumed, but with the same volume, hyperhydration was achieved with the high-sodium drink (61 mmol/L).

Adapted from S.M. Shirreffs et al., 1996, "Post-exercise rehydration in man: Effects of volume consumed and drink sodium content," *Medicine and Science in Sport Exercise* 28: 1260-1271.

Selected Recommendations on Exercise and Fluid Replacement

The following recommendations are taken from the American College of Sports Medicine Guidelines on Fluid Intake for Exercise (2002) and the Position Stand on Exercise and Fluid Replacement (2007).

Adequate fluid replacement helps maintain hydration and therefore promotes the health, safety, and optimal physical performance of people who participate in regular physical activity. The following are general recommendations on the amount and composition of fluids that should be ingested in preparation for, during, and after exercise or athletic competition.

- Individuals should consume a nutritionally balanced diet and drink adequate fluids during the 24-hour period before an event, especially during the period that includes the meal before exercise, to promote proper hydration before exercise or competition.

- Individuals should drink about 6 to 8 ml of fluid per kilogram of body weight about 2 hours before exercise to allow sufficient time for fluid absorption and allow time for excretion of excess ingested water. Consuming beverages containing sodium or drinking beverages together with eating salted snacks or small meals can help to stimulate thirst and retain needed fluids.

- During exercise, athletes should start drinking early and at regular intervals in an attempt to consume fluids at a rate sufficient to prevent excessive (reductions from baseline body weight greater than 2%) dehydration. Because people vary considerably in their rates of sweating (and, of course, sweating rate depends greatly on environmental conditions and exercise intensity), individuals should develop customized fluid replacement programs to achieve this goal. The routine measurement of preexercise and postexercise body weight is useful for determining sweat rates and establishing appropriate customized fluid replacement programs.

- Ingested fluids should be cooler than the ambient temperature (between 15 and 22 °C [59 and 72 °F]) and flavored to enhance palatability and promote fluid replacement. Fluids should be readily available and served in containers that allow adequate volumes to be ingested with ease and with minimal interruption of exercise.

- Addition of proper amounts of carbohydrates or electrolytes to a fluid replacement solution is recommended for exercise events longer than 1 hour because such additives do not significantly impair water delivery to the body and can enhance performance. For exercise of less than 1 hour, little evidence exists of physiological or physical performance differences resulting from consuming a carbohydrate–electrolyte drink compared with consuming plain water.

- During intense exercise lasting longer than 1 hour, carbohydrates should be ingested at a rate of 30 to 60 g/h to maintain oxidation of carbohydrate and delay fatigue. This rate of carbohydrate delivery can be achieved without compromising fluid delivery by drinking 600 to 1,200 ml/h of solutions containing 4% to 8% carbohydrates (g/100 ml). The carbohydrates can be sugars (glucose or sucrose) or starch (e.g., maltodextrins).

- Inclusion of sodium (500 to 700 mg/L of water) in the rehydration solution ingested during exercise lasting longer than 1 hour is recommended because it may enhance palatability, promote fluid retention, and possibly prevent hyponatremia in certain individuals who drink excessive quantities of fluid. Little physiological evidence suggests the need for sodium in an oral rehydration solution for enhancing intestinal water absorption as long as sodium is sufficiently available from the previous meal.

- After exercise, in situations in which people need rapid and complete recovery from excessive dehydration, 1.5 L of fluid should be consumed for each kilogram of body weight lost. Consuming beverages with sodium will help the attainment of rapid and complete recovery of hydration status by stimulating thirst and fluid retention.

But this increase only approaches statistical significance (compared with lemonade alone) when alcohol content is around 4% w/v. This concentration of alcohol in the rehydration drink is also associated with a slower rate of recovery of plasma volume, as shown in figure 9.22, whereas drinks containing 1% and 2% alcohol seem just as effective as lemonade alone.

In most circumstances, athletes should consume solid food as well as drink between exercise bouts, unless food intake is likely to result in gastrointestinal disturbances. In one study, the same fluid volume consumed as a meal-plus-water combination compared with a sports drink alone resulted in a smaller volume of urine produced and hence greater fluid retention (Maughan, Leiper, and Shirreffs 1996). The greater efficacy of the meal-plus-water treatment in restoring whole-body fluid balance was probably a

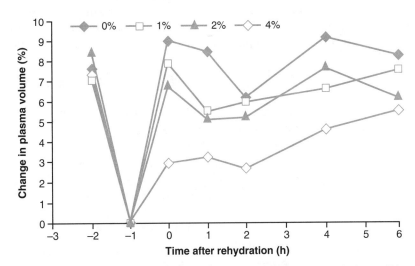

Figure 9.22 Percentage change in plasma volume with dehydration equivalent to 2% of body weight, followed by rehydration with drinks containing 0%, 1%, 2%, and 4% (w/v) alcohol in a volume equivalent to one-and-a-half times the sweat loss. Note that plasma volume restoration was delayed with the 4% alcohol drink.

Data from S.M. Shirreffs and R.J. Maughan, 1997, "Restoration of fluid balance after exercise-induced dehydration: Effect of alcohol consumption," *Journal of Applied Physiology* 83: 1152-1157. Used with permission.

Practical Application

The routine measurement of body weight in kilograms before and after exercise is useful for determining sweat rates and establishing appropriate customized fluid replacement programs. The following example illustrates how a customized fluid ingestion strategy can be established for a 70 kg male athlete:

- *Recommendation:* Drink about 6 to 8 ml of fluid per kilogram of body weight about 2 hours before exercise. *Application:* To achieve this, a 70 kg athlete would need to drink 420 to 560 ml (15 to 19 fl oz). If the fluid ingested was water, body fluid retention would be improved if a salty snack (e.g., pretzels) was eaten at the same time. Alternatively, a carbohydrate–electrolyte beverage could be ingested.

- *Recommendation:* Customize fluid ingestion during exercise according to estimated sweat loss. Approximate sweat loss during exercise under known environmental conditions could be determined from training sessions. *Application:* For example, let us say that body weight was measured and found to be 70.38 kg just before a training session begins and 68.75 kg at the end of the 90-minute session. The athlete drank 350 ml of a sports drink during the session (this volume could be estimated from weighing a drink bottle before and after the session or using a graduated drink bottle). Assuming that all weight lost during the session was from sweat, which is not unreasonable because only a small amount of weight would be lost as carbon dioxide and water in breathing, the change in body weight was 70.38 − 68.75 = 1.63 kg. We need to correct this for the additional weight of the 350 ml fluid that was ingested, which was 0.35 kg (it can be assumed that the density of the drink was 1.0 g/ml or 1 kg/L). Thus, actual weight loss if no fluid had been ingested would have been 1.63 kg + 0.35 kg = 1.98 kg. This amount of weight was lost in 90 minutes (1.5 hours), so the estimated sweating rate was 1.98/1.5 = 1.32 L/hour.

- *Recommendation:* After exercise, in situations in which people need rapid and complete recovery from excessive dehydration, 1.5 L of fluid should be consumed for each kilogram of body weight lost. *Application:* In our example, actual body weight loss during exercise was 1.63 kg. Therefore, 1.63 × 1.5 = 2.45 L of fluid should be consumed in the first hour or so after exercise to restore hydration status.

consequence of its greater total sodium and potassium content. In exercise situations in which sweat losses are large, total sodium and chloride losses are high. For example, the loss of 10 L of sweat, with a sodium concentration of 50 mmol/L, amounts to a loss of about 29 g of sodium chloride.

Obviously, food intake can be important in restoring these salt losses because most commercial sports drinks do not contain more than about 25 mmol/L of sodium. Rehydration after exercise can be achieved only if sweat electrolyte losses as well as water are replaced. One problem is that drinks with high-sodium content (i.e., 40 to 80 mmol/L) are unpalatable to some people, which results in reduced consumption. On the other hand, drinks with low-sodium content (e.g., most soft drinks) are much less effective for rehydration, and they reduce the stimulus to drink.

KEY POINTS

- High rates of sweat secretion are necessary during hard exercise to limit the rise in body temperature that would otherwise occur. If the exercise is prolonged, body-temperature increase leads to progressive dehydration and loss of electrolytes.

- A body temperature of 36 to 38 °C (96.8 to 100.4 °F) is considered the normal range at rest, and it may increase to 38 to 40 °C (100.4 to 104 °F) during exercise. When body temperature rises toward 39.5 °C (103 °F), central fatigue ensues. Further increases are commonly associated with heat exhaustion and occasionally with life-threatening heatstroke, characterized by lack of consciousness after exertion and by clinical symptoms of organ damage.

- Some people may lose up to 2 to 3 L/h of sweat during strenuous activity in a hot environment. Even at low ambient temperatures of about 10 °C (50 °F), sweat loss can exceed 1 L/h.

- Because the electrolyte composition of sweat is hypotonic to plasma, the replacement of water rather than electrolytes is the priority during exercise.

■ Fatigue toward the end of a prolonged event may result as much from the effects of dehydration as from substrate depletion. Exercise performance is impaired when a person becomes dehydrated by as little as 2% of body weight, and losses in excess of 5% of body weight can decrease the capacity for work by about 30%. Some evidence indicates that lower levels of dehydration can also impair performance even during relatively short-duration, intermittent exercise.

■ Dehydration during physical activity in the heat provokes greater performance decrements than similar activity in cooler conditions, a difference thought to be due, at least in part, to greater cardiovascular and thermoregulatory strain associated with heat exposure. Although additional research is needed to produce greater understanding of the effect of low-level dehydration on physical performance, we can generalize that when performance is at stake, being well hydrated is better than being dehydrated.

■ Oral fluid ingestion during exercise helps restore plasma volume to near preexercise levels and prevents the adverse effects of dehydration on muscle strength, endurance, and coordination. Dehydration also poses a serious health risk because it increases the risk of cramps, heat exhaustion, and life-threatening heatstroke.

■ Relying on feeling thirsty as the signal to drink is unreliable because a considerable degree of dehydration (certainly sufficient to impair athletic performance) can occur before the desire for fluid intake is evident. Ideally, athletes should consume adequate fluids during activity so that body weight remains fairly constant before and after exercise.

■ The composition of drinks to be taken during exercise should suit individual circumstances. Where rehydration is the main priority (e.g., for prolonged exercise in the heat), the solution should contain some carbohydrate as glucose or glucose polymers (20 to 60 g/L) and sodium (20 to 60 mmol/L) and should not exceed isotonicity (290 mOsmol/L).

■ Optimal rehydration after exercise can be achieved only if the sodium lost in sweat is replaced along with the water. Plasma volume is more rapidly and completely restored in the postexercise period if some sodium chloride is added to the water consumed. A volume equivalent to at least one-and-a-half times the sweat loss must be consumed to ensure that complete rehydration is achieved at the end of a 6-hour recovery period after exercise.

RECOMMENDED READINGS

American College of Sports Medicine. 2009. ACSM position stand: Exercise and fluid replacement. *Medicine and Science in Sports and Exercise* 39 (2): 377–390.

Armstrong, L.E. 2000. *Performing in extreme environments.* Champaign, IL: Human Kinetics.

Coris, E.E., A.M. Ramirez, and D.J. Van Durme. 2004. Heat illness in athletes: The dangerous combination of heat, humidity and exercise. *Sports Medicine* 34 (1): 9–16.

Judelson, D.A., C.M. Maresh, J.M. Anderson, et al. 2007. Hydration and muscular performance: Does fluid balance affect strength, power and high-intensity endurance? *Sports Medicine* 37 (10): 907–921.

Maughan, R.J. 2000. Water and electrolyte loss and replacement in exercise. In *Nutrition in sport,* ed. R.J. Maughan, 226–240.

Maughan, R.J., and L.M. Burke. 2002. Sport nutrition. *Handbook of sports medicine and sciences.* Oxford: Blackwell Science.

Maughan, R.J., and R. Murray (eds). 2000. *Sports drinks: Basic science and practical aspects.* Boca Raton, FL: CRC Press.

Maughan, R.J., and E.R. Nadel. 2000. Temperature regulation and fluid and electrolyte balance. In *Nutrition in sport,* ed. R.J. Maughan, 203–215. Oxford: Blackwell Science.

Nelson, J.L., and R.A. Rogbergs. 2007. Exploring the potential ergogenic effects of glycerol hyperhydration. *Sports Medicine* 37 (11): 981–1000.

Sawka, M.N., W.A. Latzka, and S.J. Montain. 2000. Effects of dehydration and rehydration on performance. In *Nutrition in sport,* ed. R.J. Maughan, 216–225. Oxford: Blackwell Science.

Shirreffs, S.M., L.E. Armstrong, and S.N. Cheuvront. 2004. Fluid and electrolyte needs for preparation and recovery from training and competition. *Journal of Sports Sciences* 22 (1): 57–63.

Shirreffs, S.M., and R.J. Maughan. 2000. Rehydration and recovery of fluid balance after exercise. *Exercise and Sport Sciences Reviews* 28:27–32.

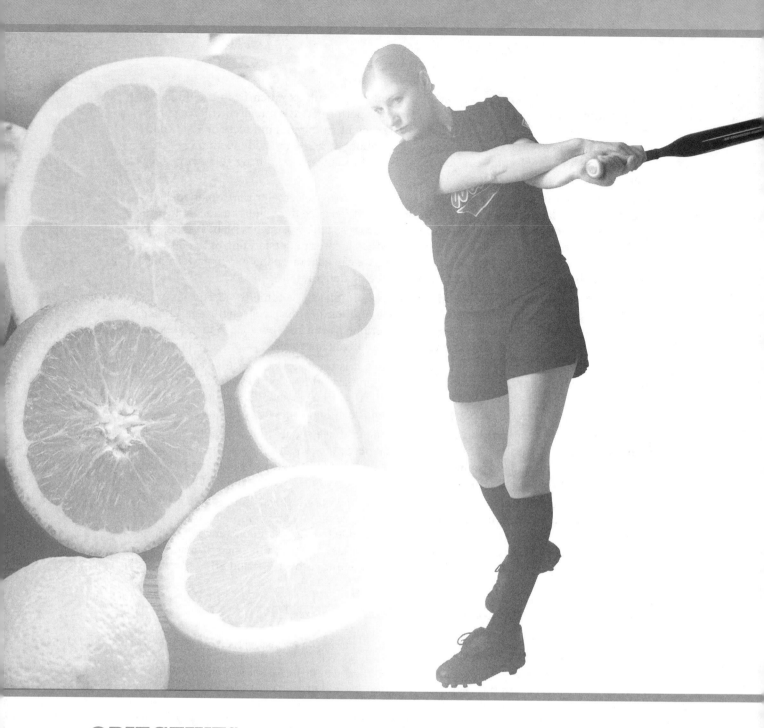

OBJECTIVES

After studying this chapter, you should be able to do the following:

- Describe the vitamins and minerals that are required to maintain a healthy body
- Describe some of the major dietary sources of essential micronutrients
- Describe the role of micronutrients in growth and repair of body tissues, in metabolism as cofactors for enzymes, in oxygen transport, in immune function, and in defense against free radicals
- Describe the effects of exercise training on micronutrient requirements
- Describe particular groups of athletes who may be at risk for micronutrient deficiencies
- Describe some of the consequences of micronutrient deficiency and excess

10

Vitamins and Minerals

Besides consuming the macronutrients (i.e., carbohydrate, fat, and protein), humans must consume relatively small amounts of certain micronutrients (i.e., organic vitamins and inorganic minerals) in the diet to maintain health. In addition to being found in foods, micronutrients are available individually or in a variety of combined preparations referred to as supplements. Many top athletes consume large quantities of vitamin and mineral supplements in the mistaken belief that they will help prevent infection or injury, speed recovery, or improve athletic performance. Some minerals are likely to do more harm than good. Although vitamin and mineral supplementation may improve the nutritional status of people who consume marginal amounts of micronutrients from food and may improve performance in athletes with deficiencies, no evidence indicates that doses in excess of the RDA improve performance.

This chapter deals with the micronutrient requirements of athletes and the problems associated with inadequate or excessive intake. Emphasis is on the vitamins and minerals that are important for athletic performance. Rather than dealing with the role and requirement for each individual vitamin and mineral, this chapter describes some of the important roles for which various vitamins and minerals are needed (e.g., in forming the building blocks of body tissues, as cofactors in enzyme catalyzed metabolic reactions, for oxygen transport and oxidative metabolism, and as antioxidants). This approach should help the reader understand (1) why micronutrients are an essential component of the diet, (2) why the requirement for some micronutrients may be greater in athletes, (3) which groups of athletes are most at risk for inadequate micronutrient intake, and (4) the scientific basis of advice given to athletes regarding their intake of vitamin and mineral supplements. Any sustained deficiency of an essential vitamin or mineral results in ill health, and an unhealthy athlete is extremely unlikely to perform to the best of his or her potential. Several micronutrients are important for the maintenance of immune function, and this important role is discussed in detail in chapter 16.

Water-Soluble and Fat-Soluble Vitamins

Vitamins are organic compounds that are needed in small quantities in the diet. They are essential for specific metabolic reactions in the body and for promoting normal growth and development.

With the exception of vitamin D, which can be synthesized in the presence of sunlight, vitamin K, and small quantities of selected B vitamins, which can be produced by the bacterial microflora of the gastrointestinal tract, vitamins are not produced by the human body and must be consumed in the diet.

Although vitamins do not directly contribute to the energy supply, they play an important role in energy metabolism as reusable coenzymes in many metabolic reactions. Many vitamins, particularly from the B group, are cofactors in the pathways of energy metabolism, including glycolysis, the β-oxidation of FAs, the tricarboxylic acid cycle, and the electron-transport chain. A deficiency of some of the B group vitamins that act as cofactors of enzymes in carbohydrate (e.g., thiamin [vitamin B_1], niacin [vitamin B_3], and pyridoxine [vitamin B_6]), fat (e.g., riboflavin [vitamin B_2], thiamin, pantothenic acid, and biotin), and protein (e.g., pyridoxine) metabolism causes premature fatigue and inability to maintain a heavy training program.

Other vitamins play a role in heme synthesis and red and white blood cell production (e.g., folic acid and cobalamin [vitamin B_{12}]) or assist in the formation of bones, connective tissue, and cartilage (e.g., vitamins C and D). Several vitamins, including A, C, and E, act as antioxidants and help protect the body tissues against the potentially damaging effects of free radicals.

Thirteen different compounds are now considered vitamins, and they are classified either as water soluble or fat soluble. The water-soluble vitamins, C (ascorbic acid), B_1 (thiamin), B_2 (riboflavin), B_3 (niacin), B_6 (pyridoxine), pantothenic acid, and biotin, are involved in mitochondrial energy metabolism. Folic acid and vitamin B_{12} (cobalamin) are mainly involved in nucleic acid synthesis and hence are important for maintaining healthy populations of rapidly dividing cells in the body (e.g., red blood cells, immune cells, and the gut mucosa). Of the fat-soluble vitamins, A (retinol), D (calciferol), E (tocopherol), and K (menadione), only vitamin E has a probable role in energy metabolism. Vitamins A, C, and E have antioxidant properties. Vitamin K is required for the addition of sugar residues to proteins to form glycoproteins, such as the blood-clotting factors. Tables 10.1 and 10.2 summarize the major roles of the vitamins and the main effects of dietary deficiency or excess.

Vitamin deficiencies inhibit body function and impair health. Indeed, most of the vitamins were first recognized by the deficiency symptoms and illnesses that arose when their intake was inadequate

■ TABLE 10.1 ■

Major Functions of Fat-Soluble Vitamins and the Effects of Dietary Deficiency or Excess

Vitamin	Major roles in body	Effects of deficiency	Effects of excess
A (retinol)	Maintains epithelial tissues in skin, mucous membranes, and visual pigments of eye; promotes bone development and immune function	Night blindness, infections, impaired growth, and impaired wound healing	Nausea, headache, fatigue, liver damage, joint pains, peeling skin, and abnormal fetal development in pregnancy
D (calciferol)	Increases calcium absorption in gut and promotes bone formation	Weak bones (rickets in children and osteomalacia in adults)	Nausea, loss of appetite, irritability, joint pains, and calcification of soft tissues (e.g., kidneys)
E (α-tocopherol)	Defends against free radicals; protects cell membranes	Hemolysis and anemia	Headache, fatigue, and diarrhea
K (menadione)	Forms blood-clotting factors	Bleeding and hemorrhage	Thrombosis and vomiting

■ TABLE 10.2 ■

Major Functions of Water-Soluble Vitamins and the Effects of Dietary Deficiency or Excess

Vitamin	Major roles in body	Effects of deficiency	Effects of excess
B_1 (thiamin)	Forms coenzyme with thiamine pyrophosphate; promotes carbohydrate metabolism and central nervous system function	Loss of appetite, apathy, depression, beriberi, and pain in calf muscles	No toxic effects
B_2 (riboflavin)	Forms coenzymes with FAD and FMN; promotes carbohydrate and fat oxidation; maintains healthy skin	Dermatitis, lip and tongue sores, and damage to cornea of eyes	No toxic effects
B_3 (niacin)	Forms coenzymes with NAD and NADP; promotes anaerobic glycolysis, carbohydrate and fat oxidation, and fat synthesis; maintains healthy skin	Weakness, loss of appetite, skin lesions, gut and skin problems, and pellegra	Headache, nausea, skin irritation, liver damage, and inhibition of lipolysis
B_6 (pyridoxine)	Forms coenzyme with pyridoxal phosphate; promotes protein metabolism, formation of hemoglobin and red blood cells, glycogenolysis, and gluconeogenesis	Irritability, convulsions, anemia, dermatitis, and tongue sores	Loss of nerve sensation and abnormal gait
B_{12} (cobalamin)	Forms coenzyme for DNA and RNA; promotes formation of red and white blood cells; maintains nerve, gut, and skin tissue	Pernicious anemia, fatigue, nerve damage, paralysis, and infections	No toxic effects
Folic acid	Forms coenzyme for DNA and RNA; promotes formation of hemoglobin and red and white blood cells; maintains gut	Anemia, fatigue, diarrhea, gut disorders, and infections	No toxic effects
Biotin	Forms coenzyme for CO_2 transfer; promotes carbohydrate, fat, and protein metabolism	Nausea, fatigue, and skin rashes	No toxic effects
Pantothenic acid	Forms coenzyme A for energy metabolism; promotes carbohydrate and fat oxidation and fat synthesis	Nausea, fatigue, depression, and loss of appetite	No toxic effects
C (ascorbic acid)	Antioxidant; promotes collagen formation, development of connective tissue, catecholamine and steroid synthesis, and iron absorption	Weakness, slow wound healing, infections, bleeding gums, anemia, scurvy	No toxic effects in smaller doses (<1,000 mg/day); diarrhea, kidney stones, and iron overload in larger doses

FMN = flavin mononucleotide.

(e.g., scurvy in vitamin C–deficient sailors; rickets in vitamin D–deficient children). Although marginal deficiencies of vitamins may have only a small effect on otherwise healthy young sedentary people, such deficiencies may crucially affect athletic performance in elite athletes. The margins between winning and coming in second can be minuscule in many sports, and a deficiency that impairs performance by only 1% could easily affect the outcome of a competitive event. Tables 10.3 and 10.4 show the amounts of vitamins normally required in adults' diet (recommended daily

■ **TABLE 10.3** ■

Major Sources of Fat-Soluble Vitamins

Vitamin	Sources	RDA or AI*
A (retinol)	Liver, fish, dairy products[a], eggs, margarine; formed in body from provitamin A (carotenoids) found in carrots, dark green leafy vegetables, tomatoes, and oranges	0.9 mg (M)[b] 0.7 mg (F)
D (calciferol)	Liver, fish, eggs, fortified dairy products, oils, and margarine; formed by action of sunlight on the skin	5 μg* (M, F)
E (tocopherol)	Liver, eggs, whole-grain cereal products, vegetable oils, seed oils, margarine, and butter	15 mg (M, F)
K (menadione)	Liver, eggs, green leafy vegetables, cheese, and butter; formed in large intestine by bacteria	120 μg* (M) 90 μg* (F)

RDA = recommended daily allowance; AI* = adequate intake. M = males; F = females.
[a]Dairy products include milk, cream, butter, and cheese.
[b]RDA for vitamin A is 0.9 mg of retinol or 5.4 mg of β-carotene for males; 80% of these values for females.

■ **TABLE 10.4** ■

Major Sources of Water-Soluble Vitamins

Vitamin	Sources	RDA or AI*
B_1 (thiamin)	Whole-grain cereal products, fortified bread, pulses, potatoes, legumes, nuts, pork, ham, and liver	1.2 mg (M) 1.1 mg (F)
B_2 (riboflavin)	Dairy products[a], meat, liver, eggs, green leafy vegetables, and beans	1.3 mg (M) 1.1 mg (F)
B_3 (niacin)	Meat, liver, poultry, fish, whole-grain cereal products, lentils, and nuts; formed in the body from essential amino acid tryptophan	16 mg (M) 14 mg (F)
B_6 (pyridoxine)	Meat, liver, poultry, fish, whole-grain cereal products, potatoes, legumes, green leafy vegetables, dairy products[a], bananas, and nuts	1.3 mg (M, F)
B_{12} (cobalamin)	Meat, fish, shellfish, poultry, liver, eggs, dairy products[a], and fortified breakfast cereals	2.4 μg (M, F)
Folic acid	Meat, liver, green leafy vegetables, whole-grain cereal products, potatoes, legumes, nuts, and fruit	400 μg (M, F)
Biotin	Meat, milk, egg yolk, whole-grain cereal products, legumes, most vegetables	30 μg* (M, F)
Pantothenic acid	Liver, meat, dairy products[a], eggs, whole-grain cereal products, legumes, and most vegetables	5 mg* (M, F)
C (ascorbic acid)	Citrus fruits, green leafy vegetables, broccoli, potatoes, peppers, and strawberries	90 mg (M) 75 mg (F)

RDA = recommended daily allowance; AI* = adequate intake. M = males; F = females.
[a]Dairy products include milk, cream, butter, and cheese.

allowances [RDA] or adequate intakes [AI]) and the major food sources from which they are obtained.

Recommended Intakes of Vitamins

Each vitamin has a minimal requirement that covers only the basic needs and is just sufficient to prevent clinical deficiency and ensuing disease symptoms. The estimated average requirement (EAR) is higher, and it ensures a safety margin. As discussed in chapter 2, the EAR represents the amount of a nutrient deemed sufficient to meet the needs of the average individual in a certain age and gender group. The recommended daily intake (RDI) or recommended dietary allowance (RDA) of any particular vitamin is defined as the intake required to meet the known nutritional needs of more than 97% of healthy people. For some vitamins, including biotin, pantothenic acid, and vitamin D, scientific evidence is currently insufficient to estimate an EAR, and in these cases an adequate intake (AI) has been set. People should use the AI as a goal for intake if no RDA exists.

This EAR is normally distributed, and the RDA recommendation is set so that it covers 97.5% of all healthy people with an ordinary (normal) diet. This coverage is achieved by adding two standard deviations to the average daily requirement. Thus, individuals who consume less than the RDA of a nutrient are not necessarily deficient in that nutrient, but the more the actual intake lies below the RDA, the greater the risk of a deficiency state that is detrimental to the health of the individual (see figure 2.1, p. 29). Note that the data used to determine the RDAs often did not include athletes, or the activity levels of the subjects were not reported. Therefore, the RDAs may not be an accurate means of evaluating the nutritional needs of those engaged in regular strenuous exercise. The RDAs are calculated from population-based data. Metabolic, environmental, and genetic factors as well as age, gender, and body mass can make individual nutrient requirements different from these estimated needs.

Although physical activity may increase the requirement for some vitamins (e.g., vitamins C, B_2, and possibly B_6, A, and E), this increased requirement typically can be met by consuming a balanced high-carbohydrate,

moderate-protein, low-fat diet. As shown for vitamin B_1 (thiamin) and vitamin C in figure 10.1, vitamin intakes in athletes are correlated with energy intakes up to 20 MJ/day (4,800 kcal/day). Thus, if energy intake matches the energy requirement and athletes consume a reasonably balanced diet, they get all the vitamins that they need from food without any need for supplements.

Individuals at risk for low vitamin intake are those who consume a low-energy or unbalanced diet. When energy intake is high (>20 MJ/day [>4,800 kcal/day]), athletes tend to consume a large number of in-between meals and high-energy sports

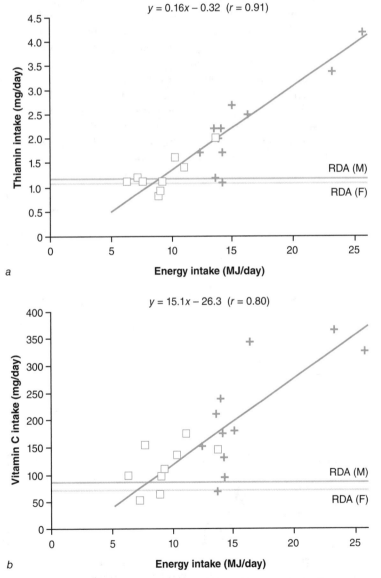

Figure 10.1 The relationship between mean intake of dietary energy and *(a)* thiamin (vitamin B_1) and *(b)* ascorbic acid (vitamin C) intake in male (crosses) and female (open squares) athletes. Each point represents a mean value for a group.

Data from van Erp-Baart et al. 1989; Fogelholm 1994.

drinks, often composed mainly of refined carbohydrate and low in protein and micronutrients; consequently, the nutrient density for vitamins drops. Vegetarian athletes obviously have problems obtaining sufficient intakes of some vitamins, particularly vitamin B_{12} [cobalamin], whose only natural dietary source is from meat. Fortunately, in Western countries, milk and several breakfast cereals are fortified with vitamin B_{12}, so this potential problem can be overcome by appropriate food selection and vitamin supplementation.

Vitamin losses in sweat are negligible, and no increased vitamin excretion in urine and feces of athletes is evident. Temporary increases in the plasma concentrations of some vitamins (e.g., vitamin C [as shown in figure 10.2], vitamin E, and vitamin B_6, as pyridoxal 5'-phosphate) have been reported after an acute bout of exercise, which may reflect a redistribution of labile pools of these vitamins. In general, however, vitamin turnover seems to be remarkably unaffected by exercise.

Physical training may increase vitamin B_2 (riboflavin) and vitamin B_6 (pyridoxine) requirements, which may be a consequence of increased retention of these vitamins in skeletal muscle. Adaptations to regular prolonged exercise include an increased number of mitochondria in skeletal muscles and increased oxidative enzyme activity, which might explain the increased retention of vitamins that are cofactors in energy metabolism within the muscle. Because of the increased free-radical production during exercise compared with the resting state, an increased intake of antioxidant vitamins (C, E, and β-carotene) may be desirable for those who engage in regular physical activity. A free radical is an atom or molecule that possess at least one unpaired electron in its outer orbit. The free radicals produced by oxidation in the mitochondria include superoxide ($\cdot O_2^-$), hydroxyl ($\cdot OH$), and nitric oxide ($\cdot NO$). These radical species are highly reactive and directly target lipid membrane structures by lipid peroxidation, causing membrane instability and increased permeability. Free radicals can also cause oxidative damage to proteins, including enzymes and DNA.

Macrominerals and Microminerals

A mineral is an inorganic compound found in nature, and the term is usually reserved for solid compounds. In nutrition, the term *mineral* usually refers to the dietary constituents essential to life processes. Minerals are classified as macrominerals or microminerals (trace elements), based on the extent of their occurrence in the body and the amounts needed in the diet. The seven macrominerals are potassium, sodium, chloride, calcium, magnesium, phosphorus, and sulfur, and each constitutes at least 0.01% of total body mass (see table 10.5).

Inadequate mineral nutrition has been associated with a variety of human diseases, including anemia, cancer, diabetes, hypertension, osteoporosis, and tooth decay. Thus, appropriate dietary intake of essential minerals is necessary for optimal health and physical performance (see tables 10.6 and 10.7). Some minerals (e.g., calcium and phosphorus) are the building blocks for body tissues, including bones and teeth. A number of minerals (e.g., magnesium, copper, and zinc) are essential for the normal function of enzymes that are involved in the regulation of metabolism, and some minerals (e.g., iron and zinc) have an essential role in the functioning of immune cells. Several other minerals (e.g., sodium, potassium, and chloride) exist as ions or **electrolytes** dissolved in the intracellular and extracellular fluids. Like vitamins, minerals cannot be used as a source of energy.

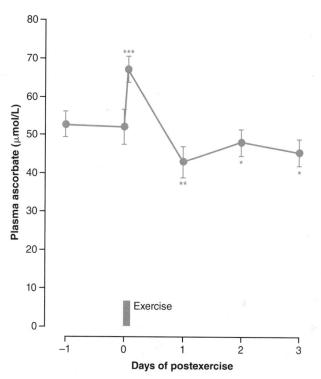

Figure 10.2 The effect of running a 21 km road race on the plasma concentration of vitamin C. Data are means ± SEM from nine subjects. Statistical significance of differences of means compared with the immediately preexercise value on day 0: $P < 0.05$, ** $P < 0.01$, *** $P < 0.001$.

Adult Total Body Content
and Body Fluid Concentrations of Macrominerals

Macromineral	Symbol	Atomic weight	Total amount in body (mg)	BODY FLUID CONCENTRATION (mg/l)		
				Plasma	Sweat	Urine
Calcium	Ca	40	1,500,000	85–105	0–40	100–180
Chlorine	Cl	35.5	75,000	3,400–3,900	700–2,100	5,000–7,500
Magnesium	Mg	24	25,000	16–30	4–15	60–100
Potassium	K	39	180,000	130–220	160–320	800–3,200
Phosphorus	P	31	850,000	20–50	3–6	20–1,100
Sodium	Na	23	65,000	3,000–3,500	460–1,840	2,500–5,000

Electrolyte concentrations in interstitial fluid are virtually identical to those in plasma.

■ TABLE 10.6 ■

Major Functions of Macrominerals
and the Effects of Dietary Deficiency or Excess

Macromineral	Major roles in the body	Effects of deficiency	Effects of excess
Calcium	Promotes bone and teeth formation, muscle contraction, membrane potentials, and nerve impulse transmission; regulates enzyme activity	Osteoporosis, brittle bones, impaired muscle contraction, muscle cramps	Impaired trace metal absorption, cardiac arrhythmia, constipation, kidney stones, and calcification of soft tissue
Chlorine	Promotes nerve impulse conduction and hydrochloric acid formation in the stomach	Convulsions	Hypertension[a]
Magnesium	Promotes protein synthesis and metalloenzyme, ATPases, and 2,3-DPG formation; bone component	Muscle weakness, fatigue, apathy, muscle tremor, and cramps	Nausea, vomiting, and diarrhea
Potassium	Promotes membrane potential, nerve impulse generation, muscle contraction, and acid–base balance	Hypokalemia, muscle cramps, apathy, loss of appetite, and irregular heart beat	Hyperkalemia, cardiac arrhythmia, and cardiac failure
Phosphorus	Promotes bone formation; buffer in muscle contraction; component of ATP, PCr, NADP, DNA, RNA, and cell membranes	Osteoporosis, brittle bones, muscle weakness, and muscle cramps	Impaired iron, zinc, and copper absorption; impaired calcium metabolism
Sodium	Promotes blood volume homeostasis, nerve impulse generation, muscle contraction, acid–base balance	Hyponatremia, dizziness, coma, muscle cramps, nausea, vomiting, loss of appetite, and seizures	Hypertension and nausea
Sulfur	Acid–base balance; liver function	Unknown and extremely unlikely to occur	Unknown

In rare instances chlorine deficiency can be caused by excess vomiting.

[a] In conjunction with excess sodium.

■ **TABLE 10.7** ■

The Major Functions of Microminerals (Trace Elements) and the Effects of Dietary Deficiency or Excess

Micromineral	Major roles in body	Effects of deficiency	Effects of excess
Chromium	Augments insulin action	Glucose intolerance and impaired lipid metabolism	Rare toxic effects
Cobalt	Forms component of vitamin B_{12} needed for red blood cell development	Pernicious anemia	Nausea, vomiting, and death
Copper	Promotes normal iron absorption, oxidative metabolism, connective tissue formation, and hemoglobin synthesis; forms cofactor with superoxide dismutase	Anemia, impaired immune function, and bone demineralization	Nausea and vomiting
Fluorine	Promotes bone and teeth formation	Dental caries	Discolored teeth, inhibited glycolysis in high doses
Iodine	Forms component of thyroid hormones T3 and T4	Goiter and reduced metabolic rate	Depressed thyroid gland activity
Iron	Transports oxygen as hemoglobin and myoglobin; forms cytochromes and metalloenzymes; promotes immune function	Anemia, fatigue, and increased infections	Hemochromatosis, liver cirrhosis, heart disease, and increased infections
Manganese	Forms cofactor with energy metabolism enzymes; promotes bone formation and fat synthesis	Poor growth	Weakness and confusion
Molybdenum	Forms cofactor with riboflavin in carbohydrate and fat metabolism enzymes	No deficiency effects	Rare toxic effects
Selenium	Forms cofactor with glutathione peroxidase	Cardiomyopathy, cancer, heart disease, impaired immune function, and erythrocyte fragility	Nausea, vomiting, fatigue, and hair loss
Zinc	Forms metalloenzymes; promotes protein synthesis, immune function, tissue repair, energy metabolism, and antioxidant activity	Impaired growth, impaired healing, increased infections, and anorexia	Impaired absorption of Fe and Cu, increased HDL cholesterol:LDL cholesterol ratio, anemia, nausea, vomiting, and impaired immunity

Recommended Intakes of Minerals

At least 20 mineral elements are known to be essential for humans, and 14 trace elements have been identified as essential for maintenance of health. Besides those listed in table 10.7, trace amounts of arsenic, nickel, silicon, tin, and vanadium may also be essential, but deficiencies or excesses (because of dietary sources) for these micronutrients are extremely rare. Deficiencies of one or more of the trace elements result in symptoms of disease, and many deficiencies are also associated with immune dysfunction and increased incidence of infection (see table 10.7).

The RDA has been established for seven minerals, and the AI is available for five others (see tables 10.8 and 10.9). Estimated mineral requirements have been proposed for potassium, sodium, and chlorine. Each of the trace elements (e.g., iron, zinc, copper, chromium, and selenium) constitutes less than 0.01% of total body mass (see table 10.10) and is needed in a quantity of less than 100 mg/day.

Sources and Recommended Daily Allowances or Adequate Intakes of Macrominerals for Adults 19 to 50 Years of Age

Macromineral	Sources	RDA or AI*	Percent absorbed
Calcium	Dairy products, egg yolk, beans and peas, dark green vegetables, and cauliflower	1,000 mg* (M, F)	30–40
Chlorine	Meat, fish, bread, canned foods, table salt, beans, and milk	2,300 mg* (M, F)	90–99
Magnesium	Seafood, nuts, green leafy vegetables, fruits, whole-grain products, milk, and yogurt	420 mg (M) 320 mg (F)	25–60
Potassium	Meat, fish, milk, yogurt, fruit, vegetables, and bread	4,700 mg* (M, F)	90–99
Phosphorus	Meat, eggs, fish, milk, cheese, beans, peas, whole-grain products, soft drinks	700 mg (M, F)	80–90
Sodium	Meat, fish, bread, canned foods, table salt, sauces, and pickles	1,500 mg* (M, F)	90–99

RDA = recommended daily allowance; AI* = adequate intake. M = males; F = females.

Also shown is the proportion of the ingested amount that is absorbed; the remainder is excreted in the feces.

Sources and Recommended Daily Allowances or Adequate Intakes of Microminerals for Adults 19 to 50 Years of Age

Micromineral	Sources	RDA or AI*	Percent absorbed
Chromium	Liver, kidney, meat, oysters, cheese, whole-grain products, beer, asparagus, mushrooms, nuts, and stainless steel cookware	35 μg* (M) 25 μg* (F)	<1
Cobalt	Meat, liver, and milk	As part of vitamin B_{12}	
Copper	Liver, kidney, shellfish, meat, fish, poultry, eggs, bran cereals, nuts, legumes, broccoli, banana, avocado, and chocolate	0.9 mg (M, F)	20–50
Fluorine	Milk, egg yolk, seafood, and drinking water	4 mg* (M) 3 mg* (F)	
Iodine	Iodized salt, seafood, and vegetables	150 μg (M, F)	
Iron	Liver, kidney, eggs, red meats, seafood, oysters, bread, flour, molasses, dried legumes, nuts, leafy green vegetables, broccoli, figs, raisins, and cocoa	8 mg (M) 18 mg (F)	10–30 (heme iron) 2–10 (nonheme iron)
Manganese	Whole grains, peas and beans, leafy vegetables, and bananas	2.3 mg* (M) 1.8 mg*(F)	
Molybdenum	Liver, kidney, whole-grain products, beans, and peas	45 μg (M, F)	
Selenium	Meat, liver, kidney, poultry, fish, dairy products, seafood, whole grains, and nuts from selenium-rich soil	55 mg (M, F)	
Zinc	Oysters, shellfish, beef, liver, poultry, dairy products, whole grains, vegetables, asparagus, and spinach	11 mg (M) 8 mg (F)	20–50

RDA = Recommended daily allowance; AI* = adequate intake. M = males; F = females.

Also shown (where known) is the proportion of the ingested amount that is absorbed; the remainder is excreted in the feces.

■ TABLE 10.10 ■
Adult Total Body Content and Body Fluid Concentrations of Microminerals (Trace Elements)

Micromineral	Symbol	Atomic weight	Total amount in body (mg)	BODY FLUID CONCENTRATION (mg/l)[a]		
				Plasma	Sweat	Urine
Chromium	Cr	52	6			
Cobalt	Co	59	<1			
Copper	Cu	64	100	0.7–1.7	0.2–0.6	0.03–0.04
Fluorine	F	19	2,500			
Iodine	I	127	11			
Iron	Fe	56	5,000	0.4–1.4	0.3–0.4	0.1–0.15
Manganese	Mn	55	12			
Molybdenum	Mo	96	9			
Selenium	Se	79	13			
Zinc	Zn	65	2,000	0.7–1.3	0.7–1.3	0.2–0.5

Electrolyte concentrations in interstitial fluid are virtually identical to those in plasma.

[a]Values only shown where concentration of mineral is greater than 0.1 mg/L.

Critical Micronutrient Functions

Micronutrients not only form the building blocks of tissues but also function as antioxidants and perform or are associated with a variety of functions essential to the maintenance of life and health, including oxygen transport, enzyme-catalyzed reactions, immunity, and electrolytes.

Micronutrients Form the Building Blocks of Tissues

Although vitamins are not structural components in body tissues, several minerals, including calcium, phosphorus, and fluorine are, particularly in bones and teeth. Vitamin D is required for the normal absorption of dietary calcium, and deficiency of this vitamin is associated with brittle bones. Vitamin C is required for normal production of collagen and hence is important for the maintenance of healthy connective tissue and cartilage.

The mineral in bone is calcium phosphate crystalline salts in the form of hydroxyapatite. Bone matrix is a mixture of collagen fibers, which resist pulling forces, and solid hydroxyapatite crys-tals, which resist compression. Bone tissue is not metabolically inert. Even in adults, bone undergoes continuous turnover and remodeling of the matrix with simultaneous release and uptake of calcium. The cells involved in bone formation are osteo-blasts, and the cells responsible for breakdown (demineralization) are osteoclasts (see figure 10.3). When the rate of demineralization exceeds the rate of bone formation, osteoporosis, a weakening of the bone structure, occurs.

The hormones calcitonin and parathyroid hormone (PTH) are principally involved in the regulation of calcium metabolism in bone tissue. Their main actions are shown in figure 10.3. PTH stimulates bone demineralization when calcium levels in blood are low. PTH and ultraviolet radiation from sunlight also stimulate production in the skin of the active form of vitamin D, which promotes the uptake of calcium in the small intestine. Calcitonin is released from the thyroid gland and stimulates bone formation when the plasma concentration of calcium rises.

Calcium intake influences the development of osteoporosis. Among different groups of athletes, calcium intake is closely related to total energy intake (see figure 10.4). Other factors that influence the development of osteoporosis are estrogen levels, alcohol and caffeine intake, family history, female gender, and the amount and type of physical activity (Aulin 2000). Emphasis in the prevention of osteoporosis should be on maximizing the body's stores of calcium at an early age and minimizing calcium loss. A calcium intake of 1,000 to 1,300 mg/day is recommended to protect against the development of osteoporosis. The performance of regular weight-bearing activity promotes the deposition of calcium in bone.

Several groups of athletes can be identified as possibly having insufficient calcium intake (see table 10.11) and hence increased risk of osteoporosis. The absence of menstruation (amenorrhea) or infrequent menstruation (oligomenorrhea), which are commonly associated with low levels of body fat, low energy intake, and high physical activity (especially gymnastics, swimming, and long-distance running) is associated with a high risk of early osteoporosis because of the chronically low plasma estrogen levels (Aulin 2000). This condition, which forms part of the female athlete triad syndrome and can be precipitated by eating disorders, is dealt with in detail in chapter 15. The steroid hormone estrogen promotes bone formation in females; in males, the hormone testosterone assumes this role. In young female athletes, amenorrhea may hinder bone growth at a time when bone should be forming at its maximum rate. Side effects, such as the increased risk of stress fractures, could hinder athletic performance as well as cause potentially debilitating problems later in life. When amenorrhea is present, increasing the consumption of calcium to 120% of the RDA appears to help bones to maintain density and develop properly.

Such nutrition guidance should be given to low-body-weight amenorrheic women. Weight-conscious athletes (e.g., gymnasts) may markedly reduce their consumption of dairy products to decrease their intake of dietary fat. But because the main sources of calcium are milk, butter, and cheese, their intake of calcium may fall considerably below the RDA. Most low-fat dairy products

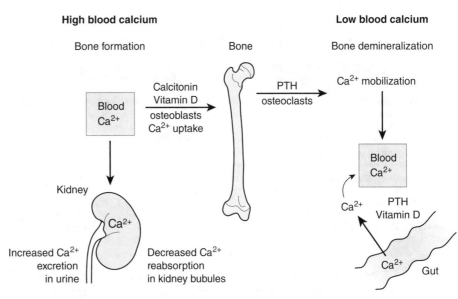

Figure 10.3 Bone formation and demineralization in calcium homeostasis.

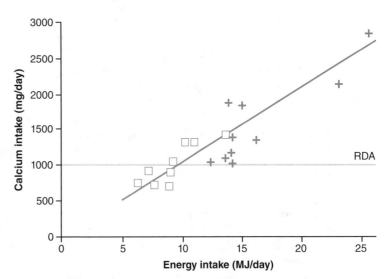

Figure 10.4 The relationship between mean intake of dietary energy and calcium intake in male (crosses) and female (open squares) athletes. Each point represents a mean value for a group.

Data from van Erp-Baart et al. 1989.

(e.g., skimmed milk) contain similar amounts of calcium as the full-fat dairy product, so athletes should be encouraged to include low-fat dairy products in their diet to preserve calcium intake.

Phosphorus, in the form of phosphate salts, is the other major inorganic constituent of bones and teeth. The adult male body contains about 850 g of phosphorus, of which 80% is found in bone. Phosphorus is also found as a component of nucleic acids (DNA and RNA) and phospholipids, which form the lipid bilayer of cell membranes. The RDA for adolescents and young adults (age 9

Risk Factors for Marginal Mineral Nutrition in Athletes

Conditions and causes	Sports
Low body weight—chronically low energy intake to achieve low body weight	Gymnastics, jockeys, ballet, ice dancing, and dancing
Making competition weight—drastic weight-loss regimens to achieve desired weight category	Weight-class sports (rowing, wrestling, boxing, and judo)
Low fat—drastic weight-loss regimens to achieve low body fat	Bodybuilding
Vegetarian diets	Endurance events
Training in hot, humid conditions	Endurance events

to 18 years) is 1,250 mg of phosphorus; for persons older than 19 years, the requirement is 700 mg. Phosphorus deficiency is rare because many food items contain substantial amounts of it.

Fluorine is necessary for the normal formation of healthy bones and teeth, and it protects against dental caries (tooth decay by oral bacteria). Frequent intakes of soft drinks and carbohydrate, particularly sugars, depress the pH in the mouth and cause a net demineralization of the teeth. Sugars in the mouth are metabolized to organic acids by bacteria in plaque. Given the relatively high intake of sugary foods and sports drinks by athletes, good oral hygiene and plaque control are important. The RDA for fluorine is 3 to 4 mg/day, and this trace element is found in milk, egg yolk, and seafood. Several toothpastes and mouth rinses contain fluorine (as sodium fluoride), and in some countries, including the United States, fluoride is added to drinking water. Excess intake of fluoride is poisonous because of its inhibitory effects on a number of enzymes, including some of the enzymes of glycolysis.

Several other trace elements have been suggested to be capable of increasing lean-body mass. Boron supplementation has been reported to increase the serum estrogen and testosterone concentrations in postmenopausal women; subsequent studies found no effect on serum testosterone, lean body mass, or muscle strength in male athletes who took boron supplements. Chromium is also claimed to increase lean body mass, through potentiating insulin action. Insulin promotes glucose and amino acid uptake into muscle and stimulates muscle protein synthesis. But most studies show that chromium supplements are not effective in increasing lean body mass, and chromium supplementation is accompanied by increased urinary excretion of chromium. Chromium stores are unlikely to be inadequate in people who consume a well-balanced diet, because chromium is widely available in fruits, vegetables, cereals, and organ meats.

Vanadium appears to increase tissue sensitivity to insulin in individuals suffering from type 2 (non-insulin-dependent) diabetes, but to date, no studies have established whether vanadium compounds exhibit insulin-like actions, such as promoting muscle protein and glycogen synthesis. A study showed no effect of vanadium on insulin sensitivity in healthy people assessed by an oral glucose tolerance test (Jentjens and Jeukendrup 2002). (See chapter 11 for details of studies that have investigated the effects of boron, chromium, and vanadium supplementation.)

Micronutrients as Antioxidants

Antioxidants prevent or limit the actions of free radicals, usually by removing their unpaired electron and thus converting them into something far less reactive. Vitamins with antioxidant properties (including vitamins C, E, and β-carotene [provitamin A]) may be required in increased quantities in athletes to inactivate the products of exercise-induced increased free-radical formation and lipid peroxidation. Free radicals damage membranes, proteins, and DNA. Damage to DNA could result in mutations that cause cancer. Several minerals (including selenium, copper, and manganese) are components of antioxidant enzymes involved in the defense against free radicals. Increased intake of antioxidant vitamins and other antioxidant compounds has been suggested to reduce the extent of exercise-induced muscle damage. Current evidence is not convincing, however, so more studies of the effects of antioxidants on exercise-induced muscle soreness and damage are needed.

Antioxidant Protection Against Exercise-Induced Skeletal Muscle Damage Unaccustomed exercise or muscle activity that involves eccentric actions (lengthening of the muscle during activation) can damage some of the myofibers. Such exercises include downhill running, bench stepping, and lowering of weights. The consequences of exercise-induced muscle damage include muscle pain, soreness, and stiffness; reduced range of motion; higher than normal blood lactate concentration and perceived exertion during exercise; and loss of strength and reduced maximal dynamic power output that can last 5 to 10 days. Exercise-induced muscle damage also impairs the restoration of muscle glycogen stores. Damaged muscle has an impaired ability to take up glucose from the blood, which is required to resynthesize glycogen in the muscle. This condition results in decreased endurance performance in subsequent exercise bouts.

A practical index of muscle damage in athletes performing heavy training is elevated muscle proteins (e.g., myoglobin, creatine kinase [CK], or lactate dehydrogenase) in the blood plasma. The damaged muscle tissue causes an initial activation of the immune system, as white blood cells are attracted to the damaged muscles to begin breakdown of damaged fibers and initiate the repair process. This process involves the production of free-radical reactive oxygen species (ROS) by the invading leukocytes. Growing evidence indicates that ROS is an underlying cause of disrupted muscle homeostasis, muscle soreness, and elevated CK activity in eccentric type exercise. ROS can also cause oxidative damage to DNA and proteins, including enzymes.

Reactive Oxygen Species and Other Free Radicals In normal cellular metabolism, small amounts of ROS are produced during the aerobic process by which humans and animals derive energy from the mitochondria. In the electron-transport chain located on the inner mitochondrial membrane, most of the oxygen consumed by cells is reduced by cytochrome oxidase to yield water (and energy that is used to resynthesize ATP from ADP and Pi). But a small proportion, most recently estimated to be about 0.15% of the total oxygen consumed at rest, can be used in an alternate pathway for the univalent reduction of oxygen; thus, ROS are produced. Note that earlier studies suggested that this proportion was as high as 3 to 5% of the total oxygen consumed (more than 10-fold higher than the current accepted value [St-Pierre et al. 2002]). One free-radical molecule can start a destructive process by removing electrons from stable compounds, such as polyunsaturated FAs, and forming large numbers of ROS, thereby transforming stable compounds into highly reactive free radicals.

Additional sources of ROS and other free radicals are ultraviolet light, alcohol, cigarette smoke, high-fat diets, and the respiratory burst of white blood cells, such as neutrophils and monocytes, that are capable of ingesting foreign material, including bacteria. The generation of ROS by the neutrophil respiratory burst is an essential mechanism of the host defense mechanism of the immune system for killing bacteria and clearing away damaged tissue. But these ROS can also initiate damaging chain reactions, such as lipid peroxidation, and the subsequent release of large numbers of ROS. In addition to the production of free radicals by the mitochondrial respiratory chain during whole-body eccentric exercise, invading neutrophils and monocytes are thought to be important sources of oxidative stress. Several inflammatory diseases have been associated with increased generation of ROS by monocytes. Migration of neutrophils into damaged muscle tissue occurs within the first hour after eccentric exercise and is followed by infiltration of monocytes and macrophages, reaching a maximum at 24 to 72 hours after exercise.

Increases in the free iron concentration of body fluids (caused, for example, by hemolysis or ischemia-reperfusion) may amplify ROS toxicity by increasing the generation of the highly reactive hydroxyl radical. Ferric iron (Fe^{3+}) ions can stimulate free-radical reactions by breaking down lipid peroxides to chain-breaking alkoxyl radicals, and ferrous (Fe^{2+}) ions can react with H_2O_2 to produce $\cdot OH$ and other highly reactive species in what is called a Fenton reaction:

$$Fe^{2+} + H_2O_2 \rightarrow Fe^{3+} + \cdot OH + OH^-$$

The hydroxyl radical can also be formed through the Haber-Weiss reaction:

$$Fe^{2+} + H_2O_2 + \cdot O_2^- \rightarrow Fe^{3+} + \cdot OH + OH^- + O_2$$

This potential is one of the reasons that iron supplements should not be recommended indiscriminately. Free radicals have been implicated in the etiology of various diseases including cancer and coronary heart disease, and an excess of iron could potentiate their adverse effects. Excess iron intake may also increase the risk of hemochromatosis.

Reactive Oxygen Species Production by Exercising Muscle The first serious studies of the generation and potential roles of ROS during exercise were carried out in the late 1970s. During the ensuing years, a great deal of research has been undertaken to try to understand the nature and sources of the species generated, the factors influencing their generation, their effects on muscle and other cells, and how these effects might be manipulated. An assumption that has underpinned much of the work since the early studies is that the species generated are essentially by-products of metabolism and are damaging to cells and tissues. Note that even the earliest studies in the area attempted to scavenge the species generated and look for potential functional benefits of such interventions. Unsurprisingly, early studies were also characterized by limitations in the analytical methods available to detect free-radical species. Nonspecific approaches—for example, the analysis of lipid peroxides such as malondialdehyde or thiobarbituric acid reactive species (TBARS) in complex biological tissues—were commonly used. The early studies reported that the predominant source for formation of free radicals during exercise is from leakage from the electron-transport chain in the mitochondria (as much as 3 to 5% of the total oxygen consumed by mitochondria was suggested to undergo one electron reduction with the generation of superoxide). It was assumed that this source of ROS production was directly related to the rate of oxygen uptake by muscle tissue, which can increase up to 100-fold during exercise compared with rest. This assumption, of course, implies that potentially a 100-fold increase in superoxide generation by skeletal muscle could occur during aerobic exercise. These assumptions became firmly rooted and extensively quoted in the subsequent literature, but the most recent research in this area has not supported them.

Since 2000 the development of improved techniques has established that the primary ROS generated by skeletal muscle are nitric oxide and superoxide. Mitochondria are cited as the major site of superoxide generation in tissues, but a number of recent findings have argued against the previously high estimates of rates of formation of superoxide within mitochondria. The most recent estimates of the rate of production of ROS by mitochondria indicate that no more than about 0.15% of the electron flow gives rise to ROS (i.e., less than 10% of the original minimum estimate), and it is becoming increasingly clear that even this low rate of production may be further reduced by intrinsic control mechanisms. As for exercise, the most recent data indicate that muscle intracellular ROS production increases by only a modest two- to fourfold during contractions (Jackson 2007),

which seems to support the suggestion that there is considerable internal control of mitochondrial ROS generation.

Studies have identified the NAD(P)H oxidase enzymes associated with the sarcoplasmic reticulum (SR) of cardiac and skeletal muscle as additional sources of ROS. The superoxide generated by these enzymes seems to influence calcium release by the SR through oxidation of the ryanodyne receptor. A NAD(P)H oxidase somewhat similar to that found in phagocytic cells of the immune system has also been described; this is located in the plasma membrane, triads, and transverse tubules of skeletal muscle and is activated by membrane depolarization. Many studies have now indicated that skeletal muscle cells release superoxide into the extracellular space and that nonmuscle cells contain other plasma membrane redox systems capable of undertaking electron transfer across the plasma membrane to effect transfer of electrons from intracellular reductants to appropriate extracellular electron acceptors. Other enzyme systems that can generate ROS in skeletal muscle tissue include phospholipases and xanthine oxidase. Skeletal muscle fibers themselves have been reported not to contain significant amounts of xanthine oxidase, although this enzyme will inevitably be present in associated endothelial cells of the blood vessels in muscle tissue.

Thus, skeletal muscle has multiple potential sites for generation of ROS, and data are increasingly casting doubt about whether mitochondria are the major dominant site for ROS generation in skeletal muscle during contractile activity. In particular, the inability to detect an increase in intracellular ROS activity at the levels predicted by the original studies of mitochondrial ROS generation and the increasing debate about the degree of internal regulation of mitochondrial ROS generation contrast sharply with the observations that superoxide is specifically generated by nonmitochondrial systems (such as the transverse tubule-localized NAD(P)H oxidase enzymes) in response to physiological stimuli. This latter ROS generation system is clearly stimulated by physiological processes and seems to be linked to signaling processes acting to modify muscle gene expression and adaptations to exercise. The various potential pathways of ROS generation within muscle are illustrated in figure 10.5. The old view that ROS are a by-product of metabolism and have only a deleterious effect on muscle function is now replaced by the concept that specific ROS are generated in a controlled manner by skeletal muscle fibers in response to physiological stimuli and play important roles in the physiological adaptations of muscle to contractions. These include optimization of contractile performance and initiation of key adaptive changes in gene expression to the stresses of contractions.

Antioxidant Mechanisms An antioxidant is a compound that protects biological systems against the harmful effects or reactions that create excessive oxidants. Dietary antioxidants significantly decrease the adverse effects of ROS. Enzymatic and nonenzymatic antioxidants prevent oxidation initiated by ROS by

- preventing ROS formation;
- intercepting ROS attack by scavenging the reactive metabolites and converting them to less-reactive molecules;
- binding transition metal ion catalysts, such as copper and iron, to prevent initiation of free-radical reactions;
- reacting with chain-propagating radicals, such as the peroxyl and alkoyl species, to prevent continued hydrogen abstraction from FA side chains; and
- providing a favorable environment for the effective functioning of other antioxidants or acting to regenerate the nonenzymatic antioxidant molecules.

Antioxidant enzymes can affect free-radical generation at both the initiation and propagation stage. The antioxidant enzymes superoxide dismutase (SOD) and catalase can inhibit the initial phase by inactivating precursor molecules of ROS production (see figure 10.6). At the propagation stage, glutathione peroxidase, another antioxidant enzyme, can scavenge · OH and lipid peroxides as described earlier. The trace elements copper and manganese are required as cofactors of SOD, and selenium is also a component of antioxidant defense because it is a cofac-

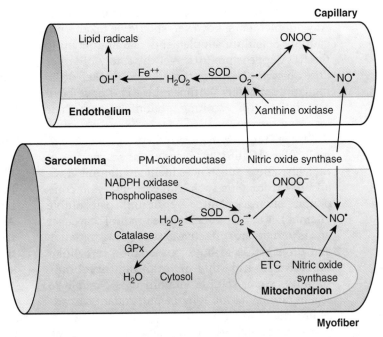

Figure 10.5 Simplified diagram of the processes contributing to ROS generation in exercising muscle.

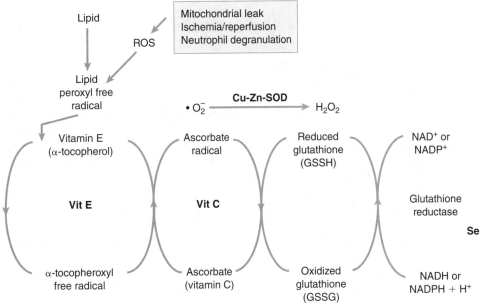

Figure 10.6 The antioxidant action cascade.

tor of glutathione peroxidase–reductase and thus influences the quenching of ROS. The effects of exercise on manganese and selenium status are presently unknown, but training is associated with an increase in levels of antioxidant enzymes, suggesting that there may be an increased requirement for these trace elements during periods of increased training. As with other minerals, losses of manganese and selenium in urine and sweat are likely higher in athletes than in nonathletes. Any supplements, however, should be taken with caution. Selenium supplements of amounts up to the RDA appear nontoxic, yet the safety of larger doses has not been confirmed, and intakes of 25 mg (approximately 40 times the RDA) have been associated with vomiting, abdominal pain, hair loss, and fatigue.

Besides the enzyme defense system, some low-molecular-weight substances act as scavengers of radicals. These substances include vitamins A, C, and E; carotenoids such as β-carotene; and compounds such as plant polyphenols. Fat-soluble vitamin E is a chain-breaking free-radical scavenger and is particularly effective at preventing initiation and propagation of lipid peroxidation in cellular membranes and thus maintaining membrane stability. Water-soluble vitamin C is capable of regenerating vitamin E in the antioxidant cascade as illustrated in figure 10.6.

Polyphenol compounds scavenge peroxyl, superoxide, and nitric oxide radicals. Rich sources of polyphenols include tea, wine (particularly red wine), fruits, and vegetables. Flavonoids, a subclass of polyphenols that includes the flavonols, flavonones, and anthocyanidins, contain a number of phenolic hydroxyl (-OH) groups attached to ring structures that confer their antioxidant activity. Differences in the antioxidant power of individual flavonoids result from the variation in the number and arrangement of the hydroxyl groups, as well as extent and nature of the glycolation of these groups. Flavonoids are reported to inhibit the enzyme lipoxygenase and to inhibit oxidant generation by neutrophils in a manner similar to vitamin E. As with vitamin E, the antioxidant power of the flavonoids results from donating a hydrogen atom from a hydroxyl moiety. But studies in chemical systems show flavonoids to be 3 to 10 times more effective than vitamin E in their scavenging abilities. In addition, they may have anti-inflammatory effects. Flavonoids are used clinically to decrease inflammation and endothelial damage in diseases in which free radicals play a major role.

Free Radicals and Antioxidants Studies in Exercise-Induced Muscle Damage

After eccentric exercise-induced damage to muscle, the phase of greatest loss of muscle force generation (sometimes referred to as the secondary injury because it follows an immediate mechanical damage to the muscle) is associated with considerable infiltration of phagocytic cells (blood neutrophils and monocytes) into the damaged fibers. This secondary damage has been mostly attributed to ROS released by these activated phagocytic invaders, and neutrophils in particular have been identified as the major contributors to the oxidative damage in muscle (Pizza et al. 2005).

Several studies have attempted to determine whether pretreatment with antioxidants can reduce or alter the time course of eccentric exercise-induced muscle damage. In an animal study, mice treated with superoxide dismutase (SOD), the antioxidant enzyme involved in the elimination of the superoxide radical, showed smaller reductions in muscle force output 3 days after eccentric exercise (Zerba et al. 1990). The finding that SOD reduced loss of muscle function supports the role of free radicals in damage induced by eccentric contraction. But muscle levels of SOD and free-radical activity were not measured in this study. Furthermore, force reduction in mice given SOD supplements was found only in older mice. Endogenous levels of protective antioxidant enzymes decline with age (Meydani et al. 1993). These studies suggest that humans and animals have increased susceptibility to muscle damage with increasing age. Similarly, Cannon et al. (1990) compared the effect of an antioxidant supplement with a placebo treatment in two age groups (younger than 30 years and older than 55 years) using downhill running as the muscle-damaging exercise protocol. The authors found that vitamin E supplementation eliminated the differences between the two age groups.

Maughan et al. (1989) measured serum lipid peroxide concentration as total thiobarituric acid-reactive substances (TBARS) and found that subjects with the greatest increase in serum CK showed the highest TBARS concentrations, suggesting that free-radical reactions and subsequent loss of membrane integrity could be responsible for the release of muscle-derived enzymes into the circulation. Although TBARS may be a useful indicator of free-radical damage, methodological difficulties mean that care should be taken when interpreting results of such studies. One of the problems of free-radical research has been the difficulty in directly measuring free-radical activity, particularly in vivo (see Duthie [1999] for a review). But these indirect measures of free-radical activity suggest that free radicals are formed during exercise.

Although free radicals are difficult to detect directly, electron spin resonance (ESR) has been used to try to measure increased free-radical production. Davies et al. (1982) observed a two- to threefold increase in ROS concentration in the muscles and liver after exercise to exhaustion in rats. More recent studies support these findings. Fielding et al. (1993) demonstrated a relationship between neutrophil infiltration, ultrastructural damage, and increased muscle membrane permeability after downhill running in humans. Postexercise muscle infiltration and in vitro neutrophil superoxide generation were closely related to the time course of release of CK into the circulation and muscle ultrastructural damage. These events may be causally related to other symptoms of muscle damage, such as loss of muscle strength and muscle soreness.

A study by Jackson (2000) reported that dietary vitamin E deficiency in rats increased the susceptibility of skeletal muscles to contractile damage as indicated by CK release, but rats supplemented with $240 \, mg \cdot kg^{-1} \cdot day^{-1}$ of vitamin E exhibited lower CK release after a downhill run. Moreover, the peak CK activity in serum was significantly correlated to neutrophil superoxide release. In contrast, Van Der Meulen et al. (1997) found that 5 to 8 days of intravenous injections in mice increased vitamin E content threefold but did not alter the extent of eccentric-exercise-induced muscle damage in situ. Moreover, vitamin E did not alter the force deficit or change the percentage of muscle fibers damaged. In the same study, however, postexercise CK levels were significantly reduced with vitamin E injections, suggesting that vitamin E may help to reduce membrane damage related to enzyme efflux but may not alter other indices of muscle damage induced by eccentric contractions. But neither antioxidant capacity nor ROS production was measured in these studies.

Warren et al. (1992) investigated rat muscle susceptibility to oxidative stress and observed lower CK release in a group given vitamin E supplements compared with a control group. Although force loss was similar in both groups, the susceptibility of the muscles to oxidant stress decreased after supplementation. The authors concluded that vitamin E supplementation may be useful in reducing free-radical damage but does not appear to alter muscle-fiber damage caused by eccentric exercise.

Several human studies have also shown contrasting findings. Cannon et al. (1990) reported that vitamin E supplementation (400 IU/day) for 48 days increased the amount of CK in the plasma of subjects older than 55 years. Moreover, plasma CK activity correlated with superoxide release from neutrophils at the time of peak CK levels; however, significant increases in plasma lipid peroxides were not observed. Cannon et al. (1990) concluded that free radicals are involved with the delayed increase in muscle-membrane permeability after damaging exercise but are not involved in the initial injury.

Meydani et al. (1993) studied the effects of a 45-minute run at 75% of maximal heart rate. The subjects were given either a placebo or vitamin E (800 IU) for 48 days before the exercise. Those given the vitamin E supplement decreased production of urinary TBARS after eccentric exercise, which suggested that vitamin E reduced free-radical-mediated damage. But the reliability of TBARS as a measure of lipid peroxidation has been questioned. Kaminiski and Boal (1992) studied the effect of vitamin C supplementation for 7 days after exercise in a double-blind crossover trial. Although this study noted that vitamin C treatment reduced muscle damage, as indicated by muscle soreness, it did not measure any biochemical markers of muscle damage, and a carryover effect from the previous bout of exercise was likely.

Studies using a well-characterized model of lengthening contractions in rodents in which a single discrete muscle (in this case the extensor digitorum longus; EDL) is damaged in a highly reproducible manner have investigated in more detail the effects of vitamin E supplementation on exercise-induced muscle damage. The findings from these studies have provided evidence that the EDL muscle was under considerable oxidative stress after lengthening contractions and that vitamin E had differential effects on individual measures of damage to muscle (van der Meulen et al. 1997). Animals subjected to a protocol of repeated lengthening contractions had a significant force deficit and morphological damage to the EDL fibers on histological examination at 3 days postexercise. This was associated with a significant elevation of serum CK activity at 3 hours and 3 days postexercise. Prior vitamin E supplementation of the rats had no effect on the loss of force generation by the EDL or on the percentage of damaged fibers but, surprisingly, prevented the rise in circulating CK activity that occurred postexercise. This apparent selective effect of vitamin E on the release of CK (a cytosolic enzyme) from the damaged muscle is consistent with previous in vitro data suggesting that vitamin E can stabilize muscle membranes by interaction with phospholipids (Phoenix et al. 1991) and may provide an explanation for at least some of the apparently discrepant data in this area.

Because of the inconsistent and often contradictory findings, whether antioxidant vitamins are helpful in reducing free-radical-mediated damage is not clear. These conflicts may be the result of different indices of muscle damage being measured, variations in mode and intensity of exercise, previous training, the dose and the length of time of supplementation, and the ages of the subjects. But antioxidants react with free radicals and deactivate them, lowering the amount of ROS produced, and therefore may reduce or prevent secondary muscle damage. In addition, any effects that they may have in reducing the initial damage will likely result in a reduction in the later infiltration of neutrophils and macrophages, with consequent attenuation of secondary damage. Caution must be exercised, however, because some studies have even reported deleterious effects on muscle function with antioxidant supplementation following exercise-induced muscle damage (e.g., Close et al. 2006).

Flavonoids and Free Radicals Some flavonoids are excellent scavengers of free radicals such as $\cdot O_2^-$ and $\cdot OH$. All subgroups of flavonoids decrease oxidant-induced lipid peroxidation and membrane permeability to potassium ions in isolated human erythrocytes (Meydani et al. 1993). Therefore, the ability of these compounds to chelate metal ions and prevent free-radical formation suggests that they may play an important protective role. In addition, flavonoids are also scavengers of the $\cdot NO$ radical. The $\cdot NO$ radical generated by inflammatory cells is reported to be toxic after reaction with the $\cdot O_2^-$ radical. Scavenging $\cdot NO$ radicals could therefore contribute to the proposed beneficial effect of the flavonoids.

Arteriosclerosis begins in a process in which $\cdot NO$ radicals play an unfavorable role, which adds additional weight to the possibility that flavonoids reduce the risk of coronary heart disease (CHD) (Acker et al. 1995). Further support for this possibility was provided by the Dutch Zutphen Elderly study, which showed an inverse correlation between intakes of flavonoids and incidence of CHD (Hertog et al. 1993). Moreover, a higher flavonoid intake from red wine may explain why the French have a lower mortality from CHD compared with the British, despite the fact that the consumption of saturated fat in France is greater than that in the United Kingdom.

But the in vivo evidence for a protective effect of increased flavonoid intake is limited. The antioxidant capacity of plasma is increased in response to the oral ingestion of phenol-rich beverages, such as red wine and teas, or phenol-rich foods, such as dark chocolate. Polyphenols are rapidly absorbed, and peak plasma concentrations are reached within 1 hour of consuming nonalcoholic red wine. In vitro studies have demonstrated that alcohol-free red wine displays a stronger antioxidant activity than does alcohol-free white wine, and the only consistent chemical difference between the two wines is the phenol content, which is 20 times higher in red wine than in white wine. The higher phenol content results from the incorporation of the grape skins into the fermented grape juice during production of red wine. White wine production does not use the grape skins, only the fermented grape juice. The biological actions of phenols may add significantly to the suggested protective effects of increased consumption of fruits and vegetables, such as the reduced risk of various cancers and CHD. Indeed, red wine inhibits LDL oxidation in vitro and reduces the susceptibility of plasma components to lipid peroxidation.

Possible Risks of High-Dose Antioxidant Supplementation Antioxidants obviously provide some defense against the damaging effects of free radicals, and the media commonly extols the potential health benefits of a high antioxidant intake. This publicity has prompted many people to take large doses of antioxidant vitamins. Excessive antioxidant ingestion, however, may not be uniformly helpful. For example, in heavy smokers, increased intake of vitamin E and β-carotene actually increases the incidence of lung cancer (Blot 1997; De Luca and Ross 1996). One possible reason for this effect is that antioxidants may interfere with important processes needed to kill cancer cells. Administration of antioxidants inhibits apoptosis (cell death), an important defense mechanism that inhibits tumor development by eliminating new mutated cells. ROS are intermediate messengers in several apoptosis signaling pathways. So excess antioxidants may effectively "shoot the messengers." Thus, in situations in which people have damaged their DNA (e.g., by heavy smoking or by exercise), the administration of antioxidants may prevent the effective removal of damaged cells.

Some side effects are associated with consuming excessive amounts of individual antioxidant vitamins. Very large doses of vitamin C are associated with urinary stone formation, impaired copper absorption, and diarrhea. Excess intakes of vitamin A by pregnant women can cause birth defects, and recent evidence suggests that high doses of vitamin A may be associated with reduced bone density and increased risk of hip fractures in postmenopausal women. Large intakes of vitamin E can impair absorption of vitamins A and K. Thus, more is not always better.

The controversy continues about whether physically active people should consume large amounts of antioxidant compounds. At present, the data are insufficient to recommend antioxidant supplements for athletes. In the last few decades, the role of ROS in exercise physiology has received considerable attention. Acute exercise has been shown to induce elevated generation of ROS in skeletal muscle through various mechanisms, and clear evidence shows that ROS formation in response to vigorous physical exertion can result in oxidative stress. But research has revealed the important role of ROS as signaling molecules that modulate contractile function and adaptive processes in skeletal muscle (Powers et al. 2007; Steensberg et al. 2007). In particular, ROS seem to be involved in the modulation of gene expression through redox-sensitive transcription pathways (Ji 2007).

This potentially represents an important regulatory mechanism, which has been suggested to be involved in the process of training adaptation. In this context, the adaptation of endogenous antioxidant systems in response to regular training reflects a potential mechanism responsible for augmented tolerance of skeletal muscle to exercise-induced stress. If so, it is likely that recommendations to athletes on antioxidant supplements may soon change. Consumption of high-dose supplements could actually impair the ability of the athlete to adapt to the training stimulus, and some evidence for this has emerged from animal and human studies (Gomez-Cabrera et al. 2005, 2008). Further research is needed to document the effects on training adaptation of long-term antioxidant use. Some facts may help athletes come to a decision about whether to supplement with antioxidants:

■ Numerous studies indicate that the body's natural antioxidant defense system is upregulated as an adaptation to exercise training.

■ Antioxidant supplementation does not improve exercise performance, and some studies indicate that antioxidant supplementation may impair the adaptive response to exercise training.

■ People who exercise regularly have a lower incidence of CHD, obesity, diabetes, and some (though not all) types of cancer compared with sedentary people, suggesting that the benefits of regular physical exercise outweigh the risks of free-radical-mediated damage.

■ Megadoses of antioxidant vitamins can have undesirable side effects in some individuals.

■ Athletes can obtain sufficient intakes of natural antioxidants by consuming a well-balanced diet that is rich in a variety of fruits and vegetables.

Oxygen Transport

Iron, as a component of hemoglobin, myoglobin, and cytochromes, is essential for oxidative metabolism. Hemoglobin is the protein in red blood cells that transports oxygen. Myoglobin is the respiratory pigment found inside the muscle fibers. The cytochromes are components of the electron-transport chain located on the inner mitochondrial membrane.

Thus, iron is essential for both oxygen transport and utilization. Besides the iron in the "functional compartment," mainly in hemoglobin and myoglobin, about one-fourth, or 1,000 mg, of the total body iron content in adult males is in storage. In contrast, iron stores are typically lower in adult women (300 to 500 mg), even lower in 18- to 21-year-old women (< 200 mg), and virtually absent in adolescents and young children. Unlike most adult male athletes, female and adolescent athletes need a regular supply of dietary iron to maintain iron balance and avoid anemia.

The gradual depletion of iron from the body when dietary intake is inadequate is commonly referred to as iron drain. This condition is thought to progress through a number of stages with different functional and diagnostic criteria, as described in table 10.12. Iron is stored in the body complexed with ferritin, a protein found mostly in the liver, spleen, and bone marrow. Soluble ferritin is released from cells into the blood plasma in direct proportion to cellular ferritin content. Hence, the plasma, or serum, ferritin concentration can be used to indicate the status of the body's iron stores.

Iron depletion (low iron stores as evidenced by a serum ferritin concentration of less than 12 μg/L) is common in female athletes (with a lesser incidence in male athletes), but whether this deficiency affects athletic performance in the absence of anemia remains controversial. Researchers have reported that depletion of the body's iron stores without anemia can be associated with increased lactate production during maximal exercise, indicative of reduced oxygen utilization by working muscle, and can also be associated with an increased subjective feeling of exercise overload in elite athletes. A few studies indicate that some performance benefits may result from iron supplementation in iron-depleted female athletes who are not anemic (Brownlie et al. 2002; Brutsaert et al. 2003). Furthermore, adaptations to endurance training, including improvements in maximal oxygen uptake and endurance performance, are enhanced by iron supplementation in iron-depleted, nonanemic women (Brownlie et al. 2002; Hinton et al. 2000).

Other studies have shown that $\dot{V}O_2$max, endurance performance, and muscle oxidative enzyme activity can be maintained even when body iron stores are severely depleted. What seems certain is that if the condition should progress to a state of iron deficiency resulting in anemia (low blood hemoglobin concentration [see table 10.12]), athletic performance is negatively affected. At this stage, not enough iron is available in the bone marrow to manufacture normal amounts of hemoglobin and red blood cells, leading to the production of small, pale red blood cells.

Anemia lowers the oxygen-carrying capacity of the blood and reduces exercise performance. In

■ **TABLE 10.12** ■

Stages of Iron Drain From Normal Iron Status Through to Iron Deficiency Anemia

DIAGNOSTIC CRITERIA

Stage	Characteristics	Blood hemoglobin (g/L)	Serum ferritin (mg/L)	Serum transferrin saturation (%)
Normal iron status	Normal iron status measurements and normal appearance of RBCs	>120 (F) >140 (M)	>30 (F) >110 (M)	20–40 (M, F)
Iron depletion	Normal hematocrit and hemoglobin but low serum ferritin with normal to high transferrin saturation	>120 (F) >140 (M)	<30 (M, F)	20–40 (M, F)
Iron deficiency	Normal hemoglobin but low serum ferritin, iron, and transferrin; low transferrin saturation	>120 (F) >140 (M)	<12 (M, F)	<16 (M, F)
Iron deficiency anemia	Low hematocrit and hemoglobin; low serum ferritin, iron, and transferrin saturation; small and pale RBCs	<120 (F) <140 (M)	<10 (M, F)	<16 (M, F)

M = males. F = females. RBCs = red blood cells (erythrocytes). Hematocrit = packed cell volume (normal = 38%–45% [F], 42%–48% [M]). Serum iron concentration is normally 0.4–1.4 mg/L. Characteristics of each stage and the associated diagnostic criteria are based on blood measures.

Adapted from V. Deakin 2000.

severe cases of anemia, affected people report sensations of breathlessness on mild exertion and generally feel so lethargic that they can no longer carry out everyday activities. Impaired functioning of several enzymes that require iron as a cofactor may result in mental dysfunction, impaired temperature control, and weakened immunity, which exacerbate the symptoms of reduced exercise tolerance.

Iron deficiency is reported to be the most widespread micronutrient deficiency in the world, and field studies consistently associate iron deficiency with increased morbidity from infectious disease. The incidence of iron-deficiency anemia is rare and is similar among athletes and the general population. The cause of anemia in athletes may be low energy intake, insufficient iron intake to maintain iron stores (see figure 10.7), or low meat intake (which provides the most readily available dietary source of iron). The routine testing of iron status in athletes is therefore recommended.

Exercise may cause some hemolysis of red blood cells, alterations of iron metabolism, and increased losses in sweat and urine. In some susceptible

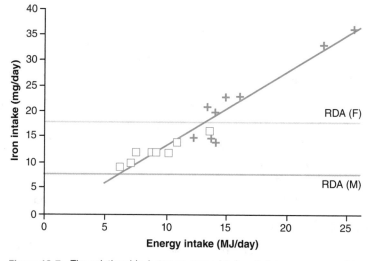

Figure 10.7 The relationship between mean intake of dietary energy and iron intake in male (crosses) and female (open squares) athletes. Each point represents a mean value for a group.

Based on van Erp-Baart et al. 1989.

individuals, additional losses caused by gastrointestinal bleeding may occur during prolonged strenuous exercise. The body adapts to endurance training by increasing the red blood cell mass and the myoglobin content of skeletal muscle. Altitude exposure causes an additional increase in red blood cell production. Hence, regular exercise increases the dietary requirement for iron.

The periodic screening of serum ferritin levels in athletes is recommended, because changes in the storage and transport of iron typically precede decreases in functional iron (hemoglobin) levels. During training, some athletes experience a transient fall in hemoglobin concentration and hematocrit, which is probably caused mostly by the increase in plasma volume that is commonly associated with the initiation of training or a sudden increase in the training load. This form of hemodilutional iron deficiency, sometimes called sports anemia, has no apparent effect on exercise performance.

About 60% of iron in animal tissues is in the heme form, that is, associated with hemoglobin and myoglobin and thus found only in animal foods. Nonheme iron is found in both animal and plant foods. Heme iron is absorbed better than nonheme iron. About 10% to 30% of ingested heme iron is absorbed in the gut, whereas only about 2% to 10% of nonheme iron is absorbed. The form in which it is consumed influences the bioavailability of iron (and many other minerals).

Some substances found in foods may promote or inhibit absorption of minerals. For example, vitamin C prevents the oxidation of ferrous iron (Fe^{2+}) to ferric (Fe^{3+}). Because ferrous iron is more readily absorbed, vitamin C facilitates nonheme iron absorption but has no effect on heme iron absorption. Thus, drinking a glass of fresh orange juice improves the absorption of iron from bread or cereals. Some natural substances found in foods such as tannins (e.g., in tea), phosphates, phytates, oxalates, and excessive fiber may decrease the bioavailability of nonheme iron. Iron absorption is also a function of storage: The larger the stores are, the poorer the absorption is, and vice versa. Thus, people with inadequate stores have better absorption, regardless of diet.

The low bioavailability of iron in vegetarian diets possibly contributes to lower serum ferritin levels in athletes who consume a modified vegetarian diet, and iron may also be short in a lactovegetarian diet because of the absence of heme iron. But a number of studies have failed to find that exercise per se decreased iron status, although this failure may be attributed to the relatively low training volumes employed. The consensus is that all athletes should include foods rich in heme iron such as lean red meat, poultry, and fish in their daily diets.

Because prolonged bouts of exercise increase the losses of iron in feces, urine, and sweat, most athletes need more iron in their diet than sedentary people. Weaver and Rajaram (1992) noted that iron losses may be around 70% higher in athletes compared with the reference value for sedentary people. Males can achieve an iron intake equivalent to twice the RDA through consumption of a well-balanced diet sufficient to meet daily energy requirements. Studies of various groups of athletes have shown that iron intake is proportional to energy intake (see figure 10.9), such that male athletes consuming in excess of 10 MJ/day (2,400 kcal/day) from a varied food base will obtain the RDA of iron. Thus, male endurance athletes who match their energy intake (from varied food sources) to their energy expenditure are likely to obtain more than enough iron. The same cannot be said for females. Without consuming iron-fortified cereals or other iron-fortified foods, it is challenging for 16- to 40-year-old females, even those consuming an energy balanced diet, to consume the RDA for iron. Those at particularly high risk for poor iron status are those athletes who consume a low-energy diet or avoid food sources rich in heme iron. Vegetarian athletes should ensure that plant food choices are iron dense (e.g., green leafy vegetables, legumes), and they should include iron-fortified products (breads, cereals, breakfast bars), whole-grain breads, and pasta in their diets.

Megadoses of iron are not advised, and routine oral iron supplements should not be taken without medical supervision following the diagnosis of iron deficiency by a physician. Only after laboratory confirmation of very low iron status or iron-deficiency anemia should iron supplements be used. Prolonged consumption of large amounts of iron can cause a disturbance in iron metabolism in susceptible individuals. Iron may accumulate in the liver, and the risk of developing hemochromatosis will increase. Hepatic iron accumulates as a compound called hemosiderin, which in excess can cause cell damage in the 0.3% of the population who are genetically predisposed. This condition causes cirrhosis and can be fatal. Excess intake of iron may also reduce absorption of other divalent cations, particularly zinc and copper. Groups at risk for insufficient iron intake who may be suitable candidates for iron supplementation include female endurance athletes, gymnasts, vegetarians, and those undergoing restricted energy intakes.

Anemia can also arise from deficiencies of vitamin B_6, vitamin B_{12}, folic acid, and copper. Vitamin B_6 is required for the synthesis of the porphyrin ring component of hemoglobin and myoglobin. Vitamin B_{12}, which contains the trace element cobalt, is required for the synthesis of nucleic

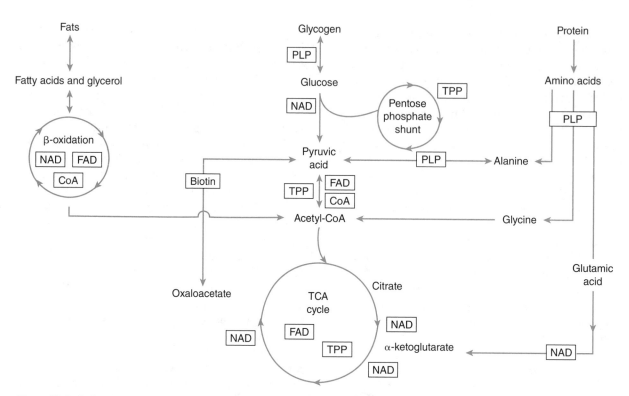

Figure 10.8 B vitamins as precursors of coenzymes in energy metabolism. CoA = coenzyme A; FAD = flavin adenine dinucleotide; NAD = nicotinamide adenine dinucleotide; PLP = pyridoxal phosphate; TPP = thiamin pyrophosphate.

acids, which are essential for the proliferation of stem cells that develop into red and white blood cells in the bone marrow. For the same reason, folic acid is also required for normal blood cell production. Deficiencies of these micronutrients are associated with megaloblastic or pernicious anemia, reduced blood leukocyte count, and impaired lymphocyte proliferation. Major food sources of vitamin B_{12} are meat, liver, and milk. Hence, athletes who avoid animal foods are at risk for cobalt and vitamin B_{12} deficiency. Some food products, notably breakfast cereals and milk, are fortified with vitamin B_{12}. For example, in the United Kingdom, 120 g of cornflakes, or 40 g of cornflakes with 150 ml of pasteurized whole milk, provides 1 µg of vitamin B_{12} (67% of the RNI). Copper is a cofactor of many enzymes and plays an important role in the formation of red blood cells.

Phosphorus, besides being a constituent of bones, teeth, and cell membranes, is a component of 2,3-diphosphoglycerate (2,3-DPG), which is found predominantly in red blood cells. 2,3-DPG alters the affinity of hemoglobin for oxygen and promotes more effective unloading of oxygen from the erythrocytes in the tissue capillaries, where the partial pressure of oxygen is lower than it is in the arteries. In response to altitude exposure, the erythrocyte concentration of 2,3-DPG increases.

Cofactors in Enzyme Catalyzed Reactions

Many of the B vitamins are reusable coenzymes in energy metabolism. Some of their roles can be seen in figure 10.8. Niacin (B_3), pyridoxine (B_6), and thiamin (B_1) are involved in carbohydrate metabolism; riboflavin (B_2), thiamin, pantothenic acid, and biotin are involved in fat metabolism; and vitamin B_6 and vitamin K are involved in protein metabolism. Niacin is the precursor of the important coenzymes nicotinamide adenine dinucleotide (NAD) and nicotinamide adenine dinucleotide phosphate (NADP); riboflavin is the precursor of flavin adenine dinucleotide (FAD) and flavin mononucleotide (FMN). These nicotinamide and flavin nucleotides are involved in oxidation and reduction reactions in energy metabolism, including some of the reactions of glycolysis, the TCA cycle, and the electron-transport chain (see figure 10.8). Pantothenic acid is the precursor of coenzyme-A (CoA), which is essential for the processes involved in both carbohydrate and fat oxidation (see chapter 3). A deficiency of these vitamins can result in premature fatigue and inability to maintain a heavy training program.

Zinc serves either a structural or a catalytic role in more than 200 human enzymes. It is a cofactor of several enzymes involved in energy metabolism and is required for normal cell replication, immune function, and wound healing. Some zinc-containing enzymes, such as carbonic anhydrase and lactate dehydrogenase, are involved in intermediary metabolism during exercise.

Studies have indicated that the intake of zinc among some groups of athletes (wrestlers, female endurance runners, and gymnasts) is considerably less than the RDA (11 mg/day and 8 mg/day for males and females, respectively). Prolonged exercise may cause significant losses of zinc and magnesium in sweat. Losses of these minerals in urine also increase as a result of intensive training. The total amount of zinc in the human body is about 2 g, and most of it is in muscle (60%) and bone (30%). Hence, measurements of zinc concentrations in blood may not be meaningful. Although losses of zinc in sweat and urine increase in physically active people, no evidence indicates that these losses are sufficient to cause concern. Small amounts of zinc are present in many foods of both animal and plant origin, and no benefit of additional zinc supplements for health or performance has been established.

Magnesium is an essential cofactor for more than 300 enzymes involved in biosynthetic processes and energy metabolism. It is essential for the normal functioning of ATPases, including myosin ATPase involved in muscle contraction, and it is involved in glycogen breakdown, protein synthesis, and fat oxidation. Magnesium is also required for the maintenance of electrical potentials in muscles and nerves, so it is important for normal neuromuscular coordination. The total body content of magnesium is about 25 g (see table 10.5). The RDA for magnesium is 420 mg/day for men and 320 mg/day for women; hence, magnesium is a macromineral rather than a trace element. The main dietary sources of magnesium are listed in table 10.8. Several studies have reported low serum magnesium concentrations in athletes, and prolonged strenuous exercise is associated with increased losses of magnesium in urine and sweat. Although, as with zinc and iron, a single bout of exercise is extremely unlikely to induce substantial magnesium losses, but a period of heavy training could induce a state of mild magnesium deficiency, particularly in a warm environment where sweat losses are high.

Magnesium deficiency in both humans and animals is associated with neuromuscular abnormalities, including muscle weakness, cramps, and structural damage of muscle fibers and organelles. The abnormalities may be caused by an impairment of calcium homeostasis secondary to an oxygen free-radical-induced alteration in the integrity of the membrane of the sarcoplasmic reticulum. Lack of magnesium may also be associated with depletion of selenium and reduced glutathione peroxidase activity, which would be expected to increase the susceptibility to damage by free radicals. Hence, magnesium deficiency possibly potentiates exercise-induced muscle damage and stress responses, but direct evidence for these is lacking. Magnesium deficiency exacerbates the inflammatory state after ischemic insult to the myocardium, which may be caused by a substance P–mediated increase in the secretion of proinflammatory cytokines in the magnesium-deficient state.

Copper is a cofactor of many enzymes, including several oxidases, and appears to be needed for the proper use of iron. Copper plays an important role in energy metabolism and the synthesis of hemoglobin, catecholamines, and some peptide hormones. Copper is also required for the normal formation of erythrocytes and the development of connective tissue. The RDA for copper for adult men and women is 0.9 mg/day. Intakes up to 10 mg/day are safe, and toxicity from dietary copper ingestion is extremely rare. The main dietary sources of copper are shown in table 10.9. Even though copper deficiency is rare in humans, athletes who take zinc supplements may compromise the gastrointestinal absorption of copper because of the similar physicochemical properties of these two minerals. Athletes should also be aware that large doses of vitamin C can limit copper absorption.

The results of changes in copper status caused by exercise and training are controversial and perhaps reflect the inadequacy of measuring techniques or redistribution of copper between body compartments, although athletes have been reported to lose copper in sweat. Compared with sedentary control subjects, several groups of athletes have similar or higher resting blood levels of copper. Thus, the copper status of athletes seems to be normal. After an acute bout of prolonged exercise, the plasma copper concentration may rise or remain unchanged. One study reported a substantial increase in plasma copper concentration during the first 8 days of a 20-day running road race, and this elevation persisted for the remainder of the race. This increase was attributed to a rise in the production of ceruloplasmin by the liver as part of the acute-phase response. Ceruloplasmin is a glycoprotein that binds copper and is thought to exert a protective effect against cellular damage caused by free radicals. As explained previously, manganese and selenium are cofactors of the antioxidant enzymes superoxide dismutase and glutathione reductase–peroxidase, respectively.

Immune Function and Resistance to Infection

Heavy exercise and nutrition exert separate influences on immune function; these influences appear to be greater when exercise stress and poor nutrition act synergistically. The poor nutritional status of some athletes very likely predisposes them to immunodepression. Several vitamins, including vitamin B_{12} and folic acid, are needed for the normal production of white blood cells that defend the body against invading pathogens. Other vitamins, including A, C, and E, are needed for normal functioning of these cells. Several minerals, including zinc, iron, copper, and selenium, are also essential for optimal immune function. The role of both micronutrients and macronutrients in immune function and resistance to infection is dealt with in detail in chapter 16.

Electrolytes in Body Fluids

An electrolyte conducts an electric current when dissolved in water. Electrolytes, which include acids, bases, and salts, usually dissociate into ions carrying either a positive charge (cation) or a negative charge (anion). The major electrolytes in the body fluids are sodium, potassium, chloride, bicarbonate, phosphate, sulfate, magnesium, and calcium. Of these, sodium, potassium, and chloride are found in the highest concentrations, although their distribution differs between the intracellular and extracellular fluids.

Sodium and chloride are found in higher concentrations in the extracellular fluid, whereas potassium is found in higher concentration inside cells. These concentration differences arise because of active transport mechanisms in cell membranes. The sodium–potassium ATPase actively pumps three sodium ions out of the cell for every two potassium ions pumped into the cell, which sets up an electrical potential (charge) difference across the cell membrane; the interior of the cell is slightly negative compared with the outside. This electrical potential difference can be measured as a voltage difference. Amounts, in most cells, are about 70 millivolts (mV). This resting membrane potential can be reversed by a sudden influx of positive ions into the cell, which is the basis of the action potential generated in nerve and muscle fibers when sodium channels in the membranes of these cells are temporarily opened.

Sodium, as the principal cation in the extracellular fluids (see table 10.5), serves primarily to maintain normal body fluid balance, osmotic pressure, and blood pressure. The role of excess sodium intake in the etiology of high blood pressure (hypertension) is discussed in chapter 2. Normal body fluid levels of sodium are critical for nerve impulse transmission and muscle contraction. The body has effective hormonal control mechanisms for dealing with wide variations in dietary sodium intake.

If the plasma concentration of sodium falls, aldosterone secretion from the adrenal glands increases, and this steroid hormone stimulates the kidney to reabsorb more sodium so that less is excreted in the urine. When the plasma concentration of sodium rises, aldosterone production falls, allowing increased urinary excretion of sodium. Other hormones, notably vasopressin or antidiuretic hormone (ADH), through its effect on water reabsorption by the kidney, help to maintain normal sodium concentration in the body fluids. During prolonged moderate exercise or short durations of high-intensity exercise, the plasma sodium concentration increases, which helps maintain blood volume. Exercise also leads to increased secretion of both aldosterone and ADH, which results in the conservation of body sodium and water.

The estimated minimum daily requirement for sodium in adults is 0.5 g (amount contained in 1.25 g of table salt), the adequate intake of sodium is 1.5 g, and the upper recommended intake of sodium is 2.4 g/day. Sodium occurs in small amounts in most natural foods, but many processed foods have substantial amounts of salt added. For example, a 180 g (5 oz) serving of cooked fresh beans contains 25 mg of sodium, whereas an equal portion of canned beans contains 750 mg of sodium. Because of health concerns, in recent years food manufacturers have reduced the salt content of processed foods. Even so, the average consumption of sodium by people in the United States is reported to be about 4.5 g/day. About one-third of this amount is from natural foods, one-half is from processed foods, and the rest is from table salt.

The typical sodium content of several foods is shown in table 10.13. Fresh meats, fruits, and vegetables generally contain relatively small amounts of sodium, whereas several processed foods such as sauces, pickles, chips, ready meals, and processed meats (e.g., sausages and burgers) contain much greater amounts of sodium.

Sodium Content of Common Food Items

Food item	Amount	Sodium content (mg)
MEAT		
Luncheon meat	1 oz (28 g)	450
Beef	1 oz (28 g)	25
Chicken	1 oz (28 g)	13
White fish	1 oz (28 g)	33
Tuna (in oil)	1 oz (28 g)	270
Salmon (canned)	1 oz (28 g)	140
Pork sausage	1 oz (28 g)	70
CEREAL AND STARCH PRODUCTS		
Bread	1 slice	130
Corn flakes	1 oz (28 g)	280
Pretzels	1 oz (28 g)	890
Chips or crisps (plain, salted)	1 oz (28 g)	195
Chips or crisps (salt and vinegar)	1 oz (28 g)	335
VEGETABLES AND FRUITS		
Beans (fresh, cooked)	1 oz (28 g)	5
Baked beans (canned)	1 oz (28 g)	150
Red kidney beans (canned)	1 oz (28 g)	85
Peas (canned)	1 oz (28 g)	55
Pickled onions	1 oz (28 g)	225
Potato (baked)	1 medium size	6
Banana	1 medium size	1
Orange	1 medium size	1
DAIRY PRODUCTS		
Milk (semiskimmed)	100 ml	120
Butter	1 teaspoon (5 g)	50
Cheese	1 oz (28 g)	445
Cottage cheese	1 oz (28 g)	20
OTHER COMMON PRODUCTS		
Margarine	1 teaspoon (5 g)	50
Spaghetti sauces	1 oz (28 g)	340
Soups	100 ml	500
Tomato ketchup	1 tablespoon (15 g)	100
Soy sauce	1 tablespoon (15 g)	1,020
Bolognese sauce	1 oz (28 g)	140
Gravy powder	1 oz (28 g)	1,620
Cakes and tarts	1 oz (28 g)	85
Isotonic sports drinks	100 ml	46
Table salt	1 teaspoon (5 g)	5,000

Deficiency of sodium is rare, partly because of the widespread availability of sodium in many food products and partly because humans have a natural appetite for salt. Nevertheless, substantial losses of sodium and chloride from the body can result from prolonged sweating. Although sweat composition is quite variable, the average amount of sodium and chloride lost in sweat is about 1.2 g/L and 1.4 g/L, respectively. Because most people sweat at a rate of 1 to 2 L/h during strenuous exercise, even in ambient temperatures around 20 °C (68 °F), salt losses can be considerable. Thus, for the athlete exercising in the heat, short-term deficiencies of sodium and chloride may be incurred, which, if not corrected in the recovery period, can have debilitating effects on subsequent exercise performance.

Low blood sodium levels (hyponatremia) can also occur with excessive consumption of water over a period of several hours, which can lead to potentially fatal water intoxication (see chapter 9). Chloride is the major anion in the extracellular fluids (see table 10.5), and, like sodium, it is involved in the regulation of body fluid balance and electrical potentials across cell membranes. Chloride ions are also a component in the formation of hydrochloric acid in the stomach, which promotes the denaturation and digestion of dietary proteins. The estimated minimum daily requirement for chloride in adults is 0.75 g, and the adequate intake is currently set at 2.30 g. The dietary intake of chloride, as might be expected, parallels that of sodium.

Potassium is the major cation found inside cells. The intracellular concentration is about 150 mmol/L compared with around 4 mmol/L in the extracellular fluids. Potassium is also involved in body fluid homeostasis and in the generation of electrical impulses in nerves, skeletal muscle, and the heart. Excretion of potassium in the urine is, like that of sodium, regulated by aldosterone. A rise in the plasma potassium concentration stimulates the secretion of aldosterone, leading to increased urinary excretion of potassium. Conversely, a fall in the plasma potassium concentration causes a reduction in aldosterone secretion from the adrenal cortex and hence greater potassium retention by the kidneys. The estimated minimum daily requirement for potassium in adults is 2.0 g, and the adequate intake is set at 4.7 g. Potassium is found in most foods and is particularly abundant in bananas, citrus fruits, vegetables, and milk (see table 10.14). Because potassium balance is tightly regulated in the body, long-term deficiencies or excesses are extremely rare. Short-term imbalances, however, may occur in certain circumstances. For example, low blood potassium levels (hypokalemia) have been reported in persons suffering from diarrhea, during prolonged fasting, and after diuretic drug administration.

Low plasma potassium concentrations can lead to muscle weakness and fatal cardiac arrest. A higher than normal blood level of potassium (hyperkalemia) is also potentially dangerous because this condition, too, can cause cardiac arrhythmias, resulting in death. For this reason, people should not take large doses of potassium supplements. During high-intensity exercise, active skeletal muscle releases potassium ions that enter the circulation and cause a temporary rise in the plasma potassium concentration. Under normal circumstances, however, normal potassium levels are rapidly restored during the recovery period. Some potassium is excreted in sweat, but these losses are relatively small (160 to 320 mg/L) compared with the losses of sodium and chloride, so potassium status can easily be restored with ingestion of a postexercise meal.

Other Tissue Functions

Calcium, besides being an important structural component of bone, is involved in nerve conduction and muscle excitation and contraction. In the sarcoplasm (cytosol) of resting muscle, the concentration of free calcium ions (Ca^{2+}) is low (about 10 nM), whereas in the extracellular fluid and sarcoplasmic reticulum (SR), the concentration is much higher; the blood plasma concentration of free calcium, for example, is about 1 mM (100,000 times higher than in the muscle sarcoplasm). Release of calcium from the SR in response to membrane depolarization after the arrival of an action potential allows the myosin and actin filaments to interact, bringing about muscle contraction (see chapter 3). Calcium is then pumped back into the SR by an active transport mechanism, which restores the low cytosolic calcium ion concentration, allowing relaxation of the muscle.

Calcium is also required for the activation of numerous enzymes involved in energy metabolism. For example, the activity of phosphorylase, the key enzyme involved in muscle glycogen breakdown, is stimulated by increased cytosolic calcium ion concentration. Several enzymes of glycolysis are also activated by increased levels of intracel-

■ TABLE 10.14 ■
Potassium Content of Common Food Items

Food item	Amount	Potassium content (mg)
MEAT		
Beef	1 oz (28 g)	100
Chicken	1 oz (28 g)	70
White fish	1 oz (28 g)	160
CEREAL AND STARCH PRODUCTS		
Bread	1 slice	65
Corn flakes	1 oz (28 g)	100
VEGETABLES AND FRUITS		
Potato (baked)	1 medium size	780
Carrot	1 medium size	275
Broccoli	1 medium size stalk	270
Banana	1 medium size	460
Orange	1 medium size	260
Apple	1 medium size	35
DAIRY PRODUCTS		
Milk (semiskimmed)	100 ml	180
Butter	1 teaspoon (5 g)	10
Cheddar cheese	1 oz (28 g)	28
Yogurt	100 g	450

lular calcium, which neatly links the provision of energy to the same process that allows the muscle to perform work.

Calcium and vitamin K (menadione) are required for normal blood clotting. Vitamin K is required for the synthesis of blood-clotting factors. This vitamin is a coenzyme in the posttranslational modification of protein structure, specifically the addition of sugar moieties to form glycoproteins.

Zinc plays a role in appetite regulation. Oral zinc supplementation has been shown to be effective in restoring normal eating behavior and body weight in patients suffering from the eating disorder anorexia nervosa (see chapter 15). Zinc has been suggested to be involved in the pathogenesis of this eating disorder. Among female athletes, gymnasts and dancers have a particularly high incidence of eating disorders, and several dietary surveys indicate that these groups consume inadequate amounts of zinc. Indeed, in a study of female adolescent dancers and gymnasts, 75% were found to consume less than two-thirds of the RDA for zinc. Thus, athletes who attempt to maintain a low body weight should be sure to consume adequate amounts of zinc.

Besides being coenzymes in energy metabolism, several of the B-complex vitamins are also required for normal neuromuscular function. For example, vitamin B_6 is needed for the synthesis and metabolism of many neurotransmitters, including norepinephrine and dopamine.

Vitamin A (retinol) forms the visual pigments of the eye and is therefore important for normal vision, particularly in fading light.

Assessing Micronutrient Status

Vitamin (and mineral) status can be estimated directly from biopsy samples of body tissues (e.g., skeletal muscle), from blood cells or plasma, or indirectly from analysis of the diet. The vitamin status of an individual, however, is difficult to determine accurately. A diagnosis of vitamin deficiency is best made by considering a variety of sources of information, including blood analysis, an assessment of dietary intake, and clinical symptoms. Most studies that have used blood analysis (either by direct measurement of the plasma concentration of the vitamin or by indirect measurement of vitamin-requiring enzyme activities) have not revealed any distinct differences between athletic people and sedentary people. Furthermore, little evidence suggests that the vitamin intakes of athletes in general are inadequate, based on the **recommended dietary allowances (RDAs)**, except in athletes with extremely low dietary energy intakes or in athletes who fail to consume a well-balanced diet.

Dietary Surveys of Vitamin Intakes in Elite Athletes

Ideally, athletes should obtain all their nutrients from food. A well-balanced diet, including foods from each of the five food groups (meat, dairy, cereal, fruit, and vegetables) should provide adequate amounts of all 13 essential vitamins. Arguably, because total energy intake of most athletes exceeds that of sedentary nonathletes, a greater amount and variety of vitamins should be available to athletes through their dietary intake. Unfortunately, surveys of the dietary habits of elite athletes indicate that they do not always consume a well-balanced diet. Elite athletes are at risk for nutrient deficiencies because of the fatiguing and time-consuming demands of training. A combination of increased vitamin turnover, additional loss of some nutrients, poor food selection, and limited time for food preparation are contributing factors.

The first two comprehensive reports on the actual dietary intakes of athletes, published in 1981, revealed inappropriate macronutrient composition of the diets, with fat and protein components being too high. In one study (Barry et al. 1981), this inadequate diet was coupled with suboptimal intakes of thiamin, niacin, and folic acid. Intakes of these vitamins among female athletes were well below the recommended daily requirements. Some dietary surveys performed on elite

endurance athletes have reported low (< 85% of the RDA) or excessively high (> 200% of the RDA) intakes of vitamins. But apart from reports of low vitamin D intake in South African runners (Peters and Goetzsche 1997) and low vitamin A intake in Dutch elite strength athletes (van Erp-Baart et al. 1989b), deficient as well as excess intakes are reported consistently only for the water-soluble vitamins. Low intakes of vitamins A and D are likely to be attributable to the restriction of dietary fat intake in weight-conscious athletes. In a national dietary survey of Dutch athletes (van Erp-Baart et al. 1989b) who participated in endurance, strength, or team sports, intakes of vitamins B_2, B_6, and C appeared to be more than adequate in endurance athletes but were marginal in some strength athletes and team games players (see figure 10.9). This difference was attributed to the higher total dietary energy intakes in the endurance athletes. Several groups of athletes in this study consumed vitamin supplements well in excess of the RDA.

In contrast, the groups most at risk for inadequate intake of vitamins (B vitamins in particular) are female adolescent athletes and athletes who are attempting to maintain low body weight (e.g., wrestlers, gymnasts, ballet dancers) by restricting their total energy intake. Clearly, these athletes need to choose foods carefully or take vitamin supplements.

Dietary Surveys of Mineral Intakes in Elite Athletes

The interpretation of dietary records for adequacy of mineral (particularly, trace element) intake should be done with some caution. This assessment is difficult because of the differences in the bioavailability of trace elements in various foods and because not all foods have been analyzed for their mineral composition. Furthermore, assessment of a person's mineral status based on a chemical analysis of blood or biopsy samples is not always possible. In many cases, the plasma concentration of a particular mineral does not accurately reflect the body stores of the mineral. Given those limitations, information based on dietary surveys of athletes and their blood chemistry suggests that iron, zinc, calcium, and magnesium status may be of some concern, especially for young athletes and female athletes of all ages.

Several groups of athletes may have low iron stores, including middle-distance and long-distance runners, female endurance athletes, and adolescent athletes. Nevertheless, the proportion of athletes with low iron stores is no greater than that found

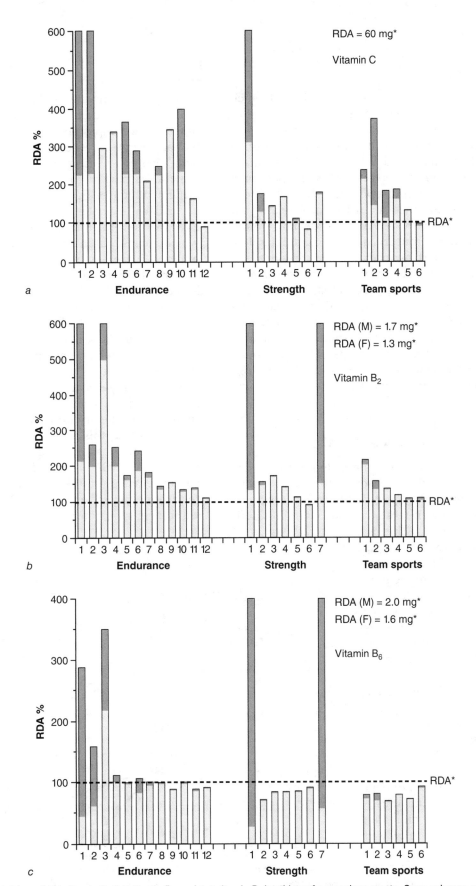

Figure 10.9 Daily intakes of *(a)* vitamin C, *(b)* vitamin B$_2$, and *(c)* vitamin B$_6$ in athletes from various sports. Open columns represent intake from food sources; filled columns indicate intake from supplements. M = males; F = females. Endurance: 1 = Tour de France M; 2 = Tour de l'Avenir M; 3 = triathlon M; 4 = cycling M; 5 = marathon speed skating M; 6 = swimming M; 7 = rowing M; 8 = running M; 9 = rowing F; 10 = cycling F; 11 = running F; 12 = subtop swimming F. Strength: 1 = body building M; 2 = judo M; 3 = weightlifting M; 4 = judo M; 5 = top gymnastics F; 6 = subtop gymnastics F; 7 = bodybuilding F. Team sports: 1 = water polo M; 2 = soccer M; 3 = field hockey M; 4 = volleyball F; 5 = field hockey F; 6 = handball F.

*These are based on RDAs in 1989, which have now changed (see appendix C).

International Journal of Sports Medicine: From A.M.J. van Erp-Baart et al., "Nationwide survey on nutritional habits in elite athletes. Part II: Mineral and vitamin intake," 1989; 10 (suppl 1): S11-S16. Reprinted by permission.

in the general U.S. population, in which the incidence of iron depletion (a serum ferritin level of less than 12 µg/L) is 21% of women and 25% of adolescent girls. The incidence of iron depletion in male athletes may be higher than it is for sedentary males, in whom iron deficiency is low (less than 2% of the male population in the United States). Males generally meet the RDA for calcium, but females, especially adolescents, do not. Young female athletes concerned with maintaining low body weight and low body fat, such as gymnasts, dancers, and runners, have low calcium intakes (Aulin 2000). The story is similar for zinc and magnesium; most male athletes appear to meet the RDA for these minerals, but many groups of female athletes do not. Limited information is available for other minerals, but reports of isolated trace element deficiencies in athletes, apart from iron and zinc, are extremely rare.

Exercise and Micronutrient Requirements

Various experimental vitamin depletion studies have determined that inadequate vitamin status is associated with impaired exercise performance, particularly when more than one vitamin is deficient in the diet. Athletes are generally assumed to need increased vitamin intake because exercise increases vitamin requirements. Theoretically, exercise can induce a marginal vitamin status (deficiency) by causing decreased absorption from the digestive tract; increased excretion in sweat, urine, and feces; increased turnover (degradation); and increased requirement (retention) because of biochemical adaptation to training (e.g., increased mitochondrial density in skeletal muscle with endurance training and muscle hypertrophy with strength training).

A temporary depression of the free (unbound) plasma concentration of some trace elements (e.g., iron, zinc,

copper) may occur after prolonged exercise, mainly because of a redistribution of the mineral to other tissue compartments (e.g., erythrocytes and leukocytes) or because of the release of proteins from liver and neutrophils that chelate (bind) the mineral as part of the acute-phase response to inflammation (see figure 10.10). Regular exercise, particularly in a hot environment, incurs increased losses of several minerals in sweat and urine, which means that the daily requirement for most minerals increases in athletes engaged in heavy training. But with the exception of iron and zinc, isolated mineral deficiencies are rare.

Iron losses in sweat may be as high as 0.3 mg iron/L of sweat (see table 10.10). When an athlete exercises hard in a hot environment, sweat production could well be about 2 L/h. If the athlete exercises for 2 hours a day in such conditions, the additional daily sweat loss is 4 L, which incurs a loss of 1.2 mg of iron. Because, on average, only about 10% of dietary iron can be absorbed in the gut, to replace this additional loss of iron, the person must consume about 12 mg of extra iron in food. The RDA for iron for men is 8 mg (18 mg for females), so the sweat losses under these conditions approximately doubles the dietary requirement for iron.

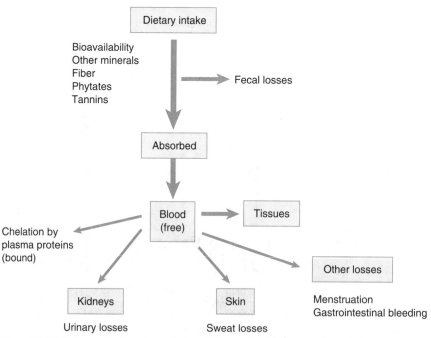

Figure 10.10 Factors affecting absorption and tissue distribution of minerals. Exercise may increase losses of minerals in urine and sweat, and several other components of the diet may interfere with mineral absorption.

But controversy exists regarding iron losses in sweat and whether athletes can lose enough iron in sweat to cause iron deficiency. In a careful study that minimized iron loss in shedded skin cells and iron contamination of skin, a much lower iron concentration in sweat (averaging only 23 µg/L) was reported (Brune et al. 1986). A subsequent study of exercising athletes (Waller and Haymes 1996) also suggested that losses of iron in sweat are modest and, furthermore, that the concentration of iron in sweat declines over time (at least during the first hour of exercise). These authors estimated that about 6% to 11% of the iron typically absorbed each day is lost in sweat during an hour of exercise and that losses for men are approximately twice those for women because of the higher sweat rate in men.

Exercise may further increase the requirement for iron because of the adaptive increase in muscle myoglobin concentration and red cell mass in response to endurance training (Eichner 2000). Some athletes are susceptible to gastrointestinal bleeding during prolonged strenuous exercise. About 20% of recreational runners are estimated to experience occult fecal blood after distance races. Bleeding may arise because of irritation of the stomach lining or superficial hemorrhage of the colon caused by ischemic insult (i.e., restricted blood supply because of constriction of blood vessels supplying the tissue). During strenuous exercise, blood is diverted to the working muscles, and when exercise is prolonged (particularly when accompanied by dehydration and hyperthermia), the restriction of blood flow to the colon may cause inflammation and blood vessel damage, a condition called segmental hemorrhagic colitis (Eichner 2000). Measurement of fecal iron loss in elite male distance runners showed that during training and racing gastrointestinal blood loss amounted to about 6 ml/day (Nachtigall et al. 1996).

Substantial amounts of magnesium are lost in sweat (see table 10.5), and increased urinary losses of both magnesium and zinc have been reported in athletes engaged in high-intensity exercise. These additional losses, if not matched by increased dietary intakes, could cause magnesium and zinc deficiency with chronic training. Several studies report lower resting serum concentrations of magnesium and zinc in athletes compared with sedentary control subjects, but serum levels of these minerals for athletes were still within the accepted normal ranges.

Ergogenic Effect of Micronutrient Supplementation

A number of papers have been written about the effects of vitamin supplementation on exercise performance. Older studies have suggested a potential ergogenic role of vitamins, based on the argument that the RDAs may not represent optimal intake. But many of the early studies that claimed to show beneficial effects of vitamin supplementation on exercise performance were poorly designed, often with no control (placebo) group against which to compare the effects of supplementation or no information about current vitamin status in the test subjects. Recent double-blind placebo-controlled studies have discredited the notion that excess vitamin intake improves exercise performance. Even so, many athletes consume relatively large amounts of vitamin and mineral supplements as a kind of insurance policy so that they feel satisfied in their own minds that they are not at risk for any vitamin deficiency.

Severe or prolonged vitamin deficiencies are, of course, deleterious to health and would therefore be expected to impair athletic performance. Vitamin and mineral supplementation may improve the nutritional status of people who consume marginal amounts of nutrients from food and may improve performance in those with deficiencies. Athletes, however, should not rely on tablets to supply them with the necessary micronutrients. Besides the established vitamins, many other compounds present in small quantities in fresh fruit and vegetables are probably needed for optimal health.

Short-term inadequacy of vitamin intake is characterized by lowered vitamin concentrations in body tissues and fluids and decreased activities of certain enzymes. But functional disturbances, including decreased $\dot{V}O_2$max or physical performance capacity, may not appear until weeks or months later. In the opposite scenario, large intakes of vitamins increase the body's vitamin stores (particularly fat-soluble vitamins) and the activity of some enzymes but will not necessarily improve physical work capacity. Furthermore, excessive intakes of the fat-soluble vitamins (A, D, E, and K) for prolonged periods can be harmful.

Some minerals are specifically promoted as potential ergogenic aids to performance. These supplements, often consumed in bulk quantities a few hours before competition, include phosphates and sodium bicarbonate. Phosphate salts are suggested as a potential ergogenic aid because these ions are an important intracellular buffer. Phosphate groups are a component of the body's energy currency, namely ATP. So phosphate loading might increase the resynthesis rate of ATP from ADP and phosphate. Another possible ergogenic mechanism could be improving oxygen extraction from the blood by muscle fibers through an elevated erythrocyte 2,3-DPG concentration. At present, however, experimental evidence for these claims is lacking.

Bicarbonate is an important extracellular buffer. Reliable evidence indicates that bicarbonate ingestion (most commonly consumed as sodium bicarbonate, although sodium itself has no independent effects in acid–base regulation) can improve performance in events in which lactic acid accumulation in the muscle is a major cause of fatigue, such as 400 to 1,500 m running (see chapter 11). But consumption of the amount of sodium bicarbonate necessary to alter blood acid–base balance sufficiently to influence performance (approximately 20 g) can cause gastrointestinal discomfort and diarrhea. Because of these unpleasant side effects, bicarbonate loading can temporarily result in inadequate absorption of essential micronutrients and carbohydrate and therefore can delay the restoration of muscle glycogen stores after exercise. The side effects and their consequences are important factors to consider for sports events involving competition on successive days. Further details of phosphate and bicarbonate loading are found in chapter 11.

Recommendations for Micronutrient Intake in Athletes

In general, supplementation with individual vitamins, including the consumption of large doses of simple antioxidant mixtures, is not recommended. Consuming megadoses of individual vitamins (common among athletes) is likely to do more harm than good. Because most vitamins function mainly as coenzymes in the body, after these enzyme systems are saturated, the vitamin in free form can become toxic. For example, extremely large doses of vitamin C are associated with urinary stone formation, impaired copper absorption, and diarrhea. Megadoses of vitamin B_6 can cause sensory neuropathy. Excess intake of vitamin A can reduce bone mineral density, and excess vitamin A

intake by pregnant women can cause birth defects. Athletes should obtain complex mixtures of antioxidant compounds from increased consumption of fruits and vegetables.

Vitamin supplements are not necessary for athletes who eat a well-balanced diet. Many athletes, however, are concerned about ensuring adequate intakes of vitamins and want to avoid the risks of oversupplementation. A daily intake of an over-the-counter multivitamin, supplying not more than the RDA, provides an adequate and safe level of vitamin intake, especially during periods of intensive training and carbohydrate loading before competition. Similarly, most athletes do not require mineral supplements because their diets are already more than adequate to meet any increased requirements resulting from the effects of regular intensive exercise.

Some groups of athletes, however, are at risk for marginal mineral intake, notably those who compete in sports events in which low body weight is essential for success (e.g., gymnasts and dancers) or compete within certain body-weight categories (e.g., boxers, wrestlers, and weightlifters). Participants in such sports often train frequently and intensively but consume low-energy diets or undergo drastic weight-loss regimens to maintain or lose body weight before competition. The low energy intakes (< 8 MJ/day [< 1,900 kcal/day]) in these situations are likely to lead to inadequate intake of essential minerals (and vitamins). Because many athletes are young and still in a period of body growth and development, they can be detrimentally affected by micronutrient deficiencies. Specific recommendations can be given to athletes to ensure an adequate calcium intake when on an energy-restricted diet:

- Include three servings per day of low-fat dairy foods.
- Include these dairy foods in high-carbohydrate meals (e.g., skimmed milk on cereal).
- Eat fish with bones (e.g., sardines).
- Include calcium-enriched soy products.
- Eat leafy green vegetables (e.g., cabbage, broccoli, spinach).

Dietary recommendations can also be given to athletes to increase available iron intake in a high-carbohydrate diet:

- Eat foods rich in heme iron at least four times a week (e.g., liver or lean red meat).

- Eat iron-fortified foods (e.g., breakfast cereal).

- Include nonheme iron food sources (e.g., dried fruit, legumes, and green leafy vegetables).

- Combine nonheme iron foods with meat or foods rich in vitamin C (e.g., orange juice) to increase iron absorption.

- Avoid drinking tea at meals.

Other athletes who are at risk for marginal mineral intake are those who abstain from normal diets (i.e., consume extremely unbalanced diets with a low micronutrient density) and vegetarians. Micronutrient supplementation is recommended for such athletes.

Amenorrheic female athletes should certainly take calcium supplements, and other female athletes should consider taking calcium supplements, to ensure adequate calcium status and maintain healthy bones. Moderately elevated intakes of calcium do not appear to be harmful, possibly because the blood calcium concentration is under tight hormonal regulation and moderate excesses can be excreted in the urine.

Athletes who train and compete in hot environments should also consider increasing their intake of minerals (particularly iron, zinc, and magnesium) because mineral losses in sweat can be considerable. Even so, daily supplements of these minerals should not exceed one to two times the RDA. As with vitamins, excessive intake of minerals can be toxic and can impair the absorption of other essential trace elements.

Poor diets are the main reason for micronutrient deficiencies found in athletes, although in certain cases, regular strenuous exercise contributes to the deficiency. Eating a well-balanced diet can easily correct micronutrient deficiencies, with the possible exceptions of iron and calcium shortfalls. Inadequate knowledge of proper dietary practices, lack of time for food preparation, misleading advertisements for micronutrient supplements, and lack of qualified dietary advice are possible reasons for suboptimal micronutrient intakes in athletes. Few studies have definitively documented beneficial effects of mineral or vitamin supplementation on exercise performance, except when supplementation was needed to correct an existing deficiency. Athletes who take micronutrient supplements are for the most part taking them to ensure good health, not to enhance sports performance. An unhealthy athlete, however, is unlikely to perform to the best of his or her potential.

KEY POINTS

- Although vitamin and mineral supplementation may improve the nutritional status of athletes who consume marginal amounts of micronutrients from food and may improve performance in athletes with deficiencies, no convincing evidence indicates that doses in excess of the RDA improve performance.

- Vitamins and minerals are needed in the body for several important processes, including the growth and repair of body tissues, as cofactors in enzyme catalyzed metabolic reactions, for oxygen transport and oxidative metabolism, for immune function, and as antioxidants. Any sustained deficiency of an essential vitamin or mineral will cause ill health, and an unhealthy athlete is extremely unlikely to perform to the best of his or her potential.

- Vitamins are organic compounds that are needed in small quantities in the diet. They are essential for specific metabolic reactions in the body and for normal growth and development. With the exception of vitamin D, which can be synthesized in the presence of sunlight, and vitamin K and some B vitamins, which can be produced by the bacterial microflora of the gastrointestinal tract, vitamins are not produced by the human body and must be consumed in the diet.

- Although vitamins do not directly contribute to energy supply, they play an important role in regulating metabolism, acting as reusable coenzymes in intermediary metabolism. A deficiency of some of the B-group vitamins, which act as cofactors of enzymes in carbohydrate (e.g., niacin, pyridoxine [B_6], and thiamin [B_1]), fat (e.g., riboflavin [B_2], thiamin, pantothenic acid, and biotin), and protein (pyridoxine) metabolism, results in premature fatigue and inability to maintain a heavy training program. Other vitamins play a role in red and white blood cell production (folic acid and cobalamin [B_{12}]) or assist in the formation of bones, connective tissue, and cartilage (e.g., vitamins C and D).

■ The water-soluble vitamins—vitamin C (ascorbic acid), thiamin, riboflavin, pyridoxine, niacin, pantothenic acid, and biotin—are involved in mitochondrial energy metabolism. Folic acid and vitamin B_{12} are mainly involved in nucleic acid synthesis and hence are important for maintaining healthy populations of rapidly dividing cells in the body (e.g., red blood cells, immune cells, and the gut mucosa). Vitamin C is also an antioxidant.

■ The fat-soluble vitamins are A (retinol), D (calciferol), E (tocopherol), and K (menadione). Of these vitamins, only vitamin E has a probable role in energy metabolism. In addition, β-carotene (provitamin A) and vitamin E have antioxidant properties. Vitamin K is required for the addition of sugar residues to proteins to form glycoproteins.

■ Although physical activity may increase the requirement for some vitamins (e.g., vitamin C, riboflavin, and possibly pyridoxine, vitamin A, and vitamin E), this increased requirement typically is met by consuming a balanced high-carbohydrate, moderate-protein, low-fat diet. Vitamin and mineral intakes in athletes are correlated with energy intakes up to 20 MJ/day (4,800 kcal/day), so if energy intake matches the energy requirement, athletes get all the micronutrients that they need from food without any need for supplements.

■ Evidence suggests that antioxidants provide an important defense mechanism in the body against the damaging effects of free radicals. Many athletes consume large doses of antioxidant vitamins (β-carotene and vitamins C and E). But excessive antioxidant ingestion may not be uniformly helpful and may impair adaptation to training. The controversy continues about whether physically active people should consume antioxidant compounds in amounts above RDA values. At present, the data are insufficient to recommend antioxidant supplements for athletes.

■ Most athletes do not require micronutrient supplements because their diets are already more than adequate to meet any increased requirements resulting from the effects of regular intensive exercise. Particular groups of athletes, however, are at risk for marginal mineral and vitamin intake. These athletes compete in sports events in which low body weight is essential for success (e.g., gymnasts and dancers) or compete within certain body-weight categories (e.g., boxers, wrestlers, and weightlifters). Participants in these sports often train frequently and intensively but consume low-energy diets or undergo drastic weight-loss regimens to maintain or lose body weight before competition.

■ Amenorrheic female athletes should certainly take calcium supplements, and other female athletes should consider taking them, to ensure adequate calcium status and maintain healthy bones. Athletes who train and compete in hot environments should also consider increasing their mineral intake (particularly iron, zinc, and magnesium) because mineral losses in sweat can be considerable. Even so, daily supplements of these minerals should not exceed one to two times the RDA. As with vitamins, excessive intakes of minerals can be toxic and can impair the absorption of other essential trace elements.

■ Although poor diets are the main reason for micronutrient deficiencies among athletes, regular strenuous exercise can contribute to deficiency. Eating a well-balanced diet can easily correct these deficiencies, with the possible exceptions of shortfalls in iron and calcium. Inadequate knowledge of proper dietary practices, lack of time for food preparation, misleading advertisements for micronutrient supplements, and lack of qualified dietary advice are possible reasons for suboptimal micronutrient intakes by athletes.

RECOMMENDED READINGS

Chen, J. 2000. Vitamins: Effects of exercise on requirements. In *Nutrition in sport,* ed. R.J. Maughan, 282–291. Oxford: Blackwell Science.

Clarkson, P.M. 1991. Minerals: Exercise performance and supplementation in athletes. *Journal of Sports Sciences* 9:91–116.

Clarkson, P.M. 2000. Trace Minerals. In *Nutrition in sport,* ed. R. J. Maughan, 339–355. Oxford: Blackwell Science.

Fogelholm, M. 2000. Vitamins: Metabolic functions. In *Nutrition in sport,* ed. R. J. Maughan, 266–280. Oxford: Blackwell Science.

Haymes, E.M. 1991. Vitamin and mineral supplementation to athletes. *International Journal of Sport Nutrition* 1:146–169.

Niess, A.M., and P. Simon. 2007. Response and adaptation of skeletal muscle to exercise—the role of reactive oxygen species. *Frontiers in Bioscience* 12:4826–4838.

Powers, S.K., K.C. DeRuisseau, J. Quindry, and K.L. Hamilton. 2004. Dietary antioxidants and exercise. *Journal of Sports Sciences* 22 (1): 81–94.

Sen, C.K., S. Roy, and L. Packer. 2000. Exercise-induced oxidative stress and antioxidant nutrients. In *Nutrition in sport,* ed. R. J. Maughan, 292–317. Oxford: Blackwell Science.

van der Beek, E.J. 1991. Vitamin supplementation and physical exercise performance. *Journal of Sports Sciences* 9:77–89.

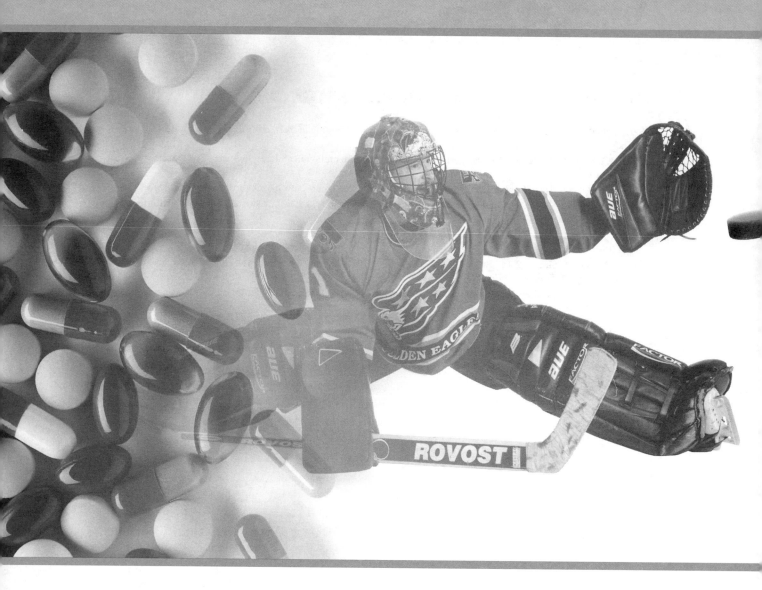

OBJECTIVES

After studying this chapter, you should be able to do the following:

- Describe various categories of nutrition supplements
- Discuss the nutrition supplements that have ergogenic properties
- Discuss the potential hazards and risks of nutrition supplements
- Understand critical analyses of research findings and reports and the importance of them

11

Nutrition Supplements

Key Terms

The use of nutrition supplements is a widespread and legitimate part of the strategy employed by many athletes in the pursuit of sporting success. The use of ergogenic aids or nutrition supplements is not new. As long ago as 500 to 400 BC, dietary fads were being used to enhance performance (Applegate et al. 1997). Many athletes today are still hopeful of finding a special beverage or pill that will improve performance.

Looking beyond genetic endowment and training, many athletes turn to ergogenic aids (Applegate 1999). Nutrition supplements by definition should be used to supplement the current diet, not substitute for it. For many modern athletes, however, sport nutrition has become synonymous with nutrition supplements. The ideas and expectations that athletes have about nutrition supplements are heavily influenced by the manufacturers and sellers of those supplements, who claim that their products increase muscle mass, improve stamina, and so on.

Weight loss and muscle gain are important concerns for many athletes as well as for people not involved in athletic training. Because achieving those goals is difficult with conventional methods (reducing energy intake and increasing energy expenditure through physical activity), these supplements sound attractive to many. Nutritional supplements are used by 40% to 100% of athletes in one form or another (Burke et al. 1993), and evidence suggests that athletes use several nutrition supplements at the same time and in extremely high doses. In this chapter we review the claims and the experimental evidence for a selection of common supplements. Because more than 800 nutrition supplements are now on the market (see the highlight box), we cannot review them all. Instead, we will focus on the most common ones.

Nonregulation of Nutrition Supplements

An abundance of information can be found in advertising and on the Internet about nutritional supplements. But most claims are not backed up by scientific studies, and many of them are unrealistic or even impossible. Claims are often based on studies in non-peer-reviewed journals or results from studies that are inappropriately extrapolated. The claims that manufacturers make about nutrition supplements are apparently difficult to regulate.

In contrast to prescription drugs, which are carefully regulated, nutrition supplements receive little governmental oversight, and retailers have enormous freedom in making marketing claims. For instance, the United States Food and Drug Administration (FDA) strictly regulates the clinical testing, advertising, and promotion of prescription drugs, which prevents retailers from making unproved claims. Nutrition supplements are

---

Common Nutritional Supplements

Acetylcholine	Coenzyme Q10	Pangamic acid*
Androstenedione	Conjugated linoleic acids	Phosphatidylserine
Arginine	Creatine (monohydrate)	Octacosanol
Bee pollen	Dessicated liver	Omega-3 fatty acids
Beta alanine	Ephedra	Royal jelly
Boron	Gamma oryzanol	Smilax
Branched-chain amino acids	Ginseng	Sodium bicarbonate
Caffeine	Glandulars	Sodium citrate
Carnitine	Glucosamine	Sodium phosphate
Carnosine	Glucose polymers	Spiruluna
Choline	Glutamine	Succinate
Chondroitin	Inosine	Vanadium
Citrulline	MCT	Wheat germ oil
Chromium picolinate		

* indicates not available for sale.

under no such regulation. Drugs are extensively tested for safety before they can be sold, but nutrition supplements are not tested. The Dietary Supplement Health and Education Act of 1994 created a new category of product called dietary supplements. These dietary supplements are treated as nutrition and are defined as "vitamins, minerals, herbs and botanicals, amino acids, and other dietary substances intended to supplement the diet by increasing the total dietary intake, or as any concentrate, metabolite, constituent or combination of these ingredients." Although manufacturers must submit information of new products (including the claims) to the FDA, this information is for notification rather than authorization (Ross 2000).

Critical Evaluation of Nutrition Supplements Studies

Athletes and others must critically examine claims made by the dietary supplements industry, including the "scientific evidence" that supports the claims. The following are some factors that should be considered when evaluating reports of scientific studies.

■ *Does the study have a clear hypothesis?* A well-designed study has a clear hypothesis and a strong theoretical basis for the expected outcome. Some studies, however, are designed with a "shotgun" approach. A supplement is given, and many variables are measured. The more variables that are examined, the greater the chance is that some of them will change. The application of study results should have a sound scientific rationale. For example, sodium bicarbonate may improve buffering capacity, which could result in improved 800 m running performance. But by no rationale can sodium bicarbonate be expected to improve Ironman triathlon performance, an event lasting 8 to 14 hours.

■ *Was the study on cells, muscle, animals, or humans?* Results are often extrapolated from findings in cell cultures. These in vitro experiments greatly help our understanding of metabolism and molecular interactions. But in vivo situations may be quite different. For instance, test tube samples are not exposed to hormonal changes that exist in living organisms. Also, muscle cells in the body may behave differently from isolated muscle cell preparations. Even if living animals are tested, the metabolism of animals may be significantly different from the metabolism of humans. Rats have relatively large stores of muscle glycogen and extremely small stores of intramuscular triacylglycerol compared with humans. High-fat diets in rats clearly improve exercise capacity (see chapter 7). But no evidence indicates that high-fat diets improve performance in humans. Thus, results from different types of studies cannot simply be extrapolated to the human athlete.

■ *Was the population for which claims are made comparable to the population in the study?* Coenzyme Q10 supplementation improves $\dot{V}O_2max$ and exercise capacity in cardiac patients but has no effect on $\dot{V}O_2max$ or exercise capacity in healthy individuals. Vanadium supplementation increases insulin sensitivity (reduces insulin resistance) in patients with type 2 diabetes but does not seem to be effective in healthy people with normal insulin sensitivity. These examples show how outcomes can differ in a target group that has different ages, sexes, body compositions, or fitness levels than the study group.

■ *Were external variables controlled?* In an ideal study, all variables and conditions are identical, so that the only difference between the trials is the treatment that each group receives. Then, all observed changes can be attributed with great certainty to the treatment. For example, if in examining the effect of caffeine on exercise performance, the environmental conditions were different in the caffeine and control trials, the observed effects might be related to environmental conditions as much as they are to caffeine.

■ *Was the study placebo controlled?* If subjects have prior knowledge or expectations with respect to a treatment or supplement, their performance could be affected. The proper choice of a placebo avoids this kind of performance bias. With some nutrition interventions, however, matching placebos are difficult to find. For example, branched-chain amino acids (BCAA) have an extremely bitter taste, and finding a placebo with a similar (horrible) taste is difficult. In this case, subjects may be aware of what they receive, possibly influencing the outcome.

■ *Were adequate techniques used?* Endurance capacity (time to exhaustion) has large day-to-day variability (Jeukendrup et al. 1996). Methods used to measure this variability may not detect small differences in performance. Similarly, some measures of body composition have a relatively large error and thus will not be able to detect small changes in fat or fat-free mass. If a treatment (supplement) is said to have no effect, perhaps the particular method used in the study was not sensitive enough to pick up small differences (Currell et al. 2008).

A small change in performance (<3%) that is undetectable in a laboratory setting may determine success or failure in a sports event (Currell et al. 2008; Hopkins 2000).

■ *Were the trials randomized?* Randomization reduces the confounding effects of variables that were not controlled or could not be controlled. When a small number of subjects are tested, a so-called counterbalanced design is preferred. If trials are randomized, eight subjects may end up in the treatment group in the first trial and only two in the control group. A counterbalanced design prevents this imbalance by appointing equal numbers of the control and treatment group to the first trial. Thus, half of the subjects will take the supplement first and the other half will take the placebo first. Failure to randomize treatments in a study may confound the outcome and hence make any conclusions untrustworthy.

■ *Was a crossover design used?* In a crossover study design the same subjects perform both the treatment trial and the placebo trial, allowing comparisons to be made within the same person. Although this type of study design can cause complications, particularly if a test substance that exerts effects in the body for a long time is given before the placebo, it is considered the ideal study design. Failure to use a crossover design may not necessarily affect the trustworthiness of the conclusions, but it is likely that variation between subjects in the measured variables will be greater than that within the same subjects. Hence, if a crossover design is not used, many more subjects will have to be studied to obtain the same degree of confidence that the conclusions are valid.

■ *Was the assignment random or was self-selection used?* If subjects are allowed to self-select their trial group, a significant bias may be introduced. For example, in a study of the effects of chromium on weight loss, subjects most motivated to lose weight would likely choose to be in the chromium group and not the placebo group.

■ *Do other studies confirm the findings?* If one study reports an ergogenic effect of a supplement, the claim may be true. But if several studies come to the same conclusion, the supplement most likely does have an ergogenic effect. The more studies that have been conducted, the larger the variety of subjects tested, and the more varied the dosages of the supplement used, the more generalizable the conclusion is.

■ *Was the study peer reviewed?* Papers sent for publication to peer-reviewed journals undergo a rigorous process whereby usually two or three referees, who are experts in the area, evaluate the paper based on specific criteria. Quality research withstands critical review and evaluation by colleagues. Articles published in popular magazines or on consumer-oriented Web sites do not undergo this extensive review process and are therefore often filled with errors and untruthful claims.

The most important supplements are discussed in this section. Table 11.1 contains a list of selected supplements, along with claims and scientific evidence for those claims. Supplements discussed in previous chapters, such as carbohydrate–electrolyte drinks (see chapter 6) and individual amino acids (see chapter 8) are not discussed.

Androstenedione

Androstenedione is one of the most popular nutrition supplements in the United States. It is believed to stimulate the endogenous synthesis of testosterone and thereby increase protein synthesis, build muscle mass, and improve recovery. Androstenedione was first developed in the former East Germany to enhance the performance of athletes. The regulations in the Dietary Supplement Health and Education Act of 1994 allow it to be sold as a food supplement, and it is available over the counter in almost any drug store or pharmacy in the United States.

If androstenedione functions as an anabolic steroid, it also has the side effects of an anabolic steroid, including acne, growth of facial and body hair, growth of the prostate, and impaired testicular function. The evidence that androstenedione has anabolic properties, however, is far from convincing. Although only a few studies have investigated the effects of androstenedione on serum testosterone concentrations and muscle strength, some conclusions can be drawn from them.

A study determined effects of short-term and long-term (8 weeks) oral androstenedione supplementation (300 mg/day) on serum testosterone and estrogen concentrations and skeletal muscle fiber size and strength in a group of people in a strength-training program (King et al. 1999). The group of 20 was randomly divided into a placebo group and an androstenedione group. No changes were observed in serum testosterone concentrations, but serum estradiol concentrations increased after androstenedione administration. Strength training resulted in increased strength, increased lean body mass, and increased cross-sectional area of type II muscle fibers after 8 weeks, but

■ TABLE 11.1 ■

Selected Nutrition Supplements, Product Claims, and Supporting Scientific Evidence

Ergogenic aids	Description	Claim	Scientific evidence
Androstenedione	Synthetic product to stimulate testosterone synthesis	Increases testosterone, increases muscle mass, and improves recovery	Does not increase testosterone; has no effect on strength
Bee pollen	Mixture of bee saliva, plant nectar, and pollen	Increases energy levels, enhances physical fitness, improves endurance, and boosts immune function	No supporting evidence
Beta-hydroxy beta methylbutyrate (HMB)	Metabolite of the essential amino acid leucine	Decreases protein breakdown, improves muscle mass, and increases strength	Possible small effects on lean body mass and strength
Boron	Trace element present in vegetables and noncitrus fruits	Improves bone density, muscle mass, and strength	Improves bone mineral density in postmenopausal women; no effect on bone density, muscle mass, or strength in men
Caffeine	Substance in coffee and chocolate	Increases performance and alertness	Improves performance in most events, except short high-intensity exercise; increases cognitive functioning during exercise
Carnitine	Vitamin-like substance important for FA transport	Improves fat oxidation, helps weight loss, and improves $\dot{V}O_2max$	Not taken up by muscle and therefore not effective
Choline	Precursor of the neurotransmitter acetylcholine	Improves performance and decreases fatigue	No supporting evidence
Chromium picolinate	Trace element that potentiates insulin action	Builds muscle and helps weight loss	No supporting evidence
Coenzyme Q10	Part of the electron-transport chain in the mitochondria	Improves $\dot{V}O_2max$, improves performance, reduces fatigue	No supporting evidence
Creatine	High-energy phosphate carrier important for direct energy	Improves strength, reduces fatigue, and increases protein synthesis	Improves performance in single and repeated sprint bouts; improves recovery between bouts; anabolic properties unclear
DHEA	A precursor of testosterone and estradiol	Improves immune function, increases lifespan, protects against cardiovascular diseases, increases lean body mass, and increases well-being	Some evidence in humans
Dihydroxyacetone	An intermediate of carbohydrate metabolism used in combination with pyruvate	Facilitates carbohydrate and fat metabolism and improves performance	Limited supporting evidence
Fish oil	Polyunsaturated fatty acids	Increases $\dot{V}O_2max$	No supporting evidence

(continued) ▶

Ergogenic aids	Description	Claim	Scientific evidence
Ginseng	Root of the *Araliaceous* plant	Improves strength, performance, stamina, and cognitive functioning; reduces fatigue	No supporting evidence, but studies poorly designed
Glutamine	An amino acid	Improves immune function, muscle glycogen resynthesis, recovery, and endurance	Does not affect immune function; possibly affects muscle glycogen resynthesis
Glandulars	Extracts of animal glands	Improves strength, performance, and stamina	No supporting evidence
Glycerol	Backbone of a triacylglycerol molecule	Induces hyperhydration, decreases heat stress, and improves performance	Induces hyperhydration and decreases heat stress during exercise; effects on performance unclear
Inosine	Nucleoside	Increases ATP stores, improves strength, training quality, and performance	No supporting evidence
Lecithin	Phosphatidylcholine	Increases $\dot{V}O_2$max and performance	No supporting evidence
Medium-chain triacylglycerols (MCT)	Synthesized from coconut oil	Supplies energy, reduces muscle glycogen breakdown, and improves performance	No supporting evidence
Pangamic acid (vitamin B_{15})	Varied composition depending on supplier	Increases oxygen delivery	No supporting evidence
Phosphate salts	Mineral	Increases ATP, provides energy, and buffers lactic acid	Possible ergogenic effects; improves performance in events 1 hour or shorter
Phosphatidylserine	Structural component of cell membranes	Reduces stress responses and improves recovery	Little supporting evidence
Polylactate	Polymer of lactate	Provides energy	No effects on performance
Pyruvate	An intermediate of carbohydrate metabolism	Improves endurance capacity, insulin sensitivity, and recovery; increases glycogen storage	Limited supporting evidence
Sodium bicarbonate	Buffer present in blood	Buffers lactic acid and improves high-intensity exercise performance	Improves high-intensity exercise performance
Sodium citrate	Buffer	Buffers lactic acid and improves high-intensity exercise performance	Can improve performance with larger doses
Vanadium	Trace element	Helps weight loss; improves insulin sensitivity and recovery	Increases insulin sensitivity in patients with insulin resistance; studies in healthy individuals lacking
Yohimbine	α_2-adrenoceptor blocker	Increases testosterone, increases fat-free mass, and improves strength	No supporting evidence
Wheat germ oil	Extracted from embryo of wheat	Improves endurance	No supporting evidence

the androstenedione group and the placebo group showed no differences. A lack of effect on serum testosterone concentrations was also reported by three other studies in which 100 to 200 mg/day were ingested for 2 days to 12 weeks (Ballantyne et al. 2000; Rasmussen et al. 2000; Wallace et al. 1999). Rasmussen et al. (2000) did not find effects on protein synthesis and breakdown or phenylalanine balance across the leg. Therefore, the conclusions that androstenedione has no effect on the plasma testosterone concentration, does not change protein metabolism, has no anabolic effect, and does not alter the adaptations to resistance training seem appropriate.

On the other hand, androstenedione may have negative health effects. A study reported a decrease in serum HDL cholesterol, a lack of which has been associated with increased risk of cardiovascular disease. Ethical issues are also involved. Androstenedione is a substance banned by the International Olympic Committee (IOC), and athletes have been disqualified and banned from their sport for using it.

Bee Pollen

Pollen is a fine, powdery substance produced by the anthers of seed-bearing plants. Bees collect it from the plants and store it in their hives. It has a rich mixture of vitamins, minerals, and amino acids and is therefore believed to be healthy, even more so because it is a natural product as opposed to some of the multivitamin and mineral supplements. Pollen is often referred to as the perfect food or complete food, and manufacturers claim that it improves endurance, reduces free-radical damage, aids in weight control, increases longevity, and prevents asthma. But no reliable information exists to prove its effectiveness as an ergogenic aid. Based on the available information on supplementation with vitamins, minerals, and amino acids (see chapters 10 and 8), ergogenic effects would not be expected. One study (Chandler et al. 1984) in which the effect of bee pollen supplementation was investigated showed no influence on maximal oxygen uptake, exercise performance, or metabolism. Bee pollen can be harmful for people who are allergic to specific pollens.

Beta Alanine and Carnosine

For sports in which glycolysis is simulated and lactic acid production is high (for example, middle-distance running), β-alanine has been suggested to be an effective supplement. During intense exercise the increased hydrogen ion (H^+) concentration is buffered by intra- and extramuscular buffering mechanisms. Sodium bicarbonate ($NaHCO_3$) is an example of extracellular buffering and will be discussed later in this chapter. Carnosine or β-alanyl-L-histidine is one of the most important intracellular buffers. Carnosine is synthesized from its precursors L-histidine and β-alanine. It is present in relatively high concentrations in skeletal muscle (5–10 mM) and is thought to be responsible for approximately 10% of the total buffering capacity of the m. vastus lateralis. Carnosine ingestion is not effective in increasing intramuscular carnosine concentration because it is broken down in the gastrointestinal tract and absorption of carnosine is poor. But recent evidence suggests that β-alanine supplementation may lead to an increase in muscle carnosine contents, which can result in enhanced intramuscular H^+ buffering. This could lead to an increase in high-intensity exercise performance.

Dosing protocols include taking a single daily dose of 3.2 g β-alanine, or up to eight daily doses of 0.4 to 1.6 g β-alanine per single dose, to reach a total daily ingestion of 3.2 to 6.4 g per day over a range of 4 to 10 weeks, which results in a 60 to 80% increase in muscle carnosine contents (Harris et al. 2006; Hill et al. 2007). It has been documented that large acute doses of β-alanine appear to induce mild pseudoallergic skin reactions of paraesthesia (mild flushing and tingling sensations) that appear to dissipate within about 2 hours. For that reason the daily dose is usually administered as four to eight small doses. Despite the relatively consistent findings that β-alanine supplementation leads to an increase in muscle carnosine, evidence for subsequent performance effects have been less clear cut. A study demonstrated that 4.8 g of β-alanine per day for 4 weeks in trained 400 m runners improved fatigue resistance in repeated bouts of exhaustive dynamic contractions. But isometric endurance and 400 m race time were not affected (Derave et al. 2007). In another study sprint performance was enhanced at the end of a simulated cycling race (Van Thienen et al. 2009).

Most studies that have used an exercise protocol in which acidosis was the primary cause of fatigue have demonstrated significant positive performance effects. Nevertheless, additional well-controlled studies need to be completed to elucidate the mechanism of action, definitive dosing tolerance and protocols, subject specificity, and effects on performance in a range of varying exercise interventions and intensities.

Beta-Hydroxy Beta Methylbutyrate

Beta-hydroxy beta methylbutyrate (HMB) is a metabolite of the essential amino acid leucine (see figure 11.1) and is synthesized in the body at an estimated rate of about 0.2 to 0.4 g/day (Nissen et al. 1996). Its use as a supplement has increased dramatically in the past few years, especially among bodybuilders, and it has become one of the most popular supplements. HMB is claimed to increase lean body mass and strength, improve recovery, improve immune function, reduce blood cholesterol, protect against stress, and reduce body fat.

The first studies of HMB were performed in rats, and the studies demonstrated that supplementing the amino acid leucine can be anticatabolic, possibly through the actions of its metabolite HMB. Later studies investigated HMB as a potential anticatabolic agent in farm animals. No effect of HMB supplementation on protein metabolism was observed in growing lambs (Papet et al. 1997). Subsequently, HMB was hypothesized to reduce protein breakdown in humans, resulting in increased muscle mass and strength. In addition, subjects given HMB supplements were believed to have a decreased stress-induced muscle glycogen breakdown. HMB thus was claimed to benefit both strength and endurance athletes.

Information about the effects of HMB in humans is scarce. Nissen et al. (1996) studied 41 untrained male volunteers who participated in a resistance-training program for 3 weeks. The program consisted of three 90-minute weightlifting sessions a week. Participants were divided into three groups, and each group received a different dose of HMB. The first group received placebo, the second group received 1.5 g/day of HMB, and the third group received 3.0 g/day of HMB. Lean tissue (determined by total-body electrical conductance, a technique with a similar principle as bioelectrical impedance analysis [BIA]) tended to increase more in the HMB groups, and this occurred in a dose-dependent matter (see figure 11.2). Total upper-body and lower-body strength also increased more in the group with the higher dose of HMB (see figure 11.3).

The group that had the largest increase in lean body mass (3.0 g/

day of HMB) was also the group with the lowest lean body mass and muscle strength to begin with. Therefore, this group would be expected to gain more than the placebo group, who already had a larger lean body mass. Also, this study had no diet control, so the leucine intake is not known.

In part 2 of the study by Nissen et al. (1996), subjects trained for 7 weeks, 6 days a week, and were given 3.0 g/day of HMB or placebo. This study showed an increase in fat-free mass in the HMB group after 14 days, but after 39 days, no

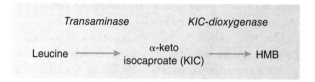

Figure 11.1 Synthesis of HMB from the amino acid leucine.

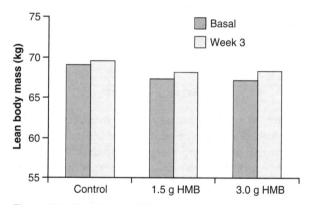

Figure 11.2 The effect of HMB supplementation on body composition.

Data from S. Nissen, 1996, "Effect of Leucine Metabolite Beta-Hydroxy-Beta-Methylbutyrate on muscle metabolism during resistance-exercise training," *Journal of Applied Physiology* 81(5): 2095-2104. Used with permission.

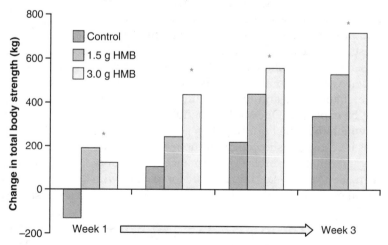

Figure 11.3 Change in body strength (total upper-body and lower-body strength) with placebo or HMB. * = indicates significant linear effect of HMB supplementation.

Data from S. Nissen, 1996, "Effect of Leucine Metabolite Beta-Hydroxy-Beta-Methylbutyrate on muscle metabolism during resistance-exercise training," *Journal of Applied Physiology* 81(5): 2095-2104. Used with permission.

differences were observed. Strength was also measured in this second study, but no differences were found in the strength measurements except for bench press. A small improvement in bench press strength occurred with HMB supplementation (2.6 kg after 7 weeks of training with HMB versus 1.1 kg with placebo). A point of criticism again is that the diet was not controlled. Since then, a number of studies have provided mixed results. Some have found an increase in lean body mass or muscle strength (Jowko et al. 2001; Nissen et al. 2000; Panton et al. 2000), whereas others have found no effect on body composition and strength (Slater et al. 2001) or signs of muscle damage after eccentric exercise (Paddon-Jones et al. 2001). In a meta-analysis, HMB was found to increase net lean mass gains by 0.28% per week and strength gains by 1.4% per week (Nissen et al. 2002). More recently it has also been suggested that HMB can increase aerobic exercise performance, although not all studies have found such improvements.

Nissen et al. (2000) collected data in nine studies ranging from 3 to 8 weeks in duration. No negative effects of 3.0 g/day of HMB were noted on organ and tissue function, emotional perception, or gastrointestinal tolerance. The authors concluded that 3.0 g/day is a safe dose. Some evidence suggests that HMB can result in increased lean body mass and muscle strength. A number of studies now show that HMB has several positive effects, but an equal number show no effect of HMB. There is now compelling evidence in clinical muscle wasting conditions that HMB can be beneficial, and some evidence for a potential mechanism is also starting to emerge. HMB seems to reduce the breakdown of protein through inhibiting proteolytic pathways and to stimulate protein synthesis through stimulation of the transcription factor mammalian target of rapamycin (mTOR) (see chapter 12). For a complete review of the effects of HMB on performance and body composition and a discussion of potential mechanisms, see the review by Wilson and colleagues (Wilson et al. 2008).

From a practical point of view, potential users should keep in mind that most of the studies have used 3 g/day (3 × 1 g/day) of HMB, whereas most recovery products currently on the market contain extremely small amounts of HMB.

Boron

The trace element boron influences calcium and magnesium metabolism (Volpe et al. 1993), steroid hormone metabolism, and membrane function. It is present in noncitrus fruits, leafy vegetables, nuts, and legumes. Although no RDA has been established for boron, the recommended daily intake is often 1 mg/day (Nielsen 1996). For humans, boron is not an essential trace element.

Boron has been studied in relation to osteoporosis. One of these studies found that boron supplementation for 48 days increased the serum estrogen and testosterone levels of postmenopausal women. It also reduced calcium, phosphorus, and magnesium excretion in urine and is therefore suggested to contribute to improved bone mineral density (Nielsen et al. 1987).

The finding that boron increased testosterone levels in postmenopausal women has been extrapolated to the claim that it may improve muscle growth and strength in strength athletes. The women in this study, however, had been deprived of boron for 4 months. Continued supplementation did not further elevate testosterone levels, and boron supplementation in men did not affect testosterone levels at all. Another placebo-controlled study investigated the effects of boron supplementation (2.5 mg/day of boron for 7 weeks) on serum testosterone, lean body mass, and strength in bodybuilders. Besides elevated plasma boron levels, no effect was found (Green et al. 1994). Therefore, although interactions are shown between boron and calcium and magnesium metabolism (Volpe et al. 1993), boron does not appear to be an ergogenic aid.

Caffeine

The use of caffeine dates back to Paleolithic times. The raw fruit of the coffee plant (Coffea arabica) was used to brew a drink with stimulant properties. This strongly caffeinated beverage was later replaced by a beverage prepared from roasted coffee beans. Caffeine originates naturally in 63 species of plants as several types of methylated xanthines. Caffeine and caffeinelike substances can be found in a variety of foods and drinks, but the main sources for these substances are coffee beans, tea leaves, cocoa beans, and cola nuts (see figure 11.4. and table 11.2). Coffee accounts for 75% of all caffeine consumption.

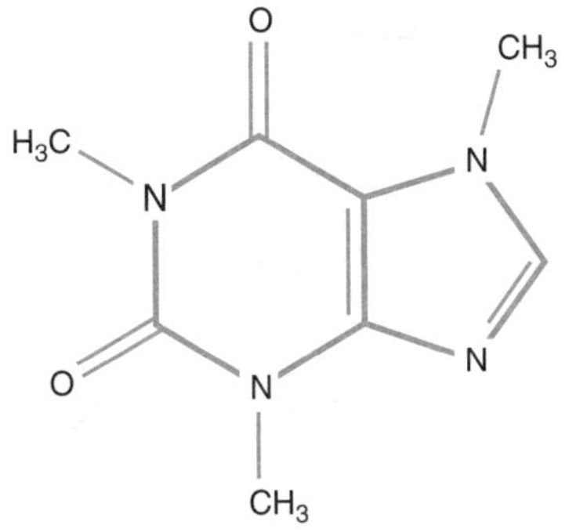

Figure 11.4 Chemical structure of caffeine and caffeine-like compounds.

Caffeine Content in Food, Beverages, and Medications

Item	Caffeine content (mg)	Item	Caffeine content (mg)
COFFEE		**PAIN RELIEVERS (PER TABLET)**	
Drip method 150 ml (5 oz)	110–150	Anacin	32
Percolated 150 ml (5 oz)	64–124	Excedrin	65
Instant 150 ml (5 oz)	40–108	Midol	32
Decaffeinated 150 ml (5 oz)	2–5	Plain aspirin	0
Starbucks grande 480 ml (16 oz)	550	Vanquish	33
Starbucks tall 360 ml (12 oz)	375	**DIURETICS**	
Starbucks short 240 ml (8 oz)	250	Aqua Ban	200
Starbucks tall latte 360 ml (12 oz)	70	Pre-Mens Forte	100
TEA		**COLD REMEDIES**	
1 min brew 150 ml (5 oz)	9–33	Coryban-D	30
3 min brew 150 ml (5 oz)	20–46	Dristan	0
5 min brew 150 ml (5 oz)	20–50	Triaminicin	30
Instant tea 150 ml (5 oz)	12–28	**WEIGHT-CONTROL AIDS**	
Iced tea 360 ml (12 oz)	22–36	Dexatrim	200
CHOCOLATE		Prolamine	140
Made from mix	6	**STIMULANTS**	
Milk chocolate (1 oz, or 30 g)	6	Pro-Plus	50
Baking chocolate	35	NoDoz	100
Chocolate bar (100 g)	12–15	**PRESCRIPTION PAIN RELIEVERS**	
SOFT DRINKS (CAN)		Cafergot	100
Mountain Dew	55	Davron compound	32
Mello Yello	52	Fiorinal	40
Coca-Cola	46	Migramal	1
Diet Coke	46		
Pepsi Cola	38		
Diet Pepsi	36		
Dr. Pepper	40		
Red Bull 250 ml (8.3 oz)	80		

Caffeine is readily absorbed after ingestion. Blood levels rise and peak after approximately 60 minutes. The half-life is reported to be between 2 and 10 hours. Caffeine is primarily degraded in the liver, and the resulting single methyl group xanthines and methyluric acids are eliminated in urine. About 0.5% to 3.5% of ingested caffeine is excreted unchanged in urine. A study showed that significant amounts of caffeine are also excreted through sweat (Kovacs et al. 1998). Caffeine remains the most widely consumed drug in Europe and America (Curatolo et al. 1983), and athletes have long used it in the belief that it improves performance. On January 1, 2004, the International Olympic Committee (IOC) took caffeine off its list of banned substances. Before January 2004, caffeine was one of the few compounds for which the IOC had set a tolerance limit. This limit was defined at a caffeine concentration in urine of 12 μg/ml. Because caffeine is a substance that can influence exercise performance, its use is a question of sports ethics.

Here we will briefly summarize the evidence that caffeine is an ergogenic aid and explain some of the proposed mechanisms. For further readings and details on caffeine metabolism and the ergogenic effects of caffeine, see Armstrong (2002), Graham et al. (1994), Spriet (1995), and Doherty and Smith (Doherty et al. 2004, 2005).

Endurance Exercise

In the late 1970s it was observed that caffeine ingested 1 hour before the start of an exercise bout increased plasma FA concentration and improved performance (Costill et al. 1977; Essig et al. 1980; Ivy et al. 1979).

Although not all studies show effects of caffeine on endurance performance, a large number of well-conducted studies have shown improved endurance capacity after ingesting caffeine at a dose of 3 to 9 mg/kg b.w. (Costill et al. 1978; Graham et al. 1991; Pasman et al. 1995; Spriet et al. 1992). More recently, studies have used smaller doses of caffeine (as little as 1–3.2 mg/kg b.w.) and still observed positive effects on performance (Cox et al. 2002; Kovacs et al. 1998) (see also the section on caffeine dosage).

At exercise intensities of about 85% of $\dot{V}O_2$max, improvements of 10% to 20% in time to exhaustion are typically found. A meta-analysis of published studies on caffeine and exercise performance (Doherty et al. 2005) suggested that the magnitude of the performance-enhancing effect increases as the duration of exercise increases. In most of these

studies, caffeine also decreased perceived ratings of exertion.

The improvement in performance was originally explained by the increased availability of plasma FAs, which supposedly resulted in a suppression of carbohydrate metabolism and consequently to a decrease in glycogen utilization. But a number of studies did see performance improvements without changes in the rate of fat oxidation, and it is highly unlikely that this mechanism is behind the observed effects. It has become clear in recent years that the effects of caffeine are due to its stimulant properties.

A given exercise thus feels easier with caffeine. The fact that not all studies found that caffeine has a performance-enhancing effect might be related to various factors, including the dosage of caffeine, the fitness level of the subjects, habitual caffeine consumption, and, perhaps most important, the type and duration of exercise.

Maximal Exercise

A few studies investigated the effects of caffeine ingestion on high-intensity exercise (about 100% of $\dot{V}O_2$max and lasting 3 to 8 minutes). Some, but not all, studies (Falk et al. 1989; Sasaki et al. 1987) demonstrated a positive effect of caffeine on exercise performance at these high intensities. Jackman et al. (1996) found that ingestion of 6 mg/kg b.w. of caffeine increased time to exhaustion at 100% of $\dot{V}O_2$max. Muscle glycogen concentrations, however, were still relatively high at exhaustion. Therefore, the authors concluded that the mechanism was not through glycogen sparing. Caffeine (150 to 200 mg) also improved 1,500 m time in well-trained runners (4:46.0 versus 4:50.2) (Wiles et al. 1992).

Generally, caffeine seems to improve performance during exercise near 100% of $\dot{V}O_2$max and lasting approximately 5 minutes. The mechanism for this improvement is unknown but has been suggested to be an effect of caffeine on the neuromuscular pathways that facilitate recruitment of muscle fibers or increase the number of fibers recruited. In addition, caffeine possibly has direct effects on muscle ion handling or enhanced anaerobic energy production or an effect on the brain that decreases sensations of effort (Spriet 1995).

Supramaximal Exercise

The effects of caffeine on short-term supramaximal exercise performance are uncertain. Williams et al. (1988) reported no effect on power output or muscular endurance during 15-second sprints after caffeine ingestion. Similar findings were reported by Collomp et al. (1991), who found that ingestion of 5 mg/kg b.w. of caffeine did not affect 30-second Wingate test performance. A study investigated the effects of caffeine ingestion on repeated Wingate exercise tests (Greer et al. 1998) and found that caffeine had no effect on the first two Wingate tests but that it decreased power output during the third and fourth tests. Caffeine, therefore, seems to have no positive effect on sprint performance. Given the limited number of studies, however, this conclusion is not definitive.

Cognitive Functioning

Caffeine has an effect on cognitive functioning. In a study by Hogervorst et al. (1999), caffeine was added to a carbohydrate–electrolyte drink, which was consumed before and during exercise. Cognitive functioning (attention, psychomotor skills, and memory) was measured immediately after a time trial (approximately 1 hour of all-out exercise). Caffeine improved all measures of cognitive functioning, and these effects were evident for the ingestion of 2 mg/kg b.w. and 3 mg/kg b.w. of caffeine. More recently, the effects of caffeine (100 mg) in an energy bar (45 g CHO) were investigated. The energy bar was ingested immediately before and after 55 and 115 minutes of exercise, which was 2.5 hours of cycling at 60% of $\dot{V}O_2$max followed by a time to exhaustion test at 75% of $\dot{V}O_2$max. The researchers found not only that time to exhaustion was extended but also that concentration, response speed and detection, and performance of complex cognitive tasks improved during and after exercise when an energy bar with caffeine was ingested. The energy bar with caffeine resulted in better cognitive function compared with an energy bar without caffeine and a control trial in which no carbohydrate or caffeine was ingested (Hogervorst et al. 2008).

Dosage

A few studies have investigated the effects of various dosages of caffeine on exercise performance (or endurance capacity). In a study by Pasman et al. (1995) cyclists received three different dosages of caffeine or placebo 1 hour before a ride to exhaustion at about 80% of $\dot{V}O_2$max. The dosages were 0, 5, 9, and 13 mg/kg b.w. With the lowest dose (5 mg/kg b.w.), endurance capacity improved by 20%, but an increase in dosage had no further effect on performance (see figure 11.5). In runners, ingestion of 3 mg/kg b.w. and 6 mg/kg b.w. of caffeine had

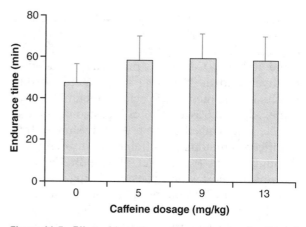

Figure 11.5 Effect of ingesting various amounts of caffeine 1 hour preexercise on time to exhaustion at about 80% of $\dot{V}O_2$max.
Data from Pasman et al. 1995.

positive effects, whereas the improvement in time to exhaustion with 9 mg/kg b.w. of caffeine did not reach statistical significance (Graham et al. 1995).

In a study by Cox et al. (2002) small amounts of caffeine (1–2 mg/kg b.w.) resulted in significant performance improvements in a time trial at the end of 2 hours of cycling. Kovacs et al. (1998) studied the effect of adding relatively small amounts of caffeine (2, 3, or 4.5 mg/kg b.w.) to a carbohydrate–electrolyte solution during prolonged exercise. Time-trial cycling performance improved with the lowest dosage of 2 mg/kg b.w. and improved more with 3 mg/kg b.w., but a higher dose did not further affect performance. These results suggest that a caffeine intake of 3 mg/kg b.w. exerts an ergogenic effect but that higher intakes will produce increased benefit.

Habitual Users

Studies have tried to address the question of whether habitual consumers of caffeine have an altered response during exercise. Although habitual caffeine users may have markedly different metabolic responses to caffeine (e.g., blunted FA response and blunted catecholamine excretion) (Dodd et al. 1991; Van Soeren et al. 1993), no studies show that changes in performance are different.

Withdrawal from caffeine for 2 to 4 days had no effect on the observed performance effect of caffeine (Van Soeren et al. 1998). Although caffeine (6 mg/kg b.w.) improved performance compared with placebo, performance did not change after 2 or 4 days of withdrawal. This study also suggested that the mechanisms by which caffeine work are not related to availability of substrate or catecholamines. No evidence suggests that habitual caffeine intake or withdrawal influences the performance effects of caffeine.

Carbohydrate Absorption

It was suggested that caffeine may also improve the absorption of carbohydrate. Van Nieuwenhoven et al. (2000) reported that caffeine (1.4 mg/kg b.w.) coingested with glucose (0.5 g/min) during 90 minutes of cycling produced higher rates of intestinal glucose absorption compared with glucose. Because absorption appears to be the rate-limiting step for exogenous carbohydrate delivery to the muscle, it was suggested that caffeine may increase exogenous carbohydrate oxidation (Yeo et al. 2005). In a study at the University of Birmingham (United Kingdom) it was shown that combined ingestion of caffeine (10 mg/kg b.w.) and glucose (0.8 g/min) resulted in 26% higher rates of exogenous carbohydrate oxidation compared with glucose (0.8 g/min). Possibly, however, this effect may be present only when a high dose of caffeine is given or when carbohydrate intake is relatively high. In a follow-up study the coingestion of caffeine (5.3 mg/kg b.w.) with carbohydrate (0.7 g/min) during exercise enhanced time-trial performance by 4.6% compared with carbohydrate and 9.0% compared with a water placebo. In this study, however, caffeine did not influence exogenous carbohydrate oxidation during exercise. So although some evidence indicates that caffeine may help carbohydrate absorption and exogenous carbohydrate oxidation, the optimal carbohydrate and caffeine intake needed to achieve this effect is uncertain.

Mechanisms of Action

Several theories of how caffeine could exert its effects have been proposed (see the highlight box). The precise mechanisms behind the ergogenic effect of caffeine are still unclear but are unlikely to be related to changes in metabolism (increased fat metabolism and decreased muscle glycogen breakdown). The most likely explanation seems to be changes in central drive, in muscle fiber recruitment, and in perceived exertion caused by central nervous system effects of caffeine.

The following are some of the mechanisms that have been suggested:

■ The traditional hypothesis for the ergogenic effect of caffeine is that caffeine stimulates lipolysis, increases fat oxidation, and thereby spares muscle glycogen, which is generally believed to improve endurance performance. Caffeine indeed stimulates lipolysis and the mobilization of FAs.

These actions might occur indirectly by increasing the circulating epinephrine levels or directly by antagonizing adenosine receptors that normally inhibit hormone-sensitive lipase and FA oxidation.

■ Another possible mechanism is a direct effect of caffeine or one of its metabolites on skeletal muscle. Possibilities include the handling of ions, inhibition of phosphodiesterase leading to an increased concentration of 3',5'-cyclic adenosine monophosphate (cAMP), and the direct effect on key regulatory enzymes such as phosphorylase. Most of these hypotheses are derived from in vitro studies in which unphysiologically high concentrations of caffeine were used, and whether similar effects would have been found with realistic physiological concentrations is unclear.

■ A third possibility, which is used to explain some of the suggested influences of caffeine on high-intensity exercise, is an increased influx of calcium from the extracellular space, increased release of calcium from the sarcoplasmic reticulum, and increased sensitivity of the myofilament to calcium, all resulting in increased excitability of the muscle fibers.

■ A fourth possible mechanism is the stimulating effect of caffeine on the central nervous system, which affects the perception of effort or affects the signal transduction from the brain to the neuromuscular junction. The cellular actions responsible for this central nervous system activation are not clear but may be related to catecholamine release and, more likely, to the release of neurotransmitters.

Caffeine Versus Coffee

Coffee accounts for 75% of all caffeine consumption. Of course, the quantity of caffeine in coffee depends on the strength and the type of bean. Robusta coffee, for example, contains about 40 to 50% more caffeine than Arabica. The caffeine content in coffee is highly variable and depends not only on the type of bean but also on the method of preparation as well as other factors. Filter coffee generally has higher caffeine content than espresso. Whatever the type of coffee bean or method of preparation, intuitively we would expect that coffee would have the same effect as caffeine if the caffeine content is comparable. Studies suggest, however, that this may not be the case. A few studies have compared coffee with an equivalent dose of caffeine alone, and one study compared decaffeinated coffee with or without added caffeine. Although some of these studies

---

Suggested Mechanisms by Which Caffeine Exerts Its Ergogenic Effect

Caffeine increases lipolysis and spares muscle glycogen.

1. Caffeine increases circulating epinephrine levels, which stimulates lipolysis.
2. Caffeine antagonizes adenosine receptors that normally inhibit hormone-sensitive lipase and FA oxidation (only shown *in vitro*).
3. Caffeine inhibits phosphodiesterase leading to an increased concentration of 3',5'-cyclic monophosphate (cAMP) (only shown *in vitro*).

Caffeine increases excitability of the muscle fibers.

1. Caffeine has a direct effect on key regulatory enzymes such as phosphorylase.
2. Caffeine increases influx of calcium from the extracellular space.
3. Caffeine increases release of calcium from the sarcoplasmic reticulum.
4. Caffeine increases the sensitivity of the myofilaments to calcium.

Caffeine influences signal transduction from the brain to the motor neuron.

1. Caffeine stimulates catecholamine release and the release of neurotransmitters (dopamine, β-endorphins), possibly resulting in decreased perception of effort.
2. Caffeine may lower the excitation threshold for motor neuron recruitment.
3. Caffeine alters excitation/contraction coupling.
4. Caffeine increases ion transport within the muscle.
5. Caffeine facilitates transmission of nervous signals.

---

reported performance benefits, some studies did not. Graham and coworkers (Graham et al. 1998) found that caffeine in coffee was less potent than caffeine given in a capsule. The differences in performance occurred despite similar plasma caffeine concentrations, and the authors therefore concluded that another component in coffee may reduce the effect of caffeine. But when McLellan and Bell (McLellan et al. 2004) gave coffee before the ingestion of a capsule of caffeine, the coffee did not seem to dampen the effect of a relatively large caffeine dose. A reasonable conclusion is that more research is needed to study whether coffee can be an ergogenic aid.

Side Effects

Caffeine use has side effects. People who normally avoid caffeine may experience gastrointestinal distress, headaches, tachycardia, restlessness, irritability, tremor, elevated blood pressure, psychomotor agitations, and premature left ventricular contractions with intake of caffeine, all caused by the effect of caffeine on the central nervous system. It is often stated that caffeine is a diuretic and therefore should not be consumed in the hours before exercise when hydration is required. Studies, however, have demonstrated that moderate intake of caffeine does not affect urine loss or hydration status (Armstrong 2002; Armstrong et al. 2005). Furthermore, during exercise, the potential diuretic effect of caffeine is counteracted by catecholamines (Wemple et al. 1997), causing constriction of renal arterioles and reducing glomerular filtration rates. The catecholamines possibly increase sodium and chloride reabsorption rates in the proximal and distal tubules by affecting aldosterone, an antidiuretic hormone, resulting in greater water retention. Caffeine has no effect on sweat rates. Thus, caffeine taken in moderate amounts may not have a diuretic effect. Extremely high intakes of caffeine have been associated with peptic ulcer, seizure, coma, and even death.

L-Carnitine

L-carnitine (carnitine), a substance present in relatively high quantities in meat (the Latin word *caro-carnis* means meat or muscle), has received much attention over the past 20 years. As a supplement, it has been popular among athletes, and it has been the focus of many studies. Carnitine became especially popular after rumors circulated that it helped the Italian national soccer team to become world champions in 1982.

Carnitine supplementation is said to increase $\dot{V}O_2$max and reduce lactate production during maximal and supramaximal exercise. But the most important claim is that carnitine improves fat metabolism, reduces fat mass, and increases muscle mass. It is generally advertised as a "fat burner." Therefore, carnitine is often used to lose weight, reduce body fat, and improve "sharpness." Endurance athletes use carnitine to increase the oxidation of fat and spare muscle glycogen.

In the Body

L-carnitine is derived from red meats and dairy products in the diet (see table 11.3) and from endogenous production in the body. Even when dietary sources are insufficient, healthy humans produce enough from methionine and lysine to maintain functional body stores. For this reason, carnitine is not regarded as a vitamin, but as a vitamin-like substance.

Carnitine is synthesized in the liver and kidney, which together contain only 1.6% of the whole-body carnitine store (about 27 g). About 98% of the carnitine of the human body is present in skeletal and heart muscle. Skeletal muscle and the heart depend on transport of carnitine through the circulation, which contains about 0.5 % of whole-body carnitine.

Muscle takes carnitine up against a very large (about 1000-fold) concentration gradient (plasma carnitine is 40 to 60 µmol/L, and muscle carnitine is 4 to 5 mmol/L) by a saturable active transport process (see figure 11.6). Carnitine is an end product of human metabolism and is only lost from the body by excretion in urine and stool. Daily losses are minimal (< 60 mg/day) and are reduced to less than 20 mg/day on meat-free and carnitine-free diets (Bremer 1983). These minimal losses imply that the rate of endogenous biosynthesis, which is needed to maintain functional body stores, is also only about 20 mg/day. The amounts lost in stool can usually be ignored except after ingestion of oral supplements.

Fat Metabolism

L-carnitine plays an important role in fat metabolism. In the overnight fasted state and during exercise of low to moderate intensity, long-chain FAs are the main energy sources used by most tissues, including skeletal muscle. The primary function of L-carnitine is to transport long-chain FAs across the mitochondrial inner membrane, because the inner membrane is impermeable to both long-chain FAs and fatty acyl-CoA esters (Bremer 1983) (see figure 7.6, p. 155). Once inside the mitochondria, FAs can be degraded to acetyl-CoA through β-oxidation. The acetyl-CoA units will then be available for the TCA cycle to provide energy.

Carnitine plays an important role in maintaining the acetyl-CoA:CoA ratio in the cell. During high-intensity exercise a large production of acetyl-CoA occurs, resulting in an increased acetyl-CoA:CoA ratio. This increased ratio, in turn, inhibits the pyruvate dehydrogenase (PDH) complex and reduces flux through the PDH complex and hence acetyl-CoA formation, resulting in increased lactate formation. Therefore, the acetyl-CoA:CoA ratio should be maintained. Acetyl-CoA reacts with free carnitine to form acetyl-carnitine and CoA.

$$\text{acetyl-CoA} + \text{carnitine} \rightarrow \text{acetyl-carnitine} + \text{CoA}$$

■ TABLE 11.3 ■
Sources of Dietary Carnitine

Source	Total L-carnitine content (mg/100g)
Sheep	210
Lamb	78
Beef	64
Pork	30
Rabbit	21
Chicken	7.5
Milk	2.0
Egg	0.8
Peanut	0.1

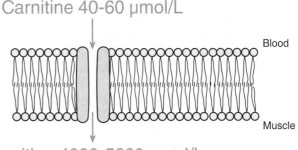

Figure 11.6 Transport of carnitine into the muscle sarcoplasm occurs against a large concentration gradient.

In theory, carnitine therefore acts as a sink for excess acetyl-CoA and blunts the accumulation of lactic acid, thereby enhancing high-intensity exercise performance.

Slimming Agent

The belief that carnitine is a slimming agent is based on the assumption that regular oral ingestion of carnitine increases the muscle carnitine concentration. Another assumption is that if carnitine concentration in the muscle increases, fat oxidation also increases, thus leading to a gradual loss of body fat stores. Several carefully conducted studies (Barnett et al. 1994; Vukovich et al. 1994; Wachter et al. 2002), however, showed that oral carnitine ingestion (daily ingestion for up to 3 months) does not change the muscle carnitine concentration. Even infusion of L-carnitine for 5 hours did not increase muscle carnitine concentration. Therefore, it seems that the reason that carnitine is unable to increase muscle carnitine concentration is partly because of poor bioavailability (20% for a 2–6 g dose) and partly because the transport of carnitine into the muscle is limited. Any claims regarding effects of carnitine on fat oxidation or weight loss are, of course, unfounded if carnitine supplementation is unable to increase the carnitine concentration in muscle. In addition, **enzyme kinetics** indicate that human muscle in resting conditions has more than enough free carnitine to allow the enzyme carnitine palmitoyl transferase I (CPT I) to function at maximal activity.

Endurance Exercise

The belief that carnitine is an ergogenic aid for endurance exercise is based on assumptions similar to the weight-loss assumptions (Wagenmakers 1991): that carnitine concentration in muscle becomes too low to allow CPT I to function at a high velocity and to support the increased rate of fat oxidation during exercise; that oral ingestion of carnitine increases the total carnitine concentration in muscle; and that the increase in muscle carnitine increases the oxidation rate of plasma FAs and intramuscular triacylglycerols during exercise, thereby reducing muscle glycogen breakdown and postponing fatigue.

During high-intensity exercise, the free carnitine concentration in muscle falls because this free carnitine reacts with acetyl-CoA. During very high-intensity exercise, the free carnitine concentration falls to extremely low levels. Studies report values as low as 0.5 mmol/kg w.w. after 3 to 4 minutes at 90% of $\dot{V}O_2$max (Constantin-Teodosiu et al. 1991).

These values approach the Km (see sidebar) of CPT I for carnitine (250 to 450 μM) measured in vitro (Bremer 1983). This decrease in free carnitine has been suggested as one of the mechanisms by which plasma FA and intramuscular triacylglycerol oxidation are reduced during high-intensity exercise (Constantin-Teodosiu et al. 1991; Timmons et al. 1996).

As discussed, however, the second assumption about carnitine as an ergogenic aid is not true because direct measurements in muscle after 14 days on 4 to 6 g/day of carnitine failed to show increases in the muscle carnitine concentration (Barnett et al. 1994; Vukovich et al. 1994). This finding implies that carnitine supplementation cannot increase fat oxidation and improve exercise performance by the proposed mechanism. Indeed, many original investigations, which are summarized in numerous reviews (Heinonen 1996; Wagenmakers 1991), have confirmed that carnitine supplementation does not increase fat oxidation and reduce glycogen breakdown and does not improve performance during prolonged cycling and running exercise.

High-Intensity Exercise

As previously indicated, carnitine may increase the availability of free CoA and maintain the acetyl-CoA:CoA ratio (see figure 11.7). This function of carnitine is especially important during maximal and supramaximal exercise such as competitive sprint and middle-distance running and 50 to 400 m swimming. If carnitine supplementation increases muscle carnitine concentration and, therefore, CoA availability in these conditions, the flux through the pyruvate dehydrogenase complex could increase and less lactic acid would be produced (see figure 11.7). Theoretically, this process could delay fatigue and improve exercise performance. But all these mechanisms are just theories because carnitine supplementation does not increase the muscle carnitine concentration. Most controlled original

---

Km

Km is the substrate concentration that results in an enzyme-catalyzed reaction proceeding at 50% of the maximum rate. So at the typical muscle carnitine concentrations of 250 to 450 μM, the reaction catalyzed by CPT I is proceeding at about 50% of its maximum rate. For further explanation about Km see appendix A.

investigations have failed to show effects of carnitine supplementation on $\dot{V}O_2max$, high-intensity exercise performance, and lactate accumulation.

New Insights

Recently some interesting discoveries were made in the lab of Dr. Greenhaff at the University of Nottingham (United Kingdom). In a series of studies it was observed that it is possible to increase muscle carnitine concentration if carnitine is given when plasma insulin concentrations are elevated. Carnitine is transported into the muscle cell by a sodium-dependent active transport process. The transport protein involved is called the organic cation transporter OCTN2, and it was hypothesized that insulin may increase the sodium-dependent transport of carnitine.

Initial studies used simultaneous infusion of insulin and carnitine and indeed observed a 15% increase in muscle carnitine (Stephens et al. 2006). Further studies revealed that a certain (fairly high) level of insulin is necessary to achieve this effect (Stephens et al. 2007b). More recently it was demonstrated that the insulin response resulting from carbohydrate feeding can be sufficient to increase the uptake of carnitine into the muscle. In this study 3 g/day of L-carnitine was ingested followed by 4 × 500 ml solution, each containing 94 g of carbohydrate. It was observed that carnitine retention improved (less carnitine excretion in urine), suggesting increased muscle carnitine (Stephens et al. 2007c). Of course, whether this strategy is practical or meaningful is questionable, especially in a weight-loss situation. If 4 × 94 g of carbohydrate has to be ingested (6,000 kJ or 1,500 kcal) to increase muscle carnitine concentration, weight gain is more likely to result than weight loss. Also, the high carbohydrate intake will suppress fat oxidation. This suppression will be greater than the possible effect of carnitine. Nevertheless, the observations are interesting and may lead to practical ways to increase muscle carnitine in the future. For now there are no reasons to recommend carnitine to athletes. An outstanding review on the topic was recently published by Stephens et al. (2007a).

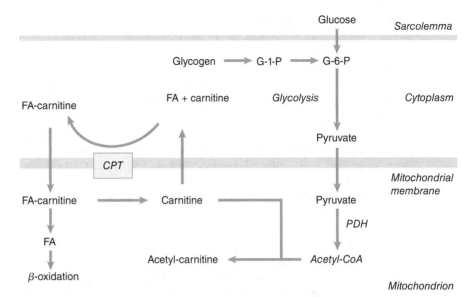

Figure 11.7 A potential link between FA uptake, carnitine, and glucose metabolism. Carnitine acts as a buffer for acetyl-CoA, thereby preventing a buildup of pyruvate and preventing lactate accumulation. This activity may, however, reduce free carnitine availability and, at least in theory, FA transport into the mitochondria. FA = fatty acid; PDH = pyruvate dehydrogenase; CPT = carnitine palmitoyl transferase.

Choline

Acetylcholine transmits the electrical potential from the neuron to the muscle cell, leading to calcium release from the sarcoplasmic reticulum and muscle contraction. Experimental studies in animals suggest that depletion of the neuromuscular transmitter acetylcholine contributes to fatigue during sustained electrical stimulation or exercise (Pagala et al. 1984). Whether this transmission defect is at the presynaptic or postsynaptic membrane or across the synapse has not been elucidated.

The precursor of acetylcholine, choline, is a normal component of the human diet, most abundant in meat and diary products. It is also an integral part of several phospholipids incorporated into cell membranes, including phosphatidylcholine (lecithin), lysophatidylcholine, and sphingomyelin (Zeisel 1998). Peak serum concentrations of choline occur several hours after ingestion of lecithin (Zeisel et al. 1991). Ingestion of choline or lecithin raises plasma choline levels in a dose-dependent matter. Based on these functions, choline supplements have been hypothesized to affect nerve transmission, increase strength, or facilitate the loss of body fat.

Strenuous exercise decreases plasma choline levels. They were reduced by 40% in participants of the 1985 Boston Marathon (Conlay et al. 1986), and similar findings were reported after the 1986 Boston Marathon (Wurtman et al. 1991). Von

Allworden et al. (1993) reported a 16.9% average decline in plasma choline concentration after 2 hours of strenuous cycling (35 km/h). Neuromuscular transmission may have been impaired before the end of marathons or during the late stages of other forms of prolonged strenuous exercise, unless choline is supplied by neuronal or muscular membrane phospholipids or ingestion. Low acetylcholine concentrations have been associated with impaired neuromuscular transmission and fatigue. The acetylcholine concentration in the brain is directly related to the plasma choline concentration. Several studies of choline uptake and distribution after intravenous administration of choline show that plasma choline and acetylcholine in kidney, liver, lung, and heart are directly proportional to the amounts administered. Haubrich et al. (1975) reported that intravenous infusion of choline in guinea pigs led to incorporation of choline into acetylcholine within minutes in a variety of tissues.

Whether this reaction is also the case for skeletal muscle in vivo is still unknown. Some evidence from in vitro studies, however, indicates that newly synthesized acetylcholine is released during neuromuscular stimulation when choline is added to the perfusion medium (Bierkamper et al. 1980). Gardiner and Gwee (Gardiner et al. 1974) infused choline in rabbits and measured an elevated choline concentration in all tissues, including muscle. Unfortunately, acetylcholine was not measured. Thus, prolonged neuromuscular efforts may conceivably result in depletion of plasma choline, which might lead to fatigue because of insufficient availability of acetylcholine. Increasing plasma choline levels, on the other hand, by ingesting choline might increase acetylcholine availability and thereby reduce fatigue.

One preliminary report showed that ingestion of choline citrate during a 20 mi (32 km) run prevented the fall in plasma choline concentration, and performance improved compared with a placebo-treated group (Sandage et al. 1992). Spector et al. (1995) reported no effect on performance after the ingestion of 4.86 g choline bitartrate. During the placebo trial, however, no fall in choline was observed and none of the subjects displayed choline depletion. In such conditions, choline ingestion is unlikely to improve performance. Interestingly, these authors reported a significant negative correlation between the decrease in choline concentration and time to exhaustion, suggesting that choline may play a role in the development of fatigue.

Von Allworden et al. (1993) gave subjects 0.2 g/kg b.w. of lecithin 1 hour before they cycled for 2 hours at 35 km/h. Lecithin ingestion increased plasma choline concentrations by 26.9%, whereas placebo ingestion decreased choline concentrations by 16.9%. Unfortunately, exercise performance was not evaluated in this study. The claims of choline as a supplement are based largely on theory and findings of in vitro studies. Although some interesting observations have been made in humans, the grounds for recommending choline as an ergogenic aid are insufficient.

Chromium

Chromium is a popular supplement because it is said to be a muscle builder and fat burner, and enormous marketing hype has surrounded this supplement over the past few years. Chromium is a trace element that is present in foods such as brewers yeast, American cheese, mushrooms, and wheat germ, and it is considered an essential nutrient. Because of insufficient methods to assess chromium status, the U.S. Food and Nutrition Board could not establish an RDA for chromium. Instead, a range of adequate intake (AI) values is recommended: 20 to 45 μg per day. Anderson and Kozlovski (Anderson et al. 1985) suggested that many people in the United States are not ingesting even 50 pg/day (picograms per day; a picogram is 10^{-12} gram) of chromium. But the AI was established using less sophisticated equipment than is available today, so the recommended values may be too high (Stoecker 1996).

Chromium potentiates insulin action, and insulin stimulates glucose and amino acid uptake by muscle cells. The stimulated amino acid uptake is thought to increase in protein synthesis and muscle mass gain. In fact, chromium supplements increase muscle mass and growth in animals (Stoecker 1996), but the effect of chromium on muscle mass in humans is less clear cut. Chromium is marketed predominantly in the form of chromium picolinate, although chromium nicotinate and chromium chloride supplements also exist. Picolinic acid is an organic compound that binds to chromium and is thought to enhance the absorption and transport of chromium (Evans 1989).

Evans (1989) was the first to report that ingesting chromium increased lean tissue in exercising humans. In those studies, untrained college students and trained football players were given 200 μg of chromium picolinate or a placebo each day for 40 to 42 days while they were on a resistance-training program. Those subjects who took chromium supplements gained significantly more lean body mass compared with the placebo group. But lean body mass was only estimated from circumference measures and the changes observed were small, so measurement error could have influenced the results.

Subsequent studies (Clancy et al. 1994; Hallmark et al. 1996; Hasten et al. 1992; Lukaski et al. 1996) have not confirmed the results of Evans (1989). In these carefully controlled studies, which used more sophisticated techniques to measure body composition, no effects were found in lean body mass.

A study investigated the effects of chromium on muscle glycogen synthesis after exercise (Volek et al. 2006). Because it has been reported that chromium may have an effect on insulin sensitivity, it was hypothesized that it may also enhance insulin sensitivity postexercise, thereby increasing glucose uptake and glycogen synthesis. Chromium supplementation for 4 weeks, however, did not augment glycogen synthesis during recovery from high-intensity exercise and high-carbohydrate feeding, although there was a trend for lower phosphoinositide-3-kinase activity (indicative of improved insulin sensitivity).

Thus, most of the studies show that chromium supplements are not effective in increasing lean body mass. Based on laboratory studies of cultured cells, chromium picolinate was suggested to accumulate in cells and cause chromosome damage (Stearns et al. 1995). Although this finding has not been confirmed in human studies (McCarty 1996), caution must be exercised in the use of chromium supplements.

Coenzyme Q10

Coenzyme Q10 (CoQ10), or ubiquinone, is an integral part of the electron-transport chain of the mitochondria. CoQ10, therefore, plays an important role in oxidative phosphorylation. In heart muscle it has been used therapeutically to treat cardiovascular disease and promote recovery from cardiac surgery. CoQ10 supplementation in patients with those conditions improves oxidative metabolism and exercise capacity (Khatta et al. 2000), and it functions as an antioxidant, promoting the scavenging of free radicals. Manufacturers extrapolated the results of improved $\dot{V}O_2$max in cardiac patients to healthy and trained athletes. CoQ10 is claimed to increase $\dot{V}O_2$max and increase stamina and energy.

A few studies have investigated the effects of CoQ10 supplementation in athletes. Although most of these studies report elevated plasma CoQ10 levels, no changes were observed in $\dot{V}O_2$max, performance, or blood lactate at submaximal workloads. Ingestion of 120 mg/day of CoQ10 for 20 days was reported to result in marked increases in plasma CoQ10 concentrations, but the muscle CoQ10 concentration was unaltered (Svensson et al. 1999). Of course, if CoQ10 supplementation does not alter muscle CoQ10 concentration, it cannot be expected to have any effects on any of the performance-related variables.

CoQ10 may even have some negative effects. It possibly augments free-radical production during high-intensity exercise when an abundance of hydrogen ions are present in the cells (Malm et al. 1997). Ironically, this effect is the opposite of what CoQ10 is claimed to do.

Creatine

Creatine became a popular supplement after the 1992 Olympics in Barcelona. Gold medal winners Linford Christie, in the men's 100 m dash, and Sally Gunnell, in the women's 400 m hurdles, supposedly used creatine supplements. By the time of the Olympic Games in Atlanta in 1996, approximately 80% of all athletes used creatine (Williams et al. 1999). The worldwide creatine consumption by athletes is now estimated to be around 3,000,000 kg/year. This section discusses the efficacy of creatine in different sports and the supposed mechanisms of action. For more detail on the role of creatine in metabolism and performance, see Casey and Greenhaff (Casey et al. 2000), Greenhaff (1998), and Terjung et al. (2000). A good and complete source of information is a book by Williams, Kreider, and Branch (Williams et al. 1999).

In the Body

Creatine, or methylguanidine-acetic acid, is a naturally occurring compound present mostly in muscle tissue. It is not an essential nutrient, because it can be synthesized within the human body. In normal, healthy people, diet and oral ingestion together provide approximately 2 g/day of creatine. At the same time and at approximately the same rate (2 g/day), creatine is broken down to creatinine and excreted in the urine.

The primary dietary sources of creatine are fish and red meat (see table 11.4). Strict vegetarians and vegans have negligible creatine intake because plants contain only trace amounts. They are, therefore, dependent on endogenous synthesis of creatine. Oral ingestion of creatine suppresses the biosynthesis. When a creatine-deficient diet is consumed, the urinary excretion of creatine and creatinine decreases.

Creatine synthesis in the human body is a two-step reaction. First, the guanidino group of arginine is transferred to glycine, forming guanidinoacetate. Second, creatine is formed by transfer of a methyl group from S-adenosylmethionine to guanidinoacetate. Most creatine synthesis in humans occurs in the liver and kidneys (see figure 11.8).

■ TABLE 11.4 ■
Sources of Dietary Creatine

Food type	Creatine content (g/100 g)
FISH	
Shrimp	Trace
Cod	0.3
Herring	0.65–0.1
Plaice	0.2
Salmon	0.45
Tuna	0.4
MEAT	
Beef	0.45
Pork	0.4
OTHER	
Milk	0.01
Cranberries	0.002

In a 70 kg (154 lb) man, the total-body creatine pool is approximately 120 g, 95% of which is in muscle (skeletal, heart, and smooth muscle). The remaining 5% is in the brain, liver, kidneys, and testes. Creatine synthesized in the liver and kidney and absorbed from the diet is transported by blood to the muscle. Muscle takes up creatine against a concentration gradient by a sodium-dependent saturable active transport process. In the muscle cell, creatine is phosphorylated, after which it is trapped within the muscle. This process helps to create a high total-creatine gradient (30 to 40 mmol/kg w.w. or 120 to 160 mmol/kg d.w. in skeletal muscle, with 60% to 70% in the form of phosphocreatine) (Wyss et al. 2000). Type I and type II muscle fibers have differing creatine content; type II fibers have about 30% more creatine than type I fibers.

Metabolic Process

The role of creatine and phosphocreatine is discussed in chapter 3 but will be briefly repeated here. As muscle contracts, adenosine triphosphate (ATP) is degraded to adenosine diphosphate (ADP) and inorganic phosphate (Pi) to provide energy:

$$ATP \rightarrow ADP + Pi + energy$$

During intense maximal exercise, ATP stores can provide energy for only 1 to 2 seconds. When the whole-muscle ATP concentration falls by about 30%, the muscle fatigues (Hultman et al. 1991; Karlsson et al. 1970). To prevent fatigue, regeneration of ATP must occur at a rate similar to that of ATP hydrolysis to maintain ATP concentration close to resting levels. An important function of phosphocreatine in muscle is to provide the high-energy phosphate group for ATP regeneration during the first seconds of high-intensity exercise, thus allowing time for glycogen breakdown and glycolysis (the other main process generating cytosolic ATP during high-intensity exercise) to speed up to the required rate. Transfer of the phosphate group from phosphocreatine to adenosine diphosphate (ADP) is catalyzed by the enzyme creatine kinase, resulting in regeneration of ATP and release of free creatine:

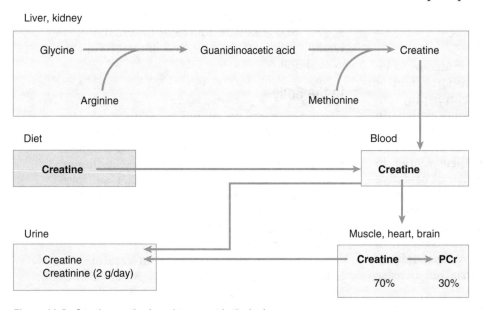

Figure 11.8 Creatine synthesis and transport in the body.

Phosphocreatine (PCr) + ADP + H$^+$ → Creatine (Cr) + ATP

PCr is present in resting muscle in a concentration that is three to four times that of ATP (see appendix A). During the 100 m sprint, 22 g of ATP is estimated to be broken down per second, or about 50% of the ATP content per kilogram of active muscle. Because fatigue occurs in human muscle when the whole-muscle ATP concentration falls by about 30%, the need for rephosphorylation of the ADP formed during contraction is obvious.

Anaerobic degradation of PCr and glycogen is responsible for the extremely high rate of ATP resynthesis during the first seconds of high-intensity exercise (Hultman et al. 1991; Karlsson et al. 1970). But the PCr store in muscle is limited and is depleted within 5 seconds of supramaximal exercise. In this manner, the concentration of skeletal muscle ATP is maintained to some degree during single bouts or repeated bouts of supramaximal exercise. Anaerobic ATP resynthesis, however, cannot be maintained at the same rate as during the first few seconds of supramaximal exercise. Consequently, over the course of 30 seconds, ATP turnover rates fall by about 20%. High PCr stores possibly reduce the need for anaerobic glycolysis and lactic acid formation during intense exercise, which might be another potential benefit of creatine supplementation.

A third important function of creatine is its potential buffering capacity for hydrogen ions because those ions are used during ATP regeneration, as shown in the previous equation. A higher creatine concentration in the muscle also implies increased flux through the creatine kinase reaction, resulting in increased PCr synthesis during recovery from high-intensity exercise. The roles of creatine listed previously suggest that elevating muscle creatine and PCr stores will benefit high-intensity exercise performance. What would be an easier way to achieve this than by simply eating creatine?

Supplementation

Harris et al. (1992) were the first to state that ingesting creatine monohydrate could increase total muscle creatine stores (creatine and phosphocreatine). In that study, ingesting 5 g of creatine four to six times a day for several days increased the total creatine concentration by an average of 25 mmol/kg d.w., and 30% of the increase in total creatine content was in the form of phosphocreatine. The authors suggested that these increases could

improve exercise performance but did not test this suggestion in their study. The first performance study was conducted by Greenhaff et al. (1993). Subjects ingested 20 g/day of creatine for 5 days, and creatine indeed improved performance by about 6% during repeated bouts of maximal knee extensor exercise. After that study, more studies were performed investigating different modes of exercise (Balsom et al. 1993a, 1993b; Birch et al. 1994; Harris et al. 1992; Volek et al. 1997). In 1999, of the 62 laboratory-based studies performed on creatine supplementation and high-intensity exercise performance, 42 reported positive effects, and the remainder showed no effects (Williams et al. 1999). Since then, the number of positive studies has accumulated.

Loading Regimens

Most studies used a creatine loading regimen of 20 g/day in four portions of 5 g each given at different times of the day for a 6-day period. This regimen has been shown to increase muscle creatine concentration, on average, by about 25 mmol/kg d.w. This increase corresponded to about 20% of the basal total muscle creatine concentration of about 125 mmol/kg d.w. Hultman et al. (1996) found that after an initial loading phase of 20 g/day for 6 days, a subsequent dose of 2 g/day was enough to maintain the high total creatine concentration for 35 days, whereas stopping creatine supplementation after 6 days caused a slow, gradual decline of the creatine concentration in muscle.

When creatine was ingested at a dose of 3 g/day, the rate of increase in muscle creatine was correspondingly lower, but after 28 days on 3 g/day the total creatine concentration was similar to the rapid-loading regimen (see figure 11.9). Therefore, a loading dose of 20 g/day for 6 days followed by a maintenance dose of 2 to 3 g/day is advised if athletes want to increase muscle creatine to maximal levels quickly, whereas a continuous dose of 3 g/day leads to the same maximal level in about 1 month. The increase in muscle PCr concentration was about 40% of the increase in total creatine concentration with both procedures.

Considerable variation exists among subjects in the initial total muscle creatine concentration. The reasons for variation are largely unknown but may be at least partly related to the habitual diet. The largest increase in muscle creatine concentration is observed in people with the lowest initial concentration, whereas those who already have high creatine concentrations benefit only marginally

(Harris et al. 1992) (see figure 11.10). A concentration of 160 mmol/kg d.w. appears to be the maximal creatine concentration achievable by creatine supplementation, but only about 20% of subjects reached this level after creatine supplementation.

Total muscle creatine can be increased more (mean increase 30 to 40 mmol/kg d.w.) when creatine (20 g/day for 5 days) is ingested in solution

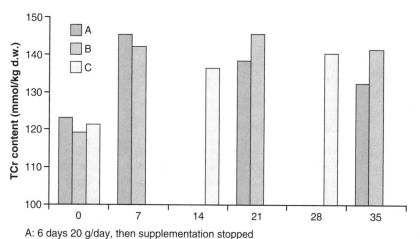

A: 6 days 20 g/day, then supplementation stopped
B: 6 days 20 g/day, then followed by 2 g/day maintenance
C: 28 days 3 g/day

Figure 11.9 Different protocols of creatine loading. TCr = total creatine.
Data from E. Hultman et al. 1996.

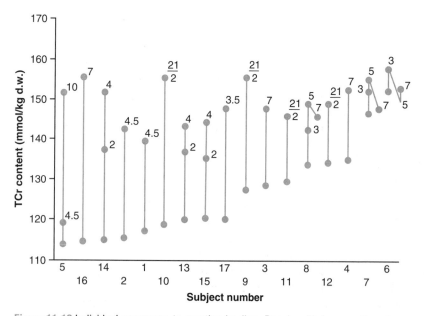

Figure 11.10 Individual responses to creatine loading. People with low creatine stores benefit most, whereas those who already have high creatine stores have minimal increases in muscle creatine. Numbers in the graph are days of supplementation at a rate of 20 to 30 g/day. 21/2 indicates subjects who ingested creatine on alternate days for 21 days.
Data from E. Hultman et al. 1996.

with simple carbohydrates (Green et al. 1995, 1996). In a study, the total muscle creatine concentration increased in most subjects close to the upper limit of 160 mmol/kg d.w. Carbohydrate ingestion is thought to stimulate muscle creatine uptake through an insulin-dependent mechanism. Insulin may stimulate the sodium–potassium pump activity and thereby the sodium-dependent muscle creatine transport.

In a study by Casey et al. (1996) the changes in performance were related to the changes in total muscle creatine content (see figure 11.11). A strong correlation was observed in that people who displayed the largest increases in total muscle creatine concentration also exhibited the largest performance benefit. A change in muscle creatine content of about 20 mmol/kg d.w. is said to be necessary before significant changes in performance are observed. About 30% of all individuals do not display such large increases in muscle creatine and therefore do not benefit. They are often referred to as nonresponders.

Weight Gain

Creatine supplementation (20 g/day for 5 to 6 days) is generally accompanied by increases in body weight of 0.5 to 3.5 kg. (For a complete overview, see Williams et al. [1999]). The average increase in body mass is about 1 kg. Theoretically, this increase in body mass and possible change in body composition results from increases in intracellular water, stimulation of protein synthesis, or a decrease in protein breakdown. Because the decrease in urine production exactly paralleled the time course of the increase in muscle creatine concentration (see figure 11.11), creatine likely causes water retention in skeletal muscle cells because of an increase of the intracellular osmolarity of the muscle fibers. Evidence suggests that some of the weight gain may be attributable to the anabolic effect of creatine (Kreider et al. 1998), although in the short term (5 to 6 days) this effect is not likely to be an important factor.

The increase in body mass may be beneficial or have no effect in some

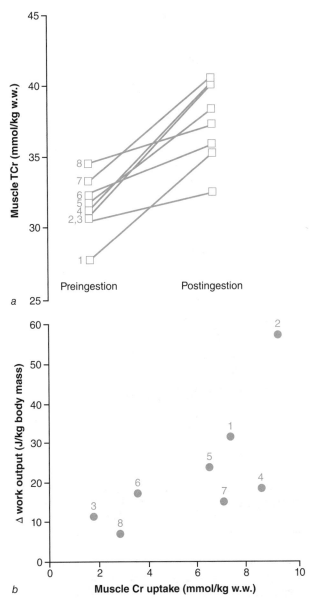

Figure 11.11 Relationship between individual changes in *(a)* mixed muscle creatine concentration and *(b)* changes in total work production after creatine loading (4 to 5 g/day for 5 days). Work production was measured during two bouts of 30 seconds of maximal isokinetic cycling exercises.

Reprinted from A. Casey et al., 1996, "Creatine ingestion favorably affects performance and muscle metabolism during maximal exercise in humans," *American Journal of Physiology* 271(1): E31-37. Used with permission.

disciplines. But in sports that involve weight-bearing activities, such as running or gymnastics, the weight gain caused by creatine supplementation could have a negative effect on performance.

High-Intensity Exercise

The findings of Greenhaff et al. (1993), who used high-intensity intermittent exercise, have been repeated by other investigations using cycle ergometry, bench press, or running as the mode of exercise. Most of these studies (about 70% of all studies) found improvements in strength, force production, or torque.

Balsom et al. (1993a) randomly assigned 16 trained subjects to a creatine group (25 g/day for 6 days) and a placebo group. One test that these subjects performed was a repeated sprint test, in which they sprinted 10 times for 6 seconds with 30 seconds of recovery between bouts. Although subjects fatigued with both creatine and placebo, after 7 sprints, fatigue was significantly greater in the placebo group. Casey et al. (1996) investigated the effect of acute creatine supplementation (20 g/day for 5 days) on isokinetic cycle performance (2 × 30 seconds with 4 minutes recovery between bouts). Increases in peak power and total work were already observed in the first of the two bouts after creatine supplementation. The improvements in total work production were positively correlated with the increased concentration of PCr in type II muscle fibers after supplementation (see figure 11.12).

Several studies investigated the effect of creatine supplementation versus placebo on 25 m, 50 m, and 100 m performance in elite swimmers performing their best stroke (Burke et al. 1996; Mujika et al. 1996; Peyrebrune et al. 1998). These studies failed to show an ergogenic effect of creatine supplementation. Two studies, however, showed improvements in 10 × 50 m or 8 × 45 m swimming velocity (Leenders et al. 1999; Peyrebrune et al. 1998). Rossiter et al. (1996) observed an ergogenic effect of creatine versus placebo supplementation on the 1,000 m performance of competitive rowers. When two groups of rugby union players received creatine or placebo, no differences were observed in body composition between the groups (Chilibeck et al. 2007). The group receiving creatine supplementation had a greater increase in the number of repetitions for combined bench press and leg press tests compared with the placebo group.

Findings suggest that creatine also improves high-intensity exercise performance in competitive squash players (Romer et al. 2001). The players fatigued less toward the end of a game when supplemented with creatine. Thus, creatine supplementation may have a positive effect on performance in competitive situations in some sports. Whether creatine has an effect may depend on the initial muscle creatine concentrations, the type of exercise, and the level of the athlete.

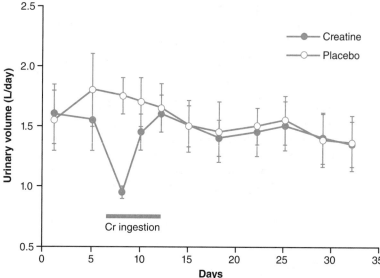

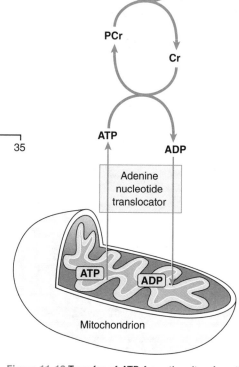

Figure 11.12 Urinary volume before and after either placebo or creatine ingestion. Creatine was administered as 5 g four times per day for 5 days. A clear relationship was found between the decreased urinary output and the increase in body mass after creatine ingestion.

Reprinted from E. Hultman et al., 1996, "Muscle creatine loading in men," *Journal of Applied Physiology* 81(1): 232-237. Used with permission.

Endurance Exercise

In endurance exercise, most ATP is resynthesized by oxidative phosphorylation in the mitochondria. Net PCr breakdown and the net contribution of PCr to energy production are minimal. But creatine and PCr provide a shuttle system for the transfer of high-energy phosphate groups from the ATP production site (the mitochondria) to the ATP consumption site (the contracting myofibrils) (see figure 11.13). A phosphate group of ATP produced in the mitochondria is donated to creatine to form phosphocreatine. From phosphocreatine, the phosphate group is donated to ADP, and ATP is formed and can be used for muscle contraction. Theoretically, creatine could, therefore, facilitate aerobic energy production and enhance performance in prolonged exercise.

Balsom et al. (1993b) investigated the effect of creatine supplementation for 6 days on endurance exercise performance in well-trained runners. No effect occurred during a supramaximal treadmill run to exhaustion in the laboratory, but a significant decrease in performance occurred during a 6 km terrain run. Subjects showed an increase in body weight of 0.5 to 1.0 kg, which possibly explains the negative result during the terrain run. In another study, 5 days of creatine supplementation (20 g/day) had no influence on oxygen uptake, respiratory gas exchange, and blood-lactate concentration

Figure 11.13 Transfer of ATP from the site of synthesis (mitochondria) to the site of usage (contractile proteins). Creatine and phosphocreatine play an important role in this process.
Adapted from Wagenmakers 1999.

during submaximal incremental treadmill exercise and recovery. These data seem to suggest that the availability of creatine and PCr is not rate limiting for the diffusion of energy-rich phosphate groups through the cytosol and that creatine supplementation, therefore, does not have an effect on muscle metabolism in endurance exercise. The studies that have investigated the effects of creatine supplementation on endurance performance generally have not reported an ergogenic effect.

Resistance Training

Vandenberghe et al. (1997) investigated the effect of creatine loading on muscle PCr phosphate concentration, muscle strength, and body composition after a 10-week resistance-training program. Compared with placebo, maximal strength of the trained muscle groups increased 20% to 25% more, maximal intermittent exercise capacity of the arm flexors increased 10% to 25% more, and fat-free mass increased by 60% more with creatine supplementation. This study and others suggest that the combination of creatine ingestion and strength training is more effective than strength training only. In addition, Wagenmakers (1999) suggested that creatine supplementation allows more repetitions and thus better quality of training and at the same time may have an anabolic effect.

Creatine causes fluid retention, which may result in muscle cell swelling. Cell swelling acts as a universal anabolic signal, causing an increase of protein synthesis and net protein deposition (Lang et al. 1998). Although several animal and clinical studies suggest that creatine ingestion has anabolic effects, no evidence in healthy individuals indicates that creatine affects protein metabolism.

Mechanisms of Action

Several mechanisms by which creatine exerts its effect have been proposed:

- The most obvious explanation is increased PCr availability, particularly in type II muscle fibers (Casey et al. 1996). Evidence indicates that increased PCr stores in the muscle improve contractile function by maintaining ATP turnover.

- Another possible mechanism is the increased rate of PCr resynthesis (Greenhaff et al. 1994), which is particularly important in short recovery periods during repeated bouts of maximal exercise.

- The increased use of PCr as an energy source could reduce anaerobic glycolysis and lactic acid formation. This activity could theoretically reduce hydrogen ion formation in the muscle and delay fatigue caused by increased muscle acidity.

- Creatine could buffer some of the hydrogen ions produced during high-intensity exercise. This process would delay fatigue in high-intensity exercise that is limited by lactic acid formation.

- As indicated in figure 11.13, creatine plays an important role in shuttling high-energy phosphates from the site of ATP production (mitochondria) to the site of ATP breakdown (myofibrils). This role of creatine was suggested as a potential mechanism for improved performance in endurance activities. But these types of activities are not affected by creatine supplementation, suggesting that this mechanism may not be important.

- Creatine may have anabolic properties.

Safety

No studies have reported detrimental health effects of creatine. According to numerous anecdotal reports, however, creatine supplementation causes ailments; gastrointestinal, cardiovascular, and muscular problems; nausea, vomiting, and diarrhea; alterations in kidney and liver function; muscle cramps; and elevated blood pressure. As pointed out in a roundtable discussion by the American College of Sports Medicine, "The evidence is not definitive and/or it is incomplete to indict the practice of creatine supplementation as a health risk; at the same time, our lack of information cannot be taken as an assurance that creatine supplementation is free from health risks. Ignorance provides little comfort of untoward effects yet to be discovered."

Dehydroepiandrosterone

Dehydroepiandrosterone (DHEA) and its sulphated ester (DHEAS) are relatively weak androgen steroid hormones synthesized primarily in early adulthood (20 to 25 years of age) by the adrenal cortex. Dehydroepiandrosterone is not present in large quantities in the diet, but when taken as a supplement it becomes a precursor for at least two hormones: testosterone and estradiol. Because DHEA is a precursor for testosterone, it is thought to increase testosterone concentration and thereby increase protein synthesis and muscle mass. DHEA is, therefore, one of the most popular supplements, especially in the United States. Synthetic DHEA is categorized as a nutrition supplement because the substance also occurs naturally. Because of its classification, the Food and Drug Administration has no control over what manufacturers say about the product. They call DHEA a superhormone that increases lean body mass, slows the aging process, boosts immune function, and protects against heart disease. Because the plasma DHEA concentration decreases with age, many studies have focused on the effects of the supplement in older individuals. Manufacturers abuse the results of this research and claim that restoring blood DHEA concentrations to youth levels slows the aging process. Little is known about the physiological role of DHEA or the cellular and molecular mechanisms of its action. But DHEA is known to interact with the receptors of the neurotransmitter γ-amino butyric acid (GABA) in the brain.

Early support for DHEA as a supplement comes from animal studies in which animals were given this hormone. The test animals showed improved immune function and resistance to arteriosclerosis, cancer, viral infections, obesity, and diabetes. Some studies even reported an extended lifespan. Rats, however, normally have extremely low DHEA levels and may respond very differently than humans. Human studies showed a decreased risk of cardiovascular diseases in men with high DHEA levels but an increased risk in women. Subsequent studies reported minimal protective effects of DHEA in men and no effects or negative effects in women (Johannes et al. 1999). In one study, DHEA supplementation resulted in enhanced protection against cardiovascular diseases (Jakubowicz et al. 1995). In general, though, the results of various studies are not consistent, and whether DHEA really protects against cardiovascular disease is difficult to determine (Sirrs et al. 1999).

Studies that investigated the effects of DHEA on body composition showed a rise in blood androgen levels after supplementation (100 to 1,600 mg/day of DHEA), but no effects on body weight or lean body mass were observed. In addition, Welle et al. (1990) did not observe effects on energy or protein metabolism. Nestler et al. (1988) reported a small decrease in fat mass without a change in total body mass, which suggests that DHEA resulted in an increase in lean body mass. In a study by Mortola and Yen (Mortola et al. 1990), 100 mg/day of DHEA for 3 months resulted in a 1% increase in lean body mass. In that study, fat mass decreased in men but increased in women. A study of obese subjects who received 1,600 mg/day of DHEA for 28 days did not report any changes in body composition. These results, although varied and not convincing, seem to indicate that DHEA has a small effect on muscle mass and immune function. Most of these studies were performed in subjects 40 to 75 years of age, and little is known about the effects in young adults.

Because so little is known about the possible side effects of DHEA, various researchers and institutions have expressed concern. DHEA is an uncontrolled substance and is readily available in pharmacies, in drugstores, and over the Internet. Clinicians fear that elevated plasma DHEA through supplementation might stimulate dormant prostate tumors or cause hypertrophy of the prostate gland itself. Ethical questions also arise about the use of hormones as ergogenic substances. Both the International Olympic Committee and the U.S. Olympic Committee have placed DHEA on the list of banned substances with zero tolerance. In March 2007 a bill introduced in the U.S. Senate attempted to classify DHEA as a controlled substance under the category of anabolic steroids.

Dihydroxyacetone

Dihydroxyacetone is an intermediate of glycolysis. Long-term ingestion of this substance in combination with pyruvate is suggested to have positive effects on both carbohydrate and fat metabolism. The studies on dihydroxyacetone and pyruvate are discussed in the section on pyruvate.

Fish Oil

Fish oil is a natural source of long-chain omega-3 FAs, including both docosahexaenoic acid and eicosapentaenoic acid. Guezennec et al. (1989) suggested that increasing the fraction of polyunsaturated FAs (PUFA) in the phospholipids of erythrocyte (red blood cell) membranes improves membrane fluidity and increases red blood cell deformability (flexibility), resulting in improved peripheral oxygen supply. They conducted a study in which 14 male subjects were divided into two groups; one group received a normal diet and the other received a diet rich in fish oil for 6 weeks. The fraction of omega-3 FAs increased in erythrocyte membranes, but no change in red blood cell deformability was seen under resting conditions. During hypobaric exercise, red blood cell deformability decreased less with consumption of fish oil.

Brilla and Landerholm (Brilla et al. 1990) studied the effects of fish oil intake and exercise training in 32 sedentary males and found that exercise training resulted in an increased $\dot{V}O_2max$, whereas fish oil supplementation had no effect. Oostenbrug et al. (1997) supplemented trained cyclists for 3 weeks with placebo or fish oil (6 g/day). Fish oil did not alter red blood cell characteristics in this study and had no effect on $\dot{V}O_2max$, maximal power output, or time-trial performance.

Physical training improves red blood cell deformability and changes the FA composition of membranes toward a higher percentage of unsaturated FAs, so the enhanced fluidity under resting conditions could be masked by physical training (Kamada et al. 1993). The enhanced membrane fluidity may be especially important when the uptake of oxygen becomes limiting, as during exercise under hypoxic conditions. The physiologic consequences of PUFA are still hypothetical, however, and further studies are necessary to evaluate the possible effects on hemorrheologic changes during exercise.

Ginseng

Ginseng, the root of the *Araliaceous* plant, is a popular supplement among athletes. It is commonly described as an "adaptogen," a substance that helps the body adapt to stress situations. Ginseng has been used for several thousand years in Asia. Its effects are said to include improved sleep, improved memory, reduced fatigue, and relief of heart pain, headache, and nausea. The known varieties of ginseng are American, Chinese, Korean, Japanese, and Siberian (see the highlight box), and the three main medicinal species are *Panax ginseng* (Chinese or Korean ginseng), *Panax japonicum* (Japanese ginseng from India, southern China, and Japan), and *Panax quinquefolium* (American ginseng). Siberian, or Russian, ginseng, although claimed to have a similar stimulant effect, is an entirely different plant, *Eleutherococcus senticosus*. It is used as a cheaper substitute of the *Panax ginseng*.

The main active constituents of the *Panax* species are triterpenoid glycosides, or saponins (also referred to as ginsenosides or panaxosides). The structure and distribution of saponins may vary with species and variety. At least 13 different saponins exist. *Panax ginseng* is believed to be the most potent form of ginseng and has become the standard. Animal studies support some of the claims about ginseng. Running performance in rats improved 132% after acute administration of ginseng and 179% after 7 days of administration. The ingestion of ginseng was accompanied by an increase in the basal ACTH and cortisol levels in rats. In humans, the effects are not clear, and several studies show inconsistent results. Most of the human studies did not have an appropriate design and were not placebo controlled or were not randomized. Some of these uncontrolled studies reported improvements in $\dot{V}O_2$max and exercise performance. In one study, five subjects ingested 2 g/day of *Panax ginseng* for 4 weeks, and six subjects acted as a control group. Measurements included substrate utilization, plasma hormone concentrations, ratings of perceived effort, and endurance capacity. No differences were found in any of these variables between the group given ginseng and the control group. Other researchers reported similar

findings (Allen et al. 1998; Engels et al. 1997). At present, little or no evidence in the literature supports the claim that ginseng is an ergogenic aid.

Glycerol

Glycerol was believed to be a substrate for gluconeogenesis and, as such, could provide fuel during exercise. More recently, a probably more important role of glycerol became apparent—a way to hyperhydrate before exercise in hot conditions. Glycerol is a three-carbon molecule that normally serves as the backbone of a triacylglycerol molecule. We therefore ingest a fairly large amount of glycerol as part of triacylglycerol, on a daily basis. Glycerol is also released into the bloodstream after lipolysis. Thus, during exercise, when lipolysis is stimulated, plasma glycerol concentrations become elevated.

Fuel Source

The studies that investigated the efficacy of glycerol as a fuel found the contribution of glycerol

---

Species of Ginseng

Russian or Siberian ginseng	*Eleutherococcus senticosus*
Chinese or Korean ginseng	*Panax ginseng*
American ginseng	*Panax quinquefolium*
Japanese ginseng	*Panax japonicum*

Glandulars

Glandulars are extracts from animal glands such as the adrenals, the thymus, the pituitary, and the testes. They are claimed to enhance the function of the equivalent gland in the human body. For example, orchic extract from the testes supposedly enhances testosterone levels (Williams 1993). But glandular extracts are degraded during the digestive process and are inactive when absorbed. Therefore, they cannot exert a pharmacological effect.

to the overall energy expenditure to be relatively small. Glycerol cannot be oxidized directly in large amounts in the muscle. Therefore, glycerol must be converted into a glucose molecule in gluconeogenesis in the liver before being used as a fuel. This process is relatively slow, and, hence, the contribution of glycerol to fuel supply during exercise is negligible.

Hyperhydrating Agent

When ingested with a relatively large volume of water (1 to 2 L), glycerol improves water absorption (Wapnir et al. 1996) and increases water retention in the extracellular space, especially in plasma (Gleeson et al. 1986; Koenigsberg et al. 1995). This action may occur through either of two mechanisms: (1) Glycerol may move to the extracellular space and, through osmosis, draw water into this compartment. In other words, glycerol acts like a sponge. (2) A small increase in the plasma osmolarity may increase ADH secretion from the posterior pituitary gland, thus decreasing urine production. Hyperhydration with glycerol before exercise decreases overall heat stress during exercise, as indicated by a lower heart rate and body temperature (Lyons et al. 1990). The recommended protocol for the intake of glycerol and water before exercise is given in table 11.5.

Although these studies look promising, several studies found no effect of glycerol on thermoregulation (Inder et al. 1998; Latzka et al. 1997, 1998). In these studies, the volume of water consumed (500 ml) may have been too small. In a study by Murray et al. (1991), no indications of hyperhydra-

tion were found. Generally, however, the ingestion of 1 g/kg b.w. of glycerol with 1 to 2 L of water seems to protect against heat stress and thus may have some health benefits for those who exercise in extreme conditions. Some studies showed that reduced cardiovascular stress and decreased body temperature resulted in improved exercise performance. This finding could not be confirmed, even though those studies reported indications of improved thermoregulation. Whether glycerol improves endurance performance remains unclear. Glycerol has significant side effects, including nausea, heartache, blurred vision, headaches, gastrointestinal problems, dizziness, and light-headedness. Also, the large volume of fluid that needs to be consumed with the glycerol causes many users to feel bloated.

Inosine

Inosine is a nucleoside, a purine base comparable to adenine, which is one of the structural components of ATP. Inosine is obtained through the diet or synthesized endogenously in the body. Manufacturers claim that inosine increases ATP stores, thereby improving muscle strength, training quality, and performance. In addition, inosine is thought to improve oxygen delivery to the cells and to improve endurance. The latter belief is based on the role that inosine plays in the formation of 2,3-diphosphoglycerate, a substance in erythrocytes that facilitates the release of oxygen to the tissues. Other suggested mechanisms for ergogenic effects of inosine include augmenting cardiac con-

■ **TABLE 11.5** ■

Recommended Protocol for Glycerol and Water Intake to Optimize Preexercise Hydration

Glycerol ingestion starts 2.5 h (150 min) before exercise	
150 min preexercise	5 ml/kg glycerol in a 20% solution
120 min preexercise	5 ml/kg water
105 min preexercise	5 ml/kg water
90 min preexercise	5 ml/kg glycerol in a 20% solution + 5 ml/kg water
60 min preexercise	5 ml/kg water
0 min	Start exercise

Stated doses are in ml per kg of body weight.

tractility, vasodilating activity, and stimulation of insulin release, increasing glucose delivery to the myocardium. The studies that have investigated the effects of inosine on strength and endurance performance do not provide support for the claims and theories.

■ In one carefully conducted study, trained men (n = 4) and women (n = 5) were administered 6 g/day of inosine or placebo for 2 days (Williams et al. 1990). No change occurred in 3 mi (5 km) treadmill run time, $\dot{V}O_2$max, or perceived exertion, and blood lactate levels were also similar. After a 30-minute break, subjects performed another run, in which speed was kept constant but the gradient gradually increased. Time to fatigue in this run decreased with inosine (i.e., it had an ergolytic effect, an effect detrimental to performance).

■ Another study investigated the effects of 5 g/day of inosine or placebo for 5 days (Starling et al. 1996). No effects were found on performance in a 30-second Wingate test or a 30-minute self-paced time trial. In addition, a supramaximal constant-load sprint test was performed, and fatigue occurred 10% earlier with inosine compared with placebo, again indicating that inosine can be detrimental to performance. No effects were observed in heart rate or ratings of perceived exertion.

■ A study investigated the effects of 10 g/day of inosine supplementation over periods of 5 days and 10 days (McNaughton et al. 1999b). Seven trained volunteers performed tests—a 5 times 6-second sprint, a 30-second sprint, and a 20-minute time trial. Inosine supplementation did not affect performance. In addition, no changes in erythrocyte 2,3-diphosphoglycerate concentrations were observed.

Inosine has adverse effects in that it increases serum uric acid levels. The levels observed by Starling et al. (1996) are often associated with gouty arthritis, particularly pain in the knee and foot joints. Inosine has no ergogenic effects and can even be ergolytic. Inosine supplements should therefore be avoided.

Lactate Salts and Polylactate

Lactate is a good fuel for the human heart, and the rate of lactate clearance and oxidation in several studies exceeded the rates achieved by glucose. Most of the lactate that appears in the blood during moderate-intensity exercise is oxidized by the active muscle fibers with a high oxidative capacity. The lactate molecule possibly serves as a shuttle for transport of glucose-derived carbon moieties between various organs and cells (e.g., from the exercising muscle to the heart, from type II fibers in an active muscle to the neighboring type I fibers in the same muscle or to the type I fibers of another active muscle) (Brooks 1986). Lactate ingestion during exercise may provide a good fuel for the muscle.

Lactate Salts

Lactate can be provided as sodium or potassium lactate. A solution containing these salts, however, has extremely high osmolarity when significant amounts of lactate must be ingested. The amounts of sodium or potassium that would also have to be ingested are large and are likely to produce severe gastrointestinal problems. Solutions of lactate salts can be taken in maximal bolus amounts of about 10 g without causing gastrointestinal problems. The performance effects of these amounts have not been investigated but are expected to be nonexistent, given the amount of endogenous lactate formed.

Polylactate

The problem of too much lactate salt could theoretically be solved by using polylactate (see the following chemical compositions), a lactate polymer, which would reduce the osmolarity yet provide relatively large amounts of lactate.

$$CH_3\text{-}CH(OH)\text{-}COOH \ CH_3\text{-}CH(OH)\text{-}COO^- \ CH_3\text{-}CH(OH)\text{-}CO[O\text{-}CH(CH_3)\text{-}CO]n\text{-}OCH(CH_3)\text{-}COOH \ (polylactate)$$

Polylactate is used as a supplement and is included in some sports drinks. It can be produced through controlled chemical synthesis. If polylactate dissolved in water and could be quickly hydrolyzed in the gastrointestinal tract of humans, similarly to glucose polymers, it could be the ideal chemical form to ingest carbohydrate. But polylactate does not normally occur in food products and does not dissolve well in water. The human body does not contain enzymes to degrade polylactate. Thus, the bioavailablity and intestinal absorption are extremely low or even zero (Wagenmakers 1999). Because of its slow biodegradability, polylactate is used by orthopedic and dental surgeons to replace steel plates in the repair of broken bones. Polylactate, in the true chemical sense, cannot function to generate lactate at a high rate and cannot function as a nutritional ergogenic aid during exercise.

Two studies (Fahey et al. 1991; Swensen et al. 1994), nevertheless, claim to have investigated the performance effects of polylactate. A careful reading of the published papers reveals that the authors appear to have investigated the effects of a commercial product called Poly-L-lactate. This supplement contains molecules of lactate bound to amino acids. Because of the much larger molecular mass of the amino acids, the lactate content of this supplement is relatively low (<50% lactate). One of the amino acids is arginine, which is known to cause gastrointestinal problems when ingested in large amounts. Swensen et al. (1994) indeed observed severe gastrointestinal distress (abdominal cramping, diarrhea, and in some cases vomiting) when Poly-L-lactate was administered in concentrations of 5% (w/v) (~2.5% w/v lactate). To prevent gastric distress, Swensen et al. (1994) added only 0.75% Poly-L-lactate to a 6.25% glucose polymer solution and compared that with a 7% glucose polymer solution. As expected, given the fact that the energy content of the drinks was almost identical, no difference occurred in time to exhaustion during exercise at 70% of $\dot{V}O_2$max. Polylactate can therefore not be considered as an ergogenic aid. The main problem with lactate supplements (in each of the available forms) is that performance effects occur only at ingestion rates that are not tolerated by the gastrointestinal tract.

Lecithin

Lecithin, or phosphatidyl choline, is a phospholipid that occurs naturally in a variety of food items, including beans, eggs, and wheat germ. It contains both choline and phosphorus and is theorized to be an ergogenic aid for those reasons. It is claimed to improve strength and reduce fatigue. A study investigated the effect of lecithin on 15-minute, all-out cycling performance after a 105-minute ride at 70% of $\dot{V}O_2$max (Burns et al. 1988). No effects of two dosages of lecithin containing 1.1 g and 1.8 g of choline were observed. The only observed change was a rise in plasma choline concentration. Lecithin, therefore, does not appear to be an ergogenic aid. (See also the sections on choline and phosphorus.)

Medium-Chain Triacylglycerol

Medium-chain triacylglycerol (MCT) is sold as a supplement to replace normal fat because MCT is said not to be stored in the body and is suggested to help athletes to lose body fat. For a while this was a popular supplement among bodybuilders. It was also used as an extra energy source in various energy bars. MCT is normally present in our diet in small quantities, and a few natural sources are available. MCT is usually synthesized from coconut oil. After hydrolysis of the oil, the medium-chain and long-chain FAs are separated, and the fraction of medium-chain FAs is subsequently esterified to form an MCT. Medium-chain FAs are used in enteral and parenteral nutrition to provide patients with a rapidly available energy source. Because of this clinical use, a possible role for medium-chain FAs in sport nutrition became the subject of investigation.

Medium-chain FAs contain 8 to 10 carbons, whereas long-chain FAs contain 12 or more carbons. Unlike most long-chain triacylglycerols (LCTs), MCTs are liquid at room temperature, partly because of the small molecular size of MCTs. MCTs are more polar and therefore more soluble in water. This greater water solubility and smaller molecular size has consequences at all levels of metabolism. MCTs are more rapidly digested and absorbed in the intestine than LCTs are. Furthermore, medium-chain FAs follow the portal venous system and enter the liver directly, whereas long-chain FAs pass into the lacteals and follow the slow lymphatic system (Bach et al. 1982; Isselbacher 1968).

MCT may therefore be a valuable exogenous energy source during exercise in addition to carbohydrates (Jeukendrup et al. 1995). In addition, MCT ingestion may improve exercise performance by elevating plasma FA levels and sparing muscle glycogen (Van Zeyl et al. 1996) because it increases the availability of plasma FAs, reduces the rate of muscle glycogen breakdown, and delays the onset of exhaustion.

MCT added to carbohydrate drinks did not inhibit gastric emptying (Beckers et al. 1992). In fact, the drinks with MCT empty faster from the stomach than isoenergetic carbohydrate drinks. In a subsequent study, the oxidation rates of orally ingested MCT were investigated (Jeukendrup et al. 1995). In a randomized crossover design, eight well-trained athletes cycled 180 minutes at 57% of $\dot{V}O_2$max. Subjects ingested carbohydrate, carbohydrate plus MCT, or MCT. During the 60- to 120-minute period, the amount of MCT oxidized was 72% of the amount ingested with carbohydrate plus MCT, whereas during the MCT trial, only 33% was oxidized. It was concluded that more MCT is oxidized when ingested in combination with carbohydrate. Data confirmed that oral MCT might serve as an energy source in addition to glucose during exercise, because the metabolic availability of MCT was high during the last hour of exercise, with oxidation rates being as high as 70% of the ingestion rate. But the maximal amount of oral MCT tolerated in the gastrointestinal tract is about 30 g, and this small amount limited the contribution of oral MCT to between 3% and 7% of total energy expenditure (see figure 11.14).

Horowitz et al. (2000) argued that MCT ingestion might be particularly effective in reducing muscle glycogen breakdown in conditions where FA availability may be limiting fat oxidation, such as during high-intensity exercise. During exercise at 85% of $\dot{V}O_2$max, plasma FAs are reduced to extremely low levels, which reduces fat oxidation (Romijn et al. 1995). Therefore, Horowitz et al. (2000) fed their subjects 25 g of MCT 1 hour before 30 minutes of exercise at 84% $\dot{V}O_2$max. Plasma β-hydroxybutyrate levels were elevated after MCT ingestion, but plasma FA concentrations remained low during exercise. Thus, the MCT feedings did not affect glycogen breakdown. Van Zeyl et al. (1996) reported a reduction in the rate of muscle glycogen oxidation when a larger amount of MCT was ingested (86 g in 2 hours). They also claimed that MCT added to a 10% (w/v) carbohydrate solution improved time-trial performance in trained cyclists compared with a 10% carbohydrate solution alone. The authors did not report gastrointestinal disturbances. The same research group repeated the study with a low dose and a high dose of MCT (27 g and 54 g, respectively,

in 2 hours) (Goedecke et al. 1999) but could not reproduce the findings by Van Zeyl et al. (1996). In fact, although MCT ingestion did not affect gastrointestinal symptoms in this study, and plasma FA and β-hydroxybutyrate levels were elevated, fuel oxidation and exercise performance were unchanged. When a large amount of MCT was ingested in a study by Jeukendrup et al. (1998) (86 g in 2 hours), subjects experienced gastrointestinal problems, and their performance did not improve. In fact, MCT ingestion caused deterioration in performance compared with the placebo (water) treatment. Angus et al. (2000) studied the effects of carbohydrate plus MCT ingestion on 100 km time-trial performance. Subjects ingested 42 g/hour of MCT during their time trials in combination with carbohydrate, but performance was not affected.

MCT is rapidly emptied from the stomach, absorbed, and oxidized, and the oxidation of exogenous MCT is enhanced when coingested with carbohydrate. Ingestion of 30 g MCT does not affect muscle glycogen breakdown, and the contribution of MCT to energy expenditure is small. Ingestion of larger amounts of MCT results in gastrointestinal distress. Therefore, MCT does not appear to have the positive effects on performance that are often claimed.

Pangamic Acid

Pangamic acid, often referred to as vitamin B_{15}, is surrounded by many unfounded claims. Most of these claims are based on anecdotal reports of athletes (or manufacturers), and they include increased maximal oxygen uptake, reduced lactate formation, and improved performance. Two studies have found no effect of pangamic acid on lactate concentration in the blood or on performance (Girandola et al. 1980; Gray et al. 1982). Pangamic acid is not a vitamin, it is not essential, and it has no known function in the human body. In contrast, synthetic pangamic acid has been shown to be harmful (Herbert 1979), and FDA guidelines forbid the sale of pangamic acid as a dietary supplement or as a drug.

Phosphatidylserine

The supplement phosphatidylserine is usually a natural soy-derived glycerophospholipid. It is a typical structural component of cell membranes, and it has been hypothesized to alter the cell membrane phospholipid composition and hence the properties of the membrane. Theoretically, when

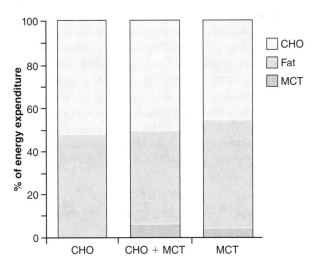

Figure 11.14 Small contribution of MCT to total energy expenditure.

phosphatidylserine is incorporated in cell membranes, it can alter the number and the affinity of various receptors. Phosphatidylserine has been suggested to alter the neuroendocrine response to stress (including exercise stress).

In one study, subjects received 800 mg/day of phosphatidylserine for 10 days (Monteleone et al. 1992). The stress response (as measured by plasma ACTH and cortisol concentration) after three 6-minute intervals of strenuous exercise was smaller than with placebo. These results agreed with earlier observations by the same researchers that phosphatidylserine injection reduced hypothalamic–pituitary–adrenal axis activation in humans (Monteleone et al. 1990). Phosphatidylserine potentially affects cognitive functioning. It reversed a memory decline that occurred in 25- to 65-year-old healthy humans (Crook et al. 1991). The authors of the study argued that phosphatidylserine is rapidly absorbed by the gut into the bloodstream and transported across the blood–brain barrier. It may also be rapidly incorporated into membranes of the central nervous system, which have naturally high phosphatidylserine content. This action could help to activate and regulate proteins involved in generation, storage, and reception of nerve impulses. Before definite conclusions can be drawn, however, more studies are needed.

Phosphatidylserine supplements that are for sale are derived from soybeans, whereas the phosphatidylserine in the previously mentioned studies was bovine derived (cerebral cortex). The possibility cannot be excluded that soy-derived phosphatidylserine has no effects or different effects than those reported in the studies. Also, whether the observed decreases in serum ACTH and cortisol concentrations are a desirable effect is not clear. Although cortisol is generally known as a catabolic hormone, and decreasing cortisol is hypothesized to decrease catabolism, no evidence supports this conclusion.

Phosphorus

The body contains about 850 g of phosphorus (phosphate salts), 80% of which is found in bone. Besides having a structural function in bone and teeth, phosphorus is a component of nucleic acids and cell membranes. Phosphorus is a component of the high-energy phosphates (ATP and PCr) and thus plays an important role in energy metabolism. It is also a cofactor or component for many B vitamins and 2,3-diphosphoglycerate (2,3 DPG)

in erythrocytes. Phosphate salts also serve as an important intracellular buffer.

Phosphorus is an essential nutrient. The RDA for males and females is 1,200 mg from 11 to 24 years of age. Persons older than 25 years have somewhat lower requirements (800 mg). Diets usually contain sufficient phosphorus because phosphorus is present in relatively large quantities in many foods.

Ingestion of larger amounts of phosphorus, or phosphate loading, has been suggested to result in improved performance. The proposed mechanisms include increased ATP synthesis (Chasiotis 1983) and improved oxygen extraction in muscle cells because of elevations of 2,3-DPG in erythrocytes. For these purposes phosphate salts are usually ingested in relative large quantities, typically 4 g/day.

Studies have found different results. An early study observed an increased $\dot{V}O_2$max and decreased lactate concentration at submaximal workload when eight cyclists ingested 4 g/day of sodium phosphate for 3 days (Cade et al. 1984). The study did not have a crossover design, but the control group, who received a placebo, did not show improvements. Three other studies reported similar findings after subjects ingested 3.6 to 4.0 g of sodium phosphate or tribasic sodium phosphate (Kreider et al. 1992, 1990; Stewart et al. 1990). In addition, improvements in 5 mi (8 km) run and 40 km time-trial performance were reported. But many studies did not find differences in $\dot{V}O_2$max, performance, or lactate concentrations (Bredle et al. 1988; Duffy et al. 1986; Galloway et al. 1996; Mannix et al. 1990).

The inconsistencies in these findings may be related to the differences in the experimental protocols (the amount of phosphate ingested, the timing of the ingestion, the type of subjects, the exercise mode, and so on). In addition, most of these studies used small numbers of subjects, which can make relatively small changes in exercise performance difficult to detect. At present, little scientific evidence indicates that phosphate loading improves exercise performance, and more studies are needed before we can confidently recommend phosphate as an ergogenic aid (Tremblay et al. 1994).

Pyruvate and Dihydroxyacetone

Pyruvate and dihydroxyacetone (DHA) are three-carbon intermediates of carbohydrate metabolism. They are formed in the glycolytic pathway. Some evidence suggests that supplementation or infusion of these metabolites can influence metabolism. Pyruvate and DHA are claimed to increase fat oxidation during exercise. They are also claimed to increase muscle glycogen storage, improve endurance capacity, and alter body composition (decrease fat mass).

Suggestions from the literature regarding the efficacy of pyruvate are based on long-term supplementation of pyruvate (7 days or more). Although only one study investigated the acute effects of pyruvate and lactate infusion, the results suggest a negative effect on running performance in rats compared with saline or glucose infusion (Bagby et al. 1978). Pyruvate infusion seemed to accelerate carbohydrate metabolism and increase both muscle and liver glycogen breakdown.

When pyruvate was given as a supplement to human subjects for 7 days, improved endurance capacity was observed in two studies from the same research group (Stanko et al. 1990a, 1990b). In the first study, subjects received 100 g/day of pyruvate-DHA or placebo (maltodextrins) for 7 days and performed arm ergometry to exhaustion before and after the supplementation period (Stanko et al. 1990b). Muscle biopsies taken from the triceps showed that muscle glycogen concentrations at rest were significantly elevated by the pyruvate-DHA supplementation (88 versus 130 mmol/kg w.w.). Endurance times increased from 133 minutes after the control diet to 160 minutes after pyruvate-DHA supplementation. In the second study, subjects consumed a high-carbohydrate diet for 7 days or a high-carbohydrate diet supplemented with 75 g of DHA and 25 g of pyruvate (Stanko et al. 1990a). Subjects performed cycling exercise to exhaustion at 70% of $\dot{V}O_2$max. Again, the supplement increased endurance time (79 minutes versus 66 minutes).

Morrison et al. (2000) administered a much smaller dose of pyruvate (7 g/day for 7 days) or placebo to seven trained cyclists in a randomized crossover trial. Subjects cycled to exhaustion at 74% to 80% of $\dot{V}O_2$max. Time to exhaustion did not increase with pyruvate, and with this smaller dose, no changes in blood pyruvate concentration were found.

No explanation is apparent for the improved endurance times reported by Stanko and colleagues (Stanko et al. 1990b). They measured fractional extraction of glucose across one leg at rest and during exercise and found that glucose uptake increased after pyruvate-DHA supplementation. They also observed that carbohydrate oxidation was unaffected, which suggests that subjects used

less muscle glycogen when supplemented with pyruvate-DHA. In the first study, muscle glycogen was not measured, and, therefore, this question could not be answered. In the second study, muscle biopsies were taken from the vastus lateralis, but no differences were found between the control diet and the pyruvate-DHA supplemented diet. Inconsistencies between the studies by Stanko et al. (1990b) and Morrison et al. (2000) may be related to the different dosages of pyruvate, the different training status of the subjects, or the coingestion of DHA in the study. More studies are needed before definitive conclusions can be drawn about the ergogenic effect of pyruvate.

Sodium Bicarbonate

When maximal exercise is performed for more than 30 seconds, most of the energy is derived from anaerobic glycolysis (see chapter 3). Lactic acid is formed at high rates, and the increased acidity of the muscle is an important limiting factor for performance in events lasting 1 to 10 minutes. Reducing the muscle acidity and increasing the buffering capacity are theoretically ways of improving performance in such events, and bicarbonate ingestion has been proposed as one of the ways to achieve these effects. A group of substances with this buffering function is the alkalinizers (e.g., sodium bicarbonate and sodium citrate). This section summarizes only the research findings on bicarbonate, but a number of detailed reviews have been published the past few years that are well worth studying (Horswill 1995; Linderman et al. 1994).

Anaerobic Glycolysis

Events of 60 seconds to 10 minutes, such as 400 m, 800 m, and 1,500 m running; track cycling events; and speed skating, rely heavily on anaerobic glycolysis for ATP regeneration. In this process, lactic acid is produced, resulting in decreased pH in the muscle cell. This increased acidity interferes with the contraction process, causing fatigue. From the moment this high-intensity exercise starts, lactic acid (hydrogen ions and lactate) builds up in the muscle and is transported into the blood. The decrease in muscle pH is therefore, with some delay, reflected by the blood pH.

The pH of blood is normally 7.4 and may decrease to 7.1 or slightly lower after high-intensity exercise. The pH of muscle is normally around 7.0 and may decrease to about 6.5. The body has several systems to adjust and regulate the acid–base balance. Chemical buffers provide an effective and rapid way of normalizing the H^+ concentration. Other systems include excretion of CO_2 by pulmonary ventilation and H^+ excretion by the kidneys.

The primary buffers in the muscle are phosphates and tissue proteins. The most important buffers in the blood are proteins, hemoglobin, and bicarbonate. During intense exercise, the intracellular buffers are insufficient to buffer all the hydrogen ions formed. The efflux of H^+ into the circulation increases, and bicarbonate has a role in buffering these H^+ ions.

$$H^+ + HCO_3^- \rightarrow H_2CO_3 \rightarrow H_2O + CO_2$$

The mechanism by which bicarbonate supposedly exerts its action is through this buffering of H^+ in the blood (not in the muscle as is often claimed). The buffering of H^+ in the blood, however, increases the H^+ gradient and increases efflux of H^+ from the muscle. Numerous studies on the effects of bicarbonate ingestion and exercise performance have yielded equivocal results.

Various studies suggest that a minimal dose of bicarbonate ingestion is needed to improve performance. Meta-analyses from the available literature suggest a dose-response relationship between the amount of bicarbonate ingested and the observed performance effect (Horswill 1995; Matson et al. 1993) (see figure 11.15). A dose of 200 mg/kg b.w. ingested 1 to 2 hours before exercise seems to improve performance in most studies, whereas 300 mg/kg b.w. seems to be the optimum dose (with tolerable side effects for most athletes). Doses of less than 100 mg/kg b.w. do not affect performance. This finding seems to make sense because a minimal amount of bicarbonate is needed to cause a significant increase in the buffering capacity of the blood. Intakes greater than

300 mg/kg b.w. tend to result in gastrointestinal problems (bloating, abdominal discomfort, and diarrhea). No studies show an effect on exercise performance in high-intensity exercise lasting less than 1 minute. Exercises such as squat, bench press, and jumping are unaffected. Also, exercise of long duration is generally unaffected. Therefore, a window for efficacy of bicarbonate has been identified between approximately 1 and 7 minutes. But a study by McNaughton et al. (1999a) showed improved performance in a 1-hour time trial, which was accompanied by higher blood pH throughout the exercise.

Side Effects

The side effects of sodium bicarbonate intake in such large doses can be severe. At doses of 300 mg/kg b.w. many athletes experience diarrhea, gastrointestinal discomfort, bloating, and cramps 1 hour after loading. The effects are dose dependent. The main causes of these problems are the large amount of sodium that is ingested with the bicarbonate and the reaction of bicarbonate with the HCl in the stomach, which generates a large volume of CO_2 that distends the stomach wall. Drinking large amounts of water during the loading is likely to alleviate some of the problems.

Sodium Citrate

Sodium citrate works similarly to bicarbonate. It increases the buffering capacity of the extracellular space to increase the efflux of hydrogen ions from the intracellular space. Sodium citrate is effective in limiting the decrease in blood pH and improving high-intensity exercise performance of 2- to 4-minute duration (McNaughton 1990; McNaughton et al. 1992). One study also showed improved performance in a 30 km cycling time trial (Potteiger et al. 1996). The typical doses for sodium citrate are 300 to 500 mg/kg b.w. Like sodium bicarbonate, sodium citrate is likely to cause gastrointestinal problems such as diarrhea, cramping, and bloating. Sodium citrate may act as a buffering agent, improving exercise performance in events up to about 10 minutes. It is said to improve high-intensity ($\sim 80\%$ $\dot{V}O_2$max) endurance performance, but this claim has not been proved.

Vanadium

Vanadium, a trace element widely distributed in nature and normally present in human tissues, has insulin-like properties. Foods that contain vana-

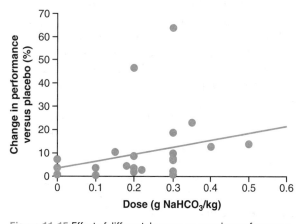

Figure 11.15 Effect of different dosages on exercise performance.
Adapted, by permission, from C.A. Horswill, 1995, "Effects of bicarbonate, citrate, and phosphate loading on performance," *International Journal of Sports Nutrition:* 5: S111-S119.

dium include cereal and grain products, dietary oils, meat, fish, and poultry. In supplements, vanadium is usually ingested as vanadyl sulphate or bis-maltolato-oxovanadium (BMOV). One of the reasons to ingest vanadium in these compounds is that less-toxic effects have been shown in rats.

The insulin-like effects of vanadium compounds are well documented in vitro and in vivo (Verma et al. 1998). In humans with type 2 diabetes mellitus (non-insulin-dependent diabetes mellitus), an increase in insulin-mediated glucose uptake (Halberstam et al. 1996), glycogen synthase activity, and glycogen synthesis has been demonstrated after vanadium administration (Cohen et al. 1995). These observations in insulin-resistant populations lead to suggestions that vanadium can help weight loss, improve insulin sensitivity, and increase muscle glycogen storage.

But no studies in healthy humans without insulin resistance are available that demonstrate insulin-like effects after acute or chronic administration of vanadium (compounds). In fact, a study did not show changes in insulin sensitivity measured with an oral glucose tolerance test in non-insulin-resistant subjects after acute or chronic (7 days) vanadyl sulphate administration (Jentjens et al. 2002). The amounts required for biological effects of vanadium in humans (1 to 2 mg · kg^{-1} · day^{-1}) obviously greatly exceeds the amounts that can be normally consumed in the diet (< 30 μg/day) (Verma et al. 1998).

Neither the short-term nor the long-term toxicity of the agents has been systematically studied in humans. Currently, no human studies are available that describe toxic effects after 2 to 10 weeks of vanadyl sulphate administration at dosages between 100 and 125 mg/day (Boden et al. 1996; Cohen et al. 1995; Halberstam et al. 1996). Some people may experience diarrhea, cramps, and nausea after intake of vanadium compounds. In rats, vanadium in excess amounts is toxic. Although some evidence indicates that vanadium can influence insulin sensitivity in patients with type 2 diabetes, such does not seem to be the case in healthy people. Thus, no evidence supports an ergogenic role of vanadium.

Wheat Germ Oil

Wheat germ oil is extracted from the embryo of wheat. It is high in linoleic acid, vitamin E, and octacosanol, a solid white alcohol that is theorized to have ergogenic effects. Wheat germ oil is advertised to increase endurance, stamina, and vigor. Several theories have been developed about the possible physiological effects of wheat germ oil, including enhanced glycogen metabolism and increased maximal oxygen uptake. Although many studies have focused on the metabolic effects of wheat germ oil, no evidence supports the contention that it is an effective ergogenic aid.

Contamination of Nutrition Supplements

Recently, speculation has arisen that some of the positive drug tests recorded in various sports have resulted from the use of nutrition supplements rather than deliberate use of banned products. Contamination of these supplements has been suggested as the reason for the positive drug tests. The supplements may have been contaminated with small amounts of prohormones or other compounds that are on the list of banned substances. The steroid nandrolone has been especially prominent. Some competitive athletes are afraid to take supplements because of uncertainty over which supplements are contaminated and which are clean.

The IOC-accredited laboratory in Cologne, Germany, reported that various steroids—including nandrolone and testosterone, as well as their precursor compounds—were found in various dietary supplements. In fact, of the 634 supplements tested, 94 of them (i.e., nearly 15%) contained enough anabolics to cause a positive result on a drug test. None of these products gave any indication on the label that they contained steroid compounds. Of the supplements made in the United States, almost 20% of the 240 tested products contained prohormones.

The substances in the following list are ingredients that have been identified in supplements and are either directly banned by the IOC or cause a positive doping outcome in some people:

- Ephedrine
- Strychnine
- Androstenedione, androstenediol, dehydroepiandrosterone (DHEA) (may lead to an elevated testosterone:epitestosterone ratio)
- 19-norandrostenedione, 19-norandrostenediol, and related compounds (may lead to a positive test for metabolites of the steroid nandrolone)

Because athletes sign a code of conduct, they are responsible for what they take, even supplements that have insufficient quality control or labeling.

Caffeine and pseudoephedrine were on this list as well, but because they have been taken off the list of banned substances and placed on a monitoring program, they will no longer cause positive doping tests.

Unfortunately, current legislation does little to protect athletes and other consumers from insufficiently labeled, mislabeled, contaminated, or even unsafe ingredients in dietary supplements. Although regulations vary widely from country to country, food supplements are never subject to the standard of manufacture and quality control that is required of foods and drugs. Also, legislation regarding product claims is less strict. Many manufacturers make claims that have never been proved scientifically. With clever marketing techniques and numerous retail outlets, supplement sellers make their products attractive and easy to obtain by athletes who do not know anything about the source or purity of the ingredients. Thus,

if an athlete decides that the benefits outweigh the risks of taking a supplement, a product from a large, respectable company is probably the best choice. Reputable brands of vitamins, minerals, and other common supplements manufactured by the major food and drug companies are normally manufactured to high standards and should be safe. Contamination is especially a problem in some smaller and more exotic companies. Companies that do not sell steroids and prohormones are less likely to have their products contaminated by those substances.

In the end, each athlete must do a cost–benefit analysis. On one side of the equation is the potential benefits of taking a product, which necessitate a thorough evaluation of the evidence to determine whether the benefits are real. On the other side is the risk, including the possibility that a seemingly innocent product may result in a positive doping test, with all the consequences that follow.

KEY POINTS

■ Nutritional supplements in one form or another are used by 40% to 100% of all athletes.

■ From a regulatory point of view, dietary supplements are treated as nutrition and are defined as vitamins, minerals, herbs and botanicals, amino acids, and other dietary substances intended to supplement the diet by increasing the total dietary intake, or as any concentrate, metabolite, constituent, or combination of these ingredients. No strict regulations apply to testing, advertising, and promoting nutrition supplements.

■ Few nutrition supplements have proved benefits in terms of performance, recovery, or effects on body weight or body composition.

■ Some evidence suggests that HMB can result in increased lean body mass and muscle strength. These findings, however, are mostly by one laboratory and need to be confirmed by others.

■ Caffeine (3 to 9 mg/kg b.w.) has an ergogenic effect in endurance exercise (1–2 hours) and exercise around 100% of $\dot{V}O_2$max lasting approximately 1 to 5 minutes as well as effects on cognitive functioning. Caffeine also has side effects that can include gastrointestinal distress, headaches, tachycardia, and restlessness.

■ Oral creatine supplementation of 20 g/day for 5 days increases total muscle creatine content in men by about 20% (30% to 40% of the increase is phosphocreatine). A subsequent daily dose of 2 g is enough to maintain this concentration. This quantity allows an increase in the amount of work performed during single and repeated bouts of short-term, high-intensity exercise but may also result in some weight gain.

■ A dose of 200 mg/kg b.w. of bicarbonate ingested 1 to 2 hours before exercise seems to improve performance in most studies, whereas 300 mg/kg d.w. seems to be the optimum dose. Side effects are diarrhea, gastrointestinal discomfort, bloating, and cramps 1 hour after loading.

RECOMMENDED READINGS

Bahrke, M.S., and C.E. Yesalis. 2002. *Performance enhancing substances in sport and exercise.* Champaign, IL: Human Kinetics.

Wagenmakers, A.J. 1999. Amino acid supplements to improve athletic performance. *Current Opinion in Clinical Nutrition and Metabolic Care* 2 (6): 539–544.

Williams, M.H. 1998. *The ergogenic edge.* Champaign, IL: Human Kinetics.

Williams, M.H., R.B. Kreider, and J.D. Branch. 1999. *Creatine: The power supplement.* Champaign, IL: Human Kinetics.

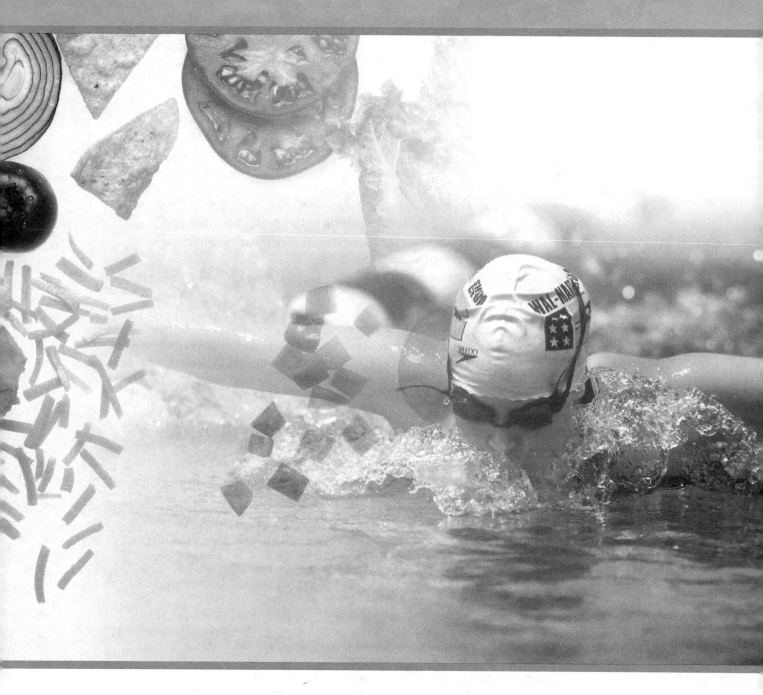

OBJECTIVES

After studying this chapter, you should be able to do the following:

- Describe the main adaptations to resistance and endurance training
- Discuss the mechanisms behind these changes and the molecular mechanisms underlying such changes
- Discuss how carbohydrate intake can influence signaling, protein synthesis, and training adaptations
- Discuss how antioxidants can influence signaling, protein synthesis, and training adaptations
- Discuss how carbohydrate intake can reduce symptoms of overreaching

12

Nutrition and Training Adaptations

Key Terms

Regular physical activity results in adaptations that eventually result in improved physiological function. **Exercise training** makes use of this principle by planning and systematically applying exercise activities with the goal to optimize those adaptations and thus improve performance. A multitude of adaptations occurs at all levels and in different organs in the body including increased capillarization, fast-to-slow muscle fiber type conversion, increased heart size, increased mitochondrial mass, increased muscle mass, and so on. Table 12.1 lists a number of adaptations to exercise (either resistance exercise or endurance exercise). Adaptations to exercise or exercise training are specific to the exercise performed. High-intensity (predominantly anaerobic) exercise will result in adaptations different from those resulting from moderate-intensity, longer-duration (aerobic) exercise. Resistance exercise typically results in a different phenotype than endurance training.

With resistance exercise, hypertrophy is one of the main adaptations, whereas endurance training will not increase muscle mass and may even decrease it. Endurance training, however, will result in greater oxidative capacity, increasing the fatigue resistance of the muscle. This chapter will review the following: How does exercise result in training adaptations? Which signals and mechanisms are involved? How is it possible that different types of exercise training result in very different training adaptations? And how can nutrition modify these adaptations? Initially we will look at the signals responsible for the changes. Then we will study the effects of exercise on a variety of proteins, and finally we will look at ways in which nutritional manipulation can alter (improve) the training adaptations.

Training Adaptations

Resistance training results in a number of adaptations in the muscle including an increase in the muscle cross-sectional area (hypertrophy) and altered neural recruitment patterns. For hypertrophy to occur, the rate of myofibrillar protein synthesis must exceed the rate of myofibrillar protein breakdown over a certain period. Myofibrillar hypertrophy can occur through two processes: an increase in the number of nuclei within each muscle fiber or an increase in the amount of contractile material supported by each nucleus. Generally, resistance training does not increase the oxidative capacity of the muscle much, although some studies have observed improvements in oxidative enzyme activity (citrate synthase). The type and intensity of resistance training and the length of the recovery intervals may determine whether such adaptations take place.

Endurance exercise training is characterized by the development of improved fatigue resistance partly because of increased mitochondrial density and thus mitochondrial protein. In addition, alterations occur in neural recruitment patterns, substrate utilization, and acid–base balance. Intramuscular glycogen stores as well as triacylglycerol stores increase after endurance training, although the amounts of both these fuel stores depend on the time since the last exercise session and the adequacy of nutrition in the postexercise period. Reliance on carbohydrate (glycogen) as a fuel decreases, and the ability to oxidize fat increases. These changes result in sparing of muscle glycogen during exercise. Endurance training does not greatly alter muscle fiber size, although an increase in the cross-sectional area of type I fibers

▪ TABLE 12.1 ▪
Training Adaptations

	Endurance training	Strength training
Capillary density	++	
Muscle glycogen	++	++
Number of mitochondria	++	+
Mitochondrial density	++	+
Resting ATP	−	+
Resting PCr	−	+
Glycolytic enzymes	−	+
Phosphofructokinase	−	+
Oxidative enzymes	++	−/+
Succinate dehydrogenase	++	+
Citrate synthase	++	+
HAD	++	+
Maximum cardiac output	++	+
Maximum oxygen uptake ($\dot{V}O_2max$)	++	+
Maximum heart rate	−	−
Plasma volume	++	
Muscle fiber size	−	++
Fat oxidation	++	+

of around 20% has been observed in some studies. Endurance training can increase the mitochondrial protein content of the muscle by 50 to 100% in 6 weeks (Hoppeler and Fluck, 2003). The training adaptation is only temporary, and if the training stimulus is not maintained mitochondrial proteins will be broken down again. Their half-life is only about 1 week. The best predictors of performance improvements are mitochondrial density and mitochondrial enzyme activity. The increase in size and number of mitochondria is usually referred to as **mitochondrial biogenesis.**

Exercise will increase net protein synthesis after both resistance and endurance exercise (see chapter 8) if dietary protein and energy intakes are adequate. Studies have typically looked at mixed muscle protein synthesis without specifically looking at which proteins are synthesized. It is likely that with resistance exercise there is synthesis of predominantly actin and myosin, whereas endurance exercise results mostly in mitochondrial biogenesis with little or no change in the synthesis of myofibrillar proteins. A study confirmed this in humans: Resistance exercise increased protein synthesis specifically in the myofibrillar fraction, and endurance exercise increased protein synthesis predominantly in the mitochondrial fraction (Wilkinson et al. 2008). The increase in protein synthesis after resistance or endurance exercise may last for up to 2 to 4 days after the last training session.

Ultimately, all adaptations, whether an increase in muscle mass or an increase in mitochondrial mass, result from increases in certain proteins. The complex process of exercise-induced adaptation in skeletal muscle starts with specific molecular events that trigger an increase in protein synthesis. More specifically, signaling mechanisms triggered by exercise stress initiate replication of deoxyribonucleic acid (DNA) genetic sequences (genes) that enable subsequent translation of the genetic code into a series of amino acids to synthesize new proteins (see appendix A for a basic description of the processes involved). The synthesis of these specific proteins ultimately results in adaptations. As discussed earlier, adaptations to training are highly specific to the type of training, suggesting that different signaling events may be involved. The signaling events and the resulting increases in messenger ribonucleic acid (mRNA), as well as the synthesis of proteins, depend on the intensity and duration of exercise, the type of exercise performed, and the intake of specific nutrients. The following section examines the molecular signaling events that underlie the training adaptations and the effects that different modes of exercise and nutrition can have on these events as well as on the outcome.

Signal Transduction Pathways

Protein synthesis is regulated by **signal transduction pathways** that sense and compute local and systemic signals and regulate various cellular functions. The main signaling mechanisms are the phosphorylation of serine, threonine, and tyrosine residues by kinases and their dephosphorylation by phosphatases. The growth, metabolism, and proliferation of muscle fibers and most other functions depend on signals like nutrient availability, pH, partial pressure of oxygen, reactive oxygen species (ROS), and mechanical stimuli. The nervous and endocrine systems provide further inputs. Cells detect this ever-changing mix of signals through specific sensor proteins. Examples of sensor proteins are cell membrane receptors and amino acid, calcium, or AMP-sensing proteins. Activation of a sensor protein will trigger a cascade of reactions. These cascades of reactions form the link between the signals and the change in cellular function.

Protein kinases are typically part of a cascade of reactions that generally follows the sequence of events depicted in figure 12.1. This model is

---

Control by Signal Transduction Pathways

Signal transduction pathways control the following processes:

1. Transcription of genes (specific sequences of DNA) into mRNA
2. Translation of mRNA into protein
3. Protein modification altering catalytic activity
4. Regulation of protein degradation
5. Regulation of cell division, proliferation, and fusion

Signal → sensor protein → kinase A → kinase B → kinase C → regulatory protein → changed cellular function

Figure 12.1 Simplified model of a typical kinase signaling pathway.

oversimplified because many signals converge or branch off.

These signal transduction pathways can then influence a number of cellular events (see the highlight box and figure 12.2) and will ultimately result in altered function. The preceding general description of signaling pathways probably applies to most cells in most situations. The details of these signaling cascades, the triggers, the proteins, and the kinases involved are different in different tissues and different situations. To understand adaptations in muscle cells in response to exercise training, the signaling pathways in muscle have to be studied in more detail.

During exercise, cellular homeostasis is disturbed and initiates a cascade of events that ultimately result in an adaptation that will cause less disturbance of homeostasis the next time that the same exercise is performed. During exercise these signals include changes in muscle stretch or tension, changes in intracellular calcium ion (Ca^{2+}) concentrations, changes in the energy charge of the cell, and changes of the redox potential. Certain hormones and other ligands that can bind to receptors on the cell surface can alter these signals. These primary messengers may then trigger a series of secondary molecular events that increase or decrease transcription or translation as described in figure 12.3. The following section looks at the primary signals in detail.

Starting a Signaling Cascade

The basis for any training adaptation is a disturbance of homeostasis. Metabolic or mechanical changes in the muscle start a signaling cascade that results in the relevant proteins being broken down and synthesized. These initial signals are discussed next.

Muscle Stretch and Tension

Mechanical perturbations of skeletal muscle cells cause activation of a number of signaling pathways. More specifically, muscle stretch or altered tension can induce activation of calcineurin, mitogen-activated protein kinase (MAPK), and insulin-like growth factor (IGF) signaling cascades.

Ca^{2+}

Neural activation of skeletal muscle generates an action potential that results in Ca^{2+} release from the T-tubules of the sarcoplasmic reticulum. When the exercise is stopped the Ca^{2+} returns back from the cytoplasm to the sarcoplasmic reticulum. The fluctuations in Ca^{2+} concentration or the release and reuptake of Ca^{2+} in the sarcoplasmic reticulum are different for different types of activities, which could at least partly explain the differences in the adaptive response to exercise. Endurance exercise, for example, results in more prolonged and moderately elevated concentrations, whereas high-intensity exercise causes shorter periods of very high Ca^{2+} concentrations. Elevations of Ca^{2+} concentration in the muscle cytoplasm activate calmodulin kinase (**CaMK**) and calcineurin (**CaN**).

Perturbations in Cellular Energy Balance

During muscle contraction, ATP is broken down to provide energy. In this process ADP and Pi are formed. ADP is then resynthesized to ATP by glycolysis or oxidative phosphorylation. Some ADP is further broken down to AMP. The ratio of metabolites ADP, AMP, and Pi relative to that of ATP is often referred to as the energy charge. If a lot of ATP is present and little of the metabolites,

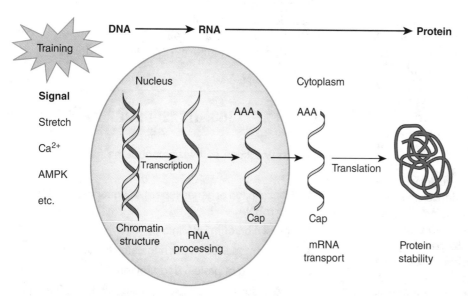

Figure 12.2 Training adaptations result from an increase in protein synthesis in response to repeated exercise sessions. It is believed that an exercise session causes a signal to transcribe DNA in the nucleus into RNA, which is then transported out of the nucleus and translated into protein. The signal caused by the exercise stimulus determines which proteins are synthesized. The amount of protein formed is determined not only by the signal, the transcription, and translation but also by the RNA processing and the stability of proteins.

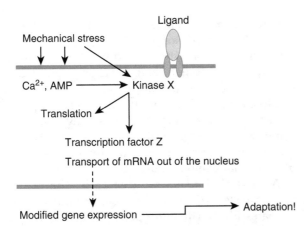

Figure 12.3 Simplified model of signal transduction in relation to exercise. Muscle contraction may result in a disturbance of homeostasis. Mechanical stress (stretch, tension), Ca^{2+}, and the accumulation of AMP or metabolites are primary signals that affect the phosphorylation state of various kinases. These kinases can influence the transcription process, the transport of mRNA out of the cell, and translation. Hormones and other ligands can influence these signals. The changes in gene expression can result in different adaptations.

the energy charge is high. If the concentration of metabolites rises, the energy charge is low. These metabolites are important regulators of metabolism, but they also serve as signaling molecules. AMP in particular can activate 5'adenosine activated protein kinase (**AMPK**), a potent secondary messenger. AMPK seems to play a role in the regulation of a variety of processes including glucose uptake, fatty acid oxidation, hypertrophy, and gene expression. The redox potential is another indicator of the energy status of the cell. If the ratio of the oxidized form of the coenzyme nicotinamide adenine dinucleotide (NAD^+) to its reduced form (NADH) is high, poor energy status is indicated. The maintenance of redox potential produces volatile free-radical oxygen molecules (reactive oxygen species, or ROS). These ROS are also thought to play a role in the exercise-induced signaling that will ultimately be responsible for training adaptations. This signaling may work by ROS acting on transcription factors like nuclear factor kappa B (NFKB) and activator protein 1 (AP1).

Hormones can affect the activation of kinases as well. The hormone or other ligand binds to a receptor, which then changes the phosphorylation state of a kinase. For example, when thyroid hormone (tri-iodothyronine, or T3) binds to its receptor, the process induces phosphorylation of AMPK in skeletal muscle.

The primary messengers activate a series of secondary messengers. These secondary messengers are often kinases and phophatases, which are

activated to pass on the exercise-induced signal. The secondary messengers often involve a complex series of reactions (cascades), which are highly regulated. Next we will discuss some of the most studied messengers.

Secondary Signals

The initial signals almost immediately trigger a secondary response. This response usually involves the phosphorylation of certain kinases (or dephosphorylation of phosphatases). These kinases will then activate or deactivate another kinase or have a direct effect on a specific protein that alters the function. Only the most relevant and most investigated signals will be discussed here.

AMPK

AMPK plays a crucial role in energy metabolism and acts as a metabolic master switch that regulates several intracellular systems including the cellular uptake of glucose, the β-oxidation of fatty acids, and the biogenesis of glucose transporter 4 (GLUT4) and mitochondria (figure 12.4). The energy-sensing capability of AMPK can be attributed to its ability to detect and react to fluctuations in the AMP:ATP ratio that take place during rest and exercise. Muscle contraction is associated with an increase in the demand for cellular ATP, which subsequently increases the AMP:ATP ratio. AMPK is activated by an increase in the AMP:ATP ratio.

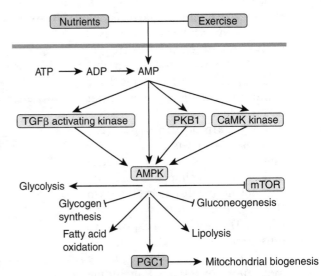

Figure 12.4 A change in the AMP:ATP ratio activates AMPK by activating AMPK kinases (LKB1, CaMK kinases, and the TGF-β activating kinase). AMPK then acts as a metabolic master switch, turning on processes that generate ATP and turning off processes that use ATP. It also causes an adaptation so that the next time the same stress is applied, the cell will be better adapted.

Acute activation of AMPK results in a response that aims to conserve energy (limit ATP use) and generate more ATP. For example, AMPK activation results in an increase in glucose uptake and an increase in fat oxidation so that ATP can be generated. When AMP is high and ATP is low, AMP activates AMPK by dislodging ATP from the α-subunit of AMPK and making it more sensitive to phosphorylation by AMPK kinases (Scott et al. 2007). In skeletal muscle, the major AMPK kinase appears to be LKB1, although the CaMK kinases and the transforming growth factor (TGF)-β activating kinase may also activate AMPK (figure 12.4).

Winder and Hardie et al. (1996) were the first to demonstrate that AMPK could be activated by exercise. They demonstrated that when rats ran at a high intensity, AMPK activity increased two-and-a-half-fold within the first five minutes and did not increase any further after 30 minutes (Winder and Hardie et al. 1996). In humans, 20 minutes of cycling at 70% of $\dot{V}O_2$max increased the activity of the α2 AMPK isoform, without altering α1 AMPK activity (Fujii et al. 2000). Cycling at a lower intensity (50% of $\dot{V}O_2$max) for the same 20 minutes did not activate either α1 or α2 AMPK. Together these data suggest that intense endurance exercise activates α2 AMPK. It has been suggested that resistance exercise may be different. In a study in which muscles were electrically stimulated, Atherton et al. (2005) showed that after endurance exercise AMPK was activated, but with resistance exercise no change in AMPK activation occurred. More recently, however, it was demonstrated that humans who are unaccustomed to resistance exercise can also show increased activation of AMPK (Coffey et al. 2006). It was also shown that endurance-trained athletes have a blunted AMPK response after endurance exercise.

Ca^{2+} Calmodulin-dependent kinases (CaMK) is a name for a family of various kinases can detect and respond to changes in calcium concentrations. It has been shown that certain isoforms of CaMK (CaMKII) can also respond to muscle stretch. After CaMK is activated, a number of other signaling molecules are activated, including nuclear factor of activated T-cells (NFAT) and histone deacetylase (HDAC). Calcineurin is another molecule that is activated by Ca^{2+}. Calcineurin is known to act as a coregulator of **muscle hypertrophy** in combination with insulin-like growth factor (IGF), but it also has a role in fiber-type transformation (fast twitch to slow twitch) and the expression of the genes of oxidative enzymes.

The insulin and insulin-like growth factor pathways play an important role in muscle hypertrophy. Contractile activity stimulates the release of IGF-1, which binds to its receptor and initiates a cascade of molecular events (figure 12.5).

After IGF binds to its receptor, insulin receptor substrate 1 (IRS1) is activated, and this in turn activates PI3K. The latter activates PDK1, which in turn phosphorylates Akt. Akt has numerous targets including those involved in protein synthesis (mTOR and tuberous scelorosis complex 2, TSC2), glycogen synthesis (glycogen synthase kinase 3, GSK3), protein degradation (forkhead Box O1, FoxO1), and glucose transport (Akt substrate of 160 kDa, AS160). There is strong evidence that the **Akt-mTOR pathway** is involved in hypertrophy through activating translation initiation as well as increasing the ribosomal protein content. The response of Akt to exercise is unclear at the moment, and studies have found either increases or no change in response to exercise. This is likely because of the central role of Akt in regulating muscle hypertrophy as well as glucose transport. The Akt response may therefore be highly specific to the type of exercise and is probably influenced by many other factors. mTOR responds to a number of different stimuli and can have effects on mRNA translation, the synthesis of ribosomes, as well as metabolism.

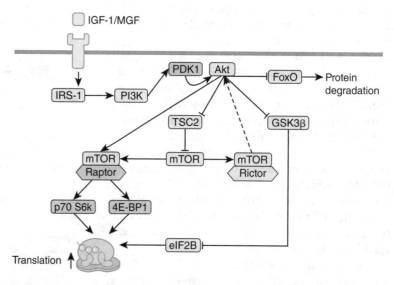

Figure 12.5 The insulin and insulin-like growth factor pathways play an important role in muscle hypertrophy through the Akt-mTOR signaling cascade.

Two mTOR protein complexes exist where mTOR binds with a G-β-L protein and either a rapamycin-sensitive raptor or a rictor protein. mTOR-raptor complex is a positive regulator of cell growth, and mTOR-rictor appears to have a key role in Akt activation and actin cytoskeleton regulation. Primary downstream targets of mTOR-raptor include p70 S6 kinase (p70 S6K), eIF4E-binding protein (4E-BP1), and eIF4B (not shown in figure 12.5). These downstream targets increase mRNA translation and increased protein synthesis. It is generally thought that mTOR plays a central role in the adaptation to resistance exercise.

PGCs

One family of transcriptional regulators in particular, the peroxisome proliferator-activated receptor γ coactivator family (**PGCs**), PGC-1α, PGC-1β, and the PGC-1 related coactivator (PRC), is important in driving mitochondrial biogenesis. The PGCs are coactivators of the peroxisome proliferator-activated receptor γ (PPAR-γ). A transcription coactivator is defined as a protein or protein complex that increases the probability of a gene being transcribed by interacting with transcription factors but does not itself bind to DNA in a sequence-specific manner. The activity and the expression of PGCs rapidly increase following a single bout of endurance exercise. PGC mRNA increases 1.5- to 10-fold following a single bout of exercise (Pilegaard et al. 2003; Baar et al. 2002; Wright et al. 2007). PGCs increase oxidative capacity and endurance performance. Therefore, the goal of endurance athletes and coaches should be to maximize the activation of PGC signaling pathways in skeletal muscle.

Consequently, it has been hypothesized that AMPK might mediate the increase in PGCs in response to training. Indeed, in humans, moderate to high intensity endurance exercise increases the amount of AMPK in muscle cells (McGee et al. 2003). These findings put AMPK directly upstream of PGCs, potentially governing the level of PGCs and therefore the metabolic state of the muscle. As a result, training that increases AMPK activity should be beneficial for endurance performance. It has also been suggested that central nervous system activity through β-adrenergic receptors may play a significant role in the activation of PGCs and the subsequent increase in mitochondria.

Time Course of Events

Typically, the initial response to exercise occurs within seconds or minutes. For example, changes in intracellular calcium are instant. Then a cascade of reaction follows. The activation of various kinases can take a bit longer, and some kinases may not reach their maximal activity until several hours after exercise. Gene expression seems to peak between 4 and 12 hours after exercise, possibly depending on the gene and the type of exercise performed. In one study, myogenic and metabolic genes peaked at 4 to 8 hours after resistance exercise. After endurance exercise, myogenic genes peaked after 8 to 12 hours (Yang et al. 2005). The changes in protein synthesis can be observed within hours after exercise but may peak many hours later. In fact, studies have demonstrated increased protein synthesis up to 48 hours after exercise. An overview of the changes is depicted in figure 12.6.

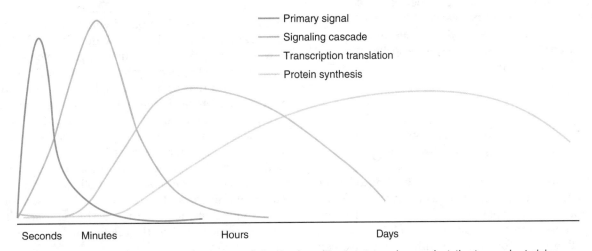

Figure 12.6 A rough overview of the time course of changes in various events causing an adaptation to exercise training.

The Link With Protein Synthesis

Several studies have investigated the signaling pathways that are activated by exercise, but few studies have linked these changes with actual changes in protein synthesis. Note that although these signals can increase the synthesis of mRNA, protein synthesis may not necessarily increase. The rate of protein synthesis depends on mRNA degradation, additional translational control mechanisms, transport of mRNA out of the nucleus, and the translation process.

Effect of Training Type

In an elegant study, Wilkinson et al. (2008) investigated changes in signaling and protein synthesis before and after a 10-week training program consisting of endurance or resistance exercise. They distinguished between mitochondrial and myofibrillar protein synthesis. They found that untrained subjects increased both mitochondrial and myofibrillar protein synthesis after a bout of resistance exercise (when fed). Endurance exercise resulted in an increase only in mitochondrial protein synthesis. After 10 weeks of training, however, the response was more specific. Resistance exercise resulted in an increase only in myofibrillar protein synthesis, and endurance training only in mitochondrial biosynthesis. Differences in translation initiation explained little of these observed differences in protein synthesis, so the mechanism for the distinctly different adaptations to resistance and endurance exercise remains unknown. Although it has been suggested that AMPK activation during endurance exercise may reduce mTOR activity and prevent muscle hypertrophy, evidence for this theory in humans is lacking. In the years to come much about these signaling pathways will be discovered. New proteins and new phosphorylation sites on existing proteins will be identified. All can play a role in the regulation of the adaptive response.

Nutrition Effects on Training Adaptations

Nutrients can have an effect on signaling and thus have the potential to regulate or alter the training adaptation. In chapter 9, for example, we discussed that the amino acid leucine not only serves as a building block for protein synthesis but also can function as a signaling molecule. This function of leucine can result in greater rates of protein synthesis. Similar functions have been suggested for muscle glycogen, reactive oxygen species, cytokines, and various inflammatory markers. Nutrition can play an important role in modulating the levels of these molecules. Here we will discuss some of these effects, starting with muscle glycogen, which has received by far the most attention.

Glycogen on the Signaling Response

A single bout of endurance exercise will increase transcription or mRNA content for various metabolic and stress-related genes. Typically, transcriptional activity peaks within the first few hours of recovery and returns to baseline within 24 hours. These findings have led to the overall hypothesis that training adaptations in skeletal muscle may be generated by the cumulative effects of transient increases in **gene transcription** during recovery from repeated bouts of exercise.

A number of studies have reported that altering substrate availability during exercise (e.g., by increasing dietary fat intake or commencing exercise with low muscle glycogen) can influence metabolic gene transcription, suggesting that modification of the training response may be possible through specific diet interventions. It has been shown that commencing endurance exercise with low muscle glycogen increases the activity of several metabolic genes and signaling proteins. In a study by Pilegaard et al. (2002), six untrained male volunteers performed 2.5 hours of cycling at 45% of $\dot{V}O_2$max. One day before the experiment, subjects performed 90 minutes of one-legged cycling to reduce the muscle glycogen content in that leg. On the day of the experiment, muscle biopsies were taken from both legs at rest before exercise, immediately postexercise, and 2 and 5 hours postexercise. Compared with the control leg, the leg that exercised the previous day had 45% lower resting preexercise muscle glycogen content. Following 2.5 hours of cycling at 45% of $\dot{V}O_2$max, it was found that transcriptional activity of pyruvate dehydrogenase kinase 4 (PDK4), uncoupling protein 3 (UCP3), and hexokinase II (HKII) was significantly higher in the leg that exercised with low muscle glycogen. Because both the control leg and the low-glycogen leg were exposed to the same systemic concentrations of metabolites, hormones, catecholamines, and cytokines, it is reasonable to assume that increased transcriptional activity was in someway directly related to low muscle glycogen content.

The role of muscle glycogen could be explained by the fact that some signaling proteins (e.g., AMPK) possess glycogen-binding domains and that when glycogen is low, these proteins are more active toward their specific targets. In support of this, Wojtaszewski et al. (2003) reported that AMPK activity was elevated when a standardized bout of exercise (1 hour of cycling at 70% $\dot{V}O_2$max) was undertaken with low muscle glycogen (160 compared with 900 mmol/kg d.w.). Elevated AMPK activity with low muscle glycogen may be beneficial to individuals undertaking exercise training because AMPK is believed to play a critical role in regulating the adaptive response. Commencing endurance exercise with low muscle glycogen has also been shown to increase the activity of p38 mitogen-activated protein kinase (p38 MAPK), and like AMPK, p38 MAPK is thought to be a regulator of mitochondrial biogenesis and endurance-training adaptations.

The aforementioned studies provide early evidence to suggest that training with low muscle glycogen might be a useful strategy to promote endurance-training adaptations. Further studies are clearly needed before this proposition can be confirmed or dismissed.

Train Low, Compete High

Only one study has determined whether long-term training with low muscle glycogen can enhance the adaptive response to endurance training. Hansen et al. (2005) recruited seven untrained males to undertake a 10-week program of knee extensor exercise. Each of the subjects' legs was trained according to a different schedule, but the total amount of work performed by each leg was kept the same. One leg was trained twice a day every second day, whereas the other leg was trained once daily. This protocol meant that the leg that trained twice every second day commenced half of the sessions with low muscle glycogen. Compared with the leg that trained with normal glycogen levels, the leg that commenced half of the training sessions with low muscle glycogen had more pronounced increases in resting muscle glycogen content and citrate synthase activity. Time to fatigue at 90% of maximal power output increased in both legs after training (figure 12.7). Performance times, however, were nearly twice as long in the leg that trained with low muscle glycogen (19.7 $\pm$ 2.4 versus 11.9 $\pm$ 1.3 minutes). These remarkable findings demonstrate that, under the specific conditions of the study, training with low muscle glycogen enhanced adaptations in skeletal muscle and improved exercise performance. But a number of details make it difficult to extrapolate these findings. First, the subjects recruited were untrained, so it is not yet known whether training with low muscle glycogen will translate into improved adaptations in well-trained athletes. Second, subjects performed a fixed amount of work even though higher glycogen

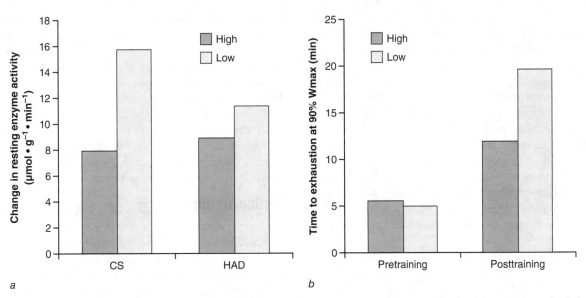

a   b

Figure 12.7 Single-leg training study in which one leg trained with low glycogen 50% of the time (low) and the other leg trained always with high glycogen (high). Training with low glycogen resulted in (a) an increase in oxidative enzymes (citrate synthase and β-hydroxyacyl-CoA dehydrogenase) and (b) improved endurance capacity after 10 weeks of knee extensor training.

Data from Hansen et al. 2005.

stores would normally allow exercise to be performed at higher intensities or longer durations. Third, it is difficult to translate the results from a single-leg kicking exercise to that of real-life sporting situations involving activities such as running, cycling, or swimming.

To take these findings to a more realistic sporting situation, researchers in Melbourne (Australia) and Birmingham (United Kingdom) investigated the effects of a 3-week training program in which all of the training was performed in the glycogen-loaded state or in which half of the training was performed in a glycogen-depleted state (Yeo et al. 2008). The performance during the self-paced training sessions in the glycogen-depleted state was significantly impaired. The subjects who always trained when glycogen loaded trained at higher absolute intensities. Despite this, however, at the end of the training period, performance improved equally in the low-glycogen group and the high-glycogen group. The metabolic adaptations in the two groups were very different though. The low-glycogen group had a greater oxidative capacity as evidenced by greater citrate synthase (TCA cycle enzyme) and β-hydroxyacyl dehydrogenase (rate-limiting enzyme of FA β-oxidation) activities as well as greater COX IV content. Fat oxidation was also enhanced in the low-glycogen group. So these findings partly confirm the findings of the single-leg study by Hansen et al. (2005). The difference is that although adaptations were observed in metabolism, no differences in performance occurred after 3 weeks. Of course, it may be that 3 weeks is sufficient to see differences in metabolism but not long enough to see improvements in performance. Future studies should investigate longer-term training protocols.

So it seems fair to conclude that endurance training in a glycogen-depleted state results in improved capacity to use fat to fuel exercise. The mechanisms behind this adaptation are unclear but may involve activation of the peroxisome proliferator-activated receptors (PPARs). The PPARs are a group of nuclear receptor proteins that function as transcription factors regulating the expression of genes. PPARs play an essential role in the regulation of metabolism as well as many other processes.

Narkar et al. (2008) recently showed that training rats on a treadmill while at the same time giving them a drug that activated a transcription factor called PPAR∂ resulted in the same changes that occur when training in the glycogen-depleted state: increased capacity to use fat as a fuel. PPAR∂

increases the concentration of the enzymes that are required for oxidizing fatty acids. The result in this study was that the rats that both got the drug and trained on the treadmill increased their ability to run at about 50% of $\dot{V}O_2$max by 70% over those that just ran on the treadmill. It is possible that exercising in a glycogen-depleted state activates PPAR∂ to a greater extent than does training in the glycogen-loaded state. PPAR∂ seems to be activated by a by-product of the breakdown of fat in muscle. As discussed earlier, exercising in the glycogen-depleted state increases both circulating FA concentration and oxidation of fat during exercise, resulting in more of the by-product and more PPAR∂ activation.

Few studies have investigated the effects of high- and low-carbohydrate diets on longer-term training adaptations. Simonsen et al. (1991) determined the effect of 4 weeks of moderate or high carbohydrate intake (5 or 10 g · kg b.w.$^{-1}$ · day^{-1}) on muscle glycogen concentration, training capacity, and exercise performance in 22 collegiate rowers (12 males and 10 females). Rowers trained twice daily throughout the 4-week period. Morning training sessions consisted of 40 minutes at 70% of $\dot{V}O_2$max, whereas evening training sessions consisted of 2,500 m time trials or high-intensity interval training (~90% of $\dot{V}O_2$max). Consuming the moderate-carbohydrate diet maintained muscle glycogen concentrations throughout the 4-week period, but consuming the high-carbohydrate diet resulted in a progressive increase in muscle glycogen concentrations, which were 65% higher by the end of the 4th week of training. Power output during 2,500 m time trials increased by 1.6% and 10.7% after 4 weeks of training with moderate- and high-carbohydrate diets, respectively. These are the first findings to demonstrate that consuming a high-carbohydrate diet can improve training adaptation and enhance performance following training.

So although the results of studies suggest that training with low glycogen could have some metabolic advantages, whether this results in improvements in performance is not clear.

Fasting Training

For many years, endurance athletes (mainly runners and cyclists) have used exercise without breakfast as a way to increase the oxidative capacity of the muscle. This protocol has often been termed *fat-burning training*. Ingesting carbohydrate in the hours before exercise will raise plasma insulin and subsequently suppress fat oxidation by up to about 35% (Achten et al. 2003). This effect of insulin on fat oxidation may last as long as 6 to 8 hours after a meal, so the highest fat oxidation rates can be achieved after an overnight fast. A study was performed at the University of Leuven in Belgium in which the effect of an endurance-training program (6 weeks, 3 days/week, 1-2 hours) in the fasted or carbohydrate-fed state was investigated (Bock et al. 2008). The investigators observed a decrease in muscle glycogen use, and the activity of various proteins involved in fat metabolism increased after training in the fasted state. But fat oxidation during exercise was the same in the two groups. It is possible, however, that small but significant changes in fat metabolism occur after fasted training, but in this study changes in fat oxidation might have been masked by the fact that these subjects received carbohydrate during their experimental trials. Note that training after an overnight fast may reduce the exercise capacity and may therefore be suitable only for low- to moderate-intensity exercise sessions. More research is needed to find out whether training in the fasted state has any advantages over training in the fed state. Note that training in the fed or fasted state is a different concept from training with low muscle glycogen. After an overnight fast, liver glycogen may be low, but muscle glycogen would be unaffected.

Carbohydrate Intake During Exercise

It has been suggested that carbohydrate intake during exercise may interfere with training adaptations. This notion is based on the observation that carbohydrate intake during exercise can reduce the expression of the mRNA of certain proteins after exercise. For example, carbohydrate ingestion has been shown to reduce carnitine palmitoyl transferase 1 (CPT1)-mRNA, mitochondrial uncoupling protein (UCP3), and the FA transporter FAT/CD36 as well as the activation of AMPK (Civitarese et al. 2005; Akerstrom et al. 2006). This finding could indicate that training adaptations could be compromised when carbohydrate is ingested during training. But another study did not show any difference in the activation of AMPK (Lee-Young et al. 2006). Although it was shown that glucose ingestion during moderate-intensity exercise reduced the expression of pyruvate dehydrogenase kinase 4 (PDK4) and UCP3, the expression of the gene for PGC-1, the PPAR-γ transcription coactivator responsible for longer-term adaptations, was not altered (Cluberton et al. 2005). From these studies that investigated the acute effects of one exercise bout, it is difficult to predict the long-term effects on protein synthesis and training adaptation.

A training study was performed in which subjects trained with or without carbohydrate ingestion in each training session for a period of 10 weeks (using a single-leg kicking model). It was found that citrate synthase and β-hydroxyacyl dehydrogenase activity and muscle glycogen increased but that there were no differences between the carbohydrate-fed and placebo-fed groups. Performance also improved after training, but the improvement was identical for the carbohydrate and placebo groups (Akerstrom et al. 2009). So the authors concluded that glucose ingestion during exercise does not alter training adaptation related to substrate metabolism, mitochondrial enzyme activity, glycogen content, or performance.

At present drawing any firm conclusions is impossible, but it seems unlikely that carbohydrate ingestion negatively influences training adaptations. Differences in the findings between acute studies and the training study described earlier may be explained by differences in the exercise protocol, including the exercise model used (one-legged kicking versus two-legged cycling exercise) and the training status of the subjects. Note that carbohydrate feeding may allow the athlete to train harder or longer; therefore, metabolic perturbations and hence changes in gene expression may be greater in that situation.

Leucine and the Signaling Response

Exercise increases muscle protein synthesis by stimulation of signaling pathways inside the contracting muscle cells. However, when no source of protein or amino acids is provided and there is no increased availability of amino acids, positive protein balance will not occur (see chapter 8). In chapter 8 we also mentioned that increased amino acid intake is necessary for two reasons: to stimulate the signaling pathways and to provide building blocks for the new proteins being synthesized. The branched-chain amino acids (BCAAs), in particular leucine, stimulate the muscles' signaling pathways.

One study is often cited to demonstrate the importance of BCAA for increasing muscle protein synthesis and ultimately the training adaptation. Anthony and colleagues (2009) studied protein synthesis in rats that ran for two hours on a treadmill. They observed that muscle protein synthesis was decreased significantly following the exercise. When leucine was given to these animals the signaling pathways were stimulated and protein synthesis increased. However, it is important to note that protein synthesis only increased to preexercise levels and this situation is very different to what is typically observed in humans. In humans exercise does not decrease muscle protein synthesis like it did in these rats. The leucine did not increase protein synthesis in these rats above preexercise levels; it merely returned muscle protein synthesis to the levels observed before the exercise. In other words, if there is a catabolic state, leucine may be effective, but whether leucine would be effective in humans where such a catabolic state cannot be observed postexercise remains unclear.

Several studies have demonstrated that signaling is increased postexercise with the ingestion of BCAA. However, no studies in humans have measured protein synthesis in combination with these measurements. It is not unlikely, however, that, although BCAAs alone can stimulate the signaling cascades, this would not result in increased protein synthesis if the amino acid building blocks are not supplied at the same time. Protein synthesis does not only depend on the activation of the protein synthetic machinery, it is also dependent on its substrate.

This line of thought led some researchers to theorize that a protein source that provides all amino acids and with a slightly higher leucine content could optimize protein balance postexercise. Koopman and colleagues (2004, 2005, 2007) demonstrated that the addition of protein to carbohydrates following resistance exercise increases muscle protein synthesis. However, when they added extra leucine to the carbohydrate–protein mixture this did not result in further improvement in protein balance (Koopman et al. 2005). It seems likely that by giving a source of protein postexercise, muscle protein synthesis is already stimulated to maximum (by the combination of exercise and protein) and leucine cannot stimulate it any further.

So although BCAAs (in particular leucine) have a role in signaling that enhances protein synthesis, it is unlikely that leucine alone will stimulate protein synthesis postexercise because the other amino acids have to be supplied as well to serve as building blocks. In some situations muscle protein synthesis may be compromised and in these situations BCAAs are more likely to have an effect. At this stage, however, the role of BCAAs and the possible effects on protein balance are not entirely clear.

Antioxidants and Training Adaptations

Skeletal muscle is repeatedly subjected to bouts of **oxidative stress** during exercise. Considerable evidence now indicates that aerobic contractile activity is associated with an increase in free-radical production in skeletal muscle. This increased production arises because a proportion of the molecular oxygen used in normal respiration undergoes one-electron reduction to produce superoxide radicals, the production of which increases with the large increase in O_2 flux in muscle mitochondria during exercise. This process leads to release of superoxide ($\cdot O_2^-$) and H_2O_2 by the muscle cell and the local formation of hydroxyl radicals ($\cdot OH$) (see chapter 10). Collectively, these are known as reactive oxygen species (ROS). Much work has been undertaken to examine the possibility that this free-radical production is the cause of exercise-induced muscle damage, and much research has focused on the detrimental effects of free radicals. But considerable evidence indicates that muscle cells adapt to this increased free-radical activity to reduce the risk of free-radical damage to the tissue. Thus, exercise training has been shown to increase the activity of several antioxidant enzymes such as superoxide dismutase and catalase in muscle and to increase muscle heat-shock protein content following exercise. It is now recognized that these adaptations can protect skeletal muscle against further bouts of (normally) damaging contractile activity.

More recently, it has become clear that physiological concentrations of free radicals may have advantageous effects. ROS and reactive nitrogen species (RNS) are involved in modulation of cell signaling pathways and the control of several (redox-sensitive) transcription factors. Although high levels of ROS may interfere with muscle function, moderate levels of ROS are essential in the development of optimal force production in muscle (Powers and Jackson 2008).

These findings also raise a number of important questions concerning the possible role of free-radical species as signals for wider adaptive responses in these and other tissues; they question the approach to protection of tissues that involves the use of widespread supplementation with antioxidant nutrients. It is entirely feasible that the adaptations to stress mediated by free radicals play an important role in maintaining cell viability in tissues routinely subjected to repeated stresses (e.g., muscle following exercise) and that increased consumption of some antioxidant nutrients might interfere with these necessary adaptive processes.

In one study, 14 men were trained for eight weeks (Gomez-Cabrera et al. 2008). Five of the men were supplemented daily with an oral dose of 1 g of vitamin C. The administration of vitamin C significantly hampered endurance capacity. The adverse effects of vitamin C may result from its capacity to reduce the exercise-induced expression of key transcription factors involved in mitochondrial biogenesis: peroxisome proliferator-activated receptor co-activator 1 (PGC1α), nuclear respiratory factor 1 (NRF1), and mitochondrial transcription factor A (Tfam). Vitamin C also prevented the exercise-induced expression of cytochrome C (a marker of mitochondrial content) and of the antioxidant enzymes superoxide dismutase and glutathione peroxidase. So the authors concluded that vitamin C supplementation decreased training efficiency because it prevented some cellular adaptations to exercise.

Much more research needs to be done to determine the exact role of ROS in training, but it seems that they may not always be damaging and that the role of ROS in modulating signaling pathways may have been ignored for a long time. It seems that supplementation with large doses of antioxidants may interfere with the function of ROS and may reduce the training adaptations.

Nonsteroidal Anti-Inflammatory Drugs and Training Adaptations

Nonsteroidal anti-inflammatory drugs (NSAIDs), including ibuprofen, aspirin (acetylsalicylic acid), naproxen, diclofenac, flurbiprofen, and ketoprofen, are perhaps the most widely known therapy in the treatment of muscle damage. Athletes often take these drugs to relieve pain or soreness following strenuous exercise. The evidence is mixed. Some studies show a reduction in muscle pain, and some studies show no change. But studies have consistently shown a reduction in the creatine kinase (CK) response after damaging exercise. The appearance of elevated levels of CK in plasma is often used as a marker of muscle damage, although it does not always correlate well with delayed-onset muscle soreness and other markers of muscle damage such as loss of strength. NSAIDs inhibit the synthesis of certain prostaglandins, which are potential mediators of edema and pain during acute inflammation. NSAIDs may therefore interfere with the normal inflammatory response after damaging exercise, and it is possible that this inflammatory response plays a role in the adaptation that occurs postexercise. Some evidence indicates that tissue protein synthesis is suppressed following high-intensity eccentric exercise as a result of over-the-counter doses of ibuprofen and paracetamol (1,200 mg and 4,000 mg daily, respectively) (Trappe et al. 2002). Animal studies also provide evidence that NSAIDs can interfere with muscle regeneration and hypertrophy. Given the equivocal acute effects of NSAIDs and their likely negative effect on training adaptation, NSAIDs should not be recommended as a strategy to treat symptoms of muscle damage. These findings provide more evidence that strategies that interfere with the normal signaling pathways have the potential to reduce training adaptations and cause training to be less effective.

Overtraining

We discussed in previous sections the role of nutrition in the development of training adaptations. Athletes often train extremely hard, even several times a day, to push their bodies to new levels. Often they push their bodies so hard that their performance deteriorates and may be substandard even after several days, weeks, or even months of rest. If recovery takes days, we generally think of this circumstance as normal; if it takes a week or more, we may call this condition overreaching, which could be regarded as an early stage of what is called the overtraining syndrome. Athletes with the overtraining syndrome (also called by some scientists the unexplained underperformance syndrome) have reduced performance and display a number of symptoms including disturbed eating, sleeping, and mood changes. The cardinal symptom of both overreaching and the overtraining syndrome is reduced performance. But because reduced performance could also be the result of fatigue, overreaching is diagnosed based on reduced performance in combination with sustained disturbances in mood state, consistent inability to perform normal training, and a prolonged recovery period.

Overreaching and the overtraining syndrome can occur when the total of all life stresses (and exercise training is only one of them) exceeds the ability of the body to cope with it. Managing overreaching means that the stresses have to be managed. Because poor nutrition is one of these stresses we will discuss here how nutrition can reduce the symptoms of overreaching and reduce the risk of developing overtraining syndrome.

Overreaching and Muscle Glycogen

Because overreaching is believed to be brought about by high-intensity training with limited recovery, it is thought that the fatigue and underperformance associated with overtraining are at least partly attributable to a decrease in muscle glycogen levels. Therefore, two studies have attempted to elucidate the role of carbohydrate and dietary intake on performance after intensified training.

Costill et al. (1988) investigated this possibility by examining the effects of 10 days of increased training volume on performance and muscle glycogen levels. Of the 12 swimmers participating in the investigation, four were unable to tolerate the increase from 4,000 to 9,000 m/day and were consequently classified as nonresponders. The group of nonresponders consumed approximately 1,000 kcal (4 MJ) per day less than their estimated energy requirement and consumed less carbohydrate than the responders (5.3 versus 8.2 g $\cdot$ kg b.w.$^{-1}$ $\cdot$ day^{-1}). Notably, however, muscular power, sprint swimming ability, and swimming endurance ability were not affected in either the responders or the nonresponders. Costill et al. (1988) concluded that the glycogen levels of the nonresponders were sufficient to maintain performance but inadequate for the energy required during training and thus fatigue resulted. Because overreaching and overtraining are primarily defined by a reduction in performance, the ability to ascertain whether the nonresponders were indeed overreached is limited.

These findings directed Snyder et al. (1995) to examine performance responses to intensified training with the addition of sufficient dietary carbohydrate in a bid to determine whether overreaching could still occur in the presence of normal muscle glycogen levels. To ensure sufficient carbohydrate intake, subjects consumed drinks containing 160 g of carbohydrate in the two hours following exercise. Subjects completed 7 days of normal training, 15 days of intensified training, and 6 days of minimal training. Resting muscle glycogen was not significantly different when compared between normal training (531 mmol/kg d.m.) and intensified training (571 mmol/kg d.m.) as determined by needle biopsy of the vastus lateralis muscle. Subjects were reported to be overreached, although maximal power output during an incremental cycle test was not statistically different after intensified training. Only four of the eight subjects demonstrated both a decline in maximal power output and an increase in responses to questionnaires about mood disturbance. Therefore, it appears that in this study only half of the subjects could be classified as overreached. From the two studies cited earlier, the role of carbohydrate intake and glycogen depletion in overreaching is unclear. Again, this is partly due to inappropriate analysis of performance.

One of the most important performance-determining factors is the resynthesis of muscle glycogen after training or competition. In a study by Costill and colleagues at Ball State University, well-trained runners ran 16 km on three consecutive days (Costill, 1971). Muscle glycogen levels decreased from 141 mmol/kg w.w. after the first run to 73 mmol/kg w.w. after the third run when a 40% to 50% carbohydrate diet was consumed (see figure 6.4). This decrease was much smaller (in fact, muscle glycogen levels were well maintained) when the runners received a high-carbohydrate diet.

Decreased glycogen levels can result in disturbances of the endocrine milieu. Glycogen depletion is related to high levels of catecholamines (epinephrine and norepinephrine), cortisol, and glucagon while insulin levels are very low. Such hormonal responses will result in changes in substrate mobilization and utilization (for instance, high epinephrine levels in combination with low insulin will increase lipolysis and stimulate the release of fatty acids).

Although insufficient carbohydrate intake (or energy intake) can contribute to the development of overtraining syndrome, overtraining may also develop when carbohydrate intake is adequate. In a study at the University of Maastricht in the Netherlands the training intensity and volume of well-trained cyclists were increased for two weeks. All cyclists showed signs of overtraining and were classified as overreached. The decrease in performance was accompanied by lower heart rates during exercise (time trial) and lower submaximal and maximal plasma lactate levels (Jeukendrup 1992). Three factors can theoretically explain lower lactate levels. First, lactate clearance may have increased. This occurrence is unlikely because normal training does not induce such an effect. A second explana-

---

Definitions of Overreaching and Overtraining

Overreaching

An accumulation of training or nontraining stress resulting in a short-term decrement in performance capacity with or without related physiological and psychological signs and symptoms of overtraining. Restoration of performance capacity may take from several days to several weeks.

Overtraining

An accumulation of training or nontraining stress resulting in a long-term decrement in performance capacity with or without related physiological and psychological signs and symptoms of overtraining. Restoration of performance capacity may take several weeks or months.

tion could be decreased glycogen concentration. When glycogen levels are low, rates of glycolysis will decrease, and, therefore, lactate formation will be reduced. But when the same research group repeated the study and provided carbohydrate supplements to avoid a decrease in muscle glycogen breakdown, the cyclists still showed signs of overreaching (Snyder et al. 1995). Submaximal and maximal lactate levels again decreased, while muscle glycogen levels remained constant. A third explanation of the lower lactate levels, therefore, could be a decreased sympathetic drive or a reduced sensitivity of adrenoceptors. This view was put forward by Barron and colleagues (Barron 1985) and can be the result of an increased stress level and increased levels of circulating catecholamines. After a while, a downregulation of receptors will occur, which results in decreased sensitivity of the target tissues (e.g., liver, muscles, heart) to catecholamines and a decreased rate of glycolysis and, hence, lower lactate levels.

Because repeated days of hard training and carbohydrate depletion seem to be linked to the development of overreaching, it is tempting to think that carbohydrate supplementation can reverse the symptoms. In a group of runners who ran 16 to 21 km on a daily basis for seven days and treated all those runs as races, performance dropped significantly when a moderate carbohydrate intake of 5.5 g · kg b.w.$^{-1}$ · day^{-1} was maintained (Achten 2003). The runners also displayed a range of symptoms indicating that they were overreached. But when the daily carbohydrate was increased to 8.5 g · kg b.w.$^{-1}$ · day^{-1}, the drops in performance were much smaller and symptoms were reduced. Recovery from this week of hard training was more complete with the high-carbohydrate treatment. In this study the dietary intake was strictly controlled and the subjects were fed to maintain energy balance. In a follow-up study subjects received a carbohydrate supplement, but their dietary intake the rest of the day was recorded but not controlled (Halson 2004). A group of well-trained cyclists were required to perform 8 days of intensive endurance training (normal training volume was doubled). This training was performed on two occasions separated by a washout, or recovery, period of at least 2 weeks. On one occasion subjects consumed a 2% carbohydrate solution before, during, and after training (moderate CHO), and on the other occasion subjects consumed a 6.4% carbohydrate solution before and during training and a 20% carbohydrate solution after training (high CHO). Total carbohydrate intake was 6.4 g · kg b.w.$^{-1}$ · day^{-1} with moderate CHO and 9.4 g · kg b.w.$^{-1}$ · day^{-1} with high CHO.

The intensified training protocol induced overreaching as indicated by a decrease in performance (time to fatigue at ~74% of $\dot{V}O_2$max), although the decrease in performance was significantly less with high CHO intake, suggesting that high-CHO diets can reduce the severity of overreaching. By forcing the subjects to consume supplements that contained a larger amount of carbohydrate, the total energy intake increased as well (13.0 versus 16.5 MJ/day for moderate CHO intake and high CHO intake, respectively). Athletes in hard training seem to reduce their spontaneous food intake, and unless they supplement with carbohydrate they may be in negative energy balance during periods of intensified training. It also appeared that the amount of carbohydrate ingested during training influenced the length of time needed for recovery. After two weeks of recovery (reduced volume and

---

Symptoms of Overtraining and Overreaching

Symptoms may be different during overreaching and overtraining and can be highly individual. Not everyone will have all symptoms, and not everyone will have the same symptoms.

- Drop in performance (note that without a decrease in performance there is no overtraining or overreaching)
- Washed-out feeling, tired, drained, lack of energy
- Mild leg soreness, general aches and pains
- Pain in muscles and joints
- Sleeping problems, insomnia
- Headaches
- Decreased immunity (increased number of colds, sore throats)
- Decrease in training capacity or intensity, inability to complete training sessions
- Moodiness and irritability
- Depression
- Loss of enthusiasm for the sport
- Decreased appetite, eating problems
- Increased incidence of injuries
- Reduced maximal lactate
- Reduced maximal heart rate
- Elevated resting heart rate, elevated sleeping heart rate
- No increase in cortisol in response to a stressful bout of exercise

intensity) from intensified training with moderate CHO intake, performance remained below that of the baseline, whereas performance improved compared with the baseline after two weeks of recovery from intensified training with high CHO intake.

Besides carbohydrate depletion, dehydration and negative energy balance can increase the stress response (increased catecholamines, cortisol, and glucagon, while insulin levels are reduced), which increases the risk of overtraining.

Glutamine and the Immune System

Increased levels of stress hormones have been associated with immunosuppression. Catecholamines can suppress the immune system but can also stimulate it. Cortisol, secreted by the adrenal cortex, has an important suppressive effect on the immune system. Changes in the hypothalamo–pituitary axis can have a distinct effect on the immune system. In general, hard training is associated with depression of immune function, and several studies that have monitored athletes during periods of hard training indicate that the incidence of infections (colds, influenza) is higher than at times when training is less intense (see chapter 16). Prolonged strenuous bouts of acute exercise are also associated with a temporary period of immune depression. For example, athletes who ran a marathon were more prone to develop symptoms of upper respiratory tract infection compared with control persons who did not run the marathon.

Glutamine is a nonessential amino acid that is an important fuel for cells of the immune system. Newsholme and colleagues suggested that hard training and overtraining result in decreased glutamine concentration in the blood (Newsholme 1987; Newsholme 1991). When the glutamine concentration decreases below a critical level, immunodepression may occur. Based on these thoughts, it is often claimed that glutamine supplements would help reduce immunodepression after strenuous exercise or periods of hard training.

But little evidence is available to support this notion. Several studies could not find decreased glutamine levels after strenuous training, and supplementation studies did not improve markers of immune function. In addition, it is unclear whether plasma glutamine levels give reliable information about body glutamine stores because 90% of all glutamine is present in the muscle. Therefore, at present, there is little reason to advise athletes to take glutamine supplements to improve immune function.

Branched-Chain Amino Acids

In the 1990s Newsholme launched another hypothesis in which the amino acid tryptophan was associated with central fatigue (Newsholme 1991). Tryptophan is the precursor of 5-hydroxytryptamine (5-HT; serotonin). During exercise the plasma concentration of the branched-chain amino acids (BCAA) leucine, isoleucine, and valine declines, while at the same time the concentration of free tryptophan increases. This is caused by an increased concentration of plasma fatty acids during exercise, which forces tryptophan to be released from its binding sites on albumin. As a result, the ratio of free tryptophan to BCAA in the plasma increases.

Because BCAA and free tryptophan use the same transport mechanism across the blood–brain barrier, they compete for transport. An increased plasma-free tryptophan:BCAA ratio allows more tryptophan to enter the brain, which could lead to increased synthesis of 5-HT. An increased concentration of this neurotransmitter in certain areas of the brain could result in fatigue. A situation like overtraining could result in chronic elevation of the free tryptophan:BCAA ratio. This circumstance may explain some of the symptoms of the overtraining syndrome. Supplementation of BCAA would reduce the free tryptophan:BCAA ratio and thereby reduce fatigue.

As discussed in chapter 8, however, it seems that BCAA supplementation has no effect on performance. Although the effect on overtraining has not been directly studied, the efficacy of BCAA feedings should be questioned.

KEY POINTS

■ Exercise leads to adaptations that eventually result in improved physiological function. Exercise training makes use of this principle by planning and systematically applying exercise activities with the goal of optimizing these adaptations and thus improving performance.

■ Adaptations to exercise or exercise training are specific to the exercise performed. Resistance exercise results in muscle hypertrophy, making the muscle stronger, and endurance training results in increased oxidative capacity, making the muscle more fatigue resistant.

- Training adaptations in skeletal muscle may be generated by the cumulative effects of transient increases in gene transcription during recovery from repeated bouts of exercise.

- The complex process of exercise-induced adaptation in skeletal muscle starts with specific molecular events that trigger an increase in protein synthesis. Signaling mechanisms triggered by exercise stress initiate replication of deoxyribonucleic acid (DNA) genetic sequences that enable subsequent translation of the genetic code into a series of amino acids to synthesize new proteins.

- Signal transduction pathways control the transcription of genes (specific sequences of DNA) into mRNA; translation of mRNA into protein; protein modification that alters catalytic activity; regulation of protein degradation; and regulation of cell division, proliferation, and fusion.

- During exercise, changes in muscle stretch or tension, changes in intracellular calcium ion concentrations, changes in the energy charge of the cell, and changes of the redox potential are primary signals that may then trigger a series of secondary molecular events, which can increase protein synthesis.

- AMPK is activated by a high AMP:ATP ratio and plays a crucial role in energy metabolism, acting as a metabolic master switch that regulates several intracellular systems including the cellular uptake of glucose, the β-oxidation of fatty acids, and the synthesis of glucose transporter 4 (GLUT4) and biogenesis of mitochondria.

- Insulin and insulin-like growth factor pathways play an important role in muscle hypertrophy through the Akt-mTOR signaling cascade.

- One family of transcriptional regulators in particular, the peroxisome proliferator-activated receptor γ coactivator family (PGCs), are important in driving mitochondrial biogenesis.

- The rate of protein synthesis depends on mRNA degradation, additional translational control mechanisms, transport of mRNA out of the nucleus, and the translation process.

- A single bout of endurance exercise will increase transcription or mRNA content for various metabolic and stress-related genes.

- Substrate availability during exercise (e.g., low muscle glycogen) can increase metabolic gene transcription, suggesting that modification of the training response may be possible with specific diet interventions.

- Although results of some recent studies suggest that training with low glycogen could have some metabolic advantages, whether this can also result in improvements in performance is not clear.

- BCAAs, in particular leucine, are signaling molecules as well as building blocks for protein synthesis. Although the BCAAs alone can stimulate signals in the muscle, this increased signaling will not result in increased synthesis if other amino acids in the blood are not available.

- Antioxidant supplementation may decrease training efficiency by preventing some cellular adaptations to exercise.

- Although a high-carbohydrate diet can maintain muscle glycogen stores and reduce or delay symptoms of overreaching during prolonged periods of intensified training, overreaching cannot be prevented by high carbohydrate intake.

RECOMMENDED READINGS

Hargreaves, M., and D. Cameron-Smith. 2002. Exercise, diet, and skeletal muscle gene expression. *Medicine and Science in Sports and Exercise* 34:1505–1508.

Hawley, J.A., K.D. Tipton, and M.L. Millard-Stafford. 2006. Promoting raining adaptations through nutritional interventions. *Journal of Sports Sciences* 24 (7): 709–721.

Hoppeler, H., and M. Fluck. 2003. Plasticity of skeletal muscle mitochondria: Structure and function. *Medicine and Science in Sports and Exercise* 35:95–104.

Spriet, L.L., and M.J. Gibala. 2004. Nutritional strategies to influence adaptations to training. *Journal of Sports Sciences* 22:127–141.

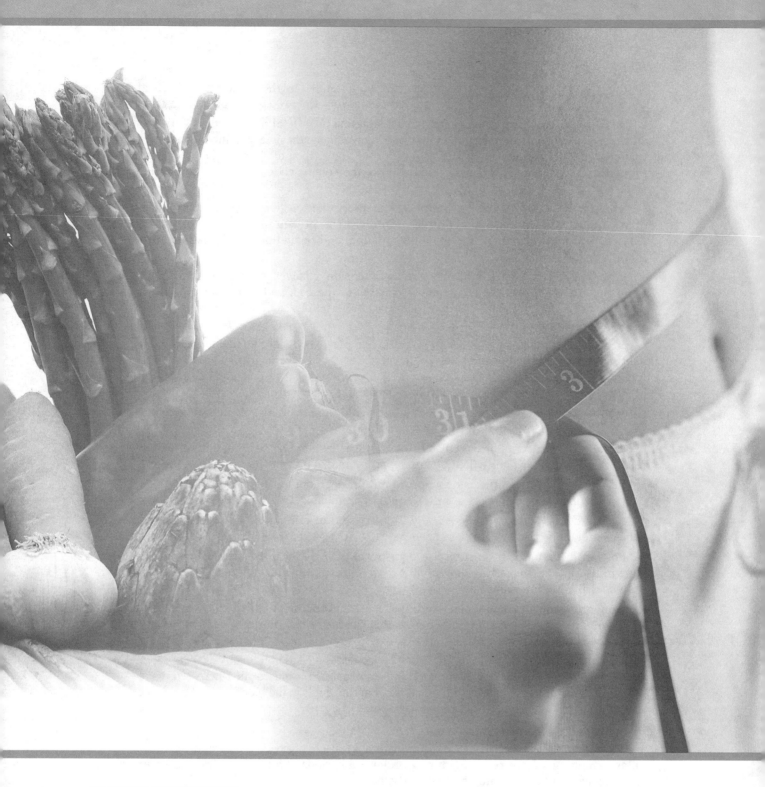

OBJECTIVES

After studying this chapter, you should be able to do the following:

- Describe the principles of methods available to measure body composition
- Compare different techniques of measuring body composition and discuss their advantages and limitations

Body Composition

Key Terms

Body weight and body composition are important determinants of performance in many sports. Some athletes try to achieve weight loss, and others try to achieve weight gain. In some sports, reducing body fat is important, whereas in other sports, increasing lean body mass is important. In most weight-bearing activities, such as running and jumping, extra weight is a disadvantage, although in some contact sports, such as American football and rugby, extra weight may be an advantage. Every sport has an optimal physique, and in some sports, a specific discipline or position requires a specific body type. For dancing and gymnastics, leanness is important, mainly for aesthetic reasons.

The desire to lose or gain weight is not limited to competitive athletes; it is also common among recreational athletes and sedentary people who wish to change their physical appearance. Although obesity is a growing problem, images in the media create continuous pressure to be lean and well proportioned. The stereotypical athlete is particularly lean and toned. Many athletes try to lose weight through either diet or exercise or both. This chapter discusses how body composition can be assessed and how it relates to performance in various sports. In the next chapter the problems associated with weight loss and weight gain and the applications in various categories of sports will be discussed.

Optimal Body Weight and Composition

Body size, structure, and composition are separate yet interrelated aspects of the body that make up the physique. Body size refers to the volume, mass, length, and surface area of the body; body structure refers to the distribution or arrangement of body parts such as the skeleton, muscle, and fat; and body composition refers to the amounts of constituents in the body. Size, structure, and composition all contribute to optimal sports performance. Evidence from sports participants in various age groups demonstrates an inverse relationship between fat mass and performance of physical activities that require translocation of body weight either vertically, such as in jumping, or horizontally, as in running. Excess fat is detrimental to performance in these types of activities because it adds mass to the body without adding capacity to produce force. In addition, acceleration is directly proportional to force but inversely proportional to mass, so excess fat, at a given level

of force application, results in slower changes in velocity and direction. Excess fat also increases the metabolic cost of physical activities that require movement of the total body mass. Thus, in most performances involving movement of body mass, a relatively low percentage body fat is advantageous both mechanically and metabolically.

By studying the anthropometry of high-level athletes, we can get an idea about optimum body size, structure, and composition for various sports. In some sports, a low percentage body fat is a requirement.

Generally, body composition of athletes can be used in three ways:

1. To track changes in body composition to monitor the effectiveness of a training program or dietary regime
2. To estimate optimal body weight or competition weight in weight-category sports such as boxing, lightweight rowing, and wrestling
3. To screen and monitor the health status of athletes to prevent disorders associated with extremely low levels of body fat

Male athletes with the lowest estimates of body fat (less than 6%) include middle-distance and long-distance runners and bodybuilders. Male basketball players, cyclists, gymnasts, sprinters, jumpers, triathletes, and wrestlers average between 6% and 15% body fat. Olympic marathon runners have 3% to 4% body fat, and Tour de France cyclists have between 4% and 6% body fat. Male athletes involved in power sports such as football, rugby, and ice and field hockey have slightly more variable levels of body fat (6% to 19%). Linebackers in American football have between 12% and 15% body fat, whereas defensive linemen have 16% body fat or more. Female athletes with the lowest estimates of body fat (6% to 15%) participate in bodybuilding, cycling, triathlons, and running events; higher fat levels (10% to 20%) are found in female athletes who participate in racquetball, skiing, soccer, swimming, tennis, and volleyball. The estimated minimal level of body fat compatible with health is 5% for males and 12% for females, but optimal body fat percentages for a particular athlete may be much higher than these minimums and should be determined on an individual basis.

Body mass may also be dramatically different in different sports. Female distance runners may weigh 50 to 55 kg (110 to 120 lb), whereas female shot putters may weigh 75 to 85 kg (165 to 185 lb).

Ballet dancers may weigh no more than 45 kg (100 lb). These body composition assessments reveal that athletes generally have physique characteristics unique to their specific sport and discipline.

Athletes who strive to maintain body weight or body-fat levels that are inappropriate, or have body-fat percentages below these minimal levels, may be at risk for an eating disorder or other health problems related to poor energy and nutrient intakes. This topic will be discussed in detail in the next chapter.

The human body is made up of various components. We can look at these components at different levels, from the molecular level to a whole-body level. In fact, in body composition research five levels are usually distinguished: atomic, molecular, cellular, tissue or organ, and whole body. For example, at the atomic level the body is mostly made up of four elements: carbon, hydrogen, oxygen, and nitrogen. Together these elements make up about 96% of the weight. The remaining 4% comes mostly from minerals (in particular, calcium in bones).

Most available techniques for measuring body composition help to quantify the most important structural components of the body: muscle, bone, and fat. Body composition measurements are usually performed at important time points in the athletic season. Often athletes and coaches discuss the measurements with a sports dietitian, a sports medic, or a sports scientist. Regular measurements (once every 3 months) are important to note trends in body composition. Changes in body composition do not occur overnight, and sufficient time must pass between measurements to allow changes to become evident. Some techniques have more variation than others, and demonstrating changes with those measurements is even more difficult. A simple way of tracking changes in body composition is to look at body fat, lean body mass, or the fat-free mass (FFM) divided by FM (fat mass). This last measure is often referred to as the FFM:FM ratio.

Body Composition Models

To understand the science of body composition assessment, it is important to understand the theoretical models that underlie these measurements of human body composition. Information about the composition of the human body has been obtained from the analysis of human cadavers, mostly in the 1950s, that quantified the total fat, protein, water,

and mineral content of the body. These studies formed the basis of body composition models that divide the body into two or more components.

Two Components

The two-component model partitions body mass into its lean (fat-free mass {FFM}) and fat (fat mass [FM]) compartments. The equation follows:

$$Body\ mass = FFM + FM$$

The term *lean body mass* is occasionally used, but *fat-free mass* is probably more appropriate. Lean body mass is a more anatomic concept that includes some essential lipids, whereas FFM is a biochemical concept. This model has had the widest application in the study of body composition, including many studies of athletes. FM is the more labile of the two compartments; it is readily influenced by diet and training. A shortcoming of the two-component model is the heterogeneous composition of FFM; it includes water, protein, mineral (bone and soft-tissue mineral), and glycogen.

Three Components

To account for interindividual differences in hydration, a three-compartment model was developed. The three-component model includes FM and partitions FFM into total body water (TBW) and fat-free dry mass (FFDM). The equation follows:

$$Body\ mass = TBW + FFDM + FM$$

Water is the largest component of body mass, and most is located in lean tissues. FFDM includes protein, glycogen, and mineral in bone and soft tissues. The use of dual X-ray absorptiometry (DXA) is based on this three-component model (see the later section about DXA).

Four Components

With the development of techniques to measure bone mineral, the four-component model is a logical extension of the preceding model. FFDM is partitioned into bone mineral (BM) and the residual. The following equation is used:

$$Body\ mass = TBW + BM + FM + residual$$

The four-component model is more accurate than the two-component model but also requires more measurements. All models measure FM, and this compartment is of particular interest in this chapter.

Normal Ranges of Body Weight and Body Fat

Body fat consists of essential body fat and storage fat. Essential body fat is present in the nerve tissues, bone marrow, and organs (all membranes), and we cannot lose this fat without compromising physiological function. Storage fat, on the other hand, represents an energy reserve that accumulates when excess energy is ingested and decreases when more energy is expended than consumed. Essential body fat is approximately 3% of body mass for men and 12% of body mass for women. Women are believed to have more essential body fat than men do because of childbearing and hormonal functions. In general, the total body-fat percentage (essential plus storage fat) is between 12% and 15% for young men and between 25% and 28% for young women (Lohman et al. 1993) (see also table 13.1). Average percentages of body fat for the general population and for various athletes are presented in tables 13.2 and 13.3.

Different sports have different requirements in terms of body composition. In some contact sports such as American football and rugby, a higher body weight is generally seen as an advantage. In sports such as gymnastics, marathon running, and other weight-bearing activities, a lower body weight and a high power-to-weight ratio are extremely important. Therefore, in these sports both low body fat and low body weight are necessary. In sports such as bodybuilding, increasing both lean body mass and body weight without increasing body fat is desirable. No accepted standards for percentage

■ **TABLE 13.1** ■

Body-Fat Percentages for Males and Females and Their Classification

Males	Females	Rating
5–10	8–15	Athletic
11–14	16–23	Good
15–20	24–30	Acceptable
21–24	31–36	Overweight
>24	>36	Obese

Note that these are rough estimates. The term *athletic* in this context refers to sports in which low body fat is an advantage.

■ **TABLE 13.2** ■

Body-Fat Percentages for the Average Population

	<30 yr	30–50 yr	>50 yr
Females	14–21%	15–23%	16–25%
Males	9–15%	11–17%	12–19%

■ **TABLE 13.3** ■

Body-Fat Percentages for the Athletic Population

Sport	Male	Female	Sport	Male	Female
Baseball	12–15%	12–18%	Rowing	6–14%	12–18%
Basketball	6–12%	20–27%	Shot putting	16–20%	20–28%
Bodybuilding	5–8%	10–15%	Skiing (cross-country)	7–12%	16–22%
Cycling	5–15%	15–20%	Sprinting	8–10%	12–20%
Football (backs)	9–12%	No data	Soccer	10–18%	13–18%
Football (linemen)	15–19%	No data	Swimming	9–12%	14–24%
Gymnastics	5–12%	10–16%	Tennis	12–16%	16–24%
High and long jumping	7–12%	10–18%	Triathlon	5–12%	10–15%
Ice and field hockey	8–15%	12–18%	Volleyball	11–14%	16–25%
Marathon running	5–11%	10–15%	Weightlifting	9–16%	No data
Racquetball	8–13%	15–22%	Wrestling	5–16%	No data

body fat exist for athletes. The ideal body composition depends largely on the particular sport or discipline, and the athlete should discuss this topic individually with the coach, a physiologist, and a nutritionist or dietitian. Body weight and body composition should be discussed in relation to functional capacity and exercise performance.

A variety of techniques have been developed to measure body composition (see table 13.4). Such measurements are more meaningful than the traditional weight and height relationship. All methods, including the simple anthropometric measurements, will be discussed in detail in the following sections.

Body Mass Index

A rough but better measure than the height–weight tables is the body mass index (BMI), also known as Quetelet index. Also derived from body mass and height, BMI is calculated thus:

$$\text{BMI} = \text{body mass in kilograms} / (\text{height in meters})^2$$

A person who is 1.76 m (5 ft 9 in) tall and weighs 72 kg (158 lb) has a BMI of $72/(1.76)^2 = 23.2$. The normal range is between 18.5 kg/m^2 and 25.0 kg/m^2. People with a BMI higher than 25 kg/m^2 are classified as overweight, and people with a BMI higher than 30 kg/m^2 are classified as obese (see the highlight box).

Even when using BMI rather than just body weight, the bodybuilder would be classified as overweight or even obese because the equation does not take into account body composition (BMI $= 100/(1.80)^2 = 30.9$) (figure 13.2). Two individuals might have the same BMI but completely different body compositions. One could achieve his or her body weight with mainly muscle mass as a result of hard training, whereas the other could achieve his or her body weight by fat deposition as a result of a sedentary lifestyle. Without information about body composition, they both might be classified as obese. In children and older people, the BMI is difficult to interpret because muscle and bone weights are changing in relationship to height.

The BMI, however, does provide useful information about risks for various diseases and is used

Anthropometry

Height–weight tables, such as the one shown in figure 13.1, provide a normal range of body weights for any given height. Such figures and tables have limitations, especially when applied to an athletic population. For instance, a bodybuilder (180 cm, 100 kg [6 ft, 220 lb]) may have very low body fat but could be classified as overweight. Clearly the "extra" weight is muscle, not body fat, which would lead to erroneous classification and possibly mistaken advice.

■ TABLE 13.4 ■
Techniques to Measure Body Composition

Method	Description
Anthropometry	Measurements of body segment girths to predict body fat
Skinfold thickness	Measurement of subcutaneous fat with a caliper that gives an estimation of lean body mass and fat mass
Hydrostatic weighing (underwater weighing or hydrodensitometry)	Underwater weighing based on Archimedes' principle to estimate lean body mass and fat mass
Air displacement plethysmography (Bod Pod)	Measurement of air displacement to estimate lean body mass and fat mass
Bioelectrical impedance analysis (BIA)	Measurement of resistance to an electrical current to estimate total-body water, lean body mass, and fat mass
Computed tomography (CT)	Computer-assisted X-ray scan to image body tissues and measure bone mass
Dual-energy x-ray absorptiometry (DEXA or DXA)	X-ray scan at two intensities to measure total-body water, lean body mass, fat mass, and bone-mineral density

Are you at a healthy weight?

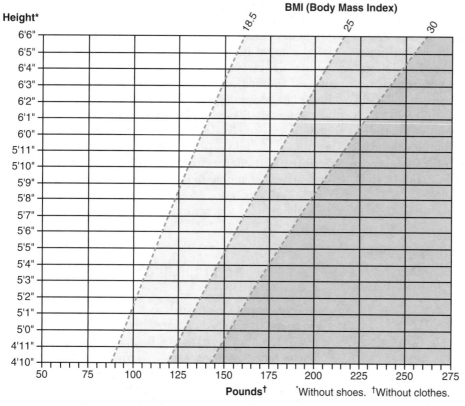

BMI measures weight in relation to height. The BMI ranges shown above are for adults. They are not exact ranges of healthy and unhealthy weights. However, they show that health risk increases at higher levels of overweight and obesity. Even within the healthy BMI range, weight gains can carry health risks for adults.

Directions: Find your weight on the bottom of the graph. Go straight up from that point until you come to the line that matches your height. Then look to find your weight group.

☐ Healthy Weight BMI from 18.5 up to 25 refers to healthy weight.

☐ Overweight BMI from 25 up to 30 refers to overweight.

☐ Obese BMI 30 or higher refers to obesity. Obese persons are also overweight.

Figure 13.1 Relationship between height, weight, and body mass index (BMI) and criteria for overweight and obesity.

Adapted from Dietary Guidelines for Americans 2000. Available from www.health.gov/dietaryguidelines/dga2000/document/frontcover.htm.

Body Mass Index Classifications

<18.5 Underweight

18.5–24.9 Normal weight

25.0–29.9 Overweight

30.0–34.9 Obesity class I

35.0–39.9 Obesity class II

>40.0 Obesity class III (extreme obesity)

in many epidemiological and clinical studies. For example, BMI correlates with the incidence of cardiovascular complications (hypertension and stroke), certain cancers, type 2 diabetes, gallstones, osteoarthritis, and renal disease (Calle et al. 1999). The BMI, however, is best used for populations rather than individuals. When used for individual assessment, BMI needs to be used in coordination with other measurements such as waist circumference, body composition, and so on.

Waist Circumference or Waist-to-Hip Ratio

The waist-to-hip ratio (WHR) measurement gives an index of body-fat distribution (figure 13.3). Because it gives an indication of the body fat distributed around the torso, it can be used to help determine obesity. The distribution of fat is evaluated by dividing waist size by hip size. A person with a 75 cm waist and 100 cm hips would have a ratio of 0.75; one with a 82 cm waist and 78 cm hips would have a ratio of 1.05. The higher the ratio is, the higher the risk of heart disease and other obesity-related disorders is. Females and males with WHRs greater than 0.80 and 0.91, respectively, have a higher risk of developing cardiovascular disease, diabetes, hypertension, and certain cancers. WHRs smaller than 0.73 for women and 0.85 for men indicate a low risk. WHR is also a better predictor of mortality in older people than waist circumference or body mass index (BMI). Other studies have found waist circumference, not WHR, to be a good indicator of cardiovascular risk factors, body fat distribution, and hypertension in type 2 diabetes. Although WHR and waist circumference are simple measures, they are of limited use to athletes.

Densitometry

Several techniques of densitometry have been developed to measure body composition and to distinguish the most important components: carbohydrate (typically < 1% of body mass), minerals (~4%), fat (~15%), protein (~20%), and water (~60%). Each of these components has a different density. Density is mass divided by volume and is usually expressed in grams per cubic centimeter (g/cm³). The density of bone, for instance, is 1.3 to 1.4 g/cm³, the density of fat is 0.9 g/cm³, and the density of fat-free (lean) tissue is 1.1 g/cm³. A lower total-body density value represents a higher fat mass.

The Greek inventor Archimedes (287 BC–212 BC) discovered a fundamental principle to assess human body composition. King Heron II of Syracuse had commissioned a goldsmith to make a crown of pure gold. When the goldsmith delivered the crown, the king noticed that the color of the gold was slightly lighter than usual. Suspecting that some of the gold had been replaced with silver, the king asked Archimedes to invent a way to measure the gold content of the crown without melting it down. Archimedes thought hard about this problem for several weeks. Then, stepping into a bath filled to the top with water and watching the overflow, he realized that he had found a way to measure the density of an object. Archimedes jumped from the bath and ran naked through the streets, shouting his famous words, "Eureka, eureka!" Archimedes had found a way to solve the mystery of the king's crown. He reasoned that a substance must have a volume proportional to its mass, and measuring the volume of an irregularly shaped object would require submersion in water and collecting the overflow. He found that pure gold with the same mass as the crown displaced less water than the crown and that silver displaced more water (see figure 13.4). He concluded that the crown was made of a mixture of gold and silver and thus confirmed the king's suspicions.

Assume that a 1,000 g crown is an alloy of 70% gold and 30% silver. Because its volume is 64.6 cm³, it displaces 64.6 g of water (water has a density of 1.00 g/cm³). The crown's apparent mass in water is thus 1,000 g minus 64.6 g, or 935.4 g. The 1,000 g of pure gold has a volume of 51.8 cm³, and so its apparent mass

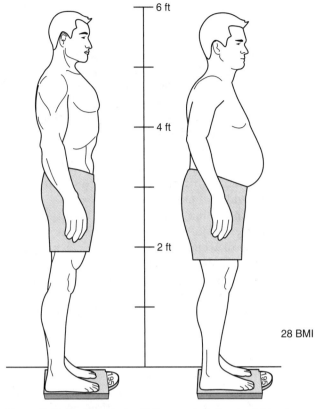

28 BMI

Figure 13.2 Two individuals with the same height and weight and therefore the same BMI but very different body compositions.

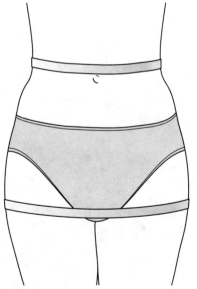

Figure 13.3 Waist-to-hip ratio

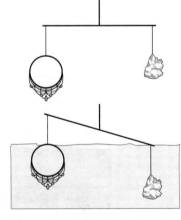

Figure 13.4 Archimedes' principle of determining the volume of an irregularly shaped object by submerging it in water and collecting the overflow. From this measurement and the weight of the object in air, the density (weight/volume) can be calculated.

in water is 1,000 minus 51.8 g, or 948.2 g. Thus, when both ends of the scale are immersed in water, the apparent mass is 935.4 g at one end and 948.2 g at the other end, an imbalance of 12.8 g. Scales from Archimedes' time could easily detect such an imbalance in mass.

The same principle can be used to distinguish between fat mass and fat-free mass in the human body (see figure 13.5). With this technique, called underwater weighing or hydrostatic weighing, a person is submerged in water and the body weight is accurately measured before and after submersion. Assume that a 75 kg (165 lb) person is submerged in water and weighs 3 kg (6.6 lb) in water. According to Archimedes' principle the loss of weight in water of 72 kg (158.4 lb) equals the weight of the displaced water.

The volume of the water displaced must be corrected for the temperature of the water at the time of weighing because water density changes with temperature. The density is 1.00 g/cm³ at 4 °C (39.2 °F), but measurements are usually performed in warmer water. Without correction, the body density in our example would be 75,000/72,000 = 1.0417 g/cm³.

Siri (1956) developed a method to estimate the percentage body fat from these measurements. The method assumes a density of 0.90 g/cm³ for the density of fat and 1.10 g/cm³ for the density of fat-free tissues. The equation for calculating the percentage body fat, often referred to as the Siri equation, is

$$\% \text{ body fat} = (495/\text{body density}) - 450$$

Using the same example of a 75 kg (165 lb) person, the percentage body fat is (495/1.0417) – 450 = 25.2%. Fat mass (FM) can then be calculated as 25.2% of 75 kg = 18.9 kg, and fat-free mass (FFM) is 75 kg – 18.9 kg = 56.1 kg.

Although this technique generally works well and is often used as the gold standard, it has several limitations. The calculations are based on a two-compartment model (fat mass and fat-free mass). The composition of the fat-free mass can change considerably after weight training. In very muscular persons, the Siri equation will overestimate body fat and underestimate fat-free mass (Modlesky et al. 1996). A slightly modified equation may give more accurate results in this population:

$$\% \text{ body fat} = (521/\text{body density}) - 478$$

Measurements are usually made after the person has made a maximal exhalation and held her or his breath under water for 5 to 10 seconds. This maximal exhalation is performed to reduce the air remaining in the lungs, which would otherwise exert a buoyant effect. Even with a maximal exhalation, however, a residual volume remains in the lungs. Therefore, residual lung volume must be

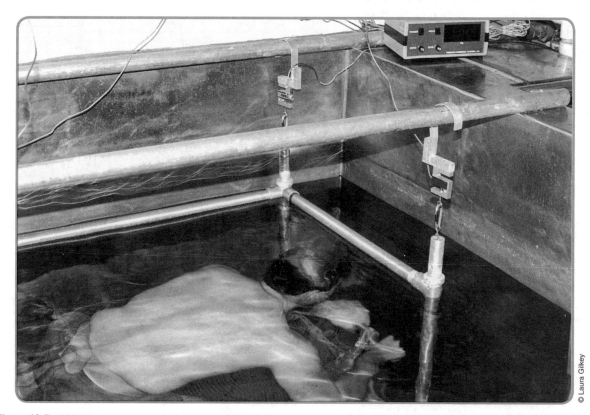

Figure 13.5 With the underwater, or hydrostatic, weighing technique, a person's body density is determined using Archimedes' principle.

measured and corrected for. Failure to correct for residual lung volume underestimates whole-body density and thus overestimates fat mass. Food intake, especially the intake of carbonated beverages, can also affect the measurement and should be avoided in the hours before measurement.

Skinfolds

The most frequently used technique to estimate body fat is measuring the thickness of skinfolds. These measurements are based on the interrelationships between the fat located underneath the skin (subcutaneous fat), internal fat, and whole-body density. Skinfolds can be measured using a caliper, which usually indicates the thickness in millimeters (see figure 13.6). The skinfold should be taken and the measurement read within 2 seconds to avoid skinfold compression. Considerable experience is necessary to produce accurate skinfold measurements. When comparing skinfold thickness, measurements should always be taken by the same person to guarantee consistency.

Several anatomical sites can be used for skinfold measurements. The four most common sites are the biceps, triceps, subscapular, and abdominal. These sites are shown in figure 13.7. Sometimes other sites on the upper thigh and chest are used. Often the sum of 4 skinfolds is chosen, but other methods take the sum of 7 or even 10 skinfolds.

The sum of skinfolds can then be used to predict body density and thence body-fat percentage. This prediction is usually based on previous research in which the skinfold measurements were compared with the results of underwater weighing. Various experimenters have put forward equations that are used either with skinfold thickness alone or in conjunction with other measurements such as body circumference or limb lengths. Two of the most common sets of equations used are attributable to Durnin and Womersley (Durnin et al. 1974) (skinfolds alone) and to Jackson and Pollock (Jackson et al. 1978) (skinfolds and body measurements).

After skinfold thickness has been measured using the sum of four skinfold measurements, body density can be calculated

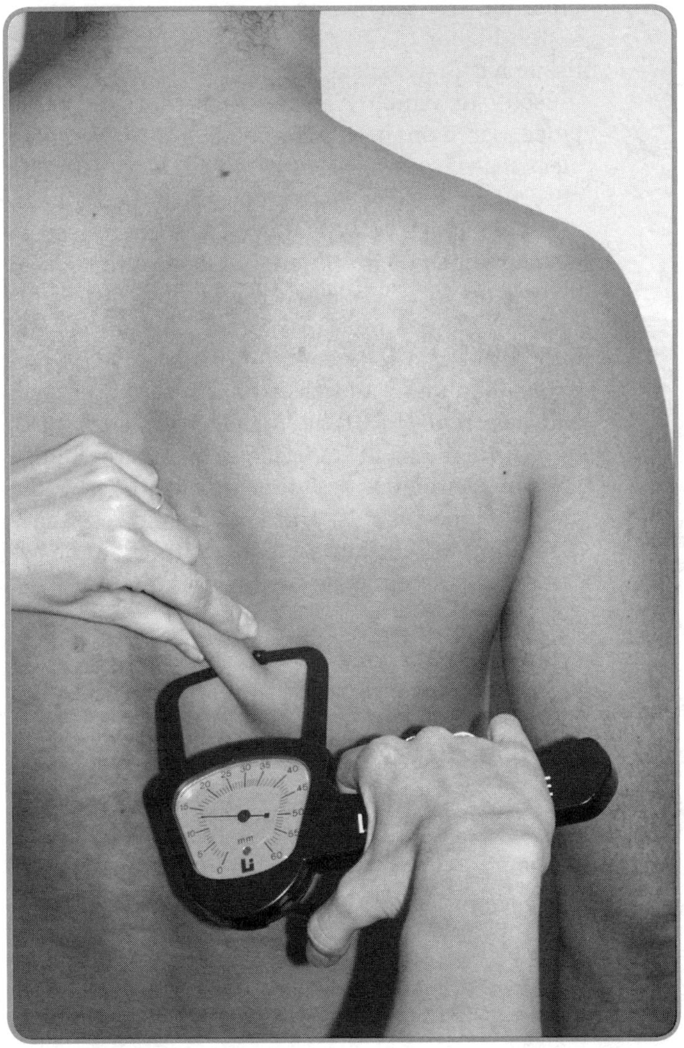

Figure 13.6 Skinfold measurement using calipers (subscapular site).

© Asker Jeukendrup

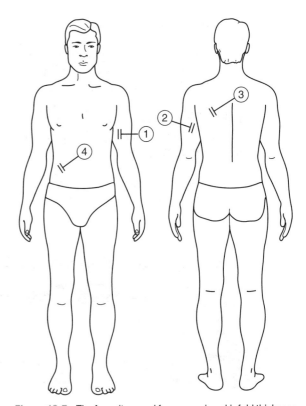

Figure 13.7 The four sites used for measuring skinfold thickness.
Based on Jackson and Pollock 1978.

based on the equation and values shown in table 13.5 (Durnin et al. 1974). The appropriate values of C and M can be read from the table, and the equation can be solved to determine body density (g/cm³) according to gender, age, and sum of the four skinfolds (in millimeters).

Percentage body fat is calculated using the Siri equation. For ease of reference, tables have also been generated for percentage body fat values for both males (see table 13.6) and females (see table 13.7) across the whole age range based on the sum of four skinfold measurements. Results are shown for each 2 mm increment of skinfold thickness.

Measurements at three skinfold sites in the body (different ones for males and females as illustrated in figures 13.8 and 13.9, respectively) can also be used to estimate percentage body fat. When using three skinfold measurements, the body density equations of Jackson and Pollock are used:

$$\text{male body density} = 1.0990750 - 0.0008209\,(X2) + 0.0000026\,(X2)^2 - 0.0002017\,(X3) - 0.005675\,(X4) + 0.018586\,(X5)$$

where $X2$ = sum of the chest, abdomen, and thigh skinfolds in millimeters; $X3$ = age in years; $X4$ = waist circumference in centimeters; and $X5$ = forearm circumference in centimeters.

$$\text{female body density} = 1.1470292 - 0.0009376\,(X3) + 0.0000030\,(X3)^2 - 0.0001156\,(X4) - 0.0005839\,(X5)$$

where $X3$ = sum of triceps, thigh, and suprailiac skinfolds in millimeters; $X4$ = age in years; and $X5$ = gluteal circumference in centimeters.

Again, percentage body fat is then calculated using the Siri equation. The correct tables must be used because the relationship between skinfold thickness and body fat may vary depending on the gender, age, and ethnicity of the individual. Estimating percentage body fat for populations other than the population that the equations were based on may result in large errors. Skinfold measurements, when properly taken, correlate highly (r = 0.83 to 0.89) with hydrostatic weighing, with a standard error of only about 3% or 4%. This error should always be kept in mind when using tables or equations to convert skinfold thickness to a percentage body fat. Sport scientists often stay with the skinfold thickness measurement rather than convert it to a percentage body fat. This method is especially useful when repeated and regular measurements are made of the same athlete.

Bioelectrical Impedance Analysis

Bioelectrical impedance analysis (BIA) is based on the principle that different tissues and substances have different impedance (resistance) to an electrical current. For example, impedance or conductivity is quite different for fat tissue and water (see figure 13.10).

Electrodes are placed on different parts of the body, often the hand and foot, and a current applied to one of those electrodes can be measured at the other electrode. The less the measured resistance is, the higher the body-water content is. Adipose tissue has high resistance, or impedance, whereas muscle—of which 75% is water—has low resistance. Based on these differential effects of applied electrical current, BIA can be used to estimate percentage body fat, percentage lean body mass, and percentage body water. BIA is often used to measure body composition, but it can also be used to estimate fluid levels in different body segments.

A simple example of a device for measuring impedance is a tube containing a highly conductive salt solution and electrodes inserted at each end (see figure 13.10a). An electrical current is sent through one of the electrodes, and resistance (Z) is measured between the two electrodes. If the length of the tube (L) and the specific resistivity (ρ) of the salt solution are known, the volume (V) can be calculated using the formula

$$V = \rho \times L^2/Z$$

◼ **TABLE 13.5** ◼

Linear Regression Equations for the Calculation of Body Density

	17–19 yr	20–29 yr	30–39 yr	40–49 yr	≥50 yr
C	1.1620 (male)	1.1631 (male)	1.1422 (male)	1.1620 (male)	1.1715 (male)
	1.1549 (female)	1.1599 (female)	1.1423 (female)	1.1333 (female)	1.1339 (female)
M	0.0630 (male)	0.0632 (male)	0.0544 (male)	0.0700 (male)	0.0779 (male)
	0.0678 (female)	0.0717 (female)	0.0632 (female)	0.0612 (female)	0.0645 (female)

Body density = C – [M($\log_{10}$ sum of all four skinfolds)]

From Durnin and Wormersley 1974.

TABLE 13.6

Percentage Body Fat for Male Subjects According to Age and Skinfold Thickness

Skinfold thickness*	AGE (YR)				
	17–19	20–29	30–39	40–49	≥50
10 mm	0.41	0.40	5.05	3.30	2.63
12 mm	2.46	2.10	6.86	5.61	5.20
14 mm	4.21	3.85	8.40	7.58	7.39
16 mm	5.74	5.38	9.74	9.31	9.31
18 mm	7.10	6.74	10.93	10.84	11.02
20 mm	8.32	7.96	12.00	12.22	12.55
22 mm	9.43	9.07	12.98	13.47	13.95
24 mm	10.45	10.09	13.87	14.62	15.23
26 mm	11.39	11.03	14.69	15.68	16.42
28 mm	12.26	11.91	15.46	16.67	17.53
30 mm	13.07	12.73	16.17	17.60	18.56
32 mm	13.84	13.49	16.84	18.47	19.53
34 mm	14.56	14.22	17.47	19.28	20.44
36 mm	15.25	14.90	18.07	20.06	21.31
38 mm	15.89	15.55	18.63	20.79	22.13
40 mm	16.51	16.17	19.17	21.49	22.92
42 mm	17.10	16.76	19.69	22.16	23.66
44 mm	17.66	17.32	20.18	22.80	24.38
46 mm	18.20	17.86	20.65	23.41	25.06
48 mm	18.71	18.37	21.10	24.00	25.72
50 mm	19.21	18.87	21.53	24.56	26.35
52 mm	19.69	19.35	21.95	25.10	26.96
54 mm	20.15	19.81	22.35	25.63	27.55
56 mm	20.59	20.26	20.73	26.13	28.11
58 mm	21.02	20.69	23.11	26.62	28.66
60 mm	21.44	21.11	23.47	27.09	29.20
62 mm	21.84	21.51	23.82	27.55	29.71
64 mm	22.23	21.90	24.16	28.00	30.21
66 mm	22.61	22.28	24.49	28.43	30.70
68 mm	22.98	22.65	24.81	28.85	31.17
70 mm	23.34	23.01	25.13	29.26	31.63
72 mm	23.69	23.36	25.43	29.66	32.07
74 mm	24.03	23.70	25.73	30.04	32.51
76 mm	24.36	24.03	26.01	30.42	32.93
78 mm	24.68	24.36	26.30	30.79	33.35
80 mm	25.00	24.67	26.57	31.15	33.75

*Sum of all four skinfolds.

TABLE 13.7

Percentage Body Fat for Female Subjects According to Age and Skinfold Thickness

Skinfold thickness*	AGE (YR)				
	17–19	20–29	30–39	40–49	≥50
10 mm	5.34	4.88	8.72	11.71	12.88
12 mm	7.60	7.27	10.85	13.81	15.10
14 mm	9.53	9.30	12.68	15.59	16.99
16 mm	11.21	11.08	14.27	17.15	18.65
18 mm	12.71	12.66	15.68	18.54	20.11
20 mm	14.05	14.08	16.95	19.78	21.44
22 mm	15.28	15.38	18.10	20.92	22.64
24 mm	16.40	16.57	19.16	21.95	23.74
26 mm	17.44	17.67	20.14	22.91	24.76
28 mm	18.40	18.69	21.05	23.80	25.71
30 mm	19.30	19.64	21.90	24.64	26.59
32 mm	20.15	20.54	22.70	25.42	27.42
34 mm	20.95	21.39	23.45	26.16	28.21
36 mm	21.71	22.19	24.16	26.85	28.95
38 mm	22.42	22.95	24.84	27.51	29.65
40 mm	23.10	23.67	25.48	28.14	30.32
42 mm	23.76	24.36	26.09	28.74	30.96
44 mm	24.38	25.02	26.68	29.32	31.57
46 mm	24.97	25.65	27.24	29.87	32.15
48 mm	25.54	26.26	27.78	30.39	32.71
50 mm	26.09	26.84	28.30	30.90	33.25
52 mm	26.62	27.40	28.79	31.39	33.77
54 mm	27.13	27.94	29.27	31.86	34.27
56 mm	27.63	28.47	29.74	32.31	34.75
58 mm	28.10	28.97	30.19	32.75	35.22
60 mm	28.57	29.46	30.62	33.17	35.67
62 mm	29.01	29.94	31.04	33.58	36.11
64 mm	29.45	30.40	31.45	33.98	36.53
66 mm	29.87	30.84	31.84	34.37	36.95
68 mm	30.28	31.28	32.23	34.75	37.35
70 mm	30.67	31.70	32.60	35.11	37.74
72 mm	31.06	32.11	32.97	35.47	38.12
74 mm	31.44	32.51	33.32	35.82	38.49
76 mm	31.81	32.91	33.67	36.15	38.85
78 mm	32.17	33.29	34.00	36.48	39.20
80 mm	32.52	33.66	34.33	36.81	39.54

*Sum of all four skinfolds.

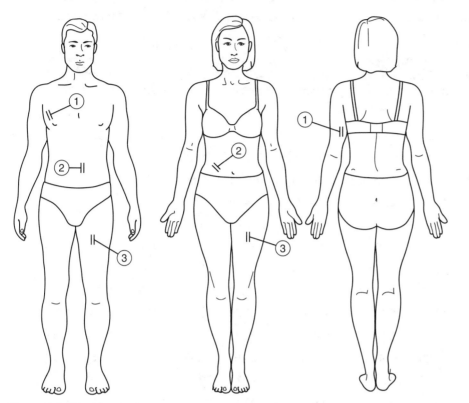

Figure 13.8 The three-site skinfold measuring system for male subjects.
Based on Jackson and Pollock 1978.

Figure 13.9 The three-site skinfold measuring system for female subjects.
Based on Jackson and Pollock 1978.

If some of the salt solution is replaced with oil, the measured resistance increases and the new volume of the salt solution is calculated. By deduction, the percentage of oil in the solution can be determined (see figure 13.10*b*). The principle is exactly the same when measuring body impedance and calculating body composition. For this purpose the measured body impedance and the subject's height are used.

Most BIA devices are tetrapolar, meaning that they have four electrodes: two that apply the current and two that receive a signal. The device applies a current of 500 μA to 800 μA at a single frequency of 50 kHz or more, too weak to be felt by the subject.

The subject lies on a nonconducting surface with arms not touching the trunk and legs at least 20 cm apart. Shoes, socks, and metal objects (jewelry) are removed. The contact surfaces on the hand and ankle should be cleaned with alcohol. The resistance measured can then be used in various formulas in a similar manner to the tube examples. The body can be viewed as five tubes: two arms, two legs, and one trunk (see figure 13.10*c*).

The example of the tubes is an oversimplification. In reality, several factors can affect impedance

and invalidate the assumptions. A larger tube increases conductivity. Warming the tube also increases conductivity. Changes in the skin temperature, in particular, alter whole-body conductivity and have a profound effect on the measurement. Higher skin temperature results in an underestimate of the body-fat content (Baumgartner et al. 1990). Often, when the measurements are performed, the subject may sweat more; a wet surface reduces impedance and underestimates body-fat content.

In humans, factors such as hydration status and distribution of water can also affect impedance. Even small changes in the hydration level can have a marked effect on the accuracy of the measurement and can influence the calculated body-fat content (Koulmann et al. 2000; Saunders et al. 1998). If a person is dehydrated, impedance decreases, whereas if a person drinks a lot of fluid before the measurement, impedance could increase. Thus, losing body water through prior exercise or voluntary fluid restriction will overestimate body-fat content. Hyperhydration has the opposite effect and will underestimate body-fat content.

Body position is important, and the fluid shifts that occur can affect impedance. The orientation of tissues can affect impedance. For example, current is more easily transported along muscle fibers than against muscle fibers. The testing conditions under which BIA is run should be extremely well controlled. Usually subjects are advised as follows:

- Abstain from alcohol for 8 to 12 hours before the measurement.

- Avoid vigorous exercise for 8 to 12 hours before the measurement.

- Measurements are performed at least 2 hours after the last meal (or drink).

- Measurements are performed within 5 minutes of lying down.

BIA seems a convenient technique, but it requires considerable experience, expertise, and control of the testing conditions. When BIA is performed in the best possible way, the results are extremely reliable, but they may not be as accurate as skinfold measurements (Broeder et al. 1997; Stolarczyk et al. 1997).

Dual-Energy X-Ray Absorptiometry

Dual-energy X-ray absorptiometry (DXA or DXA) has become the clinical standard for measuring bone density. The principle is based on absorption of low-energy X-rays. The short duration of exposure gives only a minimal radiation dose.

During the measurement, the subject lies supine on a table. A source and detector probe pass across the body at a relatively low speed (about 60 cm/min; a whole-body scan may take 6–15 minutes). The subject is exposed to these low-energy X-rays, and the loss of signal in various parts of the tissue is recorded. The measurement is performed at two intensities, so that the instrument's software can distinguish not only between soft tissues and bone-mineral content but also between fat-free mass and fat mass. The derivation of fat and fat-free soft tissue from DXA scans is based on the ratio of soft-tissue attenuation of the low-energy and high-energy photon beams as they pass through the body. The attenuation of the low-energy and high-energy soft tissues is known based on scans of pure fat and fat-free soft tissues and theoretical calculations. The DXA instrument is linked with appropriate computer algorithms to derive estimates of bone mineral, fat-free soft tissue, and fat-tissue content of the total body. The algorithms also permit division of the body into anatomic segments—arms, legs, trunk, and head—to permit estimates of regional body composition.

DXA seems to be an accurate technique that shows excellent agreement with other independent techniques to measure bone-mineral content (Going et al. 1993; Heymsfield et al. 1990). In addition, small changes in body composition can be detected with this method (Going et al. 1993).

But DXA may underestimate body-fat content somewhat compared with underwater weighing. In addition, with DXA, test conditions must be standardized (Kohrt 1995) because factors such as hydration status can influence the results (Elowsson et al. 1998). The software and hardware of the various commercially available DXA scanners are different, which is also a source of error (Van Loan et al. 1995). Although DXA has limitations,

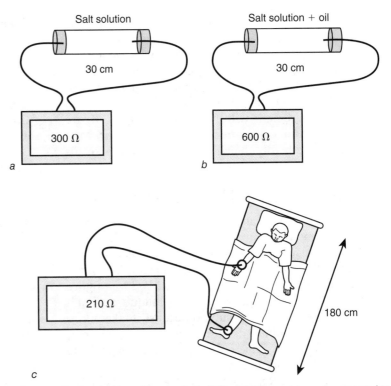

Figure 13.10 Bioelectrical impedance analysis (BIA). *(a)* If the resistance is measured to a known current in a tube with a salt solution and a known length (30 cm), the volume can be calculated. *(b)* If the same tube contains oil in addition to the salt solution, the resistance changes and a new calculation of volume is obtained. *(c)* The same principle can be applied to the human body, which can be viewed as five tubes (two arms, two legs, and one trunk).

it appears to be one of the better ways to measure body composition, and it has advantages over other methods in that it can not only distinguish lean body mass and fat mass but also assess bone density.

Computed Tomography

Computed tomography (CT) uses ionizing radiation by an X-ray beam to create images of body segments. The CT scan produces qualitative and quantitative information about the total area of the tissue investigated and the thickness and volume of tissues within an organ. With this method, fat surrounding a tissue as well as fat within a tissue can be measured.

Magnetic Resonance Imaging

With magnetic resonance imaging (MRI), pictures can be obtained from body tissues and compartments. The results are somewhat similar to those obtained by CT scan, but with MRI, electromagnetic radiation is used rather than ionizing radiation. Generally, MRI shows good agreement with other methods. A study found excellent agreement between MRI and underwater-weighing estimates in both overweight and non-overweight women, suggesting that MRI may be a satisfactory substitute for the more established methods of body-fat estimation in adult women. In fact, MRI showed the smallest day-to-day variation in measurement within an individual (see figure 13.11). But calculations of body fat from MRI scans are highly dependent on software, and this dependency can introduce error.

Air Displacement Plethysmography

A relatively new and promising method to estimate whole-body volume is a small chamber in which air displacement is measured. The technique is called air displacement plethysmography, and it is marketed commercially as Bod Pod (see figure 13.12). The advantages of this technique are that it is convenient for the subject because it takes place while the subject is sitting in a small chamber, measurements take only 3 to 5 minutes, and the reproducibility is good.

The subject is first weighed accurately outside the Bod Pod. He or she then sits in the 750 L volume Bod Pod, which consists of a dual chamber made out of fiberglass (see figure 13.12). The person's volume is the original volume in the chamber minus the air that has been displaced with the subject inside. The subject breathes into an air circuit to assess pulmonary gas volume, which,

when subtracted from measured body volume, yields true body volume. Body density can then be calculated from body mass and body volume. Although this technique has good reproducibility, it generally gives lower percentages of body fat compared with hydrostatic weighing and DXA (Collins et al. 1999; Wagner et al. 2000; Weyers et al. 2002).

Multicomponent Models

Multicomponent models use a combination of methods such as hydrostatic weighing, BIA, and DXA to reduce the errors associated with using a single method (Wagner et al. 2000). Although the traditional two-component model is based on separating fat mass and fat-free mass to determine body composition, these models assume that the density of fat-free mass is 1.1 g/cm^3 and that the components of the FFM (water, protein, and minerals) are constant for all individuals. These assumptions may not always hold true, and accuracy can therefore be improved by measuring these components. Multicomponent models can combine measures of whole-body density with measures of body-water and bone-mineral density. This approach is generally believed to give the most accurate results.

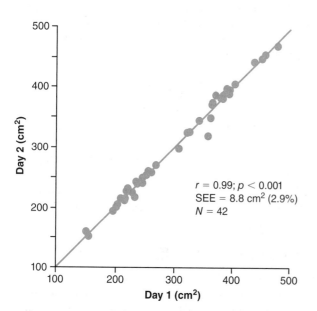

Figure 13.11 Comparison of typical in vivo magnetic resonance images obtained on two separate days from the same subject at the level of the midthigh. Regression between cross-sectional adipose tissue–free skeletal muscle (ATFSM) areas from 42 pairs of magnetic resonance images (6 subjects and 7 images each). SEE = SE of estimate; N = number of images. The solid line is the regression line.

In chart: $r = 0.99; p < 0.001$
SEE = 8.8 cm^2 (2.9%)
$N = 42$

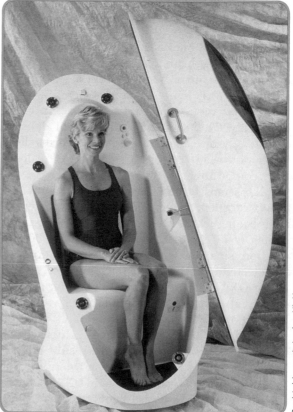

Figure 13.12 The Bod Pod.

Practical Message

Several methods are used to assess body composition. Generally, the more complex models are more accurate, but they are often unsuitable for conditions outside a laboratory or clinical setting. The gold standards are underwater weighing and DXA, but the most user-friendly method is probably skinfold measurement. Periodic measurement of body composition with the gold standard techniques is recommended to obtain accurate information about body composition. To track athletes in field conditions, the same person should collect the skinfold measurements, and the sum of skinfolds should be used as the outcome measure rather than a conversion to percentage body fat, which can be inaccurate and can cause unnecessary variation.

KEY POINTS

- Standard height–weight tables do not provide information about body composition and can be misleading when applied to individual athletes.

- Body mass index (BMI) is often used as a rough measure of body composition. Although BMI can be useful in epidemiological and clinical studies, it does not distinguish between muscle mass and fat mass.

- The technique of densitometry is based on Archimedes' principle that the loss of weight in water is equal to the volume of the displaced water. Because body fat is less dense than water, it lets the subject float, whereas fat-free mass, which is denser than water, causes the subject to sink. After correcting for residual volume, percent fat can be calculated based on underwater weight.

- The sum of skinfolds can be used to estimate body fat percentage. For accuracy, values from tables that have been established for specific populations (e.g., same gender, same age range, or same ethnicity) must be used.

- Bioelectrical impedance analysis (BIA) is a convenient technique that requires considerable experience, expertise, and control of environmental conditions to obtain reliable results. When BIA is performed in the best possible circumstances, the results may be reliable, but they may still be less accurate than skinfold measurements.

- Dual-energy X-ray absorptiometry (DEXA or DXA) is based on the principle that compartments with different densities absorb different amounts of low-energy X rays. The advantage of DXA is that it can not only distinguish fat mass and fat-free mass but also assesses bone density. DXA has become the clinical standard to measure bone density.

- Imaging technologies, such as computed tomography (CT) and magnetic resonance imaging (MRI), can visualize body fat of different parts of the body.

RECOMMENDED READINGS

Bouchard, C. 1994. Genetics of obesity: Overview and research directions. In *The genetics of obesity*, ed. C. Bouchard, 223–233. Boca Raton, FL: CRC Press.

Bouchard, C., A. Tremblay, J.P. Despres, A. Nadeau, P.J. Lupien, G. Theriault, J. Dussault, S. Moorjani, S. Pinault, and G. Fournier. 1990. The response to long-term overfeeding in identical twins. *New England Journal of Medicine* 322:1477–1482.

Flatt, J-P. 1995. Use and storage of carbohydrate and fat. *American Journal of Clinical Nutrition* 61:952S–959S.

Heymsfield, S.B., T.G. Lohman, Z. Wang, and S.B. Going. 2005. *Human body composition*. Champaign, IL: Human Kinetics.

Heyward V.H., and D.R. Wagner. 2004. *Applied body composition assessment*. Champaign IL: Human Kinetics.

Roche, A.F., S.B. Heymsfield, and T.G. Lohman. 1996. *Human body composition*. Champaign, IL: Human Kinetics.

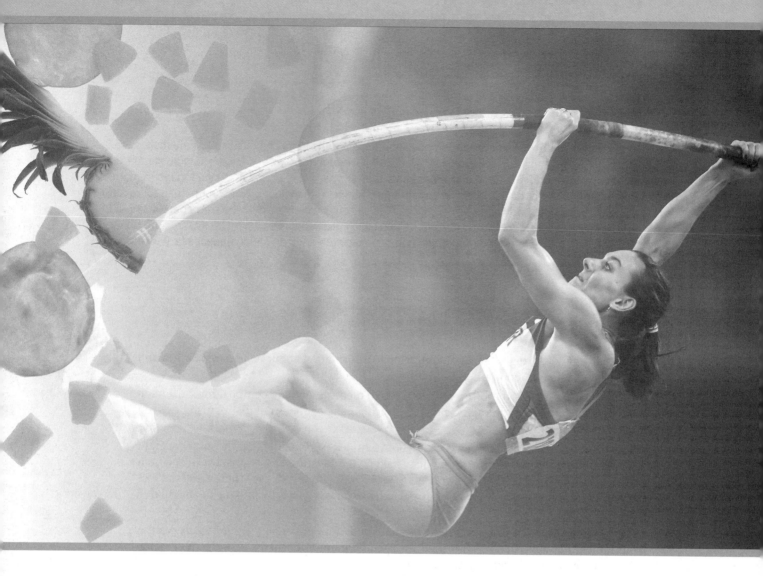

OBJECTIVES

After studying this chapter, you should be able to do the following:

- Describe the principles of methods available to measure body composition
- Compare techniques of measuring body composition and discuss their advantages and limitations
- Categorize sports and the importance of body weight or composition
- Describe ways of losing body weight by dieting
- Describe the role of exercise in losing body weight
- Describe the benefits and risks of making weight and discuss the ways of minimizing the risks

14

Weight Management

Key Terms

The desire to lose or gain weight is not limited to competitive athletes. Many recreational athletes and sedentary individuals also wish to change their physical appearance. Although obesity is a growing problem, images in the media create continuous pressure to be lean and well proportioned. The stereotypical athlete is particularly lean and toned. Many athletes try to lose weight through either diet or exercise or both. This chapter discusses the relationship between body composition and performance, techniques of assessing body composition, and the problems associated with weight loss and weight gain and applications in various categories of sport.

Body Weight and Composition in Different Sports

Body size, structure, and composition are separate yet interrelated aspects of the body that make up the physique. Body size refers to the volume, mass, length, and surface area of the body; body structure refers to the distribution or arrangement of body parts such as the skeleton, muscle, and fat; and body composition refers to the amounts of constituents in the body. Size, structure, and composition all contribute to optimal sports performance. Evidence from sports participants in various age groups demonstrates an inverse relationship between fat mass and performance of physical activities that require translocation of body weight either vertically, such as in jumping, or horizontally, as in running. Excess fat is detrimental to performance in these types of activities because it adds mass to the body without adding capacity to produce force. In addition, acceleration is directly proportional to force but inversely proportional to mass, so excess fat, at a given level of force application, results in slower changes in velocity and direction. Excess fat also increases the metabolic cost of physical activities that require movement of the total body mass. Thus, in most performances involving movement of body mass, a relatively low percentage body fat is advantageous both mechanically and metabolically.

By studying the anthropometry of high-level athletes, we can get an idea about optimum body size, structure, and composition for various sports. In some sports, a low percentage body fat is a requirement. For example, Olympic marathon runners have 3% to 4% body fat. Tour de France cyclists have between 4% and 6% body fat. Linebackers in American football have between 12% and 15% body fat, whereas defensive linemen have 16% or more of body fat.

Body mass may also be dramatically different in different sports. Female distance runners may weigh 50 to 55 kg (110 to 120 lb), whereas female shot putters may weigh 75 to 85 kg (165 to 185 lb). Ballet dancers may weigh no more than 45 kg (100 lb). These body composition assessments reveal that athletes generally have physique characteristics unique to their specific sport and discipline.

Genetics

A significant portion of the variation in body-fat levels of individuals is genetically determined. Perhaps 25% to 40% of adiposity is the result of our genes (Bouchard 1994). Evidence from both genetic epidemiology and molecular epidemiology studies suggests that genetic factors determine the susceptibility to gaining or losing body fat in response to dietary energy intake (Perusse et al. 2000). To study the influence of genetics on the effects of overfeeding, identical twins were investigated. In one study, monozygotic twins were submitted to an energy surplus of 4.2 kJ/day (1,000 kcal/day) 6 days a week for 100 days (Bouchard et al. 1990). The excess energy intake over the entire period was 353 MJ (84,000 kcal). The average gain in body mass was 8.1 kg, but considerable interindividual variation occurred. The variation between pairs was more than three times greater than the variation within pairs, suggesting an important genetic component. The variation between pairs was even greater for changes in abdominal visceral fat, indicating that the site of storage is also genetically determined.

Similarly, when identical twins completed a negative energy balance protocol by exercising over a period of 93 days without increasing energy intake, more variation occurred between pairs than within pairs. The energy deficit was estimated to be 244 MJ (58,000 kcal), and the mean body-weight loss was 5 kg. The range of weight loss, however, was 1.0 kg to 8.0 kg (see figure 14.1).

These classic early studies demonstrate a genetic factor in the development of obesity. This link has been confirmed by molecular epidemiology studies, and now more than 250 genes are believed to have the potential to influence body fatness (Rankinen et al. 2002).

Several risk factors associated with weight gain, such as a low resting metabolic rate, high reliance on carbohydrate metabolism, and a lower level of spontaneous activity, almost certainly have a genetic basis. But the relative contribution of genetic versus environmental factors is still a subject of debate.

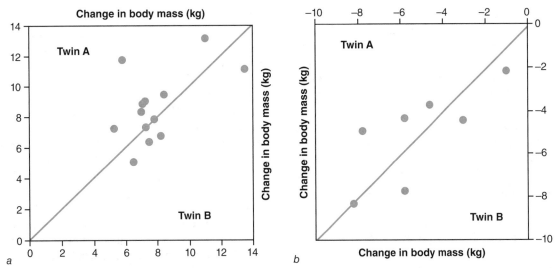

Figure 14.1 Changes in body mass in identical twins *(a)* after overfeeding and *(b)* after being subjected to a negative energy balance by exercise. Considerably more variation occurred between pairs than within pairs, strongly suggesting a genetic component in the regulation of body mass.

Based on Bouchard et al. 1990.

Energy and Macronutrient Intake

A negative energy balance is necessary to lose weight, and it can be induced by reducing energy intake, by increasing energy expenditure, or by a combination of these two. But these alterations in energy balance are just part of the picture. The macronutrient (carbohydrate, fat, and protein) intake and the expenditure of these substrates must also be considered. Excess intake of carbohydrate and protein can be converted to fat, although this process requires energy. For many years it was believed that although de novo lipogenesis did exist, it did not play an important role in human metabolism. But evidence now shows that over-feeding with carbohydrate can increase de novo lipogenesis (Aarsland et al. 1997). The liver plays only a minor role in this process, and the majority of de novo lipogenesis probably takes place in adipose tissue. The subjects in this study were overfed and received a large amount of excess energy (2.5 times their requirements). Therefore, it could be questioned whether this could occur in athletes who are in energy balance. Jeukendrup and colleagues (unpublished) performed a study in which endurance trained athletes exercised 2 hours a day at moderate intensity while maintaining energy balance, mimicking a normal training situation. Subjects stayed in a respiration chamber so that energy intake and expenditure could be accurately monitored. Subjects received two diets. One was a normal diet, and the other was a low-fat,

high-carbohydrate diet containing virtually no fat and a large amount of carbohydrate. For 10 days subjects exercised daily, and substrate use was measured during their exercise sessions as well as during the rest of the day. On the low-fat, high-carbohydrate diet, 24-hour fat oxidation exceeded fat intake, and consequently the subjects were in positive carbohydrate balance. Over a 10-day period, body composition would have to change or carbohydrate had to be turned into fat. No changes were observed in body composition after 10 days, suggesting that carbohydrate had been converted to fat. This notion was confirmed with stable isotopes; ^{13}C tracer ingested with carbohydrate was found in fatty acids in adipose tissue and plasma. It was found only in those fats that are the product of de novo lipogenesis. No such changes were observed with the control diet. These data show that even in a situation of energy balance, de novo lipogenesis can occur and that this pathway can become quantitatively important.

The body increases the oxidation rate of carbohydrate and protein immediately when excess amounts are ingested. Fat, however, is different. Generally, fat is not converted into protein or carbohydrate.

In addition, when excess amounts of fat are ingested, oxidation rates do not increase immediately, making fat more likely to be stored in adipose tissue (Abbott et al. 1988; Westerterp 1993).

The macronutrient composition of the diet, therefore, plays an important role in daily energy intake and expenditure (Westerterp et al. 1995).

These substrate balances are influenced by a variety of genetic, environmental, cultural, and socioeconomic factors (Flatt 1995). For example, dietary intake is different in different socioeconomic classes. Lower socioeconomic classes typically have a higher fat intake and lower carbohydrate intake than higher socioeconomic classes. Also, clear cultural differences exist in diets as well as in acceptability of exercise. Some African countries, for example, have a very high carbohydrate intake (>70%), whereas the carbohydrate intake in the Western world is typically around 40% to 50%.

A simple example illustrates the importance of substrate balances. Someone who eats 50 g of sugar (e.g., by drinking half a liter of a soft drink) daily in addition to the normal diet is in positive energy balance by approximately 800 kJ/day (200 kcal/day). This level of intake is 292,000 kJ (73,000 kcal) a year, which over the course of 30 years amounts to 8,760 MJ (2,190,000 kcal). Assuming an energy density of adipose tissue of 19.0 kJ/g (7.7 kcal/g), this person should experience a weight gain of 284 kg (625 lb) in those 30 years. Clearly, this amount of weight gain is not reality, and this person would probably gain only a few kilograms.

The increased body weight results in an increased metabolic rate and an increased oxidation of energy substrates. Also, some of the energy ingested as carbohydrate is lost in the conversion to fat.

Regulation of Appetite

Although both physiological and environmental factors contribute to **appetite** and eating behavior, it is widely accepted that strong social and environmental influences can easily overcome normal physiology. It is well established that the hypothalamic region of the brain plays a key role in the central regulation of eating behavior in humans (figure 14.2). The hypothalamus, in particular the arcuate nucleus, constantly receives and processes neural, metabolic, and endocrine signals from the periphery. This enables it to maintain energy homoeostasis by adjusting not only energy intake but also energy expenditure. Peripheral signals are generated mostly by the gastrointestinal tract but also by other organs such as the pancreas and the adipose tissue. In response to feeding, the gastrointestinal tract produces several appetite regulating hormones such as CCK, GLP-1, and PYY. Ghrelin produced mostly by the stomach plays an important role by stimulating appetite. Ghrelin concentrations increase before meals and stimulate food intake. After meals, ghrelin returns to baseline concentrations. Adiposity signals such as insulin and leptin act in the arcuate nuclei to provide a background tone, and this tone in turn determines the sensitivity of the brain to satiation signals that influence how much food is eaten at any one time. Note that these homeostatic mechanisms provide at most a background influence and only subtly influence intake during any given meal. Social factors, palatability, habits, stress, and many other factors are always at work, influencing not only when meals occur but also how much food is consumed. Only when extraneous factors are tightly controlled in laboratory animal experiments, or when ingestion is precisely monitored and quantified over periods of days or weeks in free-feeding humans, do the effects of these homeostatic signals become apparent.

Effect of Exercise on Appetite

Appetite and postexercise energy intake depends on many factors including the intensity, duration, and mode of exercise. Studies by King et al (1994) showed that high-intensity exercise suppressed appetite for a short period but no difference in food intake occurred when measured over 2 days. Hunger is suppressed only when the exercise is long enough (60 minutes or more) and intense enough (more than 70% $\dot{V}O_2max$). Few studies have investigated the effects of mode of exercise on appetite. King and Blundell (Blundell et al. 1995) compared treadmill exercise with cycling and did not observe a difference in appetite. Although anecdotal evidence indicates that swimming increases appetite more than other activities do, no scientific evidence backs this up. One study compared cycling submerged in cold (20 °C) water to cycling in neutral-temperature (33 °C) water and observed an increased appetite in the cold conditions, suggesting an effect of water temperature.

Evidence suggests that in the short to medium term (up to 16 days), exercise is able to produce a negative energy balance, with no substantial compensatory responses in energy intake. In the long term (more than 16 days), however, an increase in energy intake is likely to be observed. This compensation is usually partial and incomplete, generally accounting for only 30% of the energy cost associated with exercise, therefore allowing the attainment of a negative energy balance and some degree of weight loss (Blundell et al. 2003). In the short term, exercise may in fact be more effective than dieting in producing a negative energy balance. This notion is supported by the finding that an acute energy deficit created by dietary restriction (low-energy versus high-energy breakfast) induces a significant increase in subjective hunger, subsequent energy intake, and food cravings during the day. On the other hand, a similar energy deficit created by exercise failed to induce any significant change in these variables, thereby allowing the attainment of a short-term negative energy balance (Hubert et al. 1998).

Physical Activity and Energy Expenditure

Resting metabolic rate (RMR) is an important component of daily energy expenditure. It has been suggested that exercise can increase RMR and thereby increase energy expenditure during the rest of the day. The increase in RMR postexercise is often measured as postexercise oxygen consumption, or **EPOC** (Borsheim et al. 2003). It is well established that immediately after exercise, EPOC may be elevated, although this may only occur if the exercise is long enough and vigorous enough. Even if the exercise is long enough and vigorous enough, the postexercise increase in RMR seems only temporary and relatively small. After several hours RMR will return to baseline values. Suggestions that RMR is chronically increased have been refuted, and although some studies have reported an increased RMR, several other studies have even observed a decrease in RMR after training.

Another effect of exercise training could be an increase in muscle mass and thereby an increase in metabolically active tissue. This result may occur only with resistance exercise. The potential effects of resistance exercise training on weight loss will be discussed later.

So exercise may have a small, short-term effect on RMR. The longer-term effects are unclear but are unlikely to be important.

Exercise training, especially aerobic exercise, results in a shift from carbohydrate and fat metabolism. Increased mitochondrial density and increased capillarization of the muscle ensure an increase to the supply of substrates and oxygen to

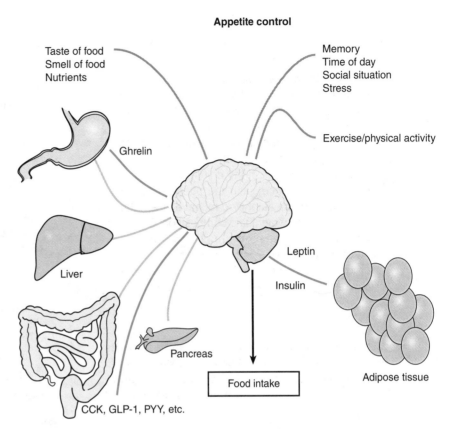

Appetite control

Taste of food
Smell of food
Nutrients

Memory
Time of day
Social situation
Stress

Exercise/physical activity

Ghrelin

Liver

Leptin

Insulin

Pancreas

Food intake

CCK, GLP-1, PYY, etc.

Adipose tissue

Figure 14.2 Appetite is sensed in the brain. The brain constantly receives and processes neural (gray lines), metabolic, and endocrine (blue lines) signals from the periphery. In addition, many other factors (pale blue lines) influence the eventual outcome (food intake).

Nutrients and Satiety

Humans eat in intervals; that is, they eat meals. Before a meal begins, the sensation of hunger rises, and this motivates food-seeking behavior. After eating starts, hunger declines, and people report that they start to feel full. The term satiation describes the processes that bring a meal to an end. An interval of time then elapses before eating begins again. **Satiety** refers to the inhibition of eating following a meal, and it is measured both by the interval between meals and by the amount consumed when food is next offered. Different macronutrients have different effects on satiety. It has been demonstrated that protein has a much stronger effect on satiety than fat and carbohydrate do. The effects of very high-protein diets on satiety and weight loss will be discussed in more detail in the section on high-protein diets and weight loss.

the muscle as well as an increase in the capacity to take up oxygen and substrates. Studies have consistently observed a decreased reliance on

Social and Behavioral Factors

Eating behavior is crucial to the maintenance of body weight, and this behavior is easily influenced by the lifestyle that athletes lead. Many sports have a specific eating culture, and in some sports, athletes are often exposed to cafeteria-type foods. In other sports, alcohol consumption is part of the culture (as a team-bonding experience), and the often-excessive consumption of alcohol can have dramatic effects on body weight and composition. On the other hand, some sports are characterized by pressure to achieve a particular low body weight or low body fat, and striving to reach that goal can result in disordered eating (see chapter 15).

Methods to Achieve Weight Loss

Dietary methods
- Fasting
- Energy restriction
- Low-fat diet
- High-protein diet
- High-carbohydrate diet
- Low-carbohydrate ketogenic diet (Atkins diet, Sugarbusters)
- Zone diet
- Food-combining diet
- Low glycemic index
- Low-energy density
- Calcium and diary products

Exercise
- Increased physical activity
- Regular exercise
- Endurance exercise

Surgical procedures
- Stomach stapling
- Removal of a section of the small intestine
- Liposuction

Pharmacological methods
- Stimulants
- Appetite suppressants
- Drugs that reduce fat absorption

carbohydrate as a fuel and an increased capacity to oxidize fat in response to as little as 4 weeks of exercise training. This increased ability to oxidize fat may help to reduce fat mass in a situation of energy restriction.

Dietary Weight-Loss Methods

Many athletes, although not overweight, seek to lose body weight, particularly body fat. For some this weight loss offers an advantage because it increases the power-to-weight ratio (particularly important in jumping events). For others, weight loss means that they can reduce their energy expenditure when competing (such as when running). Weight reduction is also common in weight-category sports in which athletes often compete well below their normal weight. Another reason that athletes want to get rid of some body fat is simply to enhance physical appearance and live up to the stereotype of the lean, toned, and strong athlete.

Weight loss is not always a good idea, and it can even be detrimental to performance. A reduction in body mass is usually accompanied by a reduction in muscle mass, and it may reduce muscle glycogen stores as well. Excessive weight loss has also been associated with chronic fatigue and increased risk of injuries. Too much emphasis on losing weight can lead to the development of eating disorders, which are discussed in chapter 15.

The various ways to lose body weight include pharmacological and surgical procedures (see the highlight box), but here we focus on the weight-loss strategies that involve diet, exercise, or a combination of the two. Several different diets exist, some of which have been commercialized. Some diets have proved to be effective, whereas others are a list of erroneous assumptions and claims. For the athlete, distinguishing between the facts and the fallacies is often difficult. This section reviews some of the most common dietary regimens and weight-loss methods.

Energy Restriction and Reduced Fat Intake

Debate continues over whether weight loss can be achieved by reducing energy intake or by reducing fat intake only. Epidemiological evidence suggests that reducing the percentage of fat in the diet is more effective in reducing body weight than is reducing the absolute amount of fat (Sheppard et al. 1991). The most important factor, however, is the reduction in energy intake. Although both energy restriction and low-fat eating result in weight loss, energy restriction usually results in a larger reduction in energy intake than does ad libitum (as desired) low-fat eating. Therefore, energy restriction may initially result in a larger weight loss, although studies show that both diets are effective over the long term (Jeffery et al. 1995; Schlundt et al. 1993).

The advantage of reduced fat intake is that relatively high carbohydrate content can be maintained, resulting in reasonable glycogen stores and better recovery. Many athletes adopt a diet that is low in fat with a small reduction in energy intake, so that they can still replenish their carbohydrate stores. This type of diet seems to be a sensible way of reducing weight, although suboptimal carbohydrate intake can still interfere with normal training. Thus, weight reduction should occur slowly and in the off-season.

Very Low-Energy Diets

Very low-energy diets (VLEDs) or very low-calorie diets (VLCDs) are used as a therapy to achieve rapid weight loss in the obese. These diets are usually in the form of liquid meals that contain the recommended daily intakes of micronutrients but only 1,600 to 3,200 kJ/day (400 to 800 kcal/day). These liquid meals contain a relatively large amount of protein to reduce muscle wasting and a relatively small amount of carbohydrate (less than 100 g/day). Such diets are extremely effective in reducing body weight rapidly. In the first week, the weight loss is predominantly glycogen and water. Fat and protein are lost as well during the initial phase, but those losses are a relatively small proportion of the total weight loss. After the initial rapid weight loss, the weight reduction is mainly from adipose tissue, although some loss of body protein occurs. The increased fat oxidation results in ketosis (formation of ketone bodies, acetoacetate, and γ-hydroxybutyrate). Ketone bodies have a specific odor that is easily detectable on the breath (bad breath). After ketosis begins, hunger feelings may decrease somewhat.

Because carbohydrate intake is low, blood glucose concentration is maintained by gluconeogenesis from various precursors (glycerol and alanine). Although increased physical activity is also encouraged when very low-energy diets are prescribed

to the obese, the diets are effective without the exercise component. Because of the associated chronic glycogen depletion, exercise capacity is severely impaired. For this reason, such diets are not advised for athletes, who would likely be unable to complete their normal training sessions. Even in the off-season such diets are not advised, because the loss of body protein can be significant. Side effects of such diets include nausea, halitosis (bad breath), hunger (which may decrease after the initiation of ketosis), light-headedness, and hypotension. Dehydration is also common with such diets, and electrolyte imbalances may occur.

Low-Fat Diets

Reducing dietary fat intake can be an effective way to reduce energy intake and promote weight loss for several reasons:

- Fat is energy dense. It has more than twice the amount of energy as the same weight of carbohydrate or protein.

- High-fat foods generally taste good, which leads to a tendency to eat more. Studies show that increasing the fat content of the diet increases the spontaneous intake of food.

- A large body of evidence has also shown that fat is less satiating than either protein or carbohydrate (de Castro 1987; de Castro et al. 1988).

- Fat is stored efficiently and requires little energy for digestion.

- Fat intake does not immediately increase fat oxidation.

Food-Combining Diets

Food-combining diets are based on a philosophy that certain foods should *not* be combined. Although many types of food-combining diets exist, most warn against the combination of protein and carbohydrate foods. Such combinations cause a "buildup of toxins" with "negative side effects such as weight gain." These diets are often tempting because they promise an easy way to rapid weight loss, and they have worked for many people. When these diets are strictly followed, energy and fat intake are likely to be reduced compared with the normal diet. The reduction in energy and fat is the reason for the success of the diet rather than the fact that certain foods were not combined. Because energy and carbohydrate intake are lower, glycogen stores decrease, and performance as well as recovery may be impaired.

High-Protein Diets

Recommendations for increased protein consumption are among the most common approaches of popular or fad diets. Some have argued that high-protein diets suppress the appetite, which might be a mechanism for facilitated weight loss. Protein also has a larger thermic effect and a relatively low coefficient of digestibility compared with a mixed, equicaloric (isoenergetic) meal. Several studies have demonstrated that increased protein content of the diet, particularly in combination with exercise training, may improve weight loss and reduce the loss of lean body mass in overweight and obese individuals during low-energy dieting (for a review, see Layman et al. 2006). Furthermore, less weight regain occurs after the energy-restricted period ends when protein intake is high compared with more normal dietary compositions (Paddon-Jones et al. 2008).

Part of the effect of protein is visible only in free-living conditions when energy intake is not controlled. This circumstance points to an effect of protein on satiety. Whereas during an isoenergetic high-protein diet, subjects did not lose body weight, during an ad libitum high-protein diet, subjects lost 4.4 to 5.4 kg and had a decrease in fat mass of 3.3 to 4.1 kg (Weigle et al. 2005). Evidence is accumulating that protein has a greater effect on satiety than the other macronutrients and that it can be helpful in a weight-loss situation.

Another effect of protein that can facilitate weight loss is its thermogenic effect. The metabolisable energy of protein as defined in the Atwater factor is 17 kJ/g (4 kcal/g). Protein, however, is particularly thermogenic, and the net metabolisable energy is actually 13 kJ/g (3.1 kcal/g), making it lower than either carbohydrate or fat (17 kJ/g [4 kcal/g] and 34 kJ/g [8.1 kcal/g], respectively). Reported values for diet-induced thermogenesis for separate nutrients are 0 to 3% for fat, 5 to 10% for carbohydrate, and 20 to 30% for protein (Tappy 1996). Thus, a high-protein diet induces a greater thermic response in healthy subjects compared with a high-fat diet. This conclusion implies even higher fat oxidation, thus a negative fat balance and a positive protein balance. The relatively strong thermic effect of protein may be mediated by the high ATP costs of postprandial protein synthesis. In one study, increasing the amount of dietary protein from 10 to 20% of total energy intake resulted in a 63 to 95% increase in protein oxidation, depending on the protein source (Pannemans et al. 1998). For example, Mikkelsen et al. (2000) observed a higher diet-induced thermogenesis with pork meat than with soy protein.

A third possible mechanism by which protein may aid weight loss is by maintaining muscle mass in an energy-restricted situation. Little evidence is available, but it seems that protein is able to prevent some of the muscle mass loss that is inevitable with energy restriction. This means that a larger muscle mass can be maintained, and because muscle is the most active tissue metabolically, RMR could increase, thus helping weight loss.

Most studies have been conducted in nonathletes and inactive populations, including elderly and obese subjects. The relevance of these findings for athletes in training is questionable. The few studies in athletes seem to provide conflicting data on the effect of increased protein intake during weight loss. One study using nitrogen balance supports the idea that increased protein intake preserves muscle during low-calorie dieting in bodybuilders (Walberg et al. 1988). But a more recent study found no effect of increased protein or branched-chain amino acid (BCAA) intake on lean body mass loss during weight loss in athletes (Mourier et al. 1997).

Overall, evidence is accumulating that protein content of a diet can be an important tool in weight management.

The Zone Diet

The Zone diet was proposed by Barry Sears in his book *The Zone: A Dietary Road Map* (Sears 1995). The diet opposes the traditional recommendations of a high-carbohydrate, low-fat diet for athletes. By reducing carbohydrate intake, insulin response decreases and a favorable insulin-to-glucagon

---

Protein in Weight Loss

Protein may be effective in supporting weight loss for several reasons:

1. Protein has a greater effect on satiety than carbohydrate or fat does.

2. Protein has a greater thermogenic effect than carbohydrate or fat does.

3. Protein may also have a role in maintaining muscle mass in a situation of energy restriction, thereby preserving metabolically active tissue.

ratio is established. The benefits are increased lipolysis and improved regulation of eicosanoids, hormone-like derivatives of FAs in the body that act as cell-to-cell signaling molecules. The diet increases the "good" eicosanoids and decreases the "bad" eicosanoids.

The good eicosanoids improve blood flow to the working muscle and enhance the delivery of oxygen and nutrients, eventually resulting in improved performance. To "enter the zone," the diet should consist of 40% carbohydrate, 30% fat, and 30% protein divided into a regimen of three meals and two snacks per day. The diet is also referred to as the 40:30:30 diet.

Although some arguments by Sears are scientifically sound, the book has problems, pitfalls, and errors in assumptions, and it contains some contradictory information. Many of the promised benefits of the Zone diet are based on selective information about hormonal influences on eicosanoid metabolism. Opposing evidence is conveniently left out.

Eicosanoid metabolism is extremely complex and highly unpredictable, and previous diet manipulation studies have been unsuccessful in stimulating the synthesis of good eicosanoids relative to bad eicosanoids. Very small changes in insulin concentration are sufficient to reduce lipolysis significantly. Such effects persist for up to 6 hours after a meal. To avoid reductions in lipolysis after a meal, carbohydrate intake must be extremely small, even less than that proposed by the Zone diet. Meals with the 40:30:30 combination are difficult to compose, unless the dieter buys the 40:30:30 energy bars marketed by Sears.

Nevertheless, the Zone diet seems to work for some people, and anecdotal evidence indicates weight loss with the diet. The successes are expected because the Zone diet is essentially low in energy (4,000 to 8,000 kJ/day [1,000 to 2,000 kcal/day]). Even for athletes who train hard, the energy intake does not increase much and they are in a relatively large energy deficit.

The principle of vasodilating muscle arterioles by altering eicosanoid production is correct in theory, but the little evidence available from human studies does not support any significant contribution of eicosanoids to active muscle vasodilation. In fact, the key eicosanoid reportedly produced in the Zone diet and responsible for improved muscle oxygenation is not found in skeletal muscle. The best available scientific evidence suggests that the Zone diet is more ergolytic than ergogenic to performance.

Low-Carbohydrate Diets

Some of the best-known low-carbohydrate ketogenic diets are the Atkins diet (Atkins 1992) and Sugarbusters (Andrews et al. 1998). These diets are based on the premise that reducing carbohydrate intake results in increased fat oxidation. Ketone body production will increase, which may suppress appetite. Ketones may also be present in urine, which could result in loss of "calories" through urine. Although all of the preceding may be true, the losses achieved in this diet are extremely small. The excretion of ketone bodies in urine is small, at most 400 to 600 kJ/day (100 to 150 kcal/day). Such diets can be effective, but they are no more effective than a well-balanced, energy-restricted diet. These low-carbohydrate diets are not recommended because of the relatively high-fat content, which may raise blood lipids. For athletes, these diets are detrimental because of reduced glycogen stores and exercise capacity. Figure 14.3 shows the effects of ad libitum energy intake (left panel) and weight of food consumed (right panel) in subjects who consume diets that have 20, 40, and 60% of their energy as fat. The left column represents the findings in carefully controlled lab conditions, and the middle column represents free-living conditions. In these two projects the energy density between diets was different. In the third study (right column), the energy density was the same despite differences in composition. Note that subjects ate a constant weight of food independent of energy and that the energy density of the meals is a major determinant of energy intake.

Manipulation of Energy Density

The **energy density** of the diet may play an important role in weight maintenance. A small quantity of food rich in fat has a very high energy content. Visual cues that may prevent a large intake of energy on a high-carbohydrate diet, which is commonly of high bulk and volume, may be absent. A number of studies have shown that subjects tend to eat a similar weight of food regardless of the macronutrient composition. Because a 500 g meal consisting mainly of carbohydrate will contain significantly less energy than a 500 g high-fat meal, lower energy intake will automatically result.

In an elegant series of studies, Stubbs et al. (1995a, 1995b, 1996) demonstrated that when subjects received a diet that contained 20%, 40%, or 60% fat and could eat ad libitum, the weight

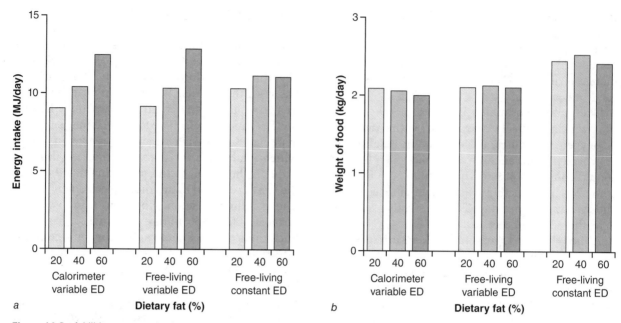

Figure 14.3 Ad libitum energy intake *(a)* and weight of food consumed *(b)* in subjects who consume diets that have 20, 40, and 60% of their energy as fat.
Based on Stubbs et al. 1995; Stubbs, Harbron, and Prentice 1996; Stubbs, Ritts et al. 1995.

of the food that they consumed was the same. Because of differences in energy density, however, the total amount of energy consumed with the higher-fat diets was greater and therefore weight gain was greater. This result happened in both controlled laboratory conditions and free-living conditions. When the fat content of the diet was altered but the energy density was kept the same, the subjects still consumed the same weight of food, but this time the energy intake was the same, independent of the fat content of the diet.

In a review, the energy intake in several longitudinal studies was plotted against energy density (figure 14.4) (Poppitt et al. 1996). It can clearly be seen that an increase in energy density results in an increase in energy intake, whereas a decrease in the energy density of the diet results in a decrease in intake.

These studies clearly demonstrate the important role of the energy density of the diet and suggest that manipulation of energy density is a good tool in weight management.

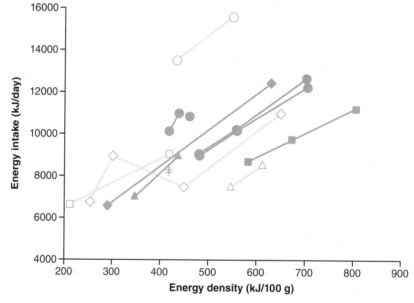

Figure 14.4 Increasing the energy density of the diet in longitudinal metabolic studies results in a corresponding increase in energy intake.
Reprinted from *Appetite*, Vol. 26, S.D. Poppitt and A.M. Prentice, "Energy density and its role in the control of food intake: Evidence from metabolic and community studies," pgs: 153-174. Copyright 1996, with permission from Elsevier.

Calcium and Dairy Products

The possible weight-reducing effect of dairy products was first observed by accident in a study in which the effects of dairy products on hypertension were investigated. As hypothesized, a higher dairy intake that provided 1,000 mg of calcium per day reduced hypertension compared with a control diet that provided 400 mg of calcium per day. But the authors were surprised to find that the subjects in the supplemented group lost 4.9 kg of body fat (Zemel et al. 2000). Similar trends were observed in several large population-based studies (NHANES, the Quebec family study, CARDIA, and the HERITAGE family study).

A suggested mechanism is that dietary calcium modulates circulating calcitriol 1,25-(OH)2-D, which regulates intracellular calcium. This intracellular calcium plays a crucial role in fat metabolism in adipocytes. It has been suggested that reducing calcitriol by increasing dietary calcium intake results in a reduction of body fat in the absence of energy restriction. In combination with energy restriction it may result in increased body fat and weight loss.

Dairy calcium appears to be more effective than just calcium, because the protein and amino acids in dairy products may have additional benefits. These could be related to the effects of protein on satiety and to the effects on angiotensin converting enzyme (ACE), which has a role in adipose tissue fat metabolism.

Although several possible mechanisms have now been proposed and some studies provide evidence of a positive effect of dairy products on weight management, debate continues about the issue. In a recent review, a large number of clinical trials were compared. Of the 49 randomized trials that assessed the effect of dairy products or calcium supplementation on body weight, 41 showed no effect, 2 demonstrated weight gain, 1 showed a lower rate of gain, and 5 showed weight loss. Four of 24 trials reported differential fat loss. Consequently, the majority of the current evidence from clinical trials does not support the hypothesis that calcium or dairy consumption aids in weight loss or fat loss.

The debate about a role for dairy and calcium will continue. For a more detailed discussion, see several reviews (Lanou et al. 2008; Zemel 2004; Zemel et al. 2005).

Nonnutritive Sweeteners

Nonnutritive sweeteners or artificial sweeteners are ecologically novel chemosensory signaling compounds that influence ingestive processes and behavior (see the highlight box). Five nonnutritive sweeteners with intense sweetening power have FDA approval (acesulfame-K, aspartame, neotame, saccharin, sucralose). These sweeteners, some of which contain hardly any energy at all, have

the potential to moderate energy intakes while maintaining diet palatability. A critical review of the literature suggests that the addition of nonnutritive sweeteners to non-energy-yielding products may heighten appetite, but this result is not observed under the common condition in which nonnutritive sweeteners is ingested in conjunction with other energy sources. Substitution of a nonnutritive sweetener for a nutritive sweetener generally results in greater energy intake in the short term, but evidence of long-term efficacy for weight management is not available. The addition of nonnutritive sweeteners to the diet poses no benefit for weight loss or reduced weight gain without energy restriction. There are long-standing and recent concerns that inclusion of nonnutritive sweeteners in the diet promotes energy intake and has contributed to the obesity problem. More research is needed to understand the underlying mechanisms and the exact effects of nonnutritive sweeteners.

Exercise for Weight Loss

Exercise is another way to create a negative energy balance. In obese people, the effectiveness of exercise programs to achieve weight loss has been questioned because of problems with motivation, compliance, and impaired ability to exercise. In athletes, these factors are unlikely to be a problem. Most athletes can include exercise sessions with the specific aim of increasing energy expenditure, and they can exercise at an intensity high enough to cause a significant increase of energy expenditure. But athletes may have different problems. For example, coaches of athletes who compete in explosive events (e.g., sprints and jumps) are often reluctant to include aerobic exercise in their training programs. Athletes may have difficulty finding time to exercise in addition to performing their normal training without compromising recovery.

Generally, however, adding exercise to a weight-loss program results in weight loss that is fat loss (Ballor et al. 1991; Kraemer et al. 1995; McMurray et al. 1985). The combination of exercise and diet is the most effective way to maintain a lower body weight after weight reduction.

Exercise Intensity

Some argue that the optimal exercise intensity is related to fat oxidation and should be the intensity with the highest fat-oxidation rates. As discussed in chapter 7, fat oxidation increases as exercise increases from low to moderate intensity, even

---

Nonnutritive Sweeteners

Natural sugar substitutes

Brazzein—protein, 800× sweetness of sucrose (by weight)

Curculin—protein, 550× sweetness (by weight)

Erythritol—0.7× sweetness (by weight), 14× sweetness of sucrose (by food energy)

Fructose—1.7× sweetness (by weight and food energy)

Glycyrrhizin—50× sweetness (by weight)

Isomalt—0.45–0.65× sweetness (by weight), 0.9–1.3× sweetness (by food energy)

Lactitol—0.4× sweetness (by weight), 0.8× sweetness (by food energy)

Lo Han Guo—300× sweetness (by weight)

Mabinlin—protein, 100× sweetness (by weight)

Maltitol—0.9× sweetness (by weight), 1.7× sweetness (by food energy), E965

Mannitol—0.5× sweetness (by weight), 1.2× sweetness (by food energy), E421

Monellin—protein, 3,000× sweetness (by weight)

Pentadin—protein, 500× sweetness (by weight)

Sorbitol—0.6× sweetness (by weight), 0.9× sweetness (by food energy), E420

Stevia—250× sweetness (by weight)

Tagatose—0.92× sweetness (by weight), 2.4× sweetness (by food energy)

Thaumatin—protein, 2,000× sweetness (by weight), E957

Xylitol—1.0× sweetness (by weight), 1.7× sweetness (by food energy), E967

Artificial sugar substitutes

Acesulfame potassium—200× sweetness (by weight), Nutrinova, E950, FDA approved 1988

Aspartame—160–200× sweetness (by weight), NutraSweet, E951, FDA approved 1981

Dulcin—250× sweetness (by weight), FDA banned 1950

Neotame—8,000× sweetness (by weight), NutraSweet, FDA approved 2002

P-4000—4,000× sweetness (by weight), FDA banned 1950

Saccharin—300× sweetness (by weight), E954, FDA approved 1958

Sucralose—600× sweetness (by weight), Splenda, Tate & Lyle, E955, FDA approved 1998

---

though the percentage contribution of fat may decrease (see figure 7.8, p. 156). Increased fat oxidation is a direct result of increased energy expenditure when going from light-intensity to moderate-intensity exercise. At high exercise intensities (>75% of $\dot{V}O_2max$), fat oxidation is inhibited, and both the relative rate and the absolute rate of fat oxidation decrease to negligible values (Achten et al. 2002). Maximal rates of fat oxidation generally occur between 55% and 65% of $\dot{V}O_2max$. Whether exercise at this intensity is more effective than exercise at other intensities remains to be determined.

Mode of Exercise

The mode of exercise also affects maximal rates of fat oxidation. For example, fat oxidation is significantly higher during uphill walking and running compared with cycling (Achten et al. 2003; Arkinstall et al. 2001; Houmard et al. 1990; Nieman et al. 1998a, 1998b). No long-term studies have been conducted to compare different types of exercise and their effectiveness in achieving or maintaining weight loss. In addition, whether exercises that optimize fat oxidation are indeed an effective way to reduce body fat remains to be determined.

Comparisons of resistance training with endurance training have demonstrated favorable effects on body composition (Broeder et al. 1997; Van Etten et al. 1994) or similar effects in facilitating body-fat loss (Ballor et al. 1991). Resistance training seems more effective in preserving or increasing fat-free mass. In turn, the amount of metabolically active tissue also increases, and the increase is suggested as one of the mechanisms by which exercise helps to maintain lower body weight after weight loss through energy restriction. The exercise preserves (or even increases) muscle mass, resulting in a smaller reduction of the RMR.

Few studies have compared the effectiveness of various types of exercise. Current evidence, however, indicates that resistance training is at least as effective as aerobic exercise in reducing body fat. One important factor, of course, is the duration of exercise, which largely determines the energy expended. Athletes who can spend more time exercising at relatively high exercise intensities have a greater opportunity to achieve a negative energy balance and thus lose body weight.

Decreased Resting Metabolic Rate With Weight Loss

It has been anecdotally reported that losing body weight becomes increasingly difficult as weight loss progresses, presumably because the body responds to weight loss by becoming more efficient. There are conflicting reports about whether resting metabolic rate adapts or decreases beyond expected values based on changes in body composition in response to energy restriction and weight loss. If RMR exhibits metabolic adaptation, this would provide evidence that metabolic changes defend a certain body weight (set point), which could partly explain why people have difficulty maintaining weight loss. Several studies have reported that RMR decreases in response to weight loss (Dulloo et al. 1998). Most studies have been performed in obese individuals. In a study, three groups of nonobese (although overweight) subjects were subjected to energy restriction for 6 months (Martin et al. 2007). One group was energy restricted by reducing food intake by 25%, one group was subjected to energy

restriction (12.5%) and an increase in physical activity by structured exercise (12.5%), and the third group served as the control group. Weight loss was similar in the two energy-restricted groups (loss of 10% of initial body weight). RMR adapted or decreased beyond values expected from changes in weight and body composition as a result of the energy deficit that was achieved through a food-based diet after 3 months and a food-based diet plus structured exercise after 6 months (Martin et al. 2007). The control group did not experience a decrease in RMR. At month 6 the combined data from the dieting groups demonstrated that RMR was lower than expected, resulting in 91 kcal/day less energy expenditure compared with control participants, even after differences in FFM were taken into consideration.

This decrease in resting metabolism is an autoregulatory feedback mechanism by which the body tries to preserve energy. This "food efficiency" may occur independently of a person's body mass or dieting history. It usually causes a plateau in weight loss and is a common source of frustration for dieters.

In a well-designed study by Leibel et al. (1995), maintenance of a 10% reduction in body weight was associated with a reduction in total energy expenditure of 25 kJ · kg FFM^{-1} · day^{-1} (6 kcal · kg FFM^{-1} · day^{-1}) in nonobese subjects (see figure

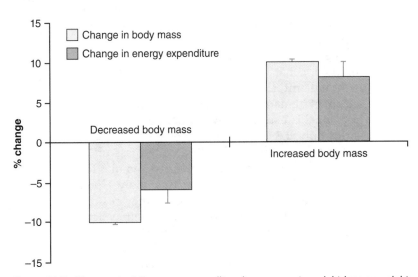

Figure 14.5 Changes in daily energy expenditure in response to weight loss or weight gain. A 10% reduction in body weight resulted in a 6% decrease in energy expenditure, and a 10% gain in body weight resulted in an 8% increase in energy expenditure. This finding shows that the body has compensatory mechanisms that try to maintain a normal body weight.

Data from Leibel, Rosenbaum, and Hirsch 1995.

14.5). Resting energy expenditure and nonresting energy expenditure each decreased 13 to 17 kJ · kg FFM^{-1} · day^{-1} (3 to 4 kcal · kg FFM^{-1} · day^{-1}). Maintenance of a 10% higher body weight was associated with an increase in total energy expenditure of 38 kJ · kg FFM^{-1} · day^{-1} (9 kcal · kg FFM^{-1} · day^{-1}). Maintenance of a reduced or elevated body weight is associated with compensatory changes in energy expenditure, which oppose the maintenance of a body weight that is different from the usual weight. This study shows that the body has compensatory mechanisms that try to maintain a normal body weight.

Female athletes, especially runners, sometimes have extremely low energy intakes. Despite their training load (30 to 90 km of running per week), they may have energy intakes similar to their sedentary counterparts (Drinkwater et al. 1984; Myerson et al. 1991). Amenorrheic runners (those whose menstrual cycles are currently absent) had a significantly lower RMR than eumenorrheic runners (those with normal monthly menstrual cycles), and their energy intake was similar, despite higher activity levels (Lebenstedt et al. 1999; Myerson et al. 1991). These findings suggest that energy efficiency or food efficiency exists. But other reasons may account for the negative energy balance or low energy intake and expenditure in these female athletes. Not all studies of these athletes have found a reduced RMR (Beidleman et al. 1995; Wilmore et al. 1992). Alternative explanations include inaccuracies and underreporting of food intake by these athletes or reduced physical activity in the hours when they are not training.

The concept of food efficiency fits in with the theory that the body has a weight set point. Although interindividual differences in body weight of humans are large, the body weight of an individual is usually fairly constant and typically varies only 0.5% over periods of 6 to 10 weeks (350 g for an individual with a body mass of 70 kg). If rats are given an energy-restricted diet for several weeks, they lose body mass rapidly. Upon being permitted to eat freely again, they restore this body mass within weeks and their weight becomes identical to their counterparts who had free access to food for the entire period. A similar change happens when rats are overfed. Evidence also exists for such a set point for body weight in humans (Keesey et al. 1997).

Weight Cycling

Often, the considerable effort applied to achieve weight loss is exceeded by the effort required to maintain the new lower body weight. After the weight is lost, it is regained in a relatively short period. This effect is usually referred to as the yo-yo effect. Studies in animals have documented this pattern of weight cycling. After a period of food restriction and weight reduction, animals tend to regain the weight quickly if they are allowed free access to food.

Several prospective studies have shown that weight fluctuation (gain–loss or loss–gain) or weight variability is associated with increased mortality, independent of the direction of weight change. When taking limited account of preexisting disease, however, studies show little evidence of negative side effects of weight cycling (Field et al. 1999; Wannamethee et al. 2002). From a public health perspective, the risks from overweight and obesity far exceed the potential risks of weight cycling.

Gender Differences in Weight Loss

Meta-analyses of studies on weight loss after aerobic exercise training showed that weight loss, although modest, was greater for males (Ballor et al. 1991). These findings confirm earlier research in males concerning exercise-training effects on body mass and body composition and extend them both to females and to a broader range of exercise types. These gender differences have been related to differences in body-fat distribution. Women store more fat in the gluteal–femoral region, whereas men store more fat in the visceral (abdominal) depot. Fat located in the upper body and abdominal regions (central fat) is more metabolically active and therefore has higher rates of lipolysis in response to adrenergic stimulation. During exercise, FAs are preferentially mobilized from these regions (Wahrenberg et al. 1991). In addition, postprandial fat storage may be higher in subcutaneous adipose tissue in women than in men. All these differences may play a role in the variation in net regional fat storage between men and women (Blaak 2001) and women's greater resistance to weight loss.

Practicalities of Weight Loss for Athletes

We have discussed the factors that influence body weight and body composition, and the research and myths that surround weight loss. But we have not yet discussed how this information can be used to achieve weight loss in athletes. Note that the studies discussed in the preceding section are predominantly performed on obese subjects and that little evidence has been obtained about athletes. These studies were concerned with longer-term weight loss. Some information is available about athlete populations, but it generally concerns short-term weight loss programs for athletes in weight-category sports. This topic will be discussed in detail in a following section. Although the information on longer-term weight loss obtained from obesity research can be informative, it is difficult to draw conclusions and come up with clear guidelines for athletes. The first step in the process should always be to define the goals: Is weight loss really required, and, if so, how much and over what period? With goals established, various strategies can be put in place to achieve the weight loss. In the process of weight management of the athlete, many mistakes can be made, and these will be discussed here as well.

Defining Goals

In conjunction with the coach and a nutritionist, weight-loss goals should be established. These goals should be carefully thought out and well defined. Whether the goal is a good idea or not depends primarily on the current body-fat percentage. Although individual differences exist, a body-fat percentage less than 5% for men and 12% for women is not recommended. As discussed earlier, some fat is essential, and people can lose only some of the storage fat without affecting physiological function.

Goals also have to be defined with a time schedule in mind. How much weight must be lost and how soon? A realistic weight loss is about a 1 kg (2 lb) every 2 weeks, so to lose 3 kg at least 6 weeks are needed. Achieving this goal means reducing energy intake by about 2,000 kJ (500 kcal) a day. Faster weight loss will make training difficult or impossible.

Defining the Strategy

The next step is to establish a strategy that will help the athlete lose weight. Following are guidelines to help athletes achieve weight loss.

- Determine a realistic body-weight goal. The help of a sports dietitian is likely needed to identify a realistic target weight.

- Do not try to lose more than about 0.5 kg/week (about 1 lb/week), and do not restrict energy intake by more than 500 to 750 kcal/day.

- Eat more fruit and vegetables.
- Choose low-fat snacks.
- Study food labels and try to find substitutes for high-fat foods. Look not only at fat content but also at the energy content per serving.
- Limit fat add-ons such as sauces, sour cream, and high-fat salad dressings, or choose the low-fat versions of these products.
- Try to structure your eating into five or six smaller meals.
- Avoid eating extremely large meals.
- Make sure that carbohydrate intake is high and consume carbohydrate immediately after training.
- A multivitamin and mineral supplement may be useful during periods of energy restriction. Seek the advice of a nutritionist or dietitian.
- Measure body weight daily and obtain measurements of body fat regularly (every 2 months). Keep a record of the changes.

Common Mistakes

When trying to lose weight, athletes make the following common mistakes:

- *Trying to lose weight too rapidly*. Like most people, athletes are impatient about weight loss. They want to see results within a couple of weeks, but unfortunately this expectation is not realistic. Although rapid weight loss is possible, this reduction is mostly dehydration, which reduces performance and the ability to train. Weight loss without performance loss has to occur slowly.

- *Trying to lose weight during the on-season*. Athletes often try to lose weight during the competitive season, and this effort may result in underperformance. Because hard training is difficult when the energy intake is reduced, weight loss is best accomplished during the off-season.

- *Not eating breakfast or lunch*. Another weight-loss approach that athletes have tried is skipping breakfast and sometimes even skipping lunch. Although this approach may work for some, it increases hunger feelings later in the day, and one large evening meal can easily compensate for the daytime reduction in food intake. In addition, exercise capacity and thus the ability to train may decrease without a breakfast, when liver glycogen stores may be low (see chapter 5).

- *Taking in too little carbohydrate*. When losing body weight (being in negative energy balance), athletes also risk losing muscle mass. But this risk can be reduced by consuming relatively large amounts of carbohydrate. Carbohydrate intake has a protein-sparing effect.

Making Weight and Rapid Weight-Loss Strategies

Sports in which **making weight** is important are those with weight categories, including judo, wrestling, rowing, and boxing. In horse racing, jockeys are weighed before and after competition to ensure that each horse carries the precise assigned weight. In these sports, weight classes are clearly defined, and to compete in a particular weight class, body weight must be within the limits for that category at the weigh-in. Rowing, for instance, has a lightweight and a heavyweight division. In the lightweight division, male athletes are not permitted to exceed 72.5 kg (160 lb) and the crew must have an average weight of 70 kg (155 lb). For females, the maximum individual weight is 59 kg (130 lb) and the crew must have an average weight of 57 kg (125 lb). Weigh-ins can take place from 30 minutes to about 20 hours before competition, although sometimes the weigh-in is performed the day before the competition. Athletes commonly compete at a weight that is 2 to 6 kg (4 to 13 lb) below their normal weight, which implies that they must lose weight rapidly in the days or weeks before competition.

Most rapid weight loss is by dehydration, and athletes use various techniques to achieve it. The most common methods are energy or fluid restriction; dehydration by exercise, sauna, hotrooms, or steam rooms; and diuretics, stimulants, and laxatives. Exercise is often performed in a hotroom, while wearing plastic or rubber garments. This rapid weight loss mainly affects body water, glycogen content, and lean body mass, and little or no loss of body fat occurs (Kelly et al. 1978; Oppliger et al. 1991). Wrestlers experience these weight-loss and weight-gain cycles about 7 to 15 times each year and approximately 100 times during a wrestling career (Tipton et al. 1993).

Rapid weight loss may result in reductions in plasma volume, central blood volume, and blood flow to active tissues and increased core temperature and heart rate. Cardiovascular changes can be observed with a weight loss of approximately 2% of body weight (see chapter 8). These rapid weight-loss strategies have also been reported to alter hormone status, impede normal growth and development, affect psychological state, impair

academic performance, and affect immune function. Severe dehydration can result in heat illness and even death.

In 1997 three previously healthy collegiate wrestlers in the United States died while engaged in rapid weight-loss programs to qualify for competition (Anonymus 1998). In the hours preceding the official weigh-in, all three wrestlers engaged in a similar rapid weight-loss regimen that promoted dehydration through perspiration and resulted in hyperthermia. The wrestlers restricted food and fluid intake and attempted to maximize sweat losses by wearing vapor-impermeable suits under cotton warm-up suits and exercising vigorously in hot environments. In response to these deaths, the National Collegiate Athletic Association (NCAA) rules were changed, and a wresting weight certification program was made mandatory to create a safer competitive environment (Davis et al. 2002). Other changes included establishing a weight-class system that better reflected the wrestling population, conducting weigh-ins close to competition (1 hour before) and for each day of a multiple-day tournament, and prohibiting use of tools that result in rapid dehydration (Davis et al. 2002). The current NCAA rules are now in line with the recommendations by the American College of Sports Medicine (ACSM) (Oppliger et al. 1996).

Weight gain is a concern for athletes in sports in which higher body weight and increased muscle mass are advantages, such as hammer throwing, discus throwing, shot put, weightlifting, American football, and rugby. The key to gaining weight is to have energy intake exceed energy expenditure. To increase lean body mass rather than just fat mass, a person must increase carbohydrate intake and not fat intake. Whereas the body counteracts a decrease in body weight that occurs with energy restriction by decreasing resting energy expenditure (see previous section), the body increases resting energy expenditure when energy intake increases in excess of expenditure. Just as expecting large weight losses in a short period is unrealistic, so is expecting large weight gains within days. Realistic weight gains are between 0.2 and 1.0 kg/week (0.4 to 2 lb/week), depending on the increase in energy intake. Protein synthesis is a slow process, and even with intake of excess amounts of protein, synthesis of muscle protein takes a long time and takes place only if combined with an adequate training program. For more information on protein synthesis and gaining muscle mass, see chapter 8.

KEY POINTS

■ An average body-fat percentage for young adults is between 12% and 15% for males and between 25% and 28% for females. Approximately 3% of body mass of males and 12% of body mass of females is essential body fat.

■ Appetite is sensed in the brain, which constantly receives and processes neural, metabolic, and endocrine signals from the periphery. In addition, a large number of external factors influence eventual food intake.

■ Negative energy balance is required to lose weight. In addition, negative fat balance will promote fat loss. The resting metabolic rate (RMR), however, decreases in response to weight loss. This effect, referred to as food efficiency, makes losing weight more difficult. A common problem is the so-called yo-yo effect, or weight cycling. After weight loss is achieved, the lost weight is often regained in a relatively short period.

■ Studies clearly demonstrate the important role of energy density of the diet for voluntary food intake and suggest that manipulation of energy density is a useful tool in weight management.

■ Common diet strategies to lose weight include very low-energy diets (VLED), low-carbohydrate diets, food combination diets, and high-protein diets. For athletes seeking to lose weight, energy restriction and reduced fat intake are recommended. This strategy allows a reasonable carbohydrate intake, enabling athletes to perform high-intensity training without major reductions in lean body mass (LBM).

■ Exercise can help to create a negative energy balance, maintain muscle mass, and compensate for the reductions in RMR seen after weight loss.

■ In weight-category sports such as judo, wrestling, rowing, and boxing, the need to make weight encourages athletes to try to lose weight in a relatively short time. Athletes should be aware of the risks of rapid weight loss. Rapid weight loss (mainly dehydration) can affect both health and performance.

■ The recommended method to gain weight is to maintain a positive energy balance without increasing fat intake. Most of the excess energy intake should come from carbohydrate.

RECOMMENDED READINGS

Blundell, J.E., R.J. Stubbs, D.A. Hughes, S. Whybrow, and N.A. King. 2003. Cross talk between physical activity and appetite control: Does physical activity stimulate appetite? *Proceedings of the Nutrition Society* 62:651–661.

Bouchard, C. 1994. Genetics of obesity: Overview and research directions. In *The genetics of obesity*, ed. C. Bouchard, 223–233. Boca Raton, FL: CRC Press.

Bouchard, C., A. Tremblay, J.P. Despres, A. Nadeau, P.J. Lupien, G. Theriault, J. Dussault, S. Moorjani, S. Pinault, and G. Fournier. 1990. The response to long-term overfeeding in identical twins. *New England Journal of Medicine* 322:1477–1482.

Flatt, J.-P. 1995. Use and storage of carbohydrate and fat. *American Journal of Clinical Nutrition* 61:952S–959S.

Lanou, A.J., and N.D. 2008. Barnard. Dairy and weight loss hypothesis: An evaluation of the clinical trials. *Nutrition Reviews* 66:272–279.

Paddon-Jones, D., E. Westman, R.D. Mattes, R.R. Wolfe, A. Astrup, and M. Westerterp-Plantenga. 2008. Protein, weight management, and satiety. *American Journal of Clinical Nutrition* 87:1558S–1561S.

Poppitt, S.D., and A.M. Prentice. 1996. Energy density and its role in the control of food intake: Evidence from metabolic and community studies. *Appetite* 26:153–174.

Roche, A.F., S.B. Heymsfield, and T.G. Lohman. 1996. *Human body composition.* Champaign, IL: Human Kinetics.

Zemel, M.B. 2004. Role of calcium and dairy products in energy partitioning and weight management. *American Journal of Clinical Nutrition* 79:907S–912S.

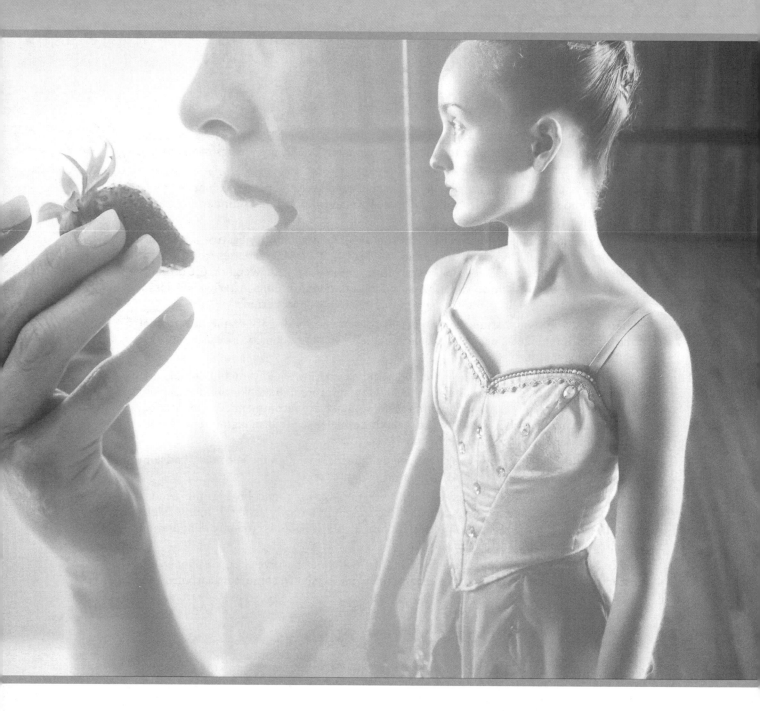

OBJECTIVES

After studying this chapter, you should be able to do the following:

- Describe the characteristics of anorexia nervosa and bulimia nervosa
- Describe the prevalence of eating disorders in athletes
- Describe the risk factors for eating disorders
- Describe the effects of eating disorders on sports performance
- Describe the effects of eating disorders on the health of the athlete
- Describe some effective strategies for the treatment and prevention of eating disorders

15

Eating Disorders in Athletes

Key Terms

For people consuming 8 to 12 MJ/day (1,900 to 2,900 kcal/day) of dietary energy, a typical pattern of eating might be two or three main meals (e.g., breakfast, lunch, and dinner), with an occasional snack (e.g., biscuit or chocolate bar) between meals. For endurance athletes with higher energy intakes (typically 15 to 20 MJ/day [3,600 to 4,800 kcal/day]), a grazing pattern of eating is common, with a substantial proportion of daily energy intake consumed between meals. In most cases, athletes are in energy balance, meaning that over the course of several days or weeks, energy intake generally matches energy expenditure. But some athletes (and nonathletes) experience eating disorders characterized by gross disturbances of eating behaviors. The major disorders are associated with abnormally low food intake or bouts of binge eating followed by purging the stomach contents. If undiagnosed and untreated, eating disorders not only can have detrimental effects on sports performance but also can have damaging, long-lasting effects on health and can even be fatal. The potentially irreversible consequences of these conditions, characterized by low energy availability, emphasize the critical need for prevention, early diagnosis, and treatment.

Evidence suggests that the prevalence of eating disorders is more common in certain athletic groups than in the general population, and the role of the sport nutritionist or dietitian working with athletes who are susceptible to eating disorders is crucial to prevention. Often the best treatment is educating athletes about the health risks of eating disorders and counseling them about wise food choices and good eating habits. This chapter reviews the characteristics of various eating disorders, the prevalence of eating disorders in various sports, risk factors for eating disorders, and the effects of eating disorders on sports performance and health. Some practical guidelines on diagnosis, treatment, and prevention of eating disorders are also given.

Types of Eating Disorders

Eating behavior can be considered as a spectrum ranging from healthy eating to overeating in one direction and clinical eating disorders in the other (figure 15.1). The major classified eating disorders include (1) anorexia nervosa, (2) bulimia nervosa, and (3) eating disorders not otherwise specified (EDNOS) (American Psychiatric Association 1994). For athletes who show significant symptoms of eating disorders but do not meet the criteria of the

Diagnostic and Statistical Manual of Mental Disorders (American Psychiatric Association 1994) for anorexia or bulimia, a subclinical eating disorder separately classified as anorexia athletica has been proposed (Sundgot-Borgen 1994a).

The major problem is low **energy availability,** which is defined not simply as low dietary energy intake but rather as the dietary energy intake minus exercise energy expenditure. Energy availability is thus the amount of dietary energy available for other body functions after exercise training. When energy availability is too low, physiological mechanisms reduce the amount of energy used for cellular maintenance, thermoregulation, growth, bone development, and reproduction. Although the compensatory mechanisms tend to restore energy balance and promote survival, health becomes impaired.

Some athletes reduce their energy availability by reducing their dietary energy intake more than their exercise energy expenditure, whereas others reduce their energy availability by increasing their energy expenditure more than their intake. Some practice abnormal eating behaviors such as fasting, binge eating, or purging. Others use drugs such as diet pills, laxatives, and diuretics to increase weight

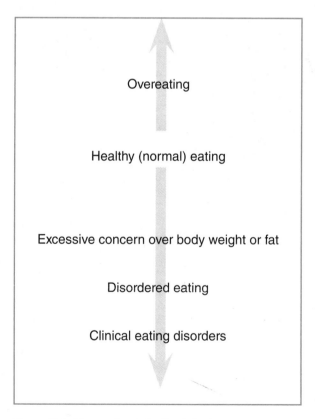

Overeating

Healthy (normal) eating

Excessive concern over body weight or fat

Disordered eating

Clinical eating disorders

Figure 15.1 The spectrum of eating behavior.

loss. Some athletes have eating disorders, which are clinical mental disorders, often accompanied by other psychiatric illnesses. These eating disorders are more common in females than in males.

Anorexia nervosa is an eating disorder characterized by an abnormally small food intake and a refusal to maintain normal body weight (according to what is expected for gender, age, and height), a distorted view of body image, an intense fear of being fat or overweight and gaining weight, or "feeling fat" when the person is at least 15% below normal weight for age and height. The absence of at least three successive **menstrual cycles** in females (amenorrhea) is a diagnostic criterion for anorexia nervosa. The physical symptoms of people who experience anorexia nervosa or anorexia athletica can be summarized as follows (Thompson and Trattner-Sherman 1993; Sundgot-Borgen 1994b):

- Weight loss beyond that normally required for adequate sports performance
- Amenorrhea or some manifestation of menstrual dysfunction
- Dehydration
- High level of fatigue (beyond that normally expected after training or competition)
- Gastrointestinal problems (e.g., constipation, diarrhea, or distress after a meal)
- Hyperactivity
- Hypothermia (lower than normal body temperature)
- Low resting heart rate
- Muscle weakness
- Susceptible to overuse injuries
- Reduced bone-mineral density and susceptibility to stress fractures
- Frequent infections, skin sores, and poor wound healing
- Low blood hemoglobin and hematocrit and low serum albumin, serum ferritin, glucose, HDL cholesterol, and estradiol levels.

The psychological characteristics of those who suffer from anorexia nervosa or anorexia athletica can be summarized as follows (Thompson and Trattner-Sherman 1993):

- General anxiety
- Avoidance of eating and absence from meal situations
- Claims of being fat or feeling fat despite being thin and underweight

- Resistance to recommendations for weight gain
- Unusual weighing behaviors (e.g., excessive weighing, avoidance of weighing, negative reaction to being weighed, or refusal to be weighed)
- Excessive training beyond that required for a particular sport or exercising while injured or when prohibited by coaching and medical staff
- Obsessed about body image and compulsive behaviors regarding eating and physical activity
- Restlessness and inability or unwillingness to relax
- Social withdrawal
- Depression
- Tiredness and irritability
- Insomnia (difficulty with sleeping)

Most people who experience anorexia do not seem to realize they have a problem and therefore are unlikely to seek treatment. Hence, for the susceptible athlete, the role of the coach, team doctor, physiologist, sport psychologist, and sport nutritionist or dietitian is crucial in identifying the problem and persuading the athlete to get medical attention. In many cases, anorexic athletes consider seeking help only when their sports performance declines.

Bulimia nervosa is an eating disorder in which affected individuals, usually in the normal weight range, repeat cycles of binge eating (consumption of large amounts of usually energy-dense foods) followed soon after by purging the stomach contents (vomiting) before many of the nutrients from the heavy meal can be absorbed. The person often eats the food in secrecy and commonly disappears from view shortly after a meal to purge the stomach contents. Bulimic athletes do not usually volunteer information about their abnormal behavior until they think that the situation is getting out of control or that their habit is detrimentally affecting their sports performance. Besides purging, other compensatory behaviors such as prolonged fasting or excessive exercise may be used. People with bulimia may also use laxatives (drugs that promote defecation) and diuretics (drugs that promote urine formation) to achieve short-term weight loss. Unlike athletes with anorexia, many athletes with bulimia are at normal body weights. Therefore, the athlete's support team must be aware of the physical symptoms and psychological characteristics associated with bulimia nervosa. The physical symptoms are as follows (Thompson and Trattner-Sherman 1993):

- Callus, sores, or abrasions on fingers or back of hand used to induce vomiting
- Dehydration
- Dental or gum problems
- Edema, complaints of bloating, or both
- Serum electrolyte abnormalities
- Gastrointestinal problems
- Low weight despite apparent intake of large amounts of food
- Frequent and often extreme weight fluctuations
- Muscle cramps, muscle weakness, or both
- Swollen parotid salivary glands
- Menstrual irregularities in females

The psychological characteristics associated with bulimia nervosa are as follows (Thompson and Trattner-Sherman 1993):

- Binge eating
- Secretive eating and agitation when bingeing is interrupted
- Disappearing after eating meals
- Evidence of vomiting unrelated to illness
- Dieting
- Excessive exercise beyond that required for the athlete's sport
- Depression
- Self-critical, especially concerning body image, body weight, and sports performance
- Substance abuse
- Use of laxatives, diuretics, or both that are unsanctioned by medical or coaching support staff

People who do not meet all criteria for anorexia nervosa or bulimia nervosa are classified as having an eating disorder not otherwise specified (EDNOS). A person may meet all the criteria for anorexia nervosa except that she has regular menses or may meet all the criteria for bulimia nervosa except that she or he binges and purges less than twice per week.

Prevalence of Eating Disorders in Athletes

Currently, data on the prevalence of eating disorders in athletes are limited and equivocal, mainly because few studies have applied strict classification criteria (such as those in the *Diagnostic and Statistical Manual of Mental Disorders* [American Psychiatric Association 1994]) to both athletes and nonathlete control subjects. Rather, most studies have looked at a limited number of symptoms of eating disorders such as a preoccupation with body weight, body image, and food intake or the use of pathogenic means of weight control.

Some athlete populations exhibit a significantly greater preoccupation with body weight than nonathlete populations, particularly in sports that emphasize body shape, leanness, or body weight (Davis 1992). Some studies have relied exclusively on the use of questionnaires, which is likely to result in underreporting of eating disorders and underreporting of the use of purging methods such as vomiting, laxatives, and diuretics (Sundgot-Borgen 1994a, 2000). Questionnaires also tend to result in overreporting of the incidence of binge eating compared with clinical evaluation by structured interviews (Sundgot-Borgen 1994a, 2000). Indeed, estimates of the prevalence of eating disorders among female athletes range from less than 1% to as high as 75% (Gadpalle et al. 1987; Burckes-Miller and Black 1988; Warren et al. 1990; Sundgot-Borgen 1994a, 1994b), and among athletic males estimates vary from 0% to 57% (Dummer et al. 1987; Burckes-Miller and Black 1988; Rosen and Hough 1988; Rucinski 1989).

Studies generally indicate a substantially higher incidence of eating disorders among athletes compared with nonathletes and greater prevalence among females compared with males. Some studies report that eating disorders are at least 10 times more prevalent among females than among males (Andersen 1995), although in recent years an increasing number of males have been diagnosed with both anorexia and bulimia among distance runners, jockeys, and lightweight rowers. Classically defined anorexia nervosa does not seem to be much more prevalent (1.3%) in the female athletic population than in the general female population (Andersen 1990), whereas bulimia nervosa (8.2%) and subclinical eating disorders (8.0%) seem to be more prevalent among female athletes than among female nonathletes. The prevalence of eating disorders appears to be higher among female athletes who compete in endurance and weight-category sports and, as can be seen in figure 15.2, is especially high in those who participate in aesthetic sports (e.g., gymnastics and dance) compared with those who compete in team game sports, power sports, and technical sports, presumably because of the relative importance of leanness to success in some sports or the perceived advantage to be gained by competing in a lower weight category.

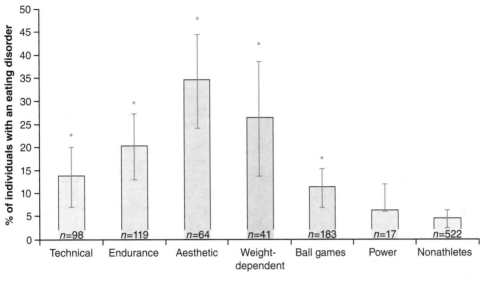

Figure 15.2 Prevalence of eating disorders among elite female athletes in various sports. Data are shown as mean and 95% confidence intervals. An asterisk (*) indicates significantly higher prevalence in athletes than in nonathletes ($P < 0.05$).

Reprinted, by permission, from J. Sundgot-Borgen, 2000, Eating disorders in athletes. In *Nutrition in sport*, (Oxford, United Kingdom: Blackwell Science), 510-522.

Risk Factors

Although the precise causes of eating disorders are unknown, several factors that increase the risk of eating disorders can be identified. These include gender, lifestyle, dieting, and certain personality traits.

Gender and Lifestyle

Clearly, the biggest risk factor is gender. Females have a 10 times greater risk of experiencing eating disorders than males (Andersen 1995). Some evidence, however, indicates that the incidence of male eating disorders is on the rise (Byrne and McLean 2002). For example, body dysmorphic disorder is a condition in which males are not happy with their bodies. They want to have more muscle and to look leaner with ripped midsections. They are quite prepared to go to excessive lengths through exercise, supplement use, and drug abuse to achieve this end.

Athletes seem to be more susceptible to eating disorders than the general population. Both male and female athletes who compete in sports that emphasize a lean body shape or low body weight have a significantly higher prevalence of eating disorders and eating-disorder symptoms than other athletes and nonathletes. But being an athlete does not place a person at increased risk for an eating disorder. The athletes who are particularly vulnerable are those who compete in sports in which

being thin is considered essential or sports in which having a low body weight is necessary to be successful (Byrne and McLean 2002). This vulnerability may be a result of the additional physical, psychological, and social stresses associated with the athletic environment and lifestyle.

Studies suggest that a high training load may induce a negative energy balance in endurance athletes, which in turn may elicit physiological and social reinforcements that lead to eating disorders. According to this hypothesis, elite athletes should be more prone to eating disorders because they do more training and are under more intense pressure to be lean than subelite athletes are. Garner et al. (1987) reported a higher prevalence of eating disorders among top-level dancers compared with dancers in lower competitive levels. But heavy training loads cannot be the prime cause of eating disorders because female cyclists, marathon runners, and triathletes expend more energy in their training than dancers and gymnasts. Nevertheless, there is no evidence to suggest that endurance athletes are more prone to developing eating disorders than dancers or gymnasts. Another possibility is that young athletes who take up serious sport at a prepubertal age may not select the sport that is most suitable for their adult body type and hence are subject to greater pressure to maintain a different (i.e., leaner, smaller) body type than is natural for them. Indeed, Sundgot-Borgen (1994b) found that athletes with eating disorders begin sport-specific training at an earlier age than athletes who did not have eating disorders.

Dieting

A large, randomized, prospective study of 1700 teenage boys and girls found that dieting and psychiatric morbidity were the most sensitive independent predictors of newly diagnosed clinical eating disorders (Patton et al. 1999). Girls who dieted at moderate and severe levels were 5 and 18 times more likely to be diagnosed with clinical eating disorders 6 months later, respectively, and girls in the highest and second highest of four psychiatric morbidity categories were 7 and 3 times more likely to be diagnosed with clinical eating disorders 6 months later, respectively. Dieting is an established risk factor for eating disorders (Polivy and Herman 1995). Sudden periods of enforced inactivity (e.g., because of injury) or longer periods of positive energy balance (e.g., during the off-season) may result in weight gain, which the athlete is then told to lose. The athlete may begin to diet excessively or may develop an irrational fear of additional weight gain. Guidance to athletes about how best to lose weight is important at this point. In some cases, athletes may be asked to lose weight rapidly to remain on the team. As a result, they may undergo periods of restricted eating and weight cycling. This type of behavior has been suggested as an important factor in triggering eating disorders in athletes (Brownell et al. 1987; Sundgot-Borgen 1994b). Nutritional counseling is also essential for preventing inadvertent low energy availability because energy deficits caused by too much exercise rather than by simple dietary restriction do not necessarily increase appetite for food (Hubert et al. 1998). Thus, in some situations, low energy availability could occur inadvertently in the absence of clinical eating disorders, disordered eating behaviors, or even dietary restriction.

Personality Traits

Certain personality traits may predispose people to eating disorders. Most affected people are reported to have low self-esteem and to be excessively self-critical, particularly about body image (Sundgot-Borgen 2000). Those with bulimia consistently show high levels of impulsivity (DaCosta and Halmi 1992), and their addictiveness scores resemble those of drug addicts (DeSilva and Eysenck 1987). Athletes, at least the most successful ones, are by nature compulsive and focused. The same traits that encourage good sports performance in many athletes—perfectionism, dedication, and

willingness to work hard and withstand discomfort—may lead to preoccupation with body image and body fat.

Exercise Dependence and Eating Disorders

Excessive exercising is widely reported to coexist with eating disorders, particularly among those who practice dietary restraint (Brewerton et al. 1995). Indeed, many of the reported characteristics of "exercise dependence" are evident in athletes with eating disorders (Touyz et al. 1987). A study described 28% of female eating-disorder patients as "compulsive exercisers" (Brewerton et al. 1995), and another study reported that the prevalence of excessive exercising among such patients was as high as 78% (Davis et al. 1994).

Overactivity among those with eating disorders appears either as deliberate exercise to increase energy expenditure and promote fat loss or as involuntary and persistent restlessness often associated with sleep disturbance (Beumont 1995). Where the former is manifest, exercise is considered a secondary symptom of the disorder, and for athletes, distinguishing this motivation to exercise from the need to train for a particular sport may be impossible. Restless hyperactivity, on the other hand, may be a central feature of the eating disorder (Kron et al. 1978). This notion is supported by evidence of reduced food consumption in rats forced to exercise excessively and increased voluntary wheel running in food-deprived rats (Epling and Pierce 1988). Accordingly, a combination of excessive exercise and food restriction may be a self-perpetuating and mutually reinforcing cycle with potentially serious consequences. Currently, the precise role of exercise in the etiology of eating disorders remains unclear. Dieting is an established risk factor for eating disorders (Polivy and Herman 1995), but high levels of physical activity may play an important role in the perpetuation of an eating disorder. Davis et al. (1994) found that 75% of eating-disorder patients were most active during the period of lowest food intake and greatest weight loss.

Effects of Eating Disorders on Sports Performance

The effect of an eating disorder on exercise performance is determined by how long the disorder has been manifest and the severity of the disorder. Whether an eating disorder affects performance in a specific sport is also determined by the nature of the sport (i.e., whether the predominant requirement of the sport is power, strength, endurance, or motor skills). In anorexia nervosa, a gradual loss of body weight may actually increase maximal oxygen uptake when expressed as milliliters per minute per kilogram of body weight (Sundgot-Borgen 2000). As in the early stages of dieting, the body adapts and uses up stored fat and certain minerals (e.g., iron) and vitamins. Decreased performance may not occur for some time, and the athlete may wrongly believe that the disordered eating behavior is harmless. But endurance performance is likely to deteriorate if liver and muscle glycogen levels are low or if the athlete becomes dehydrated or anemic (i.e., the blood hemoglobin concentration falls below normal).

Dehydration is common in both anorexia nervosa and bulimia nervosa (Sundgot-Borgen 2000), and acute dehydration has other consequences for sports performance, such as loss of motor skill and coordination (Fogelholm 1994b). Reduced plasma volume in the dehydrated state impairs the ability to thermoregulate during exercise, which can also contribute to impaired exercise performance, particularly in the heat (see chapter 9 for further details). Electrolyte disturbances are also likely to be detrimental to muscle function, and with time, a loss of lean body (muscle) mass will reduce strength and power. Both short-term anaerobic performance and muscle strength are impaired after rapid weight loss, and restoration of performance requires not 1 to 3 hours of rehydration, but 5 to 24 hours of rehydration (Fogelholm, Koskinen, et al. 1993).

Effects of Eating Disorders on the Athlete's Health

The health problems that can arise from chronic eating disorders are the effects of semistarvation in anorexia nervosa and of the binge–purge cycle in bulimia nervosa, both of which result in reduced energy availability and micronutrient deficiencies that are detrimental to the health of the athlete. For female athletes in particular, inadequate intakes of calcium, iron, and B vitamins are a serious concern. Energy and macronutrient deficiency in people with anorexia may affect mood, endocrine status, growth, reproductive function, and bone health.

Psychological Mood State

Depression is a common symptom of eating disorders (Thompson and Trattner-Sherman 1993). Increased fatigue, anxiety, anger, and irritabil-

ity are associated with low levels of energy and carbohydrate intake during periods of dieting to achieve rapid weight loss. Studies on the effects of eating disorders on mood state in athletes are currently lacking.

Growth and Maturation

Stunted growth in adolescent athletes may occur during prolonged periods of inadequate energy, protein, and micronutrient intake. The onset of puberty may be delayed in child athletes, and poor bone development can lead to increased susceptibility to fractures and problems in later life, particularly in females.

Reproductive Function

Female reproductive function is affected by the negative energy balance that results from disordered eating coupled with intense training. Psychological stress and low body-fat content can be other contributing factors that lead to amenorrhea. The pulsatile production of gonadotrophic hormones (follicle-stimulating hormone, FSH, and luteinizing hormone, LH) from the anterior pituitary gland is inhibited during prolonged energy deficits, and the ovarian production of the sex steroid hormones estrogen and progesterone drops to extremely low levels (figure 15.3). Menstrual irregularity ensues, which may be followed by amenorrhea and absence of ovulation. In this state, the female is infertile, and her endocrine status is akin to that of a postmenopausal woman. Because menstrual cycles lasting longer than 90 days are rare, amenorrhea is defined as the absence of menstrual cycles lasting more than 3 months. LH pulsatility reflects the pulsatile secretion of gonadotrophic-releasing hormone (GnRH) from the hypothalamus, and the GnRH pulse generator is influenced directly or indirectly by the levels of certain fuel substrates (glucose, free fatty acids, and ketones) and hormones (insulin, cortisol, growth hormone, and leptin). One or more of these is thought to constitute the signal to disrupt GnRH pulsatility in conditions of low energy availability. The most important of these may be leptin, which is an adipocyte-derived protein hormone that conveys a signal of the amount of energy stores in adipose tissue to the central nervous system. Recent advances in leptin physiology have established that the main role of this hormone is to signal energy availability in energy-deficient states. Leptin also plays an important role in regulating neuroendocrine function. The importance of leptin in the reproductive system has been suggested by the reproductive dysfunction associated with leptin deficiency and resistance in both animal models and humans as well as the ability of leptin to accelerate the onset of reproductive function in animals. Normal women have a pulsatile release pattern of leptin that is significantly associated with the variations in LH and estradiol levels. Studies in animals and human beings have shown that low concentrations of leptin are fully or partly responsible for starvation-induced changes in reproductive, thyroid, and insulin-like growth factor (IGF) hormones. Both anorexia nervosa and exercise-induced amenorrhea are associated with low concentrations of leptin and a similar spectrum of neuroendocrine abnormalities. It has been shown that leptin can restore ovulatory menstrual cycles and improve reproductive, thyroid, and IGF hormones and bone markers in hypothalamic amenorrhea (Chan and Mantzoros 2005).

The long-term effects of athletic amenorrhea on fertility are still unclear, although some evidence suggests that the reproductive deficiencies associated with amenorrhea are reversible when the problem is treated (Mishell 1993). Although low body-fat levels per se have not been implicated as the specific cause of menstrual dysfunction, evidence suggests that low energy availability is the major causal factor (Loucks 2006). Studies show that restricting energy intake below a critical threshold amount causes metabolic and hormonal adaptations. These changes may be mediated, at least in part, by the hormone leptin.

Athletic amenorrhea represents the extreme form of menstrual dysfunction. But even less-severe disturbances of the menstrual cycle, including reduced frequency of periods (oligomenorrhea) and luteal-phase deficiency, can result in depressed estrogen levels. Furthermore, in adolescent female athletes, the onset of puberty and menarche can be delayed (Manore 2002).

Laboratory-based studies have shown that LH pulsatility is disrupted within 5 days when energy availability of young women is reduced by more than a third from 190 kJ (45 kcal) · kg fat-free mass^{-1} · day^{-1} to 125 kJ (30 kcal) · kg fat-free mass^{-1} · day^{-1} (Loucks and Thuma 2003), which corresponds to the resting energy expenditure in healthy young adults.

Osteoporosis

Because ovarian steroid hormones, particularly estradiol, facilitate calcium uptake into bone (figure 15.3) and inhibit bone resorption, amenorrhea may predispose female athletes to osteoporosis, a pre-mature loss of bone quality and quantity. This condition can occur despite the fact that load-bearing physical activity induces greater bone-mineral density. Certain types of exercise (weight-bearing, high-impact, fast movement using a wide range of muscle groups, exceeding 70% of aerobic capacity or 70% of one-repetition maximum weightlifting) appear to be most effective for bone building. But this effect is specific to the bones that receive the most impact stress during exercise, and even this degree of protection may not be enough to prevent net demineralization of bone in the face of inadequate estrogen secretion. In fact, there seems to be a threshold of dietary calcium intake below which physical activity may have minimal effect on increasing bone mass (Bloomfield 2001). Athletes with eating disorders have decreased spinal vertebral bone mineral densities compared with normal values, but they have higher densities than nonathletes with eating disorders. Thus, exercise training may lessen the amount of bone loss, but exercise alone cannot protect the athlete from osteoporosis. Abnormal and restrictive eating behaviors seem to be related to a greater likelihood of fractures (Bennell et al. 1999; Golden 2002). Bone strength and the risk of fracture depend on the density and internal structure of bone mineral and on the quality of bone protein, which may explain why some people suffer fractures while others with the same bone-mineral density (BMD) do not.

The withdrawal of estrogens at any age is associated with bone loss and reduced BMD that could lead to osteoporosis if prolonged and is more critical than low progesterone levels for the onset of bone demineralization (Cumming 1996). The absence of menstrual cycles and the associated low plasma estradiol levels may decrease bone-mineral density to such an extent that fractures occur under minimal impact loading (Snow-Harter 1994; Cumming 1996). Bone development normally continues up to 25 years of age. After that, a gradual loss of bone occurs with advancing age.

As shown in figure 15.4, bone loss accelerates in females after menopause, when the ovaries stop producing estrogen. Thus, child and adolescent female athletes who experience eating disorders are at high risk for osteoporosis. All physically active women who lose their periods because of heavy training or eating disorders are strong candidates for premature bone loss. Typically, they lose 2% to 6% of bone each year, possibly resulting in the loss of 25% of total bone mass (Snow-Harter 1994).

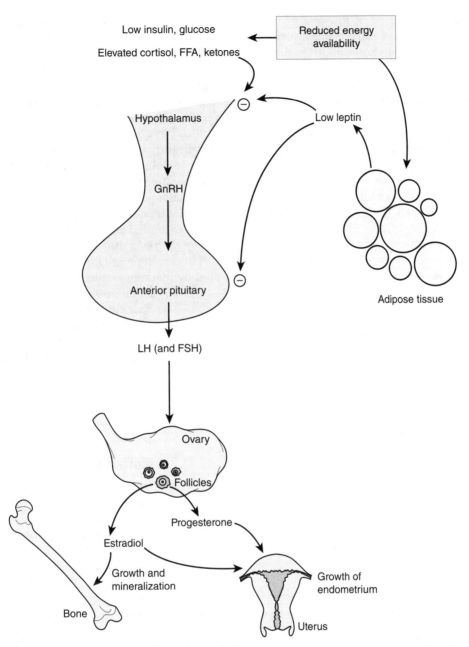

Figure 15.3 The role of hormonal disturbances in the development of amenorrhea and associated health problems such as osteoporosis. Highlighted arrows indicate the effects of reduced energy availability that lead to inhibition (−) of gonadotrophin-releasing hormone (GnRH) and luteinising hormone (LH) pulsatility. FSH = follicle stimulating hormone.

Peak bone mass is reached during the first 3 decades of life. Females attain 95% of maximum density by 18 years of age, and all women then experience age-related bone loss. Therefore, maximizing peak bone mass during the formative years is of utmost importance. Because the 2 to 3 years that constitute the pubertal growth spurt are accompanied by deposition of 60% of final bone mass, any dietary inadequacy and disrup- tion of the normal menstrual cycle may impair bone formation more severely at that time than at any other (Snow-Harter 1994; Sabatini 2001; Golden 2002). A female athlete's BMD reflects her cumulative history of energy availability and menstrual status as well as her genetic endowment and exposure to other nutritional, behavioral, and environmental factors. As is the case with suffer- ers of anorexia nervosa, athletes who experience estrogen deficiency because of low energy availability are usually chronically undernourished with inadequate protein and micronutrient intake, which further reduces the rate of bone formation. Low energy availability may also suppress bone formation by effects on other hormones, including cortisol and leptin.

The three conditions that are prevalent in female athletes—amenorrhea, disordered eating, and osteoporosis—are collectively known as the female athlete triad syndrome (see figure 15.5). Any female athlete is at risk from this triad, but women who participate in sports in which low body fat is advantageous (e.g., endurance running and gymnastics) or a requirement (i.e., weight-category sports such as rowing and martial arts) are at highest risk for the syndrome.

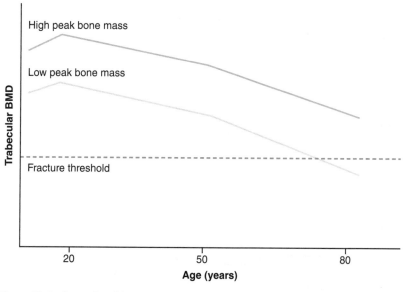

Figure 15.4 Age and peak bone mass in relation to trabecular bone-mineral density (BMD) in females. Peak bone mass is reached in the early 20s, with all women experiencing age-related bone loss after that. People with a low peak bone mass reach the critical threshold for fractures at an earlier age.

Adapted, by permission, from C.M. Snow-Harter, 1995, "Bone health and prevention of osteoporosis in active and athletic women," *Maturitas* 21(2): 159.

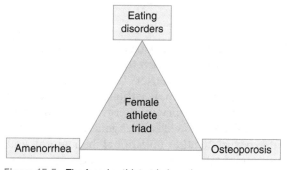

Figure 15.5 The female athlete triad syndrome.

Studies report that the total number of years of regular **menstrual cycles** predicts lumbar spine bone-mineral density more accurately than any other training, dietary, or menstrual factor (Montagnani et al. 1992; Myburgh et al. 1993). Indeed, over the past 15 years, numerous studies have reported that females with menstrual-cycle irregularities have bone-mineral density values that are significantly lower than those of normally menstruating female athletes and nonathletes (Kazis and Iglesias 2003). Consequently, the present concern is that many female athletes whose rigorous training schedules and restricted dietary practices have led to extended periods of amenorrhea may have suffered irreversible bone loss.

The development of osteoporosis is also accelerated by inadequate dietary intake of vitamin D or calcium (see chapter 10), which must be additional concerns for athletes with eating disorders (Manore 2002). When amenorrhea is present, increasing the consumption of calcium to 120% of the RDA appears to help bones maintain density and develop properly. Such nutrition guidance should be given to low-body-weight women with amenorrhea.

Mortality

Death rates from eating disorders among athletes are not known, but among patients with anorexia nervosa in the general population, increased mortality has been reported to range from less than 1% to as high as 18% (Thompson and Trattner-Sherman 1993). In patients with anorexia nervosa, death is usually caused by excessive fluid and electrolyte disturbance or is the result of suicide. Information on mortality in bulimia nervosa is not available, but clearly some deaths occur, either as a complication of vomiting behavior or as suicide. The abuse of drugs, including diuretics, laxatives, emetics (which promote vomiting), and diet pills that commonly contain stimulants (e.g., amphetamines), is frequently reported among athletes with eating disorders (Sundgot-Borgen and Larsen 1993), and excessive or inappropriate use of some of these drugs may contribute to health problems and mortality in some cases. If dehydration or electrolyte disturbances are present because of an eating disorder, the athlete is at risk for cardiac arrest during exercise.

Treatment and Prevention of Eating Disorders

Perhaps the most effective means of preventing or treating eating disorders among athletes is education of the athletes. Although educating athletes about the risks of eating disorders is only one element of a comprehensive program designed to prevent and treat disordered eating in athletes, many eating disorders may persist because of a lack of understanding of the effect that they can have on health. People with eating disorders do not seem to know what constitutes a balanced meal or a normal pattern of eating. Because of misconceptions and poor understanding of nutritional principles, athletes may have an irrational fear of admitting (even to themselves) that they have a problem. Therefore, early diagnosis is vital because eating disorders are more difficult to treat the longer that they progress. But the affected athlete does not always lack understanding, and eating disorders may persist even after appropriate education and counseling. Eating disorders are extremely complex examples of psychological dysfunction. The coexistence of exercise dependence and depression is common among athletes with eating disorders. Some evidence suggests that a coincidence of an eating disorder and depression is most effectively treated by addressing the depressive illness first by a combination of cognitive–behavioral therapy and antidepressant medication (Roth and Fonagy 1998). Managing depression is the immediate concern because it is the most life threatening. Treatment of the eating disorder would follow, generally in the form of cognitive–behavioral therapy for bulimia nervosa or interpersonal therapy for anorexia nervosa (Roth and Fonagy 1998).

For athletes with long-term conditions, the readiness to listen and accept advice should be assessed in conjunction with a mental health professional.

After the athlete's cooperation is gained, nutritional counseling can begin. The athlete's body weight and percent body fat should be measured to establish realistic goals, which also depend on the nature of the athlete's sport. An athlete who agrees to comply with all treatment regimens can continue to train and compete, but the athlete must be monitored closely, and effective treatment must always take precedence over sport.

Excessive exercising can aggravate medical complications of eating disorders (Pomeroy and Mitchell 1992) by, for example, worsening electrolyte disturbances through sweating. But exercise is employed in the treatment of depression and eating disorders in nonathletes (Beumont et al. 1994; Byrne and Byrne 1993), so a continued level of moderate exercise is preferable to stopping the athlete from exercising altogether. Nevertheless, the benefits of continued exercising should be weighed against the potential risks in each case. Furthermore, the exercise should be supervised, and signs of exercise dependence should be closely monitored. The treatment of an athlete with an eating disorder should follow a team approach, incorporating not only a physician and a dietitian but also a mental health practitioner, a physiologist, and a psychologist. Several sources thus encourage the athlete to practice healthy eating habits, and all reinforce the message that the consequences of the condition are deterioration of both health and sports performance.

According to Thompson and Trattner-Shermann (1993), athletes should maintain a minimum body weight that is not less than 90% of "ideal" health-related body weight. Athletes who have been amenorrheic for more than 6 months should be assessed for bone-mineral density and considered for hormone replacement therapy.

Affected athletes should be referred to a dietitian for nutrition counseling and to have their energy availability estimated. Adequate amounts of bone-building nutrients such as calcium (1,000–1,300 mg/day), vitamin D (400–800 IU/day), and vitamin K (60-90 μg/day) are needed, and adequacy of protein intake is another concern. Increased energy availability should continue until menses resume and are seen to be maintained during training and competition.

Coaches should understand the influence that they can have on their athletes' eating and weight-control behaviors. Although the exact causes of eating disorders remain unknown, the pressure of wanting to succeed and satisfy the coach's demands by highly motivated but uninformed young athletes seems a likely scenario that can first result in dieting followed by unhealthy eating behaviors. If such behavior is reinforced by success and praise from the coach, it could lead to a full-blown eating disorder. Coaches should therefore not comment on an athlete's body size, weight, or percent body fat. Such comments should be left to the dietitian, who at the same time can advise the athlete on healthy eating and set up a structured, supervised weight-loss program when deemed necessary.

KEY POINTS

■ Eating disorders are characterized by gross disturbances of eating behavior. The major disorders are associated with abnormally low food intake (anorexia nervosa) and bouts of binge eating followed by vomiting (bulimia nervosa). If undiagnosed and untreated, eating disorders can have detrimental effects on sports performance and damaging long-lasting effects on the health of the individual.

■ A higher incidence of eating disorders seems to occur among athletes compared with nonathletes, and female athletes have a much greater prevalence compared with male athletes. Classically defined anorexia nervosa does not seem to be much more prevalent in the female athlete population than it is in the general population, whereas bulimia nervosa and subclinical eating disorders seem to be more prevalent among female athletes than among female nonathletes.

■ The prevalence of eating disorders appears to be higher among female athletes who compete in endurance and weight-category sports and is especially high in those who participate in aesthetic sports, such as gymnastics and dance, compared with those who compete in team sports, power sports, and technical sports. Presumably, the higher prevalence is related to the importance of leanness to success in these sports or to the perceived advantage of competing in a lower weight category.

■ Risk factors for eating disorders include gender, dieting, participation in an athletic lifestyle, and certain personality traits.

■ Eating disorders are commonly associated with exercise dependence and depression.

■ The precise causes of eating disorders are not known but probably progress from an initial desire or requirement to lose weight that develops into a pathological fear of gaining weight. Highly motivated but uninformed young female athletes are probably most at risk.

■ The major problem in eating disorders is low energy availability, which is defined as the dietary energy intake minus exercise energy expenditure. When energy availability is too low, physiological mechanisms reduce the amount of energy used for cellular maintenance, thermoregulation, growth, bone development, and reproduction. Although the compensatory mechanisms tend to restore energy balance and promote survival, health becomes impaired.

■ Eating disorders are likely to be detrimental to sports performance, although this consequence depends on the severity and duration of the disorder and the nature of the sport. Athletes who experience eating disorders may have low glycogen stores, be dehydrated, or exhibit electrolyte disturbances, so both high-intensity and endurance exercise performance can be affected.

■ Prolonged episodes of negative energy balance or of bingeing and purging are likely to result in micronutrient deficiencies that are detrimental to the health of the athlete. For female athletes in particular, inadequate intakes of calcium, iron, and B vitamins are a serious concern. Energy and macronutrient deficiency are likely to affect mood, endocrine status, growth, reproductive function, and bone health in people with anorexia.

■ Athletic amenorrhea may predispose female athletes to premature osteoporosis because of the failure of the ovaries to produce estrogen. This condition can occur despite the fact that load-bearing physical activity induces greater bone-mineral density.

■ Amenorrhea, disordered eating, and osteoporosis are collectively known as the female athlete triad syndrome. Any female athlete is at risk for this syndrome, but women who participate in sports in which low body fat is advantageous or a requirement are at highest risk.

RECOMMENDED READINGS

ACSM position stand: The female athlete triad. 2007. *Medicine and Science in Sports and Exercise* 39 (10): 1867–1882.

Beals, K.A. 2004. *Disordered eating among athletes.* Champaign, IL: Human Kinetics.

Beumont, P.J.V., J.D. Russell, and S.W. Touyz. 1993. Treatment of anorexia nervosa. *Lancet* 26:1635–1640.

Brownell, K.D., and J. Rodin. 1992. Prevalence of eating disorders in athletes. In *Eating, body weight and performance in athletes: Disorders of modern society,* ed. K.D. Brownell, J. Rodin, and J.H. Wilmore, 128–143. Philadelphia: Lea and Febiger.

Byrne, S., and N. McLean. 2001. Eating disorders in athletes: A review of the literature. *Journal of Science and Medicine in Sport* 4:145–159.

Clark, N. 1993. How to help the athlete with bulimia: Practical tips and case study. *International Journal of Sport Nutrition* 3:450–460.

Garner, D.M., L.W. Rosen, and D. Barry. 1998. Eating disorders among athletes. Research and recommendations. *Child and Adolescent Psychiatric Clinics of North America* 7:839–857.

Redman, L.M, and A.B. Loucks. 2005. Menstrual disorders in athletes. *Sports Medicine* 35:747–755.

Sundgot-Borgen J. 1993. Prevalence of eating disorders in female elite athletes. *International Journal of Sport Nutrition* 3:29–40.

Torstveit, G., C.G. Rolland, and J.Sundgot-Borgen. 1998. Pathogenic weight control methods and self-reported eating disorders among elite athletes. *Medicine and Science in Sports and Exercise* 5 (suppl): 181.

Wilmore, J.H. 1991. Eating and weight disorders in female athletes. *International Journal of Sport Nutrition* 1:104–117.

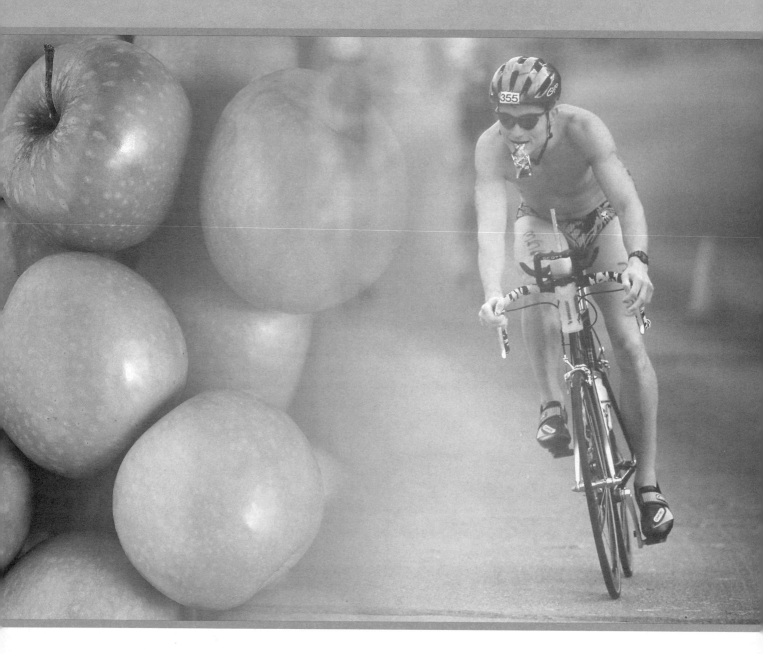

OBJECTIVES

After studying this chapter, you should be able to do the following:

- Describe the main components and functional mechanisms of the immune system

- Describe the effects of exercise and training on immune function and susceptibility to infection

- Describe the mechanisms by which nutrition may influence immune function

- Describe the roles of several vitamins and minerals that are required to maintain immune function

- Discuss nutritional strategies that may be effective in reducing exercise-induced immunodepression

- Comment on studies that have investigated the effects of nutritional supplements on exercise-induced immunodepression

- Describe particular groups of athletes who may be at increased risk for immunodepression and susceptibility to infection

16

Nutrition and Immune Function in Athletes

Key Terms

The immune system is involved in tissue repair after injury and in the protection of the body against potentially damaging (pathogenic) microorganisms such as bacteria, viruses, and fungi. In some circumstances, the immune system can become functionally depressed (known as immunodepression), which may result in an increased susceptibility to infection. Several forms of stress, including a heavy schedule of training and competition, can lead to immunodepression in athletes, placing them at greater risk for opportunistic infections, particularly upper respiratory tract infections (URTIs). An abundance of epidemiological evidence and clinical data suggests that nutritional deficiencies impair immune function and increase the risk of infection and that even medically harmless infections may significantly impair athletic performance.

Although many factors influence exercise-induced immunodepression (e.g., physical, environmental, and psychological stresses), nutrition plays a critical role. This chapter examines the role of nutrition in exercise-induced immunodepression and the effect of both excessive and insufficient nutrient intake on immune function. Because much of the present literature concerning nutrition and immune function is based on studies with sedentary subjects, the need for research that directly investigates the interrelationship between exercise immunology and nutrition is emphasized. Some important questions that must be answered include the following:

- Which aspects of nutrition are crucial to normal immune function? Are the reported dietary practices of athletes optimal for immune function?

- Do any specific nutritional practices impair immune function or exacerbate the temporary immunodepression that follows an acute bout of prolonged strenuous exercise?

- Does feeding of supplements (e.g., carbohydrate, amino acids, or vitamins) during and after prolonged exercise reduce the stress on the immune system?

- Can nutrient supplements reduce the risk of infection after heavy exertion?

Because readers of this book are unlikely to have detailed knowledge of the physiology of the immune system, the following section provides a brief summary of the main components of the immune system and their role in defending the body against pathogenic microorganisms.

Functions of the Immune System and Its Cellular Components

Simply put, the immune system recognizes, attacks, and destroys things that are foreign to the body. In actuality, the functions of this homeostatic system are far more complex, involving the precise coordination of many cell types and molecular messengers. Yet, like any other homeostatic system, the immune system is composed of redundant mechanisms to ensure that essential processes are carried out.

The immune system has two broad functions, innate (natural, or nonspecific) immunity and adaptive (acquired, or specific) immunity, which work synergistically. The attempt of an infectious agent to enter the body immediately activates the innate system. This so-called first-line of defense comprises three general mechanisms (see figure 16.1) that have the common goal of restricting microorganism entry into the body:

- Physical or structural barriers (skin, epithelial linings, and mucosal secretions)

- Chemical barriers (pH of bodily fluids and soluble factors)

- Phagocytic cells (e.g., neutrophils and macrophages or monocytes)

Failure of the innate system and the resulting infection activates the adaptive system, which aids recovery from infection. Adaptive immunity is helped greatly by T-lymphocyte and B-lymphocyte acquisition of receptors that recognize the foreign molecules (called antigens), engendering specificity and "memory" that enable the immune system to mount an augmented response when the host is reinfected by the same pathogen.

The components of the immune system comprise both cellular and soluble elements, which are listed in table 16.1. The white blood cells (leukocytes) have diverse functions, despite their common origin from the stem cells of the bone marrow. Leukocytes consist of the granulocytes (60% to 70%), monocytes (10% to 15%), and lymphocytes (20% to 25%). Various subsets of the latter can be identified through use of monoclonal antibodies, which are used to identify specific proteins (clusters of differentiation or cluster designators [CD]) that are expressed on the cell surface of a particular cell type. For example, all T-lymphocytes express the protein CD3 on the cell surface. B-lymphocytes do not express CD3 but express CD19, CD20, and CD22. A particular subset of T-lymphocytes called helper T-cells specifically express the CD4 protein, whereas the cytotoxic T-cells express CD8. T-cells recognize short peptide sequences from antigens only if they are held on the surface of the cell and complexed with a major histocompatibility complex (MHC) molecule. The characteristics of the various cells of the immune system are summarized in tables 16.2 and 16.3. The ability of the immune system to distinguish self from nonself depends largely on the MHC, a group of protein markers that is present on the surface of every cell and is slightly different in each person.

Soluble factors of the immune system activate leukocytes, neutralize (kill) foreign agents, and regulate the immune system. The factors include the cytokines, proteins that act as chemical messenger substances (like hormones) to stimulate the growth, differentiation, and functional development of immune system cells through specific receptor sites on either secretory cells (autocrine function) or on immediately adjacent cells (paracrine

function). Cytokine action is not confined to the immune system; they also influence the central nervous system and the neuroendocrine system.

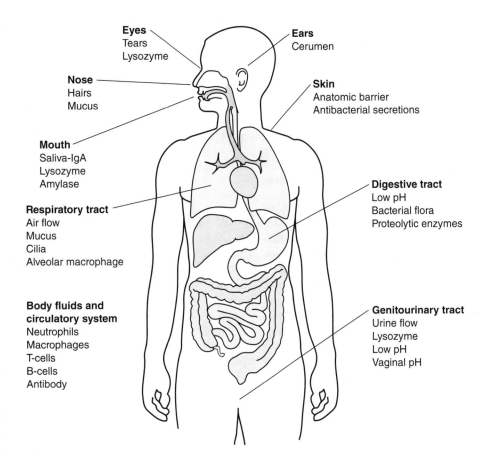

Figure 16.1 The body's barriers and innate defenses against invading microorganisms.

■ **TABLE 16.1** ■

Main Components of the Immune System

Innate components	Adaptive components
Cellular	Cellular
Natural killer cells (CD16+ and CD56+) Phagocytes (neutrophils, eosinophils, basophils, monocytes, and macrophages)	T-cells (CD3+, CD4+, and CD8+) B-cells (CD19+, CD20+, and CD22+)
Soluble	Soluble
Acute-phase proteins Complement Lysozymes Cytokines (interleukins (IL), interferons (IFN), colony-stimulating factors (CSF), tumor necrosis factors (TNF))	Immunoglobulins (IgA, IgD, IgE, IgG, and IgM)

CD = Clusters of differentiation or cluster designators.

Other soluble factors include complement, lysozyme, and the specific antibodies formed by the reaction of B-cell-derived immunoglobulins (Ig) with specific antigens. The actions of the innate soluble factors are summarized in table 16.4. The immunoglobulins are defined by the structure of the constant region of their heavy chains, which are associated with differences in biological activity and function.

General Mechanism of the Immune Response

The introduction of an infectious agent to the body initiates an inflammatory response that augments the response of the immune system. Acute inflammation increases local blood flow in the infected area, which, coupled with increased permeability of blood capillaries, facilitates the entry of leukocytes and plasma proteins into the infected tissue (see figure 16.2). The immune response itself varies according to the nature of the infectious agent (parasitic, bacterial, fungal, and viral), but a general response pattern is evident, as illustrated in figure 16.3. The key player is the macrophage, which ingests foreign material and presents antigens on its cell surface that, in turn, activates T-lymphocytes and B-lymphocytes specific for the antigen. Infectious agents also activate nonspecific (innate) host defense mechanisms, including complement, phagocytic cells (e.g., neutrophils), and natural killer (NK) cells.

The action of the macrophage on the invading microorganism initiates a chain of events. The macrophage first ingests the foreign organism and isolates it within a membranous vesicle (vacuole) inside the cell (phagocytosis). Digestive enzymes (e.g., lysozyme and elastase) and oxidizing agents (e.g., hydrogen peroxide) are secreted by the macrophage. The foreign proteins (antigens) normally found on the surface of the microorganism are digested and processed by the macrophage and incorporated into its own cell surface. The antigen can now be presented to the other cellular immune components. Helper T-cells (CD4+) coordinate the response through

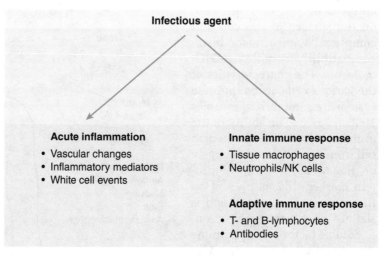

Figure 16.2 The relationship between the inflammatory and the immune response. NK = natural killer.

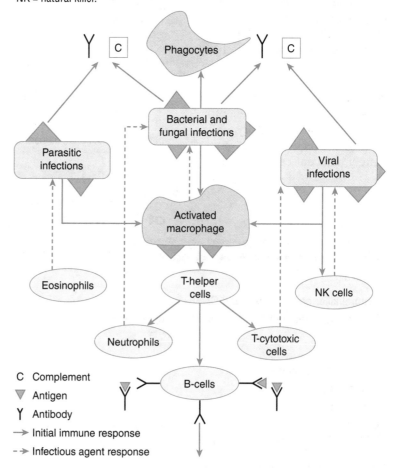

Figure 16.3 The general scheme of the immune response to various infectious agents.

Characteristics of Leukocytes

Leukocyte	Main characteristics
Granulocytes Neutrophils	• 60%–70% of leukocytes • >90% of granulocytes • Phagocytose (i.e., ingest and destroy) bacteria and other foreign material (antigens) • Have a receptor for antibody: phagocytose antibody–antigen complexes • Display little or no capacity to recharge their killing mechanisms once activated
Eosinophils	• 2%–5% of granulocytes • Phagocytose parasites • Triggered by IgG to release toxic lysosomal products
Basophils	• 0%–2% of granulocytes • Produce chemotactic factors • Tissue equivalent = the mast cell, which releases an eosinophil chemotactic factor
Monocytes or macrophages	• 10%–15% of leukocytes • Egress into tissues (e.g., liver and spleen) and differentiate into the mature form: the macrophage • Phagocytose bacteria and viruses enabling antigen presentation • Secrete immunomodulatory cytokines • Retain their capacity to divide after leaving the bone marrow
Lymphocytes	• 20%–25% of leukocytes • Activate other lymphocyte subsets • Produce lymphokines • Recognize antigens • Produce antibodies • Exhibit memory • Exhibit cytotoxicity

Lymphocyte Functions and Characteristics

Lymphocyte subset	Main function and characteristic
T-cells (CD3+) TH (CD4+)	• 60%–75% of lymphocytes • 60%–70% of T-cells • Helper T-cells • Recognize antigen to coordinate the acquired response • Secrete cytokines that stimulate T-cell and B-cell proliferation and differentiation
TC/TS (CD8+)	• 30%–40% of T-cells • TS (suppressor T-cells) involved in the regulation of B-cell and other T-cell proliferation by suppressing certain functions • TS may be important in "switching off" the immune response • TC (cytotoxic T-cells) kill a variety of targets, including some tumor cells
B-cells (CD19+, CD20+, and CD22+)	• 5%–15% of lymphocytes • Produce and secrete Ig specific to the activating antigen • Exhibit memory
Natural killer (NK) cells (CD16+ and CD56+)	• 10%–20% of lymphocytes • Large, granular lymphocytes • Express spontaneous cytolytic activity against a variety of tumor-infected and virus-infected cells • MHC independent • Do not express the CD3 cell-surface antigen • Triggered by IgG • Control foreign materials until the antigen-specific immune system responds

cytokine release to activate other immune cells. Mature B-cell stimulation results in proliferation and differentiation into immunoglobulin-secreting (antibody-secreting) plasma cells. Reaction of the immunoglobulin with a specific antigen forms an antibody–antigen complex. Antibodies are essential to antigen recognition and memory of earlier exposure to specific antigens.

Clonal Selection and Immunological Memory

An antigen that enters the body selectively activates only a tiny fraction of the quiescent lymphocytes, which then grow and divide to form a clone of identical effector cells (clonal selection). Each antigen (usually a foreign protein or lipopolysaccharide) carries several antigenic determinants, each activating a different clone, and an invading bacterium carries a number of antigens. So a particular species of bacterium invading the body activates a number of clones of lymphocytes.

The first encounter with any antigen causes the primary immune response to that antigen. After several days, clones of lymphocytes selected by the antigen multiply and differentiate to become effector B-cells and T-cells. After several more days, specific antibodies from B-cells appear in the blood, as illustrated in figure 16.4. During the lag time, pathogenic organisms may enter the body

and multiply in sufficient numbers to cause illness.

A second exposure to the same antigen (even years later) produces a much quicker, stronger, and longer-lasting secondary response. This response depends on memory cells, which are produced at the same time as effector cells during the primary response. Effector cells usually last for only a few days, but memory cells may last for decades. When a second exposure to an antigen occurs, memory cells rapidly multiply and differentiate to create a large number of effector cells and a large quantity of antibodies dedicated to attacking the antigen. This enhanced antibody response usually prevents symptoms of infection from developing (i.e., immunity to the antigen has been acquired).

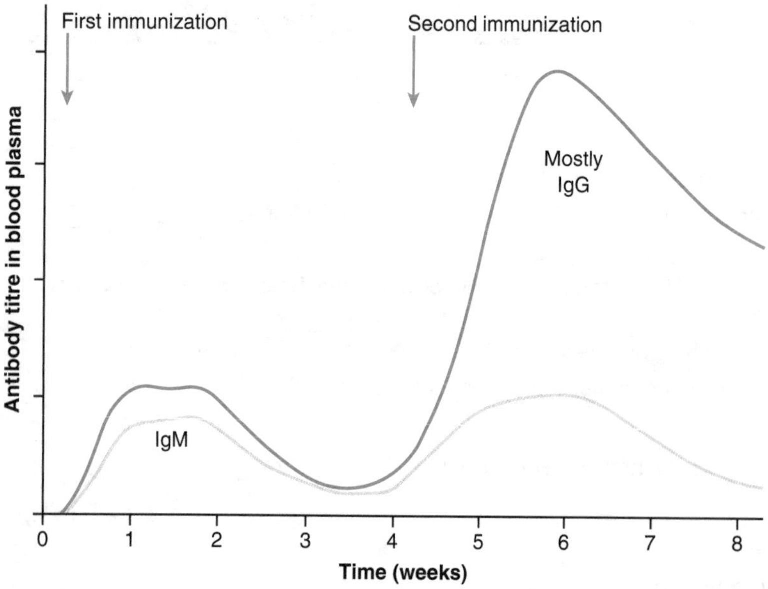

Cellular Immune Response

Many pathogens, including all viruses, are parasites that can reproduce only within host body cells. The cellular immune response fights pathogens that have already entered cells. Activated T-lymphocytes include memory cells and cytotoxic T-cells (killer cells) that attack infected host cells or foreign cells. Helper T-cells and suppressor T-cells are also important in mobilizing and regulating the whole immune response.

When helper T-cells bind to specific antigenic determinants displayed with MHC proteins on the cell surface of macrophages, the macrophage is stimulated to release a cytokine called interleukin-1 (IL-1), which causes the T-cells to grow and divide. The activated T-cells release another cytokine, IL-2, which further stimulates proliferation and growth of helper T-cells and cytotoxic T-cells (see figure 16.5). IL-2 and other cytokines from helper T-cells also stimulate B-cells to respond to specific antigens by differentiating into antibody-forming plasma cells. Cytotoxic T-cells recognize and attach to cells that have on their surface appropriate antigenic determinants coupled with the MHC complex. Cytotoxic T-cells then release perforin, a protein that causes puncture of the cell membrane so that a lethal cocktail of digestive enzymes can be passed from the T-cell into the infected cell, causing cell necrosis (death) and lysis (breakup) of the infected host cell. Natural killer (NK) cells exert cytotoxic activity in a similar way. The fragments of the lysed cell are then ingested and digested by phagocytes.

Figure 16.4 Specific antibody production (IgM and IgG subclasses) after first exposure to an antigen (at time = 0 weeks) and on subsequent exposure to the same antigen (at time = 4 weeks). Note the markedly larger and more rapid IgG response after the second exposure.

■ TABLE 16.4 ■
Producers and Actions of the Innate Soluble Factors

Soluble factor	Producers and immune actions
Cytokines IL-1	• Produced mainly from activated macrophages • IL-1α tends to remain cell associated • IL-1b acts as a soluble mediator • Stimulates IL-2 production from CD3+ and CD4+ cells • Increases IL-1 and IL-2 receptor expression • Increases B-cell proliferation • Increases TNF-α, IL-6, and CSF levels • Stimulates secretion of prostaglandins
IL-2	• Produced mainly by CD4+ cells • Stimulates T-cell and B-cell proliferation and expression of IL-2 receptors on their surfaces • Stimulates release of IFN • Stimulates NK cell proliferation and killing
IL-6	• Produced by activated helper T-cells, fibroblasts, and macrophages; also released from exercising muscle • Stimulates the differentiation of B-cells, inflammation, and the acute-phase response • Endogenous pyrogen (induces fever)
TNF-α	• Produced from monocytes, T-cells, B-cells, and NK cells • Enhances tumor cell killing and antiviral activity
Acute-phase proteins (APP)	• Made in the liver, secreted into the blood • Encourage cell migration to sites of injury and infection • Activate complement • Stimulate phagocytosis
Complement	• Found in the serum • Consists of 20 or more proteins • Stimulates phagocytosis, antigen presentation, and neutralization of infected cells • Amplifies the response

CSF = colony stimulating factor; IFN = interferon; IL = interleukin; NK = natural killer; TNF = tumor necrosis factor.

Humoral (Fluid) Immune Response

B-lymphocytes are also coated with receptors that are specific for particular antigenic determinants. Most antigens activate B-cells only when the B-cells are stimulated by cytokines from helper T-cells; they are T-cell-dependent antigens. Some antigens are T-cell independent. They usually have a repetitive structure and bind with several receptors on the B-cell surface at once (capping). As shown in figure 16.6, the antigen is taken into the cell and activates it. Exposure to an antigen causes appropriate clones of B-cells to proliferate and differentiate into memory cells and plasma cells. The latter are the effector cells of humoral immunity and are capable of secreting a large amount of antibody during their brief life of 4 to 5 days.

The antibodies circulate in the blood and lymph, binding to antigen and contributing to the destruction of the organism bearing it. Antibodies belong to a class of proteins called immunoglobulins (Ig). Each antibody molecule has the ability to bind to a specific antigen and assist with the destruction of the antigen. Every antibody has separate regions for each of these two functions. The regions that bind the antigen differ from molecule to molecule and are called variable regions. Only a few humoral effector mechanisms exist to destroy antigens, so only a few kinds of regions, the constant regions, are involved. An antibody molecule consists of two

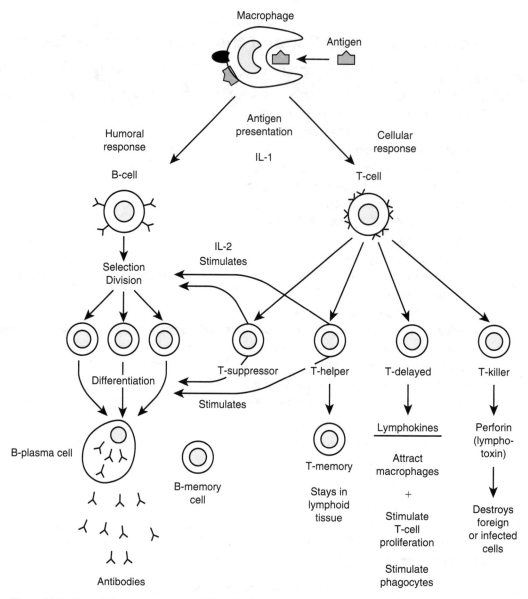

Figure 16.5 The cellular immune response (showing interaction with humoral response).

pairs of polypeptide chains: two short, identical light (L) chains and two longer, identical heavy (H) chains. The chains are joined together to form a Y-shaped molecule (see figure 16.7). The variable regions of H chains and L chains are located at the ends of the arms of the Y, where they form the antigen-binding sites. Thus, each antibody molecule has two antigen-binding sites, one at each tip of the antibody's two arms. The rest of the antibody molecule, consisting of the constant regions of the H and L chains, determines the effector function of the antibody. Along with the five types of constant region are five major classes of antibodies called IgM, IgG, IgA, IgD, and IgE. Their different roles

in the immune response are described in table 16.5. Within each class is a multitude of subpopulations of antibodies, each specific to a particular antigen.

Antibodies cannot destroy antigen-bearing invaders directly. Instead, they tag foreign molecules and cells for destruction by various effector mechanisms. Each mechanism is triggered by the selective binding of antigens to antibodies to form antigen–antibody complexes. The antibodies may simply block the potential toxic actions of some antigens (neutralization), or they may cause clumping together of antigens or foreign cells (agglutination), which can then be ingested by phagocytes (see figure 16.8). Precipitation is a similar

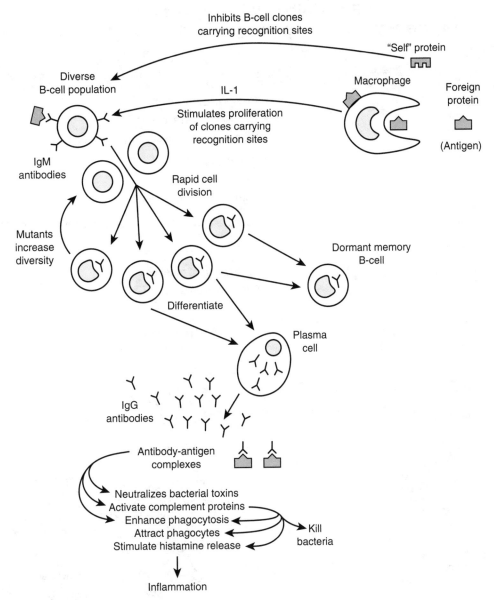

Figure 16.6 The humoral immune response.

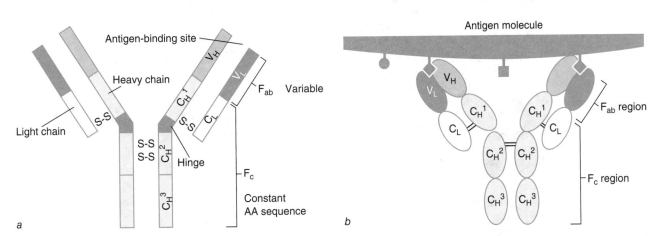

Figure 16.7 The structure of immunoglobulins or antibodies. *(a)* Antibodies are composed of two heavy polypeptide chains (H) and two light polypeptide chains (L). *(b)* Different regions within the heavy and light chains. V indicates the variable regions, and C indicates the constant regions. Antigens combine with the variable regions, as shown in *(b)*. Each antibody molecule is divided into an Fab (antigen-binding) fragment and an Fc (constant) fragment.

■ **TABLE 16.5** ■

Physiological Properties
of the Five Classes of Ig in Extracellular Fluid

Class	Mean adult serum level (g/L)	Serum half-life (days)	Physiological function
IgM	1.0	5	• Complement fixation • Early immune response • Stimulation of ingestion by macrophages
IgG	12	25	• Complement fixation • Placental transfer • Stimulation of ingestion by macrophages
IgA	1.8	6	• Localized protection in external secretions (e.g., saliva)
IgD	0.03	3	• Function unknown
IgE	0.0003	2	• Stimulation of mast cells • Parasite expulsion

 Specific antibody

 Antigen

Neutralization (of toxins)

Precipitation

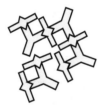

Clumps of antigen-antibody complex come out of solution

Agglutination

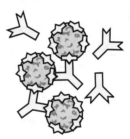

• Foreign organisms with surface antigens clump together

• Spread prevented

• Division hampered

• Phagocyte attack helper

Opsonisation

Helps phagocyte to engulf foreign organism

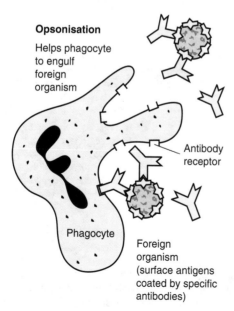

Antibody receptor

Phagocyte

Foreign organism (surface antigens coated by specific antibodies)

Complement activation

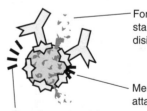

Foreign cell starts to disintegrate

Membrane attack complex

Complement proteins assembling to form membrane attack complex

Figure 16.8 Types of antibody–antigen reactions.

mechanism, in which soluble antigen molecules are cross-linked to form inactive and immobile precipitates that are captured by phagocytes. Antibody–antigen complexes on the surfaces of invading microorganisms usually cause complement activation. Complement proteins then attack the membrane of the invader or, by coating the surface of foreign material, make it attractive to phagocytes (opsonization).

Effects of Exercise on the Immune System

Athletes engaged in heavy training programs, particularly endurance events, appear to be more susceptible to infection than the general population is. For example, sore throats and flulike symptoms are more common in athletes. Some convincing evidence suggests that this increased susceptibility to infection arises because of a depression of immune system function (for detailed reviews, see Shephard [1997], Mackinnon [1999], and Gleeson and Bishop [1999]).

The main component of the immune system consists of the white blood cells, or leukocytes. The circulating numbers and functional capacities of leukocytes may be decreased by repeated bouts of intense, prolonged exercise. The cause may be increased levels of stress hormones during exercise and entry into the circulation of less mature leukocytes from the bone marrow. Drops in the blood concentration of glutamine have also been suggested as a possible cause of the immunodepression associated with heavy training, although the evidence for this is less compelling. Inflammation caused by muscle damage may be another factor.

During exercise, exposure to airborne bacteria and viruses increases because of the higher rate and depth of breathing. An increase in gut permeability may also allow entry of gut bacterial endotoxins into the circulation, particularly during prolonged exercise in the heat. Hence, the cause of the increased incidence of infection in athletes is most likely multifactorial. A variety of stressors (physical, psychological, environmental, and nutritional) suppress immune function, and these effects, together with increased exposure to potentially disease-causing pathogens, increase the athlete's susceptibility to infection (see figure 16.9).

The relationship between exercise and susceptibility to infection has been modeled in the form of a J-curve (Nieman 1994). This model suggests that although engaging in moderate activity may enhance immune function above sedentary levels,

excessive amounts of prolonged, high-intensity exercise may induce detrimental effects on immune function. Although the literature provides strong evidence in support of the latter point, relatively little evidence is available to suggest any clinically significant difference in immune function between sedentary and moderately active people. Thus, the portion of the J-curve representing this part of the relationship should perhaps be flattened out, as shown in figure 16.10. Matthews et al. (2002) reported that the regular performance of about 2 hours of moderate exercise a day was associated with a 29% reduction in risk of URTI compared with a sedentary lifestyle. This finding emphasizes that the benefit of regular, moderate exercise in improving resistance to infection is quite small.

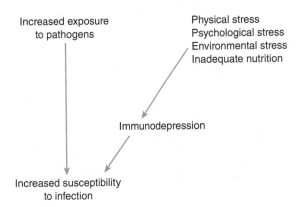

Figure 16.9 Factors contributing to infection incidence in athletes.

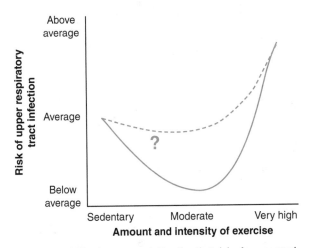

Figure 16.10 The J-curve model implies that risk of upper respiratory tract infection (URTI) is reduced by moderate activity but progressively elevated by heavier training loads. The dashed line between the two levels of exercise may be a more appropriate representation of the relationship between training load and URTI risk.

Acute Effects of Exercise on Immune Function

Prolonged strenuous exercise has a temporary depressive effect on immune function, and this effect has been associated with increased incidence of infection. For example, both Peters and Bateman (1983) and Nieman et al. (1990) described a substantially higher (two- to sixfold) frequency of self-reported symptoms of URTI in athletes who completed long-distance foot races compared with control runners who did not compete in the events.

An acute bout of physical activity is accompanied by responses that are similar in many respects to those induced by infection. A substantial increase in the number of circulating leukocytes (mainly lymphocytes and neutrophils) occurs, the magnitude of which is related to both the intensity and duration of exercise. Increases also occur in the plasma concentrations of various substances that influence leukocyte functions, including acute-phase proteins such as C-reactive protein, activated complement fragments, and inflammatory and anti-inflammatory cytokines such as interferon-γ, tumor necrosis factor-α, IL-1, IL-2, and IL-6. Hormonal changes also occur in response to exercise, including rises in the plasma concentration of several hormones (e.g., adrenaline, cortisol, growth hormone, and prolactin) that have immunomodulatory effects.

Acute exercise temporarily increases NK cell lytic activity but diminishes the proliferative response of lymphocytes to mitogens (see figure 16.11). Phagocytic neutrophils appear to be activated by an acute bout of exercise but show a diminished response to stimulation by bacterial lipopolysaccharide and reduced oxidative burst (killing capacity) after exercise, which can last for many hours (see figure 16.12).

During recovery from exercise, NK cell numbers and activity fall below preexercise levels (see figure 16.13), and if the exercise bout was high intensity or prolonged, the number of circulating lymphocytes may decrease below preexercise levels for several hours and the T-lymphocyte CD4+:CD8+ (helper:suppressor) ratio decreases. After prolonged strenuous exercise, the production of immunoglobulins by B-lymphocytes is inhibited. The plasma concentration of glutamine falls by about 20% and may remain depressed for some time.

These changes during early recovery from exercise appear to weaken the potential immune response to pathogens and possibly provide an

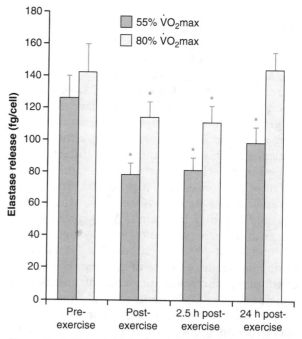

Figure 16.12 Changes in the in vitro lipopolysaccharide (LPS)-stimulated neutrophil degranulation response (elastase release per cell) after 3 hours of cycling at 55% of $\dot{V}O_2$max and after cycling to fatigue at 80% of $\dot{V}O_2$max (mean exercise duration 38 minutes) in 10 well-trained cyclists. Data are means and SEM. *$P < 0.05$ compared with preexercise. $P < 0.05$: 55% of $\dot{V}O_2$max versus 80% of $\dot{V}O_2$max.

International Journal of Sports Medicine: From P.J. Robson et al., "Effects of exercise intensity, duration, and recovery on in vitro neutrophil function in male athletes," 1999; 20: 128-135. Reprinted by permission.

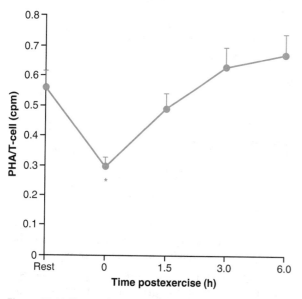

Figure 16.11 Change in phytohemaglutinin-stimulated (PHA-stimulated) lymphocyte proliferation after 2.5 hours of running.

International Journal of Sports Medicine: From D.A. Henson et al., "Carbohydrate supplementation and the lymphocyte proliferative response to long endurance running," 1998; 19: 574-580. Reprinted by permission.

open window for infection at this vulnerable time for an athlete (Pedersen and Bruunsgard 1995). Certainly, at this time, a temporary reduction in several aspects of innate immune function occurs, and athletes should be encouraged to adopt the following practices to minimize the risk of infection:

- Avoid contact with people who have symptoms of infection.
- Minimize contact with children of school age and avoid large crowds.
- Wash hands regularly, particularly after touching surfaces that are frequently handled by the public, such as doorknobs, handrails, and telephone receivers.
- Avoid hand-to-eye and hand-to-mouth contact to prevent transferring microbes to sensitive mucosal tissues.
- Maintain good oral hygiene.
- Avoid getting a dry mouth, both during competition and at rest, by drinking at regular intervals and maintaining hydration status.
- Never share drink bottles or cutlery.
- Use properly treated water for consumption and swimming.
- Avoid shared saunas, showers, and whirlpool tubs.
- Be aware of elevated vulnerability after training or competition.
- Good personal hygiene and thoughtfulness are the best defenses against respiratory infection.

Chronic Effects of Exercise Training on Immune Function

Exercise training also has a long-lasting effect on immune function. Most changes suggest an overall decrease in immune system function, particularly when training loads are high. Circulating numbers of leukocytes are generally lower in athletes at rest compared with sedentary people (see table 16.6). A low blood leukocyte count may arise from the hemodilution (expansion of the plasma volume) associated with training, or it may represent altered leukocyte kinetics, including diminished release from the bone marrow. Indeed, the large increase in circulating neutrophil numbers that accompanies a bout of prolonged exercise could, over periods of months or years of heavy training, deplete the bone marrow reserve of these important cells. The blood population of these cells seems to be less mature than that found in sedentary individuals, and the phagocytic activity of blood neutrophils

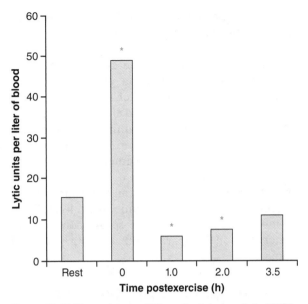

Figure 16.13 Change in natural killer cell cytotoxic activity (NKCA, expressed as lytic units per liter of blood) after 2.5 hours of running.
Data from Nieman et al. 1993.

■ **TABLE 16.6** ■

Numbers of Circulating Leukocytes in Endurance-Trained Males and Sedentary Males

Blood cell count (×10⁹/L)	Sedentary (n = 8)	Trained* (n = 8)
Leukocytes	6.62 (0.87)	4.36 (1.15)
Neutrophils	3.83 (0.86)	2.46 (0.87)
Lymphocytes	2.02 (0.27)	1.36 (0.20)

* $P < 0.01$, trained versus sedentary subjects.

Subjects were matched for age and body mass.

I don't think this is in the references. I will see if I can get an initial for the first name. - Data from Blannie et al. 1996.

Data from Blannie et al. 1996.

has been reported to be markedly lower in well-trained cyclists compared with age-matched and weight-matched sedentary control subjects.

Levels of secretory immunoglobulins, such as salivary IgA, are lower in well-trained subjects, as are T-lymphocyte CD4+:CD8+ ratios and in vitro mitogen-stimulated lymphocyte proliferation responses. Thus, with chronic periods of heavy training, both innate and adaptive immunity are depressed. Several causes of the diminution of immune function associated with heavy training are possible. One mechanism may simply be the cumulative effects of repeated bouts of intense exercise, with the consequent elevation of stress hormones, particularly glucocorticoids such as cortisol, causing temporary immunodepression. Frequently repeated exercise may not allow sufficient time for the immune system to recover fully. Furthermore, plasma glutamine levels can change substantially after exercise and may become chronically depressed after repeated bouts of prolonged strenuous training. Complement activation also occurs during exercise, and a diminution of the serum complement concentration with repeated bouts of exercise, particularly when muscle damage is incurred, can also contribute to decreased nonspecific immunity in athletes. Well-trained people have a lower serum complement concentration compared with sedentary control subjects.

Nutritional Manipulations to Decrease Immunodepression in Athletes

Poor nutritional practices may contribute to impaired immunity in athletes. Some athletes adopt diets that are extremely high in carbohydrate content at the expense of protein and fat. By avoiding foods high in animal fat, athletes are reducing their intake of fat-soluble vitamins and essential FAs. Many sports have strict weight categories, leading some competitors to follow energy-restricted diets that are often unbalanced, placing themselves at risk of several nutrient deficiencies.

Anecdotal and media reports promote the supposed performance benefits of certain vitamins and minerals, but most athletes do not realize that micronutrient supplementation is only beneficial when correcting a deficiency and that excessive intake of individual micronutrients can be toxic or can limit the absorption of other essential trace elements. Deficiencies or excesses of various dietary components have a substantial effect on immune function and may exacerbate the immunodepression associated with heavy training loads.

Mechanisms of Nutritional Influences on Immune Function in Athletes

Nutrient availability potentially affects almost all aspects of the immune system because many nutrients are involved in energy metabolism and protein synthesis. Most immune responses involve cell replication and the production of proteins with specific functions (e.g., cytokines, antibodies, and acute phase proteins). Immune system functions that may be compromised include the humoral and secretory antibody production, cell-mediated immunity, bactericidal capacity of phagocytes, complement formation, and T-lymphocyte proliferative response to mitogens.

A nutritional deficiency is said to have a direct effect when the nutritional factor has primary activity within the lymphoid system and an indirect effect when the primary activity affects all cellular material or an organ system that functions as an immune regulator. For example, carbohydrate availability directly affects a number of leukocyte functions but also indirectly affects the lymphoid system through its influence on circulating levels of the catecholamines, adrenocorticotrophic hormone (ACTH), and cortisol. Changes in plasma levels of these stress hormones are probably mostly responsible for the observed changes in immune function after an acute bout of exercise (see figure 16.14).

The effect of a nutrient deficiency on the immune system depends on the duration of the deficiency as well as on the athlete's nutritional status as a whole. The severity of the deficiency is also a factor, although even a mild deficiency of a single nutrient can alter the immune response. Because the availability of one nutrient may enhance or impair the action of another, and nutrient deficiencies often occur together, nutrient–nutrient interactions on immune function are

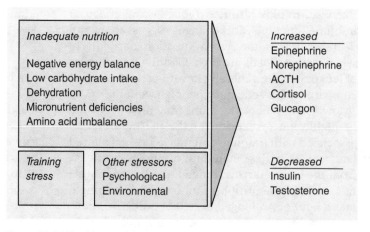

Figure 16.14 Nutrition and the stress-hormone response. Various stressors, including inadequate nutrition, prior exercise with inadequate recovery, psychological anxiety, and environmental extremes (e.g., heat and altitude) modify the hormonal response to exercise.

also an important consideration. Athletes who are training hard eat to satisfy their energy demands, consuming more macronutrients (carbohydrate, protein, and fat) and micronutrients (vitamins and minerals) than their sedentary counterparts. Therefore, they may ingest excessive amounts of some nutrients. Excessive amounts of specific nutrients (e.g., omega-3 polyunsaturated FAs, iron, and zinc) can have detrimental effects on immune function.

The 1991 Consensus Conference on Foods, Nutrition, and Sports Performance gave the following dietary advice: "In the optimum diet for most sports, carbohydrate is likely to contribute about 60% to 70% of the total energy intake and protein about 12%, with the remainder coming from fat."

Athletes are generally advised to eat a well-balanced diet consisting of a variety of foods in sufficient quantity to cover their energy expenditures. But many athletes alter their diets. They may use diets high in protein or carbohydrate or fat, very low-energy diets, fasting, or megadoses of vitamins and minerals. Such dietary extremes may in fact compromise immune function. For example, diets that are excessively high in carbohydrate, favored by many athletes to keep glycogen stores high, are generally low in meat products and thus are low in protein (an important nutrient for immune function) and vitamin B$_{12}$ (essential for DNA and RNA synthesis). Many athletes avoid dairy produce to minimize intake of saturated fat, but by doing so they are omitting from their diet major sources of vitamin D, B-group vitamins, and calcium, all of which play roles of varying importance in maintaining immune function. If fat intake is a concern, then athletes should select nonfat or low-fat dairy products that provide the same (or higher) levels of calcium, vitamin D, and vitamin B$_{12}$ as full-fat dairy products do. Only milk (regardless of fat content) is likely to be fortified with vitamin D.

Energy-restricted diets are not uncommon in sports in which leanness or low body mass confers a performance advantage (e.g., gymnastics, figure skating, and endurance running) or is required to meet certain body-weight criteria (e.g., boxing, martial arts, weightlifting, and rowing). Indeed, such demands have led to the identification of a new subclinical eating disorder, anorexia athletica, which is associated with an increased susceptibility to infection (see chapter 15). Even short-term dieting can influence immune function in athletes. For example, a loss of 2 kg of body mass over a 2-week period adversely affects macrophage phagocytic function.

Carbohydrate

The importance of adequate carbohydrate availability for maintenance of heavy training schedules and successful athletic performance is unquestionable (see chapter 6). During periods of heavy training, athletes should consume sufficient carbohydrate to cover about 60% of their energy costs. The recommended daily intake is 8 to 10 g/kg b.w. of carbohydrate for athletes who train for more than 2 hours per day. These recommendations are principally aimed at restoring muscle and liver glycogen stores to ensure sufficient carbohydrate availability for skeletal muscle contraction for training on successive days.

Glucose is also an important fuel for cells of the immune system, including lymphocytes, neutrophils, and macrophages. Phagocytes utilize glucose at a rate 10 times greater than they utilize glutamine when both substrates are present in a culture medium at normal physiological concentrations. The importance of glucose for the proper functioning of lymphocytes and macrophages is further emphasized in a study that found that mitogen-stimulated proliferation of these cells in vitro depends on a glucose concentration over the physiological range. Cells of the immune system have extremely high metabolic rates, and this finding highlights the importance of adequate nutrition for the provision of fuels to maintain immunocompetence.

Because elevated levels of stress hormones seem to cause many aspects of exercise-induced immune function impairment, nutritional strategies that effectively reduce the stress hormone response to exercise would be expected to limit the degree of exercise-induced immune dysfunction. The size of the glycogen stores in muscle and liver at the onset of exercise influence the hormonal and immune response to exercise. The amount of glycogen stored in the body is limited (usually less than 500 g) and is affected by recent physical activity and the amount of dietary carbohydrate intake. When people perform prolonged exercise following several days on very low-carbohydrate diets (typically < 10% of dietary energy intake from carbohydrate), the magnitude of the stress hormone (e.g., adrenaline and cortisol) and cytokine (e.g. IL-6, IL-1 ra, and IL-10) response is markedly higher than it is on normal- or high-carbohydrate diets, as illustrated in figure 16.15 (Gleeson et al. 1998; Mitchell et al. 1998). Furthermore, the postexercise fall in plasma glutamine concentration is greater than it is on normal- and high-carbohydrate diets.

It has been speculated that athletes deficient in carbohydrate are placing themselves at risk from the immunosuppressive effects of cortisol and reduced glutamine availability, including the suppression of antibody production, lymphocyte proliferation, and NK cell cytotoxic activity. In the study by Mitchell et al. (1998) it was observed that exercising (for 1 hour at 75% of $\dot{V}O_2$max) in a glycogen-depleted state (induced by prior exercise and 2 days on a low-carbohydrate diet) resulted in a greater fall in circulating lymphocyte numbers at 2 hours postexercise compared with the same exercise performed after 2 days on a high-carbohydrate diet. In this study the manipulation of carbohydrate status did not affect the decrease in mitogen-stimulated lymphocyte proliferation that occurred after exercise. But a more recent study by Bishop et al. (2005) showed that lymphocyte

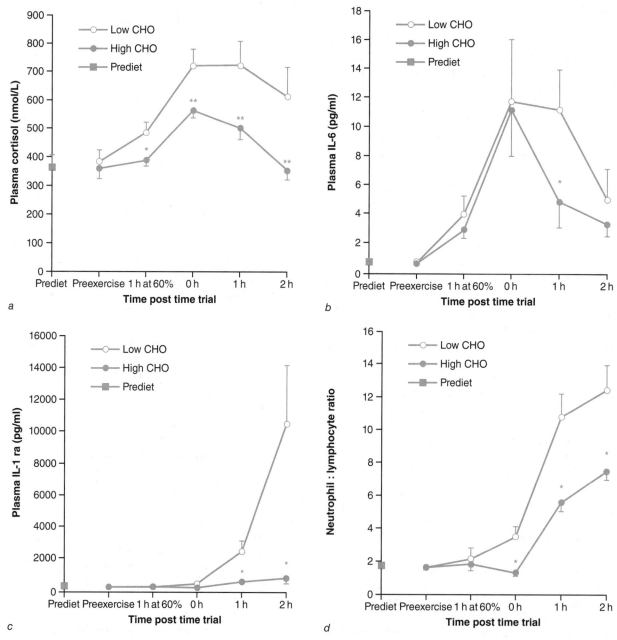

Figure 16.15 Changes in the concentrations of (a) plasma cortisol, (b) plasma interleukin-6 (IL-6), (c) plasma interleukin-1 receptor antagonist (IL-1 ra), and (d) the blood neutrophil:lymphocyte ratio after 1 hour of cycling at 60% of $\dot{V}O_2$max immediately followed by a half-hour time trial (work rate around 80% of $\dot{V}O_2$max). For the 3 days before the exercise trial, subjects (n = 12) consumed either a high-carbohydrate (CHO) diet (open circles) or a low-carbohydrate diet. Data are presented as mean and SEM. Significantly different from low carbohydrate, *P < 0.05, **P < 0.01. Unpublished observations.

proliferation responses to mitogen and influenza were lower 24 hours following a 90-minute intermittent high-intensity exercise bout when subjects consumed a placebo beverage compared with a carbohydrate beverage before, during, and following the exercise bout (figure 16.16). These differences were independent of changes in the plasma cortisol concentration, implying that these carbohydrate effects were mediated by a different mechanism.

Consumption of carbohydrate during prolonged exercise attenuates rises in plasma epinephrine, cortisol, and cytokines (Nehlsen-Cannarella et al. 1997); attenuates the trafficking of most leukocyte and lymphocyte subsets, including the rise in the neutrophil:lymphocyte ratio (see figure 16.17); prevents the exercise-induced fall in neutrophil function (see figure 16.18); and reduces the extent of the diminution of mitogen-stimulated T-lymphocyte proliferation (on a per cell basis) after prolonged exercise (Henson et al. 1998) (see figure 16.19). It was shown that consuming 30 to 60 g of carbohydrate per hour during 2.5 hours of strenuous cycling prevented both the decrease in the number and percentage of interferon-gamma (IFN-γ) posi-

tive T lymphocytes and the suppression of IFN-γ production from stimulated T-lymphocytes (figure 16.20) observed on the placebo control trial (Lancaster et al. 2005). IFN-γ production is critical to

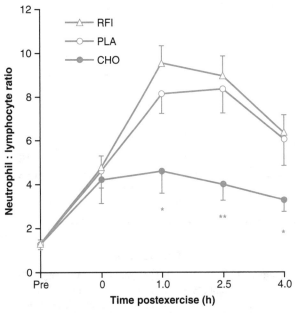

Figure 16.17 Changes in the neutrophil:lymphocyte ratio after 2 hours of cycling at 60% of V̇O₂max when fed a 6% w/v carbohydrate solution (closed circles), the same volume of an artificially sweetened placebo solution (open circles), or a restricted fluid intake (open triangles). Significantly different from placebo trial, *P < 0.05, **P < 0.01.

Data from Bishop et al., 1999b.

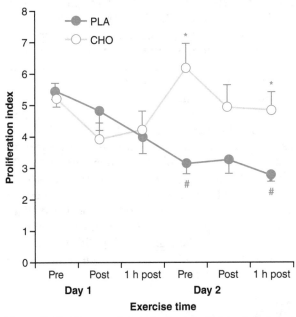

Figure 16.16 Mitogen (phytohemagglutinin)-stimulated T-lymphocyte proliferative response (fold increase relative to unstimulated cells) before and after two bouts of high-intensity intermittent exercise performed on consecutive days with either carbohydrate (CHO, 6.4% w/v) or placebo (PLA) beverage ingestion before, during, and after exercise bout. *significantly higher than PLA, P < 0.05. **significantly lower than preexercise on day 1 (PLA only), P < 0.05.

Data from Bishop et al., 2005.

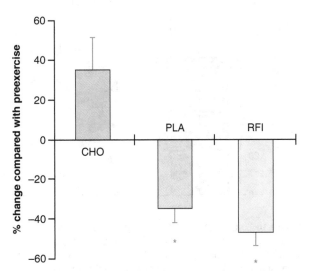

Figure 16.18 Percentage change (compared with preexercise) in the lipopolysaccharide-stimulated neutrophil degranulation response immediately after 2 hours of cycling at 60% of V̇O₂max when fed a 6% w/v carbohydrate solution (CHO), the same volume of an artificially sweetened placebo solution (PLA), or a restricted fluid intake (RFI). Significant change from preexercise, *P < 0.05.

Data from Henson et al. 1998.

antiviral defence and it has been suggested that the suppression of IFN-γ production may be an important mechanism leading to increased risk of infection after prolonged exercise bouts (Konig et al. 1997).

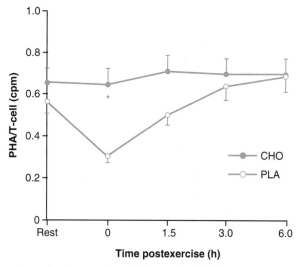

Figure 16.19 Change in phytohemaglutinin-stimulated (PHA-stimulated) lymphocyte proliferation after 2.5 hours of running when fed a 6% w/v carbohydrate (CHO) solution (closed circles) or the same volume of an artificially sweetened placebo (PLA) solution (open circles). Significantly different from PLA, *P < 0.05.
Data from Henson et al., 1998.

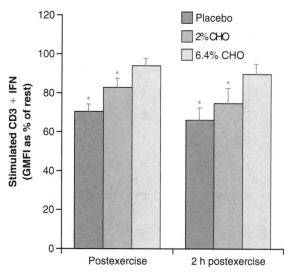

Figure 16.20 Consumption of 30 to 60 g of carbohydrate per hour as a 6.4% w/v beverage during 2.5 hours of strenuous cycling exercise prevents the suppression of interferon (IFN)-γ production from stimulated T-lymphocytes observed on the placebo control trial. *significantly lower than preexercise, P < 0.05. Note that ingesting a small amount of carbohydrate as a 2% w/v beverage is not as effective. The volume of drinks consumed was 500 ml immediately preexercise and 200 ml every 20 minutes during exercise.
Data from Lancaster et al., 2005.

The consumption of carbohydrate in beverages during exercise may have the additional benefit of helping to maintain saliva flow rate during exercise. Saliva contains several proteins with antimicrobial properties, including IgA, lysozyme, and β-amylase. During periods of heavy training, athletes have lower levels of IgA in their saliva and this condition may contribute to their increased incidence of URTI (Mackinnon 1999; Neville et al. 2008). Saliva secretion is under neural control. The sympathetic nervous system stimulation that occurs during exercise causes vasoconstriction of the blood vessels to the salivary glands and results in a reduction in saliva secretion. Regular fluid intake during exercise prevents this effect, and a study (Bishop et al. 2000) has confirmed that regular consumption of carbohydrate-containing drinks helps maintain saliva flow rate and, hence, saliva IgA secretion rate during prolonged exercise.

Although carbohydrate feeding during exercise appears to be effective in minimizing some of the immune perturbations associated with prolonged strenuous exercise, it does not prevent the fall in the plasma glutamine concentration and seems less effective for less-demanding exercise such as football (Bishop et al. 1999c) or rowing (Nieman et al. 1999) training. Carbohydrate feeding is not as effective in reducing immune-cell trafficking and functional depression when exercise is performed to the point of fatigue (Bishop et al. 2001). Preexercise feeding of carbohydrate is not effective in limiting exercise-induced changes in leukocyte trafficking or depression of neutrophil function. Evidence that the beneficial effect of carbohydrate feeding on immune responses to exercise translates to reduced incidence of URTI after prolonged exercise such as marathon races is currently lacking. Although a trend for a beneficial effect of carbohydrate ingestion on postrace URTI was reported in a study of 98 marathon runners (Nieman et al. 2002), this finding did not achieve statistical significance. Larger-scale studies are needed to investigate this possibility.

Fat

The International Consensus Conference on Foods, Nutrition, and Sports Performance advised athletes that 20% of energy intake should come from fat, whereas the *2005 Dietary Guidelines for Americans* recommended that total fat intake should be between 20% and 35% of total energy intake. The type of dietary fat is also important. In 1994 the UK Department of Health recommended that saturated fats contribute no more than 10% of daily energy intake, and the *2005 Dietary Guidelines for Americans* made an identical recommendation, advising that the remainder of fat intake be provided by monounsaturated FAs (15%), polyunsaturated FAs (6%), linoleic acid (1%), linolenic acid (0.2%), and *trans* FAs (< 2%). Two groups of polyunsaturated FAs (PUFAs) are essential to the body: the omega-6 (*n*-6) series, derived from linoleic acid, and the omega-3 (*n*-3) series, derived from linolenic acid. Adequate intakes of these FAs for adult men and women are 17 and 12 g/day, respectively, for *n*-6 FAs, and 1.6 and 1.1 g/day, respectively, for *n*-3 FAs (USDA 2006). These FAs cannot be synthesized in the body and therefore must be derived from the diet. Diets rich in either of these PUFAs improve the conditions of patients suffering from diseases characterized by an overactive immune system, such as rheumatoid arthritis. These PUFAs thus have immunomodulatory functions.

Although FAs are utilized as fuels by lymphocytes, their oxidation does not appear to be crucial for lymphocyte function, because the inhibition of FA oxidation does not affect the ability of lymphocytes to proliferate in response to mitogens. FAs exert either direct effects (by altering cell membrane fluidity) or indirect effects (as precursors of cell-signaling molecules called eicosanoids) on immune function, generally resulting in reduced IL-2 production and suppressed mitogen-induced lymphocyte proliferation. But supplementation with vitamin E or vitamin C appears to provide partial protection against some of these immunosuppressive effects.

Relatively little is known about the potential contribution of FAs to the regulation of exercise-induced modification of immune function. Although no study has been done in athletes, excessive intake of PUFA could possibly further potentiate the exercise-induced suppression of IL-2 production and lymphocyte proliferation. High intakes of arachidonic acid relative to intakes of FA of the *n*-3 group may also exert an undesirable influence on inflammation and immune function during and after exercise. Alteration of essential FA distribution through dietary changes or nutritional supplementation is already being applied in the treatment of chronic inflammatory diseases. More research is needed on the effects of altering essential FA intake on immune function after exercise and during periods of heavy training. A study that investigated the effects of endurance training for 7 weeks on carbohydrate-rich (65% of dietary energy) or fat-rich (62% of dietary energy)

diets concluded that diet during training may influence natural immunity because NK cell activity increased on the carbohydrate-rich diet compared with the fat-rich diet (Pedersen et al. 2000). The results of this study suggest that a fat-rich diet is detrimental to immune function compared with a carbohydrate-rich diet but do not clarify whether this effect is the result of a lack of dietary carbohydrate or an excess of a specific dietary fat component.

Protein and Amino Acids

The daily protein requirement of athletes is approximately twice that of the sedentary population. An intake of less than $1.6 \text{ g} \cdot \text{kg b.w.}^{-1} \cdot \text{day}^{-1}$ of protein is likely to be associated with a negative nitrogen balance in athletes who are training hard, particularly endurance athletes. If athletes consume a well-balanced diet that meets their requirement for energy, the increased requirement for protein will be met. Those at greatest risk for protein deficiency are athletes who are undertaking a program of food restriction to lose weight, vegetarian athletes, and athletes who are consuming unbalanced diets (e.g., with an excessive amount of carbohydrate at the expense of protein).

Inadequate intake of protein impairs host immunity, with particularly detrimental effects on the T-cell system, resulting in increased incidence of opportunistic infections. One of the most dramatic manifestations of this development is widespread atrophy of lymphoid tissue. In humans, protein-energy malnutrition (PEM) depresses the number of mature, fully differentiated T-lymphocytes and the in vitro response to T-lymphocyte mitogens, although the latter is reversible with nutritional repletion. Additionally, the T-lymphocyte CD4+:CD8+ ratio is markedly decreased in PEM. Essentially all forms of immunity are affected by PEM in humans, depending on the severity of the protein deficiency relative to energy intake. These effects include impaired phagocytic cell function, decreased cytokine production, and reduced complement formation. Although athletes are unlikely to reach a state of extreme malnutrition unless dieting very severely, some impairment of host-defense mechanisms is observed even in moderate protein deficiency.

Excessive dietary protein could also be harmful to immune function. A diet rich in protein (24% protein, 72% fat, and 3% carbohydrate) consumed for 4 days caused a 25% lowering of muscle and plasma glutamine levels. This decline was attributed to increased renal uptake of glutamine to reestablish normal acid–base balance because a high intake of protein combined with a low intake of carbohydrate induces chronic metabolic acidosis. Furthermore, falls in the plasma glutamine concentration after prolonged strenuous exercise are greater when consuming a low-carbohydrate diet compared with a normal diet. Ingesting carbohydrate during exercise, however, does not prevent the postexercise fall in plasma glutamine.

Glutamine is the most abundant free amino acid in human muscle and plasma, and it is utilized at extremely high rates by leukocytes to provide energy and optimal conditions for nucleotide biosynthesis. Indeed, glutamine is important, if not essential, to lymphocytes and other rapidly dividing cells, including the gut mucosa and bone marrow stem cells. Glutamine is also required for optimal macrophage phagocytic activity. Prolonged exercise is associated with a fall in the plasma concentration of glutamine, and such a decrease has been hypothesized to impair immune function. The overtraining syndrome is associated with a chronic reduction in plasma glutamine levels, which may be partly responsible for the immunodepression apparent in this condition. Interestingly, evidence indicates that an additional intake of 20 to 30 g/day of protein can restore depressed plasma glutamine levels in overtrained athletes.

Several scientists have suggested that exogenous provision of glutamine supplements may be beneficial by preventing the impairment of immune function after prolonged exercise. But the evidence that oral glutamine supplements reduce the incidence of URTI after endurance events is limited (Castell et al. 1996). Several studies that have investigated the effect of glutamine supplementation during and after exercise on various indices of immune function have failed to find any beneficial effect. A glutamine solution (0.1 g/kg b.w.) given at 0 minutes, 30 minutes, 60 minutes, and 90 minutes after a marathon race prevented the fall in the plasma glutamine concentration but did not prevent the fall in mitogen-induced lymphocyte proliferation and lymphocyte-activated NK cell activity (Rohde et al. 1998). Similarly, maintaining the plasma glutamine concentration by consuming glutamine in drinks taken both during and after 2 hours of cycling at 60% of $\dot{V}O_2$max did not affect leukocyte subset trafficking or prevent the exercise-induced fall in neutrophil function (Walsh et al. 2000). Unlike carbohydrate consumed during exercise, glutamine supplements do not seem to affect immune function perturbations, and a review article (Hiscock and Pedersen 2002) concluded that

falls in plasma glutamine are not responsible for exercise-induced immunodepression.

Bassit and colleagues (2002) reported that supplementation of BCAAs (6 g/day for 15 days) before a triathlon or 30 km run prevented the approximately 40% decline in mitogen-stimulated lymphocyte proliferation observed in the placebo control group after exercise. BCAAs are precursors for glutamine, and BCAA supplementation prevented the postexercise fall in plasma glutamine concentration and was associated with increased IL-2 and interferon production. More research is needed to resolve these conflicting findings of BCAA and glutamine supplementation on immune responses to exercise.

Alcohol and Caffeine

Increasing evidence suggests that consumption of light to moderate amounts of polyphenol-rich alcoholic beverages like wine or beer could have health benefits. Scientists have long debated the effects of alcohol on immune function, showing on the one hand that high doses of alcohol consumption can directly suppress a wide range of immune responses and that alcohol abuse is associated with an increased incidence of a number of infectious diseases. On the other hand, moderate alcohol consumption seems to have a beneficial effect on the immune system compared with alcohol abuse or abstinence, and epidemiological studies have indicated that moderate alcohol consumption is associated with lower morbidity (Romeo et al. 2007). Therefore, the link between alcohol consumption, immune response, and infectious and inflammatory processes remains incompletely understood. Of course, other factors, unrelated or indirectly related to immune function, like drinking patterns, beverage type, amount of alcohol, or gender differences, may well affect the influence that alcohol consumption has on the immune system. Thus, the ethanol in alcoholic beverages may have some detrimental effects, whereas some of the polyphenol compounds present in wine and beer may have anti-inflammatory effects. Clearly though, with alcoholic beverage consumption, more is not better, and all people should be aware of the serious health risks of consuming more than two drinks per day.

Caffeine is the most widely consumed drug in Europe and America (Curatolo and Robertson 1983), and athletes have long used it in the belief that it improves performance. In 2004 caffeine was taken off the list of banned substances by the International Olympic Committee (IOC). The effect of caffeine on exercise performance is dealt with in chapter 11. Caffeine originates naturally in 63 species of plants as several types of methylated xanthines. Caffeine and caffeinelike substances can be found in a variety of foods and drinks (now including several sports drinks and energy drinks), but the main sources for these substances are coffee beans, tea leaves, cocoa beans, and cola nuts. Coffee accounts for 75% of all caffeine consumption. Caffeine is an adenosine receptor antagonist, and several immune cell types including neutrophils and lymphocytes express adenosine receptors. Furthermore, caffeine ingestion results in elevated circulating epinephrine (adrenaline) concentration both at rest and during exercise and so could affect immune cell functions indirectly through actions on adrenoreceptors. At present, little information is available about the effects of caffeine on immune function at rest. Addition of pharmacological doses of caffeine to cell culture media has been associated with dose-dependent suppression of in vitro mitogen-stimulated lymphocyte proliferative responses in humans (Rosenthal et al. 1992). But in vivo administration of 18 mg · kg^{-1} · day^{-1} of caffeine in rats was associated with a significant increase in mitogen-stimulated T-cell proliferation (Kantamala et al. 1990). In the same study, B-cell proliferative responses to mitogen significantly decreased following administration of 6 mg kg^{-1} · day^{-1} of caffeine.

Recent exercise studies have demonstrated that caffeine compared with placebo ingestion 1 hour before a bout of intensive endurance exercise was associated with greater perturbations in numbers of circulating lymphocytes, CD4+ cells, and CD8+ cells. Moreover, caffeine ingestion was associated with an increased percentage of CD4+ and CD8+ cells expressing the early activation marker CD69 in vivo before and after exercise (Bishop et al. 2005). Furthermore, the postexercise fall in stimulated neutrophil oxidative burst responses was attenuated by caffeine ingestion (Walker et al. 2006). It is thought that these effects may be largely mediated through the action of caffeine as an adenosine receptor antagonist.

Vitamins

Vitamins are essential organic molecules that cannot be synthesized in the body and therefore must be obtained from food (see chapter 10). Several vitamins are essential for normal immune function: fat-soluble vitamins A and E and water-soluble vitamins B_{12} and C. Other vitamins (e.g., B_6 and folic acid) also play important roles in immune function, but dietary deficiencies of these vitamins in humans are extremely rare.

No indications in the literature suggest that vitamin intake among athletes in general is insufficient. Athletes tend to ingest above-average quantities of these micronutrients, and as with dietary protein requirements, increased dietary intake may satisfy any increase in need. On the other hand, the requirement for most vitamins may simply not increase in athletes. For example, vitamin loss through sweat during exercise is negligible.

Antioxidant Vitamins Vitamins with antioxidant properties, including vitamins C, E, and β-carotene (provitamin A), may be required in increased quantities in athletes to inactivate the products of exercise-induced lipid peroxidation (Packer 1997). Oxygen free-radical formation that accompanies the dramatic increase in oxidative metabolism during exercise (see chapter 10) could potentially inhibit immune responses.

Reactive oxygen species (ROS) inhibit locomotory and bactericidal activity of neutrophils, reduce the proliferation of T-lymphocytes and B-lymphocytes, and inhibit NKCA. Sustained endurance training appears to be associated with an adaptive upregulation of the antioxidant defense system. Such adaptations, however, may be insufficient to protect athletes who train extensively, and these individuals should consider increasing their intakes of nutritional antioxidants such as vitamins C, E, and β-carotene to reduce free-radical damage.

Vitamin C (ascorbic acid) occurs in high concentration in leukocytes and is implicated in a variety of anti-infective functions, including promotion of T-lymphocyte proliferation, prevention of corticosteroid-induced suppression of neutrophil activity, production of interferon, and inhibition of virus replication. It is also a major water-soluble antioxidant that is effective as a scavenger of ROS in both intracellular and extracellular fluids. It can act as an antioxidant both directly (e.g., in the prevention of auto-oxidative dysfunction of neutrophil bactericidal activity) and indirectly through its regeneration of reduced vitamin E (α-tocopherol). Vitamin C occurs in high concentration in the adrenal glands and is necessary for the production of several hormones that are secreted in response to stress, such as epinephrine, norepinephrine, and cortisol.

Studies report that daily supplementation of large doses of vitamin C reduced the incidence of symptoms of URTI in athletes after they participated in ultramarathon races (Peters et al. 1993, 1996). The results of one of these studies are illustrated in figure 16.21, which also shows that the supplementation of additional dietary antioxidants (vitamin E and β-carotene) does not confer any additional beneficial effect. The doses of vitamin C used in these studies (600 to 1,000 mg/day) are considerably higher than the daily dosage of 200 mg that is associated with accelerated clinical improvement in elderly patients hospitalized with acute respiratory infection after 4 weeks of daily supplementation (Hunt et al. 1994). In a more recent randomized, double-blind, placebo-controlled study, intake of 1,500 mg/day of vitamin C for 7 days before an ultramarathon race and consumption of vitamin C in a carbohydrate beverage during the race (subjects in the placebo group consumed the same carbohydrate beverage without added vitamin C) did not affect oxidative stress, cytokine, or immune function measures during and after the race (Nieman et al. 2002). In contrast, it has been reported (Fischer et al. 2004) that 4 weeks of combined supplementation of vitamin C (500 mg/day) and vitamin E (400 IU/day) before a 3-hour knee extension exercise protocol reduced muscle IL-6 release and reduced the systemic rise in both circulating IL-6 and cortisol (figure 16.22). Some degree of blunting of the plasma cortisol response to exercise and better-maintained neutrophil function after exercise was reported in a placebo-controlled study that used the same daily dose of vitamin C and E supplements and examined immunoendocrine responses to 2.5

hours of cycling after 4 weeks of supplementation (Davison et al. 2007). Furthermore, administration of the antioxidant N-acetyl-L-cysteine (a precursor of glutathione) to mice prevented the exercise-induced reduction in intracellular glutathione concentration and markedly reduced postexercise apoptosis in intestinal lymphocytes (Quadrilatero and Hoffman-Goetz 2004). Thus, although some inconsistencies are seen in the literature regarding antioxidant supplementation and immune responses to exercise, some basis is present for believing that such supplementation could have beneficial effects in alleviating exercise-induced immunodepression through the mechanisms summarized in figure 16.23.

The most recent Cochrane meta-analysis examined the evidence that daily doses of more than 200 mg vitamin C were more effective than placebo in preventing or treating the common cold (Douglas et al. 2007). Twenty-nine trial comparisons involving 11,077 study participants contributed to this meta-analysis on the relative risk (RR) of developing a cold while taking prophylactic vitamin C. The pooled RR was 0.96 (95% CI 0.92 to 1.00). A subgroup of six trials that involved physically active subjects (a total of 642 marathon runners, skiers, and soldiers on subarctic exercises) reported a pooled RR of 0.50 (95% CI 0.38 to 0.66). Thirty comparisons that involved 9,676 respiratory epi-

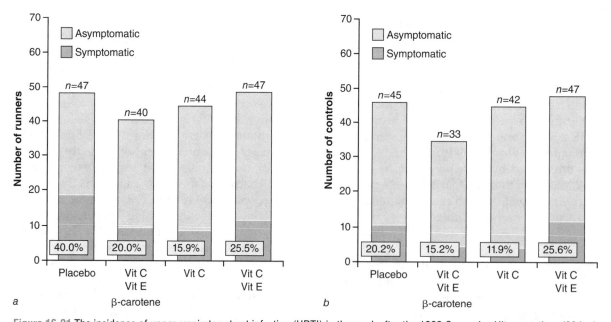

Figure 16.21 The incidence of upper respiratory tract infection (URTI) in the week after the 1993 Comrades Ultramarathon (90 km) in South Africa. Different groups of runners (see (a)) or control subjects (see (b)) received different combinations of antioxidant supplements or placebo for 3 weeks before the ultramarathon.

Adapted, by permission, from E.M. Peters et al., 1996, "Vitamin C as effective as combinations of anti-oxidant nutrients in reducing symptoms of upper respiratory tract infections in ultramarathon runners," *South African Journal of Sports Medicine* 11: 23-27.

sodes contributed to the meta-analysis on common cold duration during vitamin C or placebo supplementation. A consistent benefit of vitamin C was observed, representing a reduction in cold duration of 8% (95% CI 3% to 13%) for adult participants and 13.5% (95% CI 5% to 21%) for child participants. Fifteen trial comparisons that involved 7,045 respiratory episodes contributed to the meta-analysis of severity of episodes experienced while on prophylaxis, and the results revealed a benefit of vitamin C when days confined to home and off work or school were taken as a measure of severity. A limited number of trials had examined cold duration and severity during therapy with vitamin C that was initiated after the onset of cold symptoms, and no significant differences from placebo were found. The authors concluded that the failure of vitamin C supplementation to reduce the incidence of colds in the normal population indicates that routine mega-dose prophylaxis is not generally justified but that individuals subjected to brief periods of severe physical exercise or cold environments may well gain some benefit.

But even if high-dose antioxidant supplementation offers some protective effect on infection risk, athletes need to consider the risks, which may include the blunting of some of the adaptations to training. Chapter 12 discusses this issue in detail.

Animal studies show an increased oxidation of vitamin E during exercise that could result in reduced antioxidant protection. Dietary vitamin E stimulates mononuclear cell production of IL-Iβ through its influence on the arachidonic acid metabolic pathways, and cytokine production is further facilitated by a vitamin E–influenced inhibition of PGE2 production. Severe vitamin E deficiency results in impaired cell-mediated immunity and decreased antibody synthesis.

Vitamin A is also essential for immunocompetence. Vitamin A deficiency in animals and humans results in atrophy of the thymus, decreased lymphocyte proliferation in response to mitogens, increased bacterial binding to respiratory tract epithelial cells, and impaired secretory IgA production.

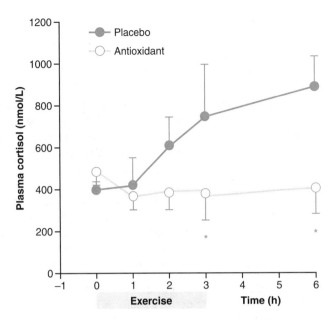

Figure 16.22 The effect of 4 weeks of antioxidant supplementation (500 mg/day of vitamin C and 400 IU/day of vitamin E) compared with placebo on plasma cortisol responses to 3 hours of dynamic knee extensor exercise.

Data from Fischer et al., 2004.

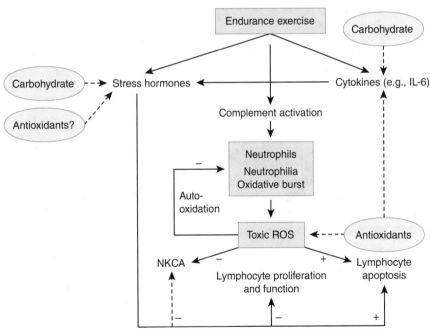

Figure 16.23 The possible mechanisms by which dietary antioxidant supplementation reduces stress-induced or exercise-induced immunodepression.

Consequently, vitamin A–deficient humans have a higher incidence of spontaneous infection. Vitamin A–deficient experimental animals also demonstrate reduced NKCA, lower production of interferon and antibodies, impaired delayed cutaneous hypersensitivity, and less-effective macrophage activity.

β-carotene (provitamin A) acts as an immunostimulant, increasing the number of CD4+ helper T-cells in healthy human volunteers and stimulating NKCA when added in vitro to human lymphatic cultures. Furthermore, elderly men who had been taking β-carotene supplements (50 mg on alternate days) for 10 to 12 years were reported to have significantly higher NKCA than did elderly men on placebo. β-carotene also functions as an antioxidant; thus, the requirement may increase in athletes who are involved in heavy training schedules that stimulate increased production of ROS. But supplementing ultramarathon runners with β-carotene had an insignificant effect on the incidence of URTI after the 90 km Comrades Ultramarathon in South Africa (see figure 16.21).

Vitamin B₁₂ and Folic Acid Vitamin B_{12} and folic-acid deficiencies have profound effects on immune function. Both of these vitamins are essential for the synthesis of nucleic acids and hence are required for the normal production of red and white blood cells in the bone marrow. Vitamin B_{12} can be absorbed from the gut only in the presence of the glycoprotein intrinsic factor. Lack of this factor or deficiency of vitamin B_{12} causes pernicious anemia, which has detrimental effects on immune function. For example, impaired lymphocyte proliferative responses to mitogens and a modest reduction in the phagocytic and bactericidal capacity of neutrophils have been reported in people with primary pernicious anemia. The only natural sources of vitamin B_{12} are of animal origin. As such, vegetarian athletes and athletes who are avoiding dairy produce to minimize saturated fat intake are at high risk for deficiency of this vitamin. If fat intake is a concern, then athletes should select nonfat or low-fat dairy products that provide the same (or higher) level of B_{12} as full-fat dairy products.

Vitamin Supplements and Megadoses In general, supplementation with individual vitamins or consumption of large doses of simple antioxidant mixtures is not recommended. Athletes should obtain complex mixtures of antioxidant compounds from consumption of fruits and vegetables. A suitable alternative is commercially available capsules of dried fruit and vegetable juice.

Consuming megadoses of individual vitamins is likely to do more harm than good. Because most vitamins function mainly as coenzymes in the body, after the enzyme systems are saturated, the vitamins in free form can have toxic effects. For example, 300 mg of vitamin E (as α-tocopherol acetate), given daily to 18 men for 3 weeks, produced a significant depression in the bactericidal activity of peripheral blood leukocytes and mitogen-induced lymphocyte proliferation. Some people suffer from diarrhea following ingestion of large doses of vitamin C, and prolonged intake of very large doses (>1,000 mg/day) of vitamin C is associated with kidney oxalate stone formation, impaired absorption of copper, and, in susceptible individuals, excessive absorption of iron and predisposition to gout. These side effects, however, seem to be rare. Consuming megadoses of vitamin A may impair the inflammatory response and complement formation as well as have other pathological effects, including causing fetal abnormalities when consumed by pregnant women and reducing bone mineral density.

Minerals

Minerals are classified as macrominerals or microminerals (trace elements), based on the extent of their occurrence in the body (see chapter 10). Of importance here are the trace elements that constitute less than 0.01% of total body mass, of which 14 have been identified as essential for maintenance of health. Of these 14, several are known to exert modulatory effects on immune function, including zinc, iron, selenium, and copper (see table 16.7). Yet with the exception of zinc and iron, isolated deficiencies are rare. Indeed, iron deficiency is reported to be the most widespread nutrient deficiency in the world, and field studies consistently associate iron deficiency with increased morbidity from infectious disease. Exercise has a pronounced effect on both zinc and iron metabolism.

Zinc The role of zinc in immune function has received increasing attention in recent years. Zinc is essential for the development of the immune system, and more than 100 metalloenzymes are dependent on it, including those involved in the transcription of DNA and synthesis of proteins. For example, zinc is a cofactor for the enzyme terminal deoxynucleotidyl transferase, which is required by immature T-cells for their replication and functioning. The effects of zinc deficiency on immune function include lymphoid atrophy, decreased delayed-hypersensitivity cutaneous responses, decreased IL-2 production, impaired mitogen-stimulated lymphocyte proliferative responses, and decreased NKCA. Zinc availability affects superoxide free-radical production by stimulated phagocytes, although in the laboratory this effect seems to depend on the actual molecular form of zinc.

Vegetarian athletes are at risk for zinc deficiency because meat and seafood are the richest zinc sources (see table 16.8). Although nuts, legumes, and whole grains are good sources of zinc, the high levels of fiber in these foods can decrease zinc absorption. Zinc deficiency can also be a problem for athletes in sports in which a low body mass confers a performance advantage. Very low-energy or starvation-type diets may induce significant zinc losses. Because zinc is lost from the body mainly

■ TABLE 16.7 ■

Roles of Minerals in Immune Function and the Effects of Dietary Deficiency or Excess

Mineral	Role in immune function	Effect of deficiency	Effect of excess
Iron	Oxygen transport and cofactor of metalloenzymes	Anemia and increased infections	Hemochromatosis, liver cirrhosis, heart disease, and increased infections
Zinc	Cofactor of metalloenzymes, protein synthesis, and antioxidant	Impaired growth, healing, increased infections, and anorexia	Impaired absorption of Fe and Cu, increased HDL cholesterol:LDL cholesterol ratio, anemia, nausea, vomiting, and immune system impairment
Selenium	Cofactor of glutathione peroxidase (antioxidant)	Cardiomyopathy, cancer, heart disease, impaired immune function, and erythrocyte fragility	Nausea, vomiting, fatigue, and hair loss
Copper	Promotes normal iron absorption and cofactor of superoxide dismutase (antioxidant)	Anemia and impaired immune function	Nausea and vomiting
Magnesium	Protein synthesis and cofactor of metalloenzymes	Muscle weakness, fatigue, apathy, muscle tremor, and cramp	Nausea, vomiting, and diarrhea

■ TABLE 16.8 ■

Dietary Sources and Daily RDA or AI of Important Minerals for Immune Function

Mineral	Source	RDA or AI*	Absorbed (%)
Iron	Liver, kidney, eggs, red meats, seafood, oysters, bread, flour, molasses, dried legumes, nuts, leafy green vegetables, broccoli, figs, raisins, and cocoa	8 mg (M) 18 mg (F)	10–30 (heme iron); 2–10 (nonheme iron)
Zinc	Oysters, shellfish, beef, liver, poultry, dairy products, whole grains, wheat germ, vegetables, asparagus, and spinach	11 mg (M) 8 mg (F)	20–50
Selenium	Meat, liver, kidney, poultry, fish, dairy produce, seafood, and whole grains and nuts from selenium-rich soil	55 mg (M, F)	Unknown
Copper	Liver, kidney, shellfish, meat, fish, poultry, eggs, bran cereals, nuts, legumes, broccoli, banana, avocado, and chocolate	0.9 mg (M, F)	20–50
Magnesium	Seafood, nuts, green leafy vegetables, fruits, whole-grain products, milk, and yogurt	420 mg (M) 320 mg (F)	25–60
Manganese	Whole grains, peas and beans, leafy vegetables, and bananas	2.3 mg* (M) 1.8 mg* (F)	Unknown

RDA = Recommended daily allowance; AI* = adequate intake. M = males; F = females.

■ TABLE 16.9 ■
Body Content and Body Fluid Concentrations of Important Minerals for Immune Function

Mineral	Symbol	Total amount in body (mg)	BODY FLUID CONCENTRATION (mg/l)		
			Plasma	Sweat	Urine
Iron	Fe	5,000	0.4–1.4	0.3–0.4	0.1–0.15
Zinc	Zn	2,000	0.7–1.3	0.7–1.3	0.2–0.5
Selenium	Se	13	0.05–0.10	<0.01	<0.01
Copper	Cu	100	0.7–1.7	0.2–0.6	0.03–0.04
Magnesium	Mg	25,000	16–30	4–15	60–100
Manganese	Mn	12	0.02	<0.01	<0.01

in sweat and urine (see table 16.9) and these losses are increased by exercise, a heavy schedule of exercise training could induce a zinc deficiency in athletes. Certainly, highly trained women have significantly higher urinary zinc excretion compared with untrained control subjects, and in well-trained male games players an acute bout of high-intensity exercise increases daily urinary zinc excretion by 34% compared with resting values.

Male and female athletes have lower plasma zinc concentrations than untrained people. Studies concerning the relationship between immune function, exercise, and zinc status in athletes are lacking. But a study of male runners found that 6 days of zinc supplementation (25 mg of zinc and 1.5 mg of copper, twice a day) inhibited the exercise-associated increase in superoxide free-radical formation by activated neutrophils (as shown in figure 16.24) and exaggerated the exercise-induced suppression of T-lymphocyte proliferation in response to mitogens. Such effects might temporarily predispose athletes to opportunistic infection. Megadoses of zinc have further detrimental effects on immune function. The administration of zinc (150 mg twice a day) to 11 healthy males for 6 weeks was associated with reduced T-lymphocyte proliferative responses to mitogen stimulation and impaired neutrophil phagocytic activity. Hence, megadoses of zinc are not recommended. Athletes should be encouraged to consume zinc-rich foods (e.g., poultry, meat, fish, and dairy products). Vegetarians have been advised to take a 10 to 20 mg supplement of zinc daily (the RDA is 10 mg and 12 mg for females and males, respectively), but in view of the findings just discussed, supplements at

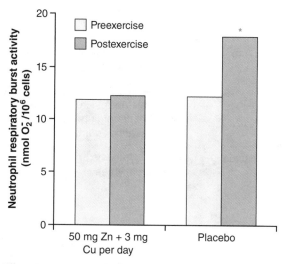

Figure 16.24 The effect of zinc and copper supplementation versus placebo on the exercise-induced change in neutrophil respiratory burst activity.
Data from Singh et al. 1994.

the lower end of this range may be more suitable for vegetarian athletes.

The efficacy of zinc supplementation as a treatment for the common cold has been investigated in at least 11 studies published since 1984. The findings have been equivocal, and several reviews of this topic conclude that further research is necessary before the use of zinc supplements to treat the common cold can be recommended (Macknin 1999; Marshall 2000). Although only limited evidence suggests that taking zinc supplements reduces the incidence of URTI (McElroy and Miller 2002), in the studies that have reported a beneficial effect of zinc in treating the common cold (i.e., reduction of symptom duration, severity, or both), zinc had to be taken within 24 hours of the onset of symptoms to be of any benefit. Potential problems with zinc supplements include nausea, bad taste reactions, lowering of HDL cholesterol, depression of some immune cell functions (e.g., neutrophil oxidative burst), and interference with the absorption of copper (Gleeson 2000).

Iron Iron deficiency is prevalent throughout the world. By some estimates, as much as 25% of the world's population is iron deficient. Endurance athletes risk potential iron deficiency because of increased iron losses in sweat, urine, and feces. The incidence of iron depletion among athletes, however, is no greater than that in the general population. Nevertheless, exercise may contribute to an iron-depleted state. The acute-phase host response to stress (including exercise) involves the depression of circulating free iron levels. Stress-induced elevation of IL-1 causes granulocyte release of the iron-binding protein lactoferrin within the circulation. Lactoferrin is then thought to bind (chelate) iron from transferrin, forming lactoferrin-iron complexes, and leading to a depression of plasma iron concentration that is independent of plasma volume changes.

The immune system itself appears to be particularly sensitive to the availability of iron, although iron deficiency has neither completely harmful nor enhancing effects on immune function. On the one hand, free iron is necessary for bacterial growth. Removal of iron with the help of chelating agents such as lactoferrin reduces bacterial multiplication, particularly in the presence of a specific antibody. A study reported that iron-deficient mice had a lower mortality after infection with *Salmonella* compared with iron-replete mice. Thus, iron deficiency may protect an individual from infection, whereas supplementation may predispose the individual to infectious disease, particularly because iron catalyzes the production of hydroxyl free radicals, and high intake of iron can impair gastrointestinal zinc absorption. On the other hand, iron deficiency depresses various aspects of immune function, including macrophage IL-1 production, the lymphocyte proliferative response to mitogens, NKCA, neutrophil phagocytic activity, and delayed cutaneous hypersensitivity (an index of cell-mediated immune function).

A number of causes of iron deficiency in endurance athletes involved in heavy training have been suggested. Exercise may cause reductions in gastrointestinal iron absorption, and iron is lost in sweat, which contains 0.3 mg/L (see table 16.9). This process can cause losses of up to 1.0 mg/day

of iron in athletes who are training extensively. Because only about 10% of dietary iron is absorbed, such losses increase the dietary requirement by about 10 mg/day, which is approximately double the normal daily iron requirement (the RDA is 15 mg for females and 10 mg for males). In addition, some damage to red blood cells (hemolysis) may occur in runners and games players because of foot strike and in swimmers because of body friction in moving through the water. Subsequently, loss of hemoglobin in the urine will occur, although this loss is thought to be a negligible drain on iron stores. Some athletes are also susceptible to gastrointestinal bleeding during exercise, which may increase fecal iron losses.

The bioavailability of iron is lower in vegetarian diets because of the lack of heme iron, which is more easily absorbed. The consensus is that all athletes should be aware of foods rich in heme iron such as lean red meat, poultry, and fish and include them in the daily diet. Iron requirements in endurance athletes may be double the RDA, although these requirements can be met through the diet without the need for artificial supplements. Vegetarian athletes should ensure that plant food choices are iron dense (e.g., green leafy vegetables, legumes, whole-grain breads and pasta, and iron-fortified products). Some breakfast cereals, bars, and breads are fortified with iron and provide a good source, though usually in amounts less than the RDA. Megadoses of iron are not advised, and routine oral supplements of iron should not be taken without medical advice.

Selenium Selenium deficiency can affect all components of the immune system. Selenium is a cofactor of glutathione peroxidase and reductase and thus influences the quenching of ROS. As such, the requirement for selenium may increase in athletes involved in regular intensive training programs. But any selenium supplement should be taken with caution. Supplements with doses up to the RDA appear nontoxic, but the safety of larger doses has not been confirmed. Intakes of 25 mg (approximately 40 times the RDA) have been associated with vomiting, abdominal pain, hair loss, and fatigue.

Copper The effects of copper deficiency on immune function include impaired antibody formation, inflammatory response, neutrophil phagocytosis, NKCA, and lymphocyte stimulation responses. The results of changes in copper status because of exercise and training are controversial, perhaps reflecting the inadequacy of techniques used to measure copper status. With exercise some redistribution of copper between body compartments may occur, and athletes have been reported to lose copper in sweat collected after exercise. Although copper deficiency is rare in humans, athletes who take zinc supplements may compromise the gastrointestinal absorption of copper because of the similar physicochemical properties of these two minerals.

Magnesium Magnesium is an essential cofactor for many enzymes involved in biosynthetic processes and energy metabolism and is required for normal neuromuscular coordination. The total-body content of magnesium is about 25 g (see table 16.9). The RDA for magnesium is 350 mg/day for men and 280 mg/day for women; hence, magnesium is classified as a macromineral rather than a trace element. The main dietary sources of magnesium are listed in table 16.8. Most studies of dietary habits in athletes suggest that magnesium intake exceeds the RDA. But the data used to determine RDAs for micronutrients often did not include athletes, or the activity levels of the subjects were not reported. Therefore, although the RDAs may apply to the sedentary population, they may not be an accurate means of evaluating the nutritional needs of athletes.

Several studies report low serum magnesium concentrations in athletes, and prolonged strenuous exercise is associated with increased losses of magnesium in urine and sweat. As with zinc and iron, a single bout of exercise is unlikely to induce substantial magnesium losses, but a state of mild magnesium deficiency may be induced during a period of heavy training, particularly in a warm environment where sweat losses are high.

Magnesium deficiency in both humans and animals is associated with neuromuscular abnormalities, including muscle weakness, cramps, and structural damage of muscle fibers and organelles. The structural damage may be caused by an impairment of calcium homeostasis secondary to an oxygen free-radical-induced alteration in the integrity of the membrane of the sarcoplasmic reticulum. A lack of magnesium may also be associated with a depletion of selenium and reduced glutathione peroxidase activity, which increases the susceptibility to damage by free radicals. Hence, magnesium deficiency may potentiate exercise-induced muscle damage and stress responses, but direct evidence for this effect is lacking.

Manganese Manganese is a cofactor of the enzyme superoxide dismutase, which aids in protection against free radicals. The RDA for manganese is 2.0 to 5.0 mg/day. Sources are whole-grain products, dried peas and beans, leafy vegetables, and bananas. The effects of exercise on manganese status are presently unknown, but training is associated with an increase in levels of antioxidant enzymes, suggesting an increased requirement for manganese during periods of increased training. As with other trace elements, losses of manganese in urine and sweat are likely higher in athletes than in nonathletes.

Cobalt Cobalt as a component of vitamin B_{12} promotes the development of red and white blood cells in the bone marrow. Deficiencies are associated with pernicious anemia, reduced blood leukocyte counts, impaired lymphocyte proliferation, and impaired bactericidal capacity of neutrophils. Major food sources of cobalt are meat, liver, and milk. Hence, athletes who avoid animal foods are at risk for cobalt and vitamin B_{12} deficiency.

Fluorine Although not directly required for normal immune function, fluorine is needed for the normal formation of healthy bones and teeth, and it protects against dental caries (tooth decay by oral bacteria). Given the relatively high intake of sugary foods and sports drinks by athletes, good oral hygiene is important in maintaining healthy teeth. Frequent intakes of soft drinks and carbohydrates, particularly sugars, depress the oral pH with a resultant net demineralization of the teeth. Sugars are metabolized to organic acids by the bacteria in the plaque on teeth and gums. Therefore, all sports people should maintain good plaque control. The RDA for fluorine is 1.5 to 4.0 mg/day, and this trace element is found in milk, egg yolk, seafood, and drinking water. Several toothpastes and mouth rinses contain fluorine (as sodium fluoride), and in some countries, including the United States, fluoride is added to drinking water.

Dietary Immunostimulants

Certain supplements may boost immune function and reduce infection risk in immunocompromised people, including athletes engaged in heavy training and competition. Many nutritional supplements are on the market besides the amino acids (e.g., glutamine), vitamins (e.g., vitamin C), and minerals (e.g., zinc) already mentioned in this chapter that are claimed to boost immunity. These include β-glucans, bovine colostrum, probiotics, and herbals such as echinacea, ginseng, and curcumin. The claims for many of these supplements are often based on selective evidence of efficacy in animals, in vitro experiments, children, the elderly, or clinical patients in severe catabolic states. Direct evidence for their efficacy for preventing exercise-induced immune depression or improving immune system status in athletes is usually lacking. In recent years, however, the effects of some of these supplements on immune function or infection incidence have been evaluated in physically active populations.

Echinacea Several herbal preparations are reputed to have immunostimulatory effects, and consumption of products containing *Echinacea purpurea* is widespread among athletes. But few controlled studies have examined the effects of dietary immunostimulants on exercise-induced changes in immune function. In a double-blind, placebo-controlled study, the effect of a daily oral pretreatment for 28 days with pressed juice of *Echinacea purpurea* was investigated in 42 triathletes before and after a sprint triathlon. A subgroup of athletes was also treated with magnesium as a reference for supplementation with a micronutrient important for optimal muscular function. During the 28-day pretreatment period, none of the athletes in the *Echinacea* group fell ill, but 3 subjects in the magnesium group and 4 subjects in the placebo group became ill. Pretreatment with *Echinacea purpurea* appeared to reduce the release of soluble IL-2 receptor before and after the race and to increase the exercise-induced rise in IL-6.

Numerous experiments have shown that *Echinacea purpurea* extracts exert significant immunomodulatory effects. Among the many pharmacological properties reported, macrophage activation has been demonstrated most convincingly. Phagocytotic indices and macrophage-derived cytokine concentrations have been shown to be *Echinacea* responsive in a variety of assays, and activation of polymorphonuclear leukocytes and NK cells has also been reasonably demonstrated (Barrett 2003). Changes in the numbers and activities of T-cell and B-cell leukocytes have been reported but are less certain. Despite this cellular evidence of immunostimulation, pathways leading to enhanced resistance to infectious disease have not been adequately described. Several dozen human experiments, including a number of blind, randomized trials, report health benefits. The most robust data come from trials testing *Echinacea purpurea* extracts in the treatment of acute URTI. Although suggesting a modest benefit, these trials are limited both in size and in methodological quality. In a randomized, double-blind, placebo-controlled trial, administering unrefined *Echinacea* at the onset of

symptoms of URTI in 148 college students did not provide any detectable benefit or harm compared with placebo (Barrett et al. 2002).

In a meta-analysis of trials on *Echinacea* (Linde et al. 2006) that included 19 well-controlled trials, 3 trials investigated prevention of colds and 16 trials tested treatment of colds. A variety of *Echinacea* preparations were used. None of the 3 comparisons in the prevention trials showed an effect of *Echinacea* over placebo. In comparing an *Echinacea* preparation with placebo as a treatment for colds, a significant beneficial effect was reported in 9 comparisons, a trend in 1, and no difference in 6. The authors' main conclusions were that *Echinacea* preparations tested in clinical trials differ greatly but that preparations based on the aerial parts of *Echinacea purpurea* might be effective for the early treatment of colds in adults, although results are not fully consistent. Beneficial effects in preventing colds have not been shown in independently replicated, rigorous, randomized trials. Hence, although a great deal of moderately good-quality scientific data regarding *Echinacea* has been gathered, its effectiveness in treating illness or in enhancing human health has not yet been proved beyond a reasonable doubt. Even so, preparations of *Echinacea* are widely used in some European countries and in North America for common colds. Most consumers and physicians, however, are probably not aware that products available under the term *Echinacea* differ appreciably in their composition, mainly because of the use of variable plant material, extraction methods, and addition of other components.

Probiotics Probiotics are food supplements that contain "friendly" gut bacteria. Regular consumption of probiotics (i.e., strains that are proved to survive gut transit) modifies the intestinal microbiota such that the number of beneficial bacteria increases and the number of species considered harmful usually decreases. This circumstance has been associated with a range of potential benefits to the health and functioning of the digestive system, as well as modulation of immune function. Probiotics have many mechanisms of action. By their growth and metabolism, they help inhibit the growth and reduce any harmful effects of other bacteria, antigens, toxins, and carcinogens in the gut. In addition, probiotics are known to interact with the gut-associated lymphoid tissue, leading to positive effects on the innate and even the acquired immune system. This result is possible because the gut, as the largest surface area of the body, has a significant role to play in immunity because every day it must deal with three different immune challenges. First, it must differentiate and tolerate the large commensal microbiota; otherwise, inflammation will occur. Second, it must tolerate the food antigens. Third, the gut must be able to mount a defense against any potential pathogens when required. The need to perform these functions explains why 85% of the body's lymph nodes are located in the gut and why probiotics, as functional foods that target the gut, are able to affect the health of the whole body and parts of the body outside the gut.

Studies have shown that probiotic intake can improve rates of recovery from rotavirus diarrhea, increase resistance to enteric pathogens, and promote antitumor activity. Some evidence even suggests that probiotics may be effective in alleviating some allergic and respiratory disorders in young children (Kopp-Hoolihan 2001). Although to date there are few published studies of the effectiveness of probiotic use in athletes, interest is beginning to grow, mostly in examining their potential in maintaining overall general health, enhancing immune function, or reducing exercise-induced immunodepression.

In a double-blind, placebo-controlled, crossover trial in which healthy elite distance runners received the probiotic *Lactobacillus (L.) fermentum* or placebo daily for 28 days with a 28-day washout period between the initial treatment and the second treatment, athletes who took a daily probiotic (*n* = 20) suffered fewer days of respiratory illness and lower severity of respiratory illness symptoms (Cox et al. 2008). A significant change also occurred in the whole-blood culture IFN-γ production; the probiotic treatment elicited a twofold greater change in whole-blood culture IFN-γ production compared with placebo, which may be one mechanism underpinning the positive clinical outcomes. It has also been reported that athletes presenting with fatigue and impaired performance and who had clinical characteristics consistent with reactivation of Epstein-Barr viral infection exhibited significantly less secretion of IFN-γ from blood CD4+ (T-helper) cells than healthy control athletes did (Clancy et al. 2006). This apparent T-cell defect in fatigued athletes was reversed following a 1-month course of daily probiotic *(L. acidophilus)* ingestion. Another small study found that consumption of a *L. casei* probiotic yogurt drink for 1 month limited the observed decrease in natural killer cell activity after an exercise stress test (Pujol et al. 2000).

Another probiotic supplement was investigated in 141 marathon runners who were recruited for a randomized, double-blind intervention study in which they received *L. rhamnosus* GG (LGG) or placebo daily for a 3-month training period and then participated in a marathon race with a 2-week follow-up of illness symptoms (Kekkonen et al. 2007). Although no differences were found in the number of respiratory infections or gastrointestinal (GI)-symptom episodes, the duration of GI-symptom episodes in the LGG group was shorter than in the placebo group during the training period (2.9 versus 4.3 days) and during the 2 weeks after the marathon (1.0 versus 2.3 days). In a study on the effect of a *L. casei* probiotic supplement on respiratory tract infection and immune and hormonal changes in soldiers participating in 3 weeks of commando training followed by a 5-day combat course, no difference in infection incidence between groups receiving daily probiotic or placebo was reported (Tiollier et al. 2007). Among the immune parameters investigated, the major finding was a significant decrease in salivary immunoglobulin A (IgA) concentration after the combat course in the placebo group. No change occurred over time in the probiotic group. Others have also reported increased levels of salivary IgA and increased numbers of circulating CD4+ cells and an increased CD4+:CD8+ (T-helper:T-suppressor) ratio after a few weeks of consuming a probiotic *L. casei* fermented milk drink.

Probiotics have also been shown to help reduce stress-induced changes in the gut, such as may be experienced by sportspeople. Stress can negatively affect both the gut flora and gut permeability, which might lead to an increase in levels of systemic blood endotoxin (the lipopolysaccharide component of the Gram-negative bacterial cell wall). This result seemed to be the case in a study of seven mountaineers on an expedition to the Himalayas in Nepal, who were found to have gut-related changes that could have health consequences (Kleessen et al. 2005). Their gut flora had lower levels of bifidobacteria and other species, and higher levels of potential pathogens including species of Enterobacteriaceae such as *E. coli,* and there was evidence of endotoxemia. This might all contribute to the higher risk of GI disorders and infection that mountaineers experience, which is likely due to a combination of altitude and exercise-induced stress. From the research reviewed here, we cannot reach a solid conclusion of probiotic benefit for sportspeople, but we have sufficient understanding of the mechanism of action of certain probiotic strains and enough evidence from trials with athletes and sportspeople to recognize that this area of research is promising.

Colostrum Bovine colostrum is the first collection of a thick creamy yellow liquid produced by the mammary gland of a lactating cow shortly after birth of her calf, usually within the first 36 hours. Colostrum contains antibodies, growth factors, enzymes, gangliosides (acid glycosphingolipids), vitamins, and minerals and is commercially available in both liquid and powder forms. Numerous health claims have been made for colostrum, ranging from performance enhancement to preventing infections, but well-controlled studies in athletes are rare. The gangliosides in colostrum may modify the gut microbial flora and act as decoy targets for bacterial adhesion as well as have some direct immunostimulatory properties (Rueda 2007). A few studies suggest that several weeks of bovine colostrum supplementation can elevate levels of antibodies in the circulation and saliva. Secretory IgA in saliva (s-IgA) is a potential mucosal immune correlate of upper respiratory tract infection (URTI) status. Thus, nutritional supplements that improve mucosal immunity could be beneficial to athletes who are at increased risk of URTI. In a study of 35 middle-aged distance runners who consumed a supplement of either bovine colostrum or placebo for 12 weeks, median levels of s-IgA increased by 79% in the colostrum group after the 12-week intervention whereas no change occurred in the placebo group (Crooks et al. 2006). Although this result was statistically significant, its physiological interpretation must be viewed with caution because of the small numbers in the study and the large variability in s-IgA levels. Further studies are needed to confirm this effect on s-IgA and to establish whether bovine colostrum can reduce the incidence of upper respiratory tract infection in athletes.

β-Glucans β-glucans are present not only as major structural components of the cell walls of yeast, fungi, and some bacteria but also, in the diet, as part of the endosperm cell wall in cereals such as barley and oats. β-glucans are carbohydrates consisting of linked glucose molecules and differ in macromolecular structure depending on the source. β-glucans from bacteria are unbranched 1,3 β-linked glycopyranosyl residues. The cell wall β-glucans of yeast and fungi consists of 1,3 β-linked glycopyranosyl residues with small numbers of 1,6 β-linked branches, whereas oat and barley cell walls contain unbranched β-glucans with 1,3 and 1,4 β-linked glycopyranosyl residues. The specific characteristics of the various β-glucans may influence their immune-modulating effects. For example, Brown and Gordon (2003) have suggested that high-molecular-weight or particulate β-glucans from fungi directly activate leukocytes, whereas low-molecular-weight β-glucans from fungi modulate the response of cells only when they are stimulated (e.g., with cytokines). This implies that the addition of β-glucans to the diet may be used to modulate immune function and so might improve the resistance against invading pathogens in humans.

To date, the evidence for immune-promoting effects of orally administered oat β-glucans in animals and humans is limited. Intragastric administration of oat β-glucans in mice enhanced resistance to bacterial and parasitic infections (reviewed by Volman et al. 2008). Furthermore, Davis et al. (2004) demonstrated that daily ingestion of oat β-glucan counteracted the decrease in macrophage antiviral resistance induced by exercise stress in mice. Results both from in vitro studies from animals treated with β-glucans suggest that β-glucans enhance the immune response in leukocytes and epithelial cells. In the in vivo situation substantial evidence now indicates that these effects ultimately translate into enhanced survival after infection with pathogens (Volman et al. 2008). In this respect, effects are observed irrespective of the β-glucan source or route of administration. It has been suggested that the protective effects of orally administered 1,3 β-glucans are mediated through receptor-mediated interactions with Microfold cells—specialized epithelial cells for the transport of macromolecules in the Peyer's patches—which lead to increased cytokine production and enhanced resistance to infection. Therefore, it might be possible to modulate immune function by increasing the dietary β-glucan intake, perhaps by developing functional foods. This approach may have benefits for specific target populations such as the elderly or type 2 diabetes patients as well as for athletes who are involved in heavy training because all these populations are characterized by a suppressed (Th1) immune response. Further clinical trials are needed in humans to evaluate this possibility.

Other Supplements Studies in exercising rodents have suggested possible beneficial effects of some other supplements including curcumin and quercitin, and a few recent studies have appeared in the literature about the effectiveness of these compounds in humans. Quercitin, a type of flavonoid polyphenol, did not alter exercise-induced changes in immune function in cyclists, but it significantly reduced URTI incidence in the 2 weeks following a short intense training period (Nieman et al. 2007). Curcumin (diferuloylmethane) is an orange yellow component of turmeric, a spice often found in curry powder. Traditionally known for its anti-inflammatory effects, curcumin has been shown to be a potent immunomodulatory agent that can modulate the activation of T-cells, B-cells, NK cells, neutrophils, macrophages, and dendritic cells (Jagetia and Aggarwal 2007). Curcumin can also downregulate the expression of various pro-inflammatory cytokines including TNF, IL-1, and IL-2, most likely through inactivation of the transcription factor NF-kappaB. At low doses, however, curcumin can also enhance antibody responses (Jagetia and Aggarwal 2007).

Conclusions and Recommendations

Both heavy exercise and nutrition exert separate influences on immune function; these influences appear to be greater when exercise stress and poor nutrition act synergistically. Exercise training increases the body's requirement for most nutrients, and in many cases, these increased needs are countered by increased food consumption. But some athletes adopt an unbalanced dietary regimen, and many surveys indicate that few athletes follow the best dietary pattern for optimal sport nutrition. Despite an abundance of studies investigating the effects of nutrition on immune function and the effects of nutrition on physical performance, relatively few have investigated the interrelationships between nutrition, performance, and immune function concurrently. Therefore, some of the conclusions drawn in this chapter remain speculative, relying on generalizations between sedentary and athletic populations. The poor nutritional status of some athletes, however, likely predisposes them to immunodepression. Although countering the effects of all of the factors that contribute to exercise-induced immunodepression is impossible, minimizing many of the effects is possible. Athletes can help themselves by eating

---

Practical Strategies to Minimize Risks of Infection

- Allow sufficient time between training sessions for recovery. Include 1 or 2 days of resting recovery in the weekly training program; more training is not always better.
- Avoid extremely long training sessions. Restrict continuous activity to less than 2 hours per session. For example, a 3-hour session might be better performed as two 1.5-hour sessions, one in the morning and one in the evening.
- Avoid training monotony by ensuring variation in the day-to-day training load. Follow a hard training day with a light training day.
- When increasing the training load, do so on the hard days. Do not eliminate recovery days.
- When recovering from overtraining or illness, begin with very light training and build gradually.
- Monitor and record mood, feelings of fatigue, and muscle soreness during training; decrease the training load if the normal session feels harder than usual.
- Keep other life, social, and psychological stresses to a minimum.
- Get regular and adequate sleep (at least 6 hours per night).
- Maintain good oral hygiene by brushing teeth regularly and consider using an antiseptic mouthwash. Wash hands regularly and do not use towels that other people have used.
- Increase rest as needed after travel across time zones to allow circadian rhythms to adjust.
- Eat a well-balanced diet to obtain all the necessary vitamins and minerals, but if dieting to lose weight or if fresh fruit and vegetables are not readily available, consider multivitamin supplements.
- Ensure adequate total dietary energy, carbohydrate, and protein intake. Be aware that periods of carbohydrate depletion are associated with immunodepression.
- Drink carbohydrate sports drinks before, during, and after prolonged workouts to reduce some of the adverse effects of exercise on immune function.
- Consider discussing vaccination with your coach or doctor. Influenza vaccines require 5 to 7 weeks to take effect. Intramuscular vaccines may have a few small side effects, so receiving vaccinations out of season is best. Do not get a vaccination before a competition or if symptoms of illness are present.

well-balanced diets that include adequate carbohydrate, protein, and micronutrients.

Consumption of carbohydrate drinks during training and competition is recommended because this practice appears to attenuate some of the immunosuppressive effects of prolonged exercise. *Echinacea* supplements may provide some boost to immune function, but more studies are needed to confirm that taking this supplement can reduce the number of training days lost to infection.

The dangers of oversupplementation of vitamins and minerals should be emphasized because many micronutrients given in quantities beyond a certain threshold reduce immune responses. Other factors that may lower infection risk in athletes include reducing other life stresses, maintaining good oral and skin hygiene, obtaining adequate rest, and spacing prolonged training sessions and competitions as far apart as possible. The practices listed in the highlight box are recommended.

KEY POINTS

- The immune system protects the body against potentially damaging microorganisms.

- Athletes engaged in heavy endurance training programs often have depressed immune function and suffer from an increased incidence of URTIs. Training and competitive surroundings may increase the athlete's exposure to pathogens and provide optimal conditions for pathogen transmission.

- Heavy, prolonged exertion is associated with numerous hormonal and biochemical changes, many of which potentially have detrimental effects on immune function. Improper nutrition can compound the negative influence of heavy exertion on immunocompetence.

- An athlete who exercises in a carbohydrate-depleted state experiences larger increases in circulating stress hormones and a greater perturbation of several immune-function indices.

- Consuming carbohydrate (but not glutamine) during exercise attenuates rises in stress hormones such as cortisol and appears to limit the degree of exercise-induced immunodepression.

- The poor nutritional status of some athletes may predispose them to immunodepression. For example, dietary deficiencies of protein and specific micronutrients are associated with immune dysfunction.

- An adequate intake of iron, zinc, and B vitamins is particularly important, but the dangers of oversupplementation should also be considered. Many micronutrients given in quantities beyond a certain threshold reduce immune responses and may have other toxic effects.

- Sustained endurance training appears to be associated with an adaptive upregulation of the antioxidant defense system. But such adaptations may be insufficient to protect athletes who train extensively, and these individuals should consider increasing their intake of nutritional antioxidants.

- In general, supplementation of individual micronutrients or consumption of large doses of simple antioxidant mixtures is not recommended. Athletes should obtain complex mixtures of antioxidant compounds from consumption of fruits and vegetables. Consuming megadoses of individual vitamins is likely to do more harm than good.

- Although countering the effects of all the factors that contribute to exercise-induced immunodepression is impossible, minimizing many of the effects is possible. Athletes can help themselves by eating a well-balanced diet that includes sufficient protein and carbohydrate to meet their energy requirements. Such a diet ensures an adequate intake of trace elements without the need for special supplements.

- By adopting sound nutritional practice, reducing life stresses, maintaining good hygiene, obtaining adequate rest, and spacing prolonged training sessions and competitions as far apart as possible, athletes can reduce their risk of infection.

RECOMMENDED READINGS

Calder P.C., C.J. Field, and H.S. Gill. 2002. *Nutrition and immune function.* Oxford: CABI.

Chandra, R.K. 1997. Nutrition and the immune system: An introduction. *American Journal of Clinical Nutrition* 66:460S–463S.

Douglas R.M., H. Hemila, E. Chalker, and B. Treacy. 2007. Vitamin C for preventing and treating the common cold. *Cochrane Database of Systematic Reviews,* Issue 3: CD000980.

Gleeson M., ed. 2005. *Immune function in sport and exercise.* Edinburgh: Elsevier.

Gleeson, M., and N.C. Bishop. 2000. Elite athlete immunology: The importance of nutrition. *International Journal of Sports Medicine* 21 (supplement 1): S44–S50.

Gleeson M., G.I. Lancaster, and N.C. Bishop. 2001. Nutritional strategies to minimise exercise-induced immunosuppression in athletes. *Canadian Journal of Applied Physiology* 26 (supplement): 635–647.

Konig, D., A. Berg, C. Weinstock, J. Keul, and H. Northoff. 1997. Essential fatty acids, immune function and exercise. *Exercise and Immunology Review* 3:1–31.

Nieman, D.C., and B.K. Pedersen, eds. 2000. *Nutrition and exercise immunology.* Boca Raton, FL: CRC Press.

Pedersen B.K., K. Ostrowski, T. Rohde, and H. Bruunsgaard. 1998. Nutrition, exercise and the immune system. *Proceedings of the Nutrition Society* 57:43–47.

Peters, E.M. 1997. Exercise, immunology and upper respiratory tract infections. *International Journal of Sports Medicine* 18 (1 supplement): S69–S77.

Scrimshaw, N.S., and J.P. SanGiovanni. 1997. Synergism of nutrition, infection and immunity: An overview. *American Journal of Clinical Nutrition* 66:464S–477S.

Key Concepts in Biological Chemistry Relevant to Sport Nutrition

The study of sport nutrition requires an understanding of some simple biochemistry and physiology. The major components that make up the body and the diet—carbohydrates, lipids, proteins, and nucleic acids—are themselves composed of smaller building blocks. This appendix contains a short review of important chemical concepts, interactions, and processes involving biomolecules, together with a brief summary of membrane transport mechanisms, enzyme actions, the structure and function of the various cellular organelles, and the characteristics of the four major tissue types found in the human body. This appendix can be used as a reference, but an understanding of what is covered is essential to most of the principles and mechanisms discussed elsewhere in this book. This appendix may be particularly useful for those who have little background in biology and chemistry. We begin with the smallest unit that any substance can be broken down to: the atom.

Matter, Energy, Atoms, and Molecules

The human body consists only of matter and energy in their various forms. Indeed, the same can be said of the entire universe. Matter occupies space and has a mass that represents the quantity of matter that is present. We often equate mass with weight, which is the force that gravity exerts on the mass, but technically the two are different. The quantity or mass of an object does not change, regardless of its location, but its weight will vary according to the pull of gravity. For example, a rock weighing 6 kg (13.2 lb) on Earth weighs only about 1 kg (2.2 lb) on the surface of the Moon because the gravitational force of the Moon is only about one-sixth of that of Earth. Of course, matter itself remains matter whether on Earth or on the Moon.

Many thousands of types of matter exist, and all can be reduced into smaller units. The smallest units into which a substance can be broken down chemically are the elements, each of which has different and unique properties. At least 94 elements are presently known to exist, but only about 12 are common in living organisms. The most abundant elements are oxygen, carbon, hydrogen, and nitrogen (in that order). These 4 elements compose 96% of the mass of a human.

Energy is the capacity of any system, including the living body, to do work (i.e., to produce a change of some sort in matter). Energy can exist in several forms, including light, heat, electrical, mechanical, and chemical energy. Energy can be transformed from one form to another. In the body, the potential chemical energy stored in foodstuffs is transformed to do various forms of work such as movement or the synthesis of large molecules from small molecules. Matter and energy are interrelated by Einstein's famous equation:

$$E = mc^2$$

where E is energy, m is mass, and c is the speed of light (about 299,792 km/s). Nothing is capable of moving faster than light. Einstein's equation can, in principle, go in either direction. Thus, energy can be transformed into matter, and matter can be transformed into energy.

Atoms are the smallest unit of an element that retains all the properties of the element. The atoms of all elements can be broken down physically into the same subatomic particles: protons, neutrons, and electrons. Hence, the atoms of the various elements differ only in the numbers of protons, neutrons, and electrons that they contain. Protons, which possess a positive charge, and neutrons, which are electrically neutral, are held together to form the nucleus of an atom. Electrons, which have negligible mass (only about 1/8,000 of that of a proton or a neutron) and possess a negative charge, spin around the atomic nucleus in discrete orbitals that may be spherical or dumbbell shaped. Some electrons move in orbitals close to the nucleus; others move in orbitals farther away. Electrons that are farther from the nucleus have more energy than those close to the nucleus; thus, the orbitals can be thought of as energy levels. Electrons normally stay at their particular energy level, but by gaining or losing energy, they jump from one energy level to another. Although electron orbitals can vary in shape, electrons at each energy level are usually depicted diagrammatically as moving in concentric and circular orbits, or shells, around the nucleus. A maximum of 2 electrons can be held in the innermost shell. The second and third shells can each hold up to 8 electrons. The fourth shell can hold up to 18 electrons.

The number of electrons is equal to the number of protons in the nucleus, resulting in an electrically neutral atom. The smallest atom is that of hydrogen, which is composed of just one proton and one electron (see figure A.1a). The carbon atom consists of six protons, six neutrons, and six electrons, whereas an oxygen atom is made up of eight protons, eight neutrons, and eight electrons. Both oxygen and carbon have two electrons in their inner shells, but they differ in the number of electrons in the second shell. Oxygen has six electrons in the second shell, and carbon has four (see figures A.1, b and c).

The chemical properties of an element and the way that it reacts with other elements depend on the number of electrons in its outer shell. If this shell is full, the element does not react with others and is said to be inert. Helium, with 2 electrons in its outer shell, and neon, with 18 electrons in its outer shell, are examples of inert elements. Atoms whose outer shells are not full tend to move toward a more stable configuration by losing or gaining electrons or sharing electrons with other atoms. The atoms are bound together by attractive forces called chemical bonds. These bonds are a source of potential chemical energy. Breaking chemical bonds releases some energy that can be used to do work.

Nearly all the mass of an atom is in its protons and neutrons, so the combined number of these particles is the atomic mass of the element. The mass of an element is indicated by a superscript in front of the element (e.g., ^1H, ^{12}C, ^{16}O). The number of protons in an atom is its atomic number, which is indicated as a subscript in front of the symbol for the atom (e.g. ^1_1H, $^{12}_6C$, $^{16}_8O$).

All atoms of a given element contain the same number of protons and electrons (which determines the chemical properties of the element), but in some elements the number of neutrons in the nucleus and, hence, the atomic mass (but not the atomic number) varies. Atoms of an element that have a different number of neutrons are called isotopes. Some isotopes are unstable and emit radiation in the form of gamma rays, electrons, or a helium nucleus (two protons and two neutrons). This radiation can be measured, and some unstable isotopes have proved useful as tracers. For example, normal carbon has an atomic mass of 12, but the radioactive isotope of carbon has a mass of 14. Glucose, a simple sugar, can be prepared using $^{14}_6C$, and its metabolism in the body can be followed by identifying the presence of $^{14}_6C$ in intermediate compounds and in expired carbon dioxide. Nowadays, the presence and quantity of stable isotopes (those that do not decay by the emission of radiation) such as $^{13}_6C$ can be detected, and these isotopes are increasingly used in place of the more dangerous radioactive isotopes in human metabolic studies.

Most elements in the body are not present as free atoms but are combined with other atoms to form molecules. For example, a molecule of water contains 1 atom of oxygen bound to 2 atoms of hydrogen, symbolized as H_2O (see figure A.2). Even the oxygen in the air that we breathe is made of molecular oxygen consisting of 2 atoms of oxygen bound together, symbolized as O_2. A molecule of glucose, a simple hexose sugar, contains 24 atoms: 6 of carbon, 12 of hydrogen, and 6 of oxygen. This formula can be expressed as $C_6H_{12}O_6$, which is known as the empirical chemical formula of glucose. The molecular mass is obtained by adding the atomic masses present in the molecule. Thus, for glucose, we have

$$6 \times {}^{12}C + 12 \times {}^1H + 6 \times {}^{16}O$$
$$= 72 + 12 + 96 = 180.$$

The molecular mass of a substance in grams is equal to 1 mole of that substance, and the number of molecules in

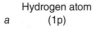
○ Proton
○ Neutron
○ Electron

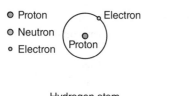

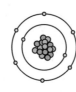

Electron

Proton

| Hydrogen atom | Carbon atom | Oxygen atom |
| a (1p) | b (6p, 6n) | c (8p, 8n) |

Figure A.1 Atoms of (a) hydrogen, (b) carbon, and (c) oxygen.

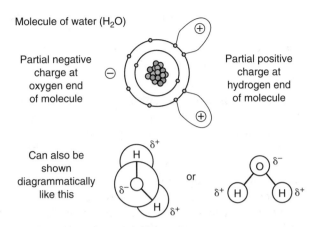

Molecule of water (H₂O)

Partial negative charge at oxygen end of molecule

Partial positive charge at hydrogen end of molecule

Can also be shown diagrammatically like this

Figure A.2 A molecule of water indicating the distribution of partial charges.

a mole of any substance is the same and known as Avogadro's number, which is 6.022×10^{23}.

One mole of a substance dissolved in enough water to make 1 liter is known as a 1-molar (1.0 M) solution. Biochemists usually deal with smaller concentrations such as millimoles per liter (1 mM = 1×10^{-3} M) because many substances that are dissolved in the body fluids are found in this concentration range. For example, the concentration of glucose in blood is about 5 mM.

Chemical Bonds, Free Energy, and ATP

This section provides a brief review of chemical bonds, emphasizing bonds between the six major elements found in the living body: hydrogen (H), carbon (C), nitrogen (N), oxygen (O), phosphorus (P), and sulfur (S).

■ Covalent bonds hold together two or more atoms by the interaction of their outer electrons. Covalent bonds are the strongest chemical bonds. The energy of a typical covalent bond is approximately 330 kilojoules per mole (330 kJ/mol [79 kcal/mol]), but this energy can vary from 210 kJ/mol to 460 kJ/mol (50 kcal/mol to 110 kcal/mol), depending on the elements involved. Once formed, covalent bonds rarely break spontaneously because the thermal energy of a molecule at room temperature (20 °C or 293 °K [68 °F]) is only about 2.5 kJ/mol (0.6 kcal/mol), much lower than the energy required to

break a covalent bond. Covalent bonds are either single, double, or triple bonds (see table A.1).

■ Carbon–carbon bonds are particularly strong and stable covalent bonds. The major organic elements have standard bonding capabilities: C, N, and P can form up to four covalent bonds with other atoms, O and S can form two covalent bonds, and H can form only one covalent bond. In solution, O and S can lose a proton (or hydrogen ion, H⁺), leaving the O or S with a negative charge (see figure A.3). Covalent bonds have partial charges when the atoms involved have different electronegativities. Water is one example of a molecule with partial charges. The symbols delta+ (δ+) and delta– (δ–) are used to indicate partial charges (see figure A.2). Oxygen, because of its high electronegativity, attracts the electrons away from the hydrogen atoms, resulting in a partial negative charge on the oxygen and a partial positive charge on each of the

TABLE A.1

Single, Double, and Triple Covalent Bonds

Bond number	Example	Energy (kJ/mol [kcal/mol])
Single	H—C—H (with H above and below C)	330 (79)
Double	H—C=C—H (with H above and below each C)	630 (150)
Triple	H—C≡C—H	840 (200)

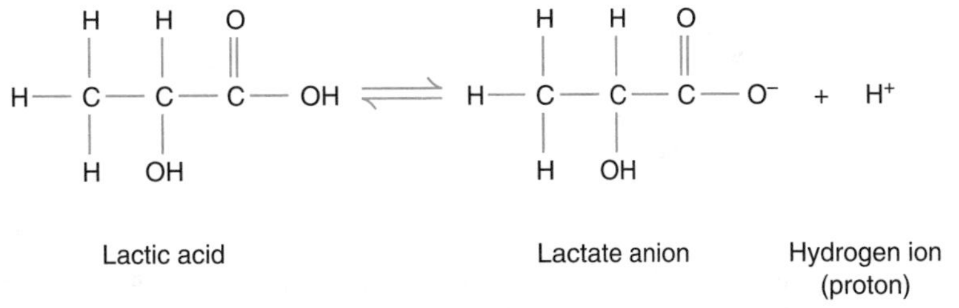

Lactic acid ⇌ Lactate anion + Hydrogen ion (proton)

Figure A.3 Dissociation of a proton (H⁺ ion) from lactic acid, leaving an oxygen (O) with a negative charge.

hydrogens. The possibility of hydrogen bonds is a consequence of these partial charges.

■ Hydrogen bonds (H-bonds) are weak intramolecular or intermolecular attractions between a hydrogen atom and an electronegative atom possessing a lone pair of electrons (e.g., oxygen or nitrogen atoms). Hydrogen bonds are formed when a hydrogen atom is shared between two molecules (see figure A.4). Hydrogen bonds have polarity. A hydrogen atom covalently attached to a very electronegative atom (N, O, or P) shares its partial positive charge with a second electronegative atom (N, O, or P). Hydrogen bonds are 21 kJ/mol (5 kcal/mol) in strength. These bonds are frequently found in proteins and nucleic acids, and by reinforcing each other they keep the protein (or nucleic acid) structure secure. But because the hydrogen atoms in the protein can also form H-bonds with the surrounding water, the relative strength of protein-protein H-bonds versus protein-H_2O bonds is smaller than 21 kJ/mol.

■ Ionic bonds are formed when a complete transfer of electrons from one atom to another occurs. The valence (outer shell) electrons are either lost or gained, resulting in two ions, one positively charged and the other negatively charged. The ions, which are oppositely charged, are held together by electrostatic forces. For example, when a sodium atom (Na) donates the one electron in its outer valence shell to a chlorine atom (Cl), which needs one electron to fill its outer valence shell, NaCl (salt) results. The symbol for sodium chloride is Na^+Cl^-. Ionic bonds are 17 to 30 kJ/mol (4 to 7 kcal/mol) in strength.

■ Nonpolar molecules cannot form H-bonds with water and are therefore poorly soluble in water. These molecules are called hydrophobic (water-hating) molecules, as opposed to hydrophilic (water-loving) molecules, which can form H-bonds with water. Hydrophobic molecules tend to aggregate together in avoidance of water molecules, such as when a drop of oil is placed on water. The oil forms a thin layer over the surface of the water. If mixed together vigorously, the oil forms small globules but does not dissolve in the water. To understand the energetics driving this interaction, visualize the water molecules surrounding a single "dissolved" molecule attempting to form the greatest number of H-bonds with each other. The best energetic solution involves forcing all the nonpolar molecules together, thus reducing the total surface area that breaks up the H-bond matrix of the water.

During biochemical reactions that involve the breaking of chemical bonds, energy is released, some of which is available to do work. Some energy is also released as heat, which cannot be used to do work in the body because body temperature is regulated within a narrow range. The free energy

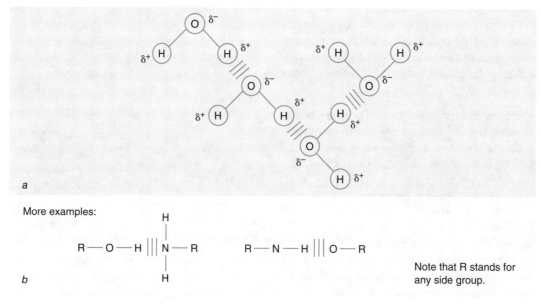

More examples:

Note that R stands for any side group.

Figure A.4 *(a)* Hydrogen bonding between water molecules. A hydrogen atom covalently attached to a very electronegative atom (N, O, or P) shares its partial positive charge with a second electronegative atom (N, O, or P). *(b)* More examples of hydrogen bonding.

released during the breaking of bonds, usually signified by the symbol G, can be used to do work because some of it is stored in the compound adenosine triphosphate (ATP). The free energy released when an inorganic phosphate group (Pi) is broken off ATP to form adenosine diphosphate (ADP) is used to drive several energy-requiring processes in the body, including the synthesis of macromolecules from smaller molecules (e.g., synthesis of proteins from free amino acids), membrane transport work (e.g., the movement of sodium ions out of a cell against the prevailing concentration gradient), and mechanical work (e.g., muscle contraction). Reactions involving the breaking of phosphate bonds and the liberation of Pi are catalyzed by enzymes called kinases. In the case of ATP breakdown, these kinases are commonly abbreviated as ATPases.

ATP is the only form of chemical energy that is convertible into other forms of energy used by living cells. Essentially, ATP is the energy currency of the cell. Fats and carbohydrates are the main storage forms of energy in the body, and when they are broken down by oxidation reactions to carbon dioxide and water, the energy released is used to resynthesize ATP from ADP and Pi.

All biochemical reactions are inefficient, which means that not all the energy released can be conserved or used to do work. Some energy is always lost as heat. This release of heat helps maintain body temperature at about 37 °C (98.6 °F). During exercise, when the rate of catabolic reactions is markedly increased in the active muscles to provide energy for contraction, the rate of heat production also increases substantially and muscle temperature rises by 1 °C to 5 °C (1.8 °F to 9 °F).

Although ATP is considered the energy currency of the cell, it cannot be accumulated in large amounts, and the intramuscular ATP concentration is only about 5 mmol/kg of muscle tissue. During maximal exercise, ATP is sufficient to fuel about 2 seconds of muscle force generation. Experiments have shown that the muscle ATP store never becomes completely depleted, because it is efficiently resynthesized from ADP and Pi at the same rate at which it is degraded. During submaximal steady-state exercise, ATP resynthesis is achieved by mitochondrial oxidation of carbohydrates and lipids. This process is commonly referred to as aerobic metabolism because it requires oxygen. At the onset of exercise and in high-intensity exercise, however, ATP resynthesis is principally anaerobic (without the use of oxygen). Further details of

the metabolic pathways involved can be found in chapter 2.

Chemical Reactions in the Body

A variety of different types of chemical reactions take place in the body. These reactions are defined in the following section and are accompanied by a few illustrative examples.

- Oxidation is a reaction involving the loss of electrons from an atom. It is always accompanied by a reduction (a reaction in which a molecule gains electrons). For example, pyruvate is reduced using hydrogen donated from the reduced form of the coenzyme nicotinamide adenine dinucleotide (NADH) to form lactate. In the reverse reaction, lactate is oxidized by NAD^+ (the oxidized form of the coenzyme) when pyruvate is reformed. This reaction is also known as dehydrogenation because it is a form of oxidation that involves the loss of hydrogen atoms:

$$\text{Pyruvate CH}_3\text{-CO-COOH} + \text{NADH} + \text{H}^+$$
$$\leftrightarrow \text{Lactate CH}_3\text{-CHOH-COOH} + \text{NAD}^+$$

- Hydrolysis is a reaction in which an organic compound is split by interaction with water into simpler compounds. An example is the hydrolysis of phosphocreatine (PCr) to creatine (Cr) and phosphate, which is coupled to the resynthesis of ATP from ADP using the phosphate group liberated from phosphocreatine:

$$\text{PCr} + \text{H}_2\text{O} \rightarrow \text{Cr} + \text{P}$$
$$\text{P} + \text{ADP} + \text{H}^+ \rightarrow \text{ATP} + \text{H}_2\text{O}$$

- Phosphorylation is the addition of a phosphate (PO_3^{2-}) group to a molecule. Many enzymes are activated by the covalent bonding of a phosphate group. The phosphorylation of ADP forms ATP:

$$\text{ADP} + \text{Pi} \rightarrow \text{ATP} + \text{H}_2\text{O}$$

- Condensation is the union of two or more molecules with the elimination of a simpler group such as H_2O. An example is the joining of two amino acid molecules to form a dipeptide.

- Hydroxylation is the addition of a hydroxyl (OH) group to a molecule.

- Carboxylation is the addition of CO_2, catalyzed by an enzyme using biotin as its prosthetic group.

- Deamination is the loss of an amino (NH_2) group, liberating free ammonia (NH_3). This is important in the metabolism of amino acids such as alanine:

Alanine → Pyruvate + NH_3

■ Transamination is the transfer of an amino (NH_2) group from an amino acid to a keto-acid. An example is the transfer of an amino group from the amino acid glutamate to the keto-acid pyruvate, forming a new amino acid alanine and another keto-acid α-ketoglutarate:

Glutamate + Pyruvate → Alanine + α-ketoglutarate

■ Denaturation is the alteration of the physical properties and three-dimensional structure of a protein by a chemical or physical treatment that does not disrupt the primary structure but generally results in the inactivation of the protein (e.g., the inactivation of an enzyme by the addition of a strong acid or excessive heat).

Hydrogen Ion Concentrations and Buffers

Free hydrogen ions are produced in many chemical reactions in the body. Problems such as decreased activity or even complete inactivation of enzymes and inhibition of several biological processes, including muscle contraction, can arise when free hydrogen ions accumulate inside cells. Hence, the body has several mechanisms that help to limit changes in the free hydrogen ion concentration in the fluids inside and outside cells.

An acid is a compound able to donate a hydrogen ion (H^+); examples include hydrochloric acid (HCl), carbonic acid (H_2CO_3), and lactic acid (CH_3-CHOH-COOH). A base is a compound able to accept a hydrogen ion; examples are hydroxyl ions (OH^-) and bicarbonate ions (HCO_3^-). The pH is a measure of the concentration of hydrogen ions. These values are derived, for example, from the dissociation of an acid, such as HCl, when it is dissolved in water (HCl → H^+ + Cl^-). The pH value is defined as the negative decimal logarithm of the free H^+ concentration or [H^+]; that is, pH = $-\log_{10}$[H^+], where [H^+] is expressed in moles per liter (mol/L or M), so the concentration of free H^+ increases 10-fold for each decrease of 1 pH unit. The [H^+] in pure water is 10^{-7} mol/L. Therefore, the pH of pure water is

$$pH = -\log_{10} (10^{-7}) = - (-7) = 7$$

pH 7 is often referred to as neutral pH. Everything below pH 7 has a higher concentration of H^+ and is considered acidic. Everything above pH 7 has a lower concentration of H^+ and is considered basic (you can also think of this as a higher concentration of OH^-). Most body fluids are close to neutral pH. For example, blood plasma has a pH of 7.4, and resting muscle intracellular fluid (sarcoplasm) has a pH of 7.0. The pH of the body fluids is tightly regulated, and even in the most severe metabolic disturbances, such as high-intensity exercise, the pH of blood does not change by more than about 0.3. Even in the exercising muscle where the additional hydrogen ions are first appearing because of the increased lactic acid production, the pH does not fall below 6.5. As previously mentioned, this stability is important because if the pH falls too low, the activity of enzymes can be inhibited, which can have fatal consequences for the cell.

Buffers act as a reservoir for hydrogen ions and thus limit, or buffer, changes in free H^+ concentration. Buffering is passive and virtually instantaneous. A buffer consists of a weak acid and its conjugate base. In solution, some, but not all, molecules of the weak acid dissociate into the conjugate base and hydrogen ions:

$$BH \leftrightarrow B^- + H^+$$

where BH is the weak acid and B^- is its conjugate base. The relationship between the concentrations of weak acid, base, and hydrogen ions can be expressed as an equation:

$$K_a.[BH] = [H^+].[B^-]$$

where K_a is the dissociation constant of the acid, that is, the concentration of H^+ at which the concentrations of the base and acid are equal. The equation can be rearranged to give the Henderson equation:

$$[H^+] = K_a.[BH]/[B^-]$$

Alternatively, by taking the negative logarithm of each side of the equation, it becomes the Henderson-Hasselbalch equation:

$$-\log_{10}[H^+] = -\log_{10}K_a + \log_{10}[B^-]/[BH]$$

which is the same as

$$pH = pK_a + \log_{10}[B^-]/[BH]$$

which tells us that optimal buffering (minimum change in pH when H^+ ions are added) occurs at pH = pK_a and that this effect occurs when the concentrations of weak acid (BH) and base (B^-) are equal.

Carbonic acid/bicarbonate (H_2CO_3/HCO_3^-) is the most important extracellular buffer, with a pK_a of 6.1. Hemoglobin and other proteins and peptides containing the amino acid histidine (pK_a usually 6.0 to 8.0) and phosphates (HPO_4^{2-}/$H_2PO_4^-$), whose pK_a is 6.8, are important intracellular buffers.

Because the pH of most body fluids is about 7.4, buffers with a pK$_a$ of between 6 and 8 are the most effective.

In exercising muscle, large amounts of hydrogen ions are produced from the dissociation of lactic acid to H$^+$ and the lactate anion (see figure A.3). The resting intracellular pH of muscle is 7.0. A large fall in pH is undesirable because it would denature enzymes and is prevented by the presence of intracellular buffers, including carnosine (a dipeptide consisting of alanine and histidine), phosphocreatine, phosphates, and histidine-containing proteins. As the hydrogen ions diffuse out of the muscle into the blood, they are buffered by bicarbonate (in plasma) and hemoglobin (in the red blood cells). An increase in the blood lactic acid concentration of 10 mmol/L changes the blood pH by only about 0.1; this concentration of lactic acid dissolved in water alone causes the pH to drop from 7.0 to 2.0. Clearly, the body's buffer systems are very effective.

Enzymes

Enzymes act as controllable catalysts. These proteins speed up the rate of specific chemical reactions and allow them to be regulated in ways that permit the body to control the interactions between the different metabolic pathways. The direction in which the reactions proceed and the equilibrium point that is reached in a nonbiological system are governed by the laws of thermodynamics. The characteristics of enzymes that allow them to act as catalysts are briefly described.

Mechanisms of Enzyme Action and Enzyme Kinetics

The laws of thermodynamics tell us that chemical reactions proceed spontaneously only in the direction that results in the products of the reaction having a lower energy status than the substrates (see figure A.5). Enzymes act as reusable catalysts, which involves the formation of an enzyme substrate complex as an intermediate step in the reaction. The formation of this substrate lowers the energy of activation. Because less energy is now needed, the reaction is more likely to proceed. Although the enzyme participates in the reaction, it is not consumed and is therefore required only in small amounts.

The energetics of formation of the enzyme substrate complex are not well understood, but clearly some kind of weak bond forms between the

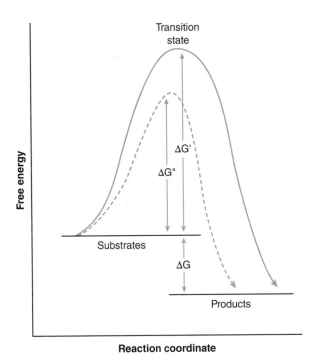

Figure A.5   Energy status of substrates and products.

substrate and the enzyme. This bond involves one or more active sites on the enzyme, and these sites have a particular shape and charge distribution that allows them to interact with the substrate. These characteristics allow enzymes to promote the rates of specific reaction in a number of ways. Where two or more substrates are involved, attachment to binding sites on the enzyme allows the substrates to be brought into close proximity in the correct orientation, thus increasing the chances that a reaction will take place. Alternatively, binding to the enzyme can cause changes in the shape of the substrate molecule that increase its susceptibility to reaction.

Enzyme Kinetics

Enzyme kinetics is the measurement of the change in substrate or product concentration as a function of time. The first stage in an enzyme-catalyzed reaction is the binding of the substrate (S) to the active site of the enzyme (E) to form an enzyme-substrate complex (ES). The substrate then reacts to form the product (P), which is released. Release of the product restores the enzyme to its original free form:

$$E + S \leftrightarrow ES \rightarrow E + P$$

The assumption is that the first stage of the process is reversible but the second is not. In almost all reactions, the substrate concentration is far in excess of the enzyme concentration. This difference means that formation of the ES complex does not result in an appreciable change in the substrate concentration but does reduce the concentration of the free enzyme.

The progress curve for the reaction is initially linear, decreasing in slope as the reaction proceeds and substrate is used up, as shown in figure A.6. The initial velocity during the linear part of the curve is called V_0. The relationship between V_0 and the substrate concentration ([S]) is described by the Michaelis-Menten equation:

$$V_0 = V_{max} [S] / K_m + [S]$$

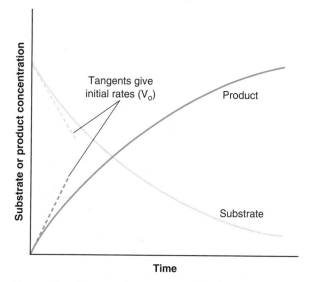

Figure A.6 Progress of an enzyme-catalyzed reaction.

where V_{max} is the maximum velocity of the reaction at infinite [S], and K_m is the Michaelis constant, equivalent to the substrate concentration in which the initial reaction velocity (V_0) is equal to one-half the maximal velocity (i.e., $K_m = [S]$ where $V_0 = V_{max}/2$). This relationship is depicted graphically in figure A.7 and clearly shows that at low concentrations of substrate, the initial reaction rate increases linearly in response to increasing substrate concentration, but the rate approaches a limit above which it is constant and independent of substrate concentration. At this point, all of the enzyme molecules are effectively saturated with substrate. The V_{max} is, therefore, a function of the amount of enzyme present.

When the substrate concentration is equal to K_m, the reaction rate is equal to half of the V_{max}. The K_m value is, therefore, equal to the substrate concentration that will result in the reaction proceeding at one-half of the maximum rate. A high

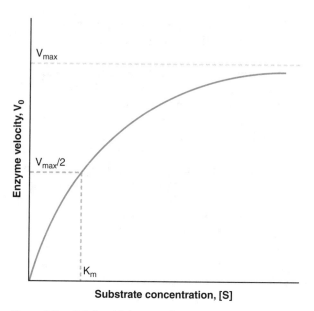

Figure A.7 Relationship between the initial reaction velocity and substrate concentration for an enzyme-catalyzed reaction.

K_m value is, therefore, an indication of low affinity of the enzyme for its substrate. A high substrate concentration is necessary to achieve a reaction rate equal to one-half the maximum rate. High reaction rates are only achieved when the substrate concentration is relatively high. If [S] is equal to 10 times the K_m, substituting these values into the Michaelis-Menten equation tells us that the reaction rate is 91% of V_{max}, and 99% of the maximum rate will be achieved only when the substrate concentration is 100 times the K_m.

Factors Influencing Enzyme Activity

The activity of enzymes can be assessed by the rate of substrate utilization or product formation under standardized conditions. The most common unit of measurement is the International Unit (IU or U). This measure is the amount of enzyme that converts 1 μmole of substrate to product in 1 minute under the conditions specified for that reaction. Although this measure is generally used among physiologists, the appropriate SI unit should be used. This unit is the katal (kat), which is the amount of enzyme that converts 1 mole of substrate to product in 1 second under optimum conditions. At least part of the reason for the persistence of the IU is the difficulty in defining optimum conditions for the activity of individual enzymes.

Effects of Temperature and pH Enzyme activity is particularly sensitive to temperature and increases as the temperature increases. Any expression of enzyme activities must therefore specify the temperature at which measurements are made. Temperatures of 25 °C and 37 °C (77 °F and 98.6 °F) are normally used as standards. At high temperatures, however, enzyme activity falls sharply and irreversibly because of structural changes caused by denaturation of the protein, as shown in figure A.8. Although body core temperature is usually about 37 °C (98.6 °F), the temperature of muscle tissue may be as low as 30 °C (86 °F) in a resting person on a cold day and can rise to 42 °C (108 °F) during high-intensity exercise. Hence, warming up before an event has important implications for maximizing reaction rates and optimizing muscle performance. Except in extreme cases of heat illness, body core temperature seldom exceeds 41 °C (106 °F), but this temperature is close to the level at which some enzymes and other proteins are affected.

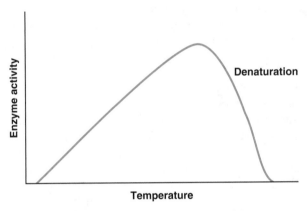

Figure A.8   Effect of temperature on enzyme activity.

Changes in the ionization state of an enzyme caused by a change in pH of the cell affects its affinity for its substrate because of changes in structure or charge distribution at the active site, as illustrated in figure A.9. The local pH may also affect the ionization state of the substrate. All enzymes have an optimum pH (where enzyme activity is at its highest, as shown in figure A.10), but optimum pH differs among different enzymes and may also be influenced by the presence of other activators and inhibitors. Variations in pH are generally small in most tissues, and skeletal muscle shows the largest changes in response to very high-intensity exercise: pH may fall from the resting value of about 7.0 to 6.5 or even less. Many enzymes normally function in an environment that is close to their pH optimum. For example, pepsin, which has a pH optimum of about 2.0, seems well adapted for the acid conditions of the stomach, where it hydrolyzes proteins into smaller fragments (peptides) and amino acids that can be absorbed in the small intestine. Some enzymes, however, have a pH optimum, at least in their isolated and purified form, that is far from their normal environment. Glycerol kinase has maximum activity at a pH of 9.8, a condition that is never reached in the cell.

Coenzymes, Prosthetic Groups, Cofactors, and Activators   Many enzymes require the presence of one or more coenzymes if the reaction is to proceed. For example, the conversion of lactate to pyruvate involves the removal of two hydrogen atoms from lactate and is catalyzed by lactate dehydrogenase, which requires that the coenzyme nicotinamide adenine dinucleotide (NAD$^+$) participates

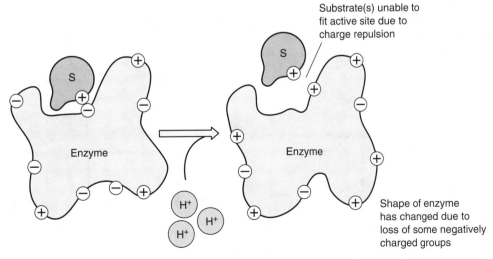

Figure A.9   Change in charge distribution of enzyme molecules caused by change in pH.

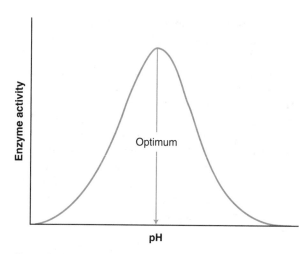

Figure A.10 Effect of pH on enzyme activity.

in the reaction. Coenzymes are chemically altered by participation in the reaction, in this case by conversion of NAD^+ to its reduced form, NADH. The coenzyme is, therefore, essentially a substrate for or product of the reaction, but a characteristic of coenzymes is that they are readily regenerated by other reactions within the cell. Some coenzymes, such as NAD^+, are loosely bound to the enzyme, but others, such as biotin, are tightly bound and are referred to as prosthetic groups.

Many enzymes have low activities in the absence of cofactors, and the presence of one or another metal ion, especially the divalent metals calcium, magnesium, manganese, and zinc, is essential for activation of many enzymes. Binding to these ions alters the charge distribution and shape of the active site of the enzyme. For example, the release of calcium into the cytoplasm in response to the nerve impulse is important in the activation of phosphorylase, which allows acceleration of the glycolytic pathway.

Competitive and Noncompetitive Inhibition Substances with a chemical structure similar to that of the normal substrate may also bind to the active site on the enzyme and thus interfere with enzyme function by reducing the number of active sites available to the proper substrate. These substances compete with the substrate for access to the active site and are, therefore, known as competitive inhibitors. The effect of competitive inhibition is to increase K_m. Increasing the concentration of substrate to a sufficient level will, however, swamp the effects of the inhibitor, and V_{max} is not affected by competitive inhibition.

Noncompetitive inhibitors bind to the enzyme at other sites, leaving the active site of the enzyme available to the substrate, but they have the effect of altering the conformation of the protein and thus reducing the catalytic activity of the active site. The V_{max} is reduced, but the same substrate concentration still produces one-half of the new maximum activity (i.e., K_m remains unchanged).

Allosteric and Covalent Modulation Allosteric modulation of enzyme activity is the reversible binding of small molecules to the enzyme at sites other than the active site, producing a conformational change in the structure of the enzyme molecule. This change in shape and charge distribution results in a change (either an increase or a decrease) in the affinity of the enzyme for its substrates or products and, hence, in its activity (see figure A.11a). The effect may either increase the activity of the enzyme, speeding up the rate of the reaction it catalyzes, or inhibit the activity of the enzyme, essentially preventing the reaction it catalyzes from taking place. Covalent modulation involves phosphorylation or dephosphorylation (i.e., the addition or removal of a phosphate group, respectively) of an enzyme, usually affecting the hydroxyl (-OH) group of a serine residue in the polypeptide chain (see figure A.11b). As with allosteric effects, covalent modulation may either activate or inhibit enzyme activity. A good example

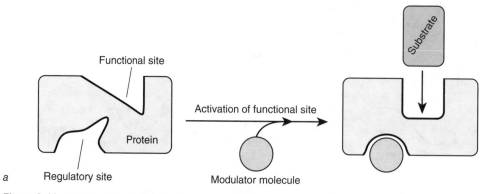

Figure A.11 *(a)* Allosteric modulation of enzyme activity.

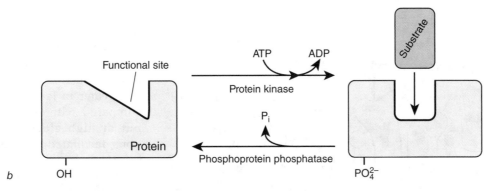

Figure A.11 *(b)* Covalent modulation of enzyme activity.

is the activity of glycogen phosphorylase, which catalyzes the breakdown of muscle glycogen. This enzyme needs to be activated at the onset of exercise to allow the muscle glycogen store to be used as an energy source, and this increase in enzyme activity is achieved by the covalent attachment of a phosphate group by a protein kinase that was itself activated by a rise in the intracellular calcium ion concentration (for further details, see chapter 3).

Enzyme Isoforms

Some enzymes exist in more than one form. These isoforms catalyze the same reaction but are generally found in different tissues and may have different specificities or catalytic capabilities. Lactate dehydrogenase exists in two forms, each made up of four subunits. The subunits exist in one of two forms: the H form, predominantly in cardiac muscle, and the M form, predominantly in skeletal muscle. Five different combinations of these subunits are possible. In muscle, the H form is associated with tissues having a high capacity for oxidative metabolism and that, therefore, have a high capacity for lactate oxidation, whereas the M form is associated with tissues having a high anaerobic capacity relative to their oxidative capability. The M form favors the conversion of pyruvate to lactate, whereas the H form favors the conversion of lactate to pyruvate. Many other enzymes exist in a variety of isoforms, but their functional significance is not well understood.

Membrane Structure and Transport

Membranes set the limits of cell boundaries. To enter a cell from the extracellular fluid, a substance must pass through the cell membrane. For example, the simple sugars that are formed from the breakdown of complex carbohydrates in the gastrointestinal tract can get into the bloodstream only by passing through the cells that line the gut. The properties of cell membranes and the components within them determine which substances can and cannot enter or leave a cell.

Cell membranes are composed of a lipid bilayer containing mostly phospholipids and some cholesterol. Within these lipids are proteins, some of which are restricted to one side of the bilayer and some of which are embedded within the membrane from one side to the other (see figure A.12). These proteins have important structural roles as receptors, channels, or transporters.

Dissolved substances (solutes) move across these semipermeable membranes by simple diffusion, facilitated diffusion, or active transport. Osmosis is the movement of water across membranes.

Simple Diffusion

Solutes move from high to low concentration only by diffusion. Simple diffusion involves the movement of the solute across the lipid bilayer and hence is to a large degree influenced by the solubility of the substance in lipid. Most water-soluble substances (e.g., glucose) and charged particles (e.g., sodium ions) are poorly soluble in lipid. Large molecules such as proteins cannot pass across membranes. Very small molecules (e.g., O_2, CO_2, H_2O, and NH_3) diffuse easily across cell membranes. Rates of diffusion are affected by temperature and the concentration difference on either side of the membrane.

Facilitated Diffusion

In facilitated diffusion, solutes move only from high to low concentration by diffusion but use a specific protein carrier molecule to pass through the membrane. The protein may be a mobile

Extracellular fluid

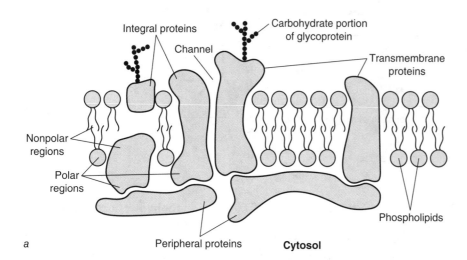

Integral proteins

Channel

Carbohydrate portion
of glycoprotein

Transmembrane
proteins

Nonpolar
regions

Polar
regions

Peripheral proteins

Phospholipids

a

Cytosol

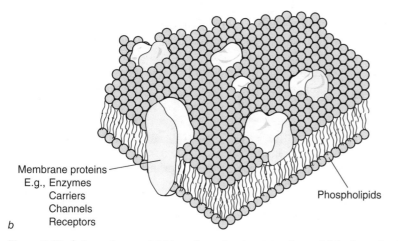

Membrane proteins
E.g., Enzymes
Carriers
Channels
Receptors

Phospholipids

b

Figure A.12 Cell membranes. *(a)* A two-dimensional cross section and *(b)* a three-dimensional view.

carrier or a gated channel, as illustrated in figure A.13. As shown in the example of glucose membrane transport in figure A.14, the rate of transport across the membrane is far greater in facilitated diffusion compared with simple diffusion, but at high glucose concentrations, facilitated transport exhibits saturation kinetics. The maximum speed of facilitated transport (V_{max}), indicated by the dashed line, is limited by the number of protein transporters available in the membrane. When all the transporters are full, additional movement can occur only by simple diffusion. In muscle, glucose is transported into the fibers by a protein carrier called GLUT4. The number of GLUT4 transporters in the muscle fiber membrane is influenced by exercise and the hormone insulin.

Active Transport

In active transport, substances are moved against their concentration gradient by a specific protein carrier and energy supplied directly by ATP or indirectly by ion electrochemical gradients. The sodium–potassium pump, or Na^+–K^+–ATPase pump, is a good example of an active cellular transport mechanism and is illustrated in figure A.15. Energy released from the hydrolysis of ATP moves sodium and potassium ions

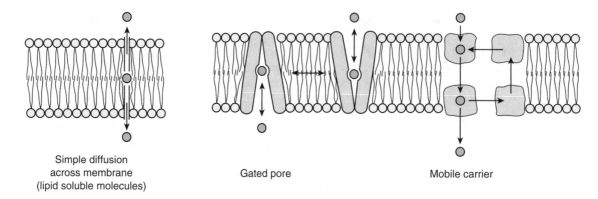

Simple diffusion
across membrane
(lipid soluble molecules)

Gated pore

Mobile carrier

Facilitated diffusion using a protein channel or transporter

Figure A.13 Diffusion and facilitated diffusion of substances across cell membranes. In both cases, net movement of the solute molecules occurs from a high concentration of solute to a low concentration of solute.

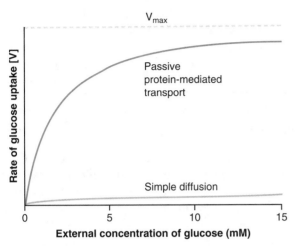

Figure A.14 Relative rates of glucose uptake into cells by simple diffusion and facilitated diffusion using a protein transporter in relation to the glucose concentration of the extracellular fluid.

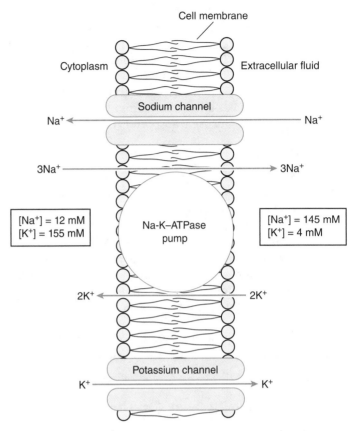

Figure A.15 The sodium–potassium ATPase pump. Energy released from the hydrolysis of ATP is used to move sodium and potassium ions across the cell membrane, against the prevailing concentration gradients.

across the cell membrane against the prevailing concentration gradients. For each molecule of ATP hydrolyzed to ADP, three sodium ions (Na^+) are transported out of the cell and two potassium ions (K^+) are transported into the cell. Because more positively charged ions are moved out of the cell than are transported in, an electrochemical gradient is established. Inside the cell becomes negative relative to outside, with a difference in electrical potential of about 70 millivolts. Inside the cell the Na^+ concentration is maintained at about 12 mM, whereas outside, it is about 145 mM. The K^+ concentration inside the cell is about 155 mM, whereas outside it is only 4 mM. The presence of separate sodium and potassium ion channels in the membrane is also shown in figure A.15. When these channels are open, the ions move by diffusion from high to low concentration. The selective opening of sodium channels (allowing a rapid influx of positively charged Na^+ ions) causes a temporary change in the resting membrane potential called depolarization. Depolarization is important in the generation and propagation of action potentials in excitable cells such as nerve and muscle.

Cotransport (or symport) mechanisms use the electrochemical gradient set up by the Na^+–K^+–ATPase pump to transport a substance against its concentration gradient. For example, the inward transport of dietary glucose from the gut lumen into intestinal epithelial cells

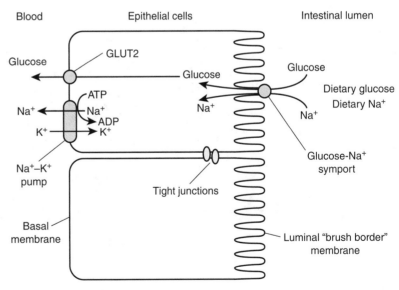

Figure A.16 Cotransport (symport) of glucose and sodium from the gut lumen into epithelial cells of the small intestine, followed by separate transport across the basal membrane into the blood by the action of a glucose transporter (GLUT2) and the sodium–potassium–ATPase pump.

is coupled to that of Na$^+$, as depicted in figure A.16. The Na$^+$–K$^+$–ATPase pump generates a large concentration difference for sodium across the membrane. The glucose–sodium symport protein uses that sodium gradient to transport glucose into the cell, followed by separate transport of glucose across the basal membrane into the blood by the action of a glucose transporter (GLUT2).

Osmosis

Water can readily diffuse across membranes, both through the lipid bilayer and through protein pores or channels in the membrane. Osmosis is the net movement of water as a consequence of a total-solute particle concentration difference across a membrane. Water moves across a semipermeable membrane from a region of low total-solute particle concentration (osmolarity) to a region of high total-solute particle concentration, until the total-solute particle concentration is equal on each side of the membrane (see figure A.17) or its movement is counteracted by the buildup of hydrostatic pressure.

Cells and Organelles

All tissues in the body are made of cells. Each cell contains several internal structures called organelles. These orgenelles include the nucleus, the mitochondrion, and other structures that are briefly described in this section. Not all cells contain all structures, because some cells are specialized for particular functions. For example, mature red blood cells are specialized for the transport of the respiratory pigment hemoglobin and oxygen and do not contain a nucleus or any mitochondria.

A typical cell is shown in figure A.18. The average diameter of a cell in the human body is about 10 μm (1/100th of a millimeter), although a wide variety of cell shapes and sizes exists. The cell is compartmentalized, and the organelles are distinct subcellular structures. In total, the adult human body contains about 10^{14} cells. Most cells (apart from those in adipose tissue) are 70% to 80% water.

■ The nucleus is the largest organelle. It is usually round or oval shaped and surrounded by a nuclear envelope composed of two phospholipid membranes. This envelope contains pores through which messenger molecules pass to the cytoplasm. The nucleus stores genetic information in the form of deoxyribonucleic acid (DNA). That genetic information passes from the nucleus to the cytoplasm, where amino acids are assembled into proteins. The nucleolus is a densely staining region of the nucleus that expresses information required by ribosomal proteins.

■ The rough granular endoplasmic reticulum is an extensive network of folded, sheetlike membranes that has ribosomes attached to its surface. Proteins are synthesized on the ribosomes. The smooth (agranular) endoplasmic reticulum is a highly branched tubular network that does not have attached ribosomes. It contains enzymes for fatty acid synthesis and stores and releases calcium, a process important in the regulation of contraction. The specialized smooth endoplasmic reticulum in muscle is called the sarcoplasmic reticulum.

■ The Golgi apparatus is a series of cup-shaped flattened membranous sacs associated with numerous vesicles. It concentrates, modifies, and sorts newly synthesized proteins before their distribution, by way of vesicles, to other organelles, to the plasma membrane, or to secretions from the cell.

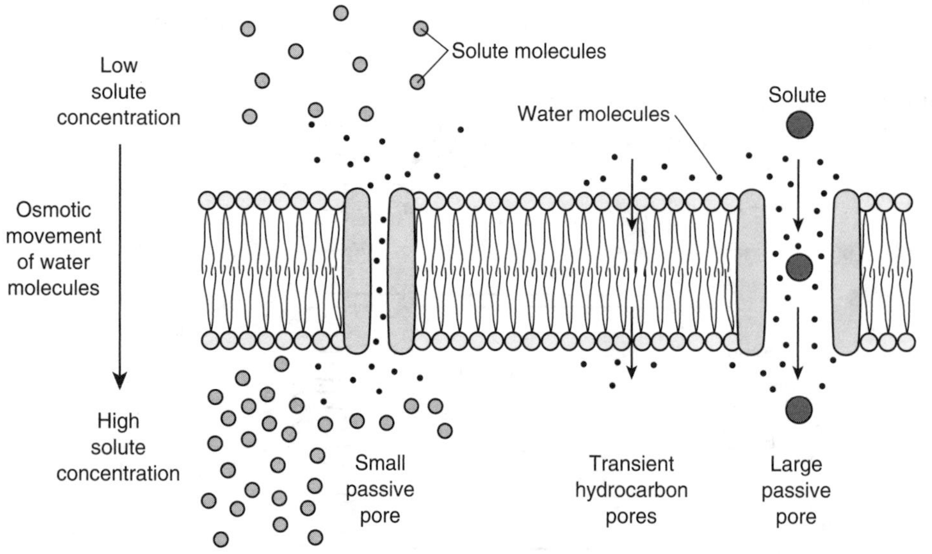

Figure A.17 Possible mechanisms for permeation of cell membranes by water. Water is a small molecule and thus permeates through the spaces between hydrophobic lipid molecules, specific water pores, or other pores (e.g., ion channels). Water molecules always move in the direction of a higher solute (dissolved particle) concentration.

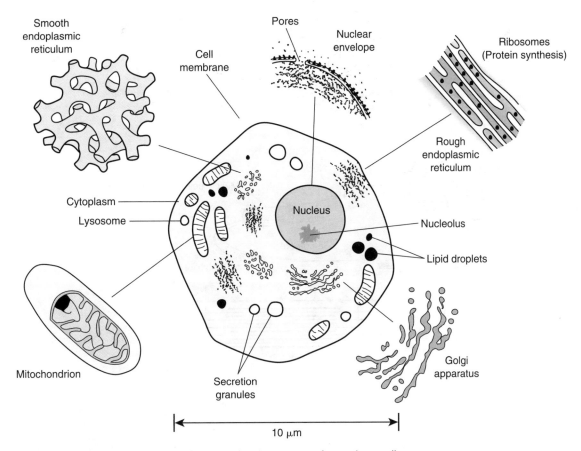

Figure A.18 A typical cell in cross section, showing the structure of several organelles.

■ The mitochondrion is an oval-shaped body surrounded by two membranes. The inner membrane folds into the matrix of the mitochondrion, forming cristae. This location is the major site of ATP production, oxygen utilization, and carbon dioxide production. It contains the enzymes of fatty acid oxidation, the tricarboxylic acid (Krebs) cycle, and the electron-transport chain.

■ Lysosomes are small membranous vesicles containing digestive enzymes. After injury, these enzymes may be activated and cause necrosis (death) of the cell.

■ The cytoplasm, or cytosol, is the fluid portion of the cell surrounding all the organelles. It stores energy in the form of glycogen granules and lipid droplets and contains the enzymes of anaerobic glycolysis.

Although the cell shape and size as depicted in figure A.18 is typical of many cells, other cells are distinctly specialized for the function they perform. For example, skeletal muscle cells are long, cylindrical striated fibers (see figure A.19). The cytoplasm of muscle fibers is the sarcoplasm, and the plasma membrane is the sarcolemma. Myofibrils are the contractile elements, composed of chains of sarcomeres containing thin (actin) and thick (myosin) filaments arranged in a regular array. Surrounding the myofibrils is the sarcoplasmic reticulum, an elaborate baglike membranous structure. Its interconnecting tubules lie in the narrow spaces between the myofibrils, surrounding and running parallel to them. It plays an important role in contraction by storing calcium ions, which, when released into the sarcoplasm, initiate muscle contraction. Numerous mitochondria are located near the plasma membrane, mostly around the outer circumference of the muscle fiber, close to the oxygen supply from the blood capillaries. Muscles contain a mixture of fiber types, classified according to their contractile speed and metabolic characteristics. Further details can be found in chapter 3.

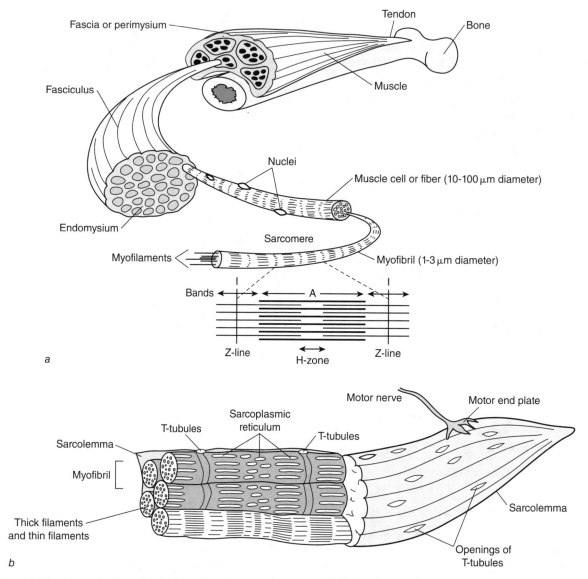

Figure A.19 *(a)* The structure of skeletal muscle and *(b)* the ultrastructure of a skeletal muscle fiber showing the location of the myofibrils (contractile proteins) and the sarcoplasmic reticulum.

Tissues, Organs, and Systems

The cells of the body form larger structures called tissues (e.g., muscle) and organs (e.g., heart, lungs, and liver). A tissue is a group of similar cells specialized to carry out particular functions. An organ is a distinct body part formed from the combination of all four major tissue groups and designed to carry out a more general function than the tissues within it.

Although all somatic cells of the body, except the germ cells (sperm in males, oocytes in females), contain the same genetic information, not all of this information in the DNA is expressed in the form of protein. Cellular specialization is possible

because of the selective expression of genes by different cells. This specialization is what makes, for example, a skeletal muscle cell different from a nerve cell or a white blood cell. Cells can generally be classified as belonging to one of four groups of tissues: epithelial, connective, nerve, and muscle.

■ Epithelial tissue generally forms sheets that protect against abrasion and the entry of potentially harmful substances or microorganisms. Epithelial tissue comprises the skin surface, the internal linings of the gastrointestinal tract, blood and lymph vessels, the respiratory tract, kidney tubules, ureters, and bladder. Parts of many glands are also formed from epithelial tissue. Some epithelial tissues synthesize and release secretions, and others absorb nutrients.

■ Connective tissue connects various body parts and forms supportive or protective structures within and around tissues and organs. Connective tissue forms cartilage and bone, holds bones together, and attaches skeletal muscles to bones and skin. Most connective tissue consists of cells surrounded by an organic, semifluid fibrous matrix. The latter is formed mostly from collagen, a fibrous protein that is synthesized and secreted by specialized epithelial cells called fibroblasts. Blood is a form of connective tissue. Normally the blood cells circulate within a fluid plasma, but after injury to a blood vessel, the plasma forms an insoluble clot by activating an insoluble fibrous protein called fibrinogen.

■ Nerve tissue initiates and carries electrical signals that control the actions of many body tissues and organs. Nerve tissue is found in the brain, spinal cord, and nerves. Motor (efferent) nerves convey information from the central nervous system (brain and spinal cord) to the periphery. Information about changes in pressure, chemical composition, and temperature is conveyed from sensory organs in the periphery to the central nervous system by sensory (afferent) nerves.

■ Muscle tissue is specialized to exert force by contracting (shortening in length). The three different types of muscle are skeletal muscle, smooth muscle, and cardiac muscle. Skeletal muscle produces body movement through its link to the bones of the skeleton and is under voluntary control. Skeletal muscle cells are long, striated, multinucleated fibers. Smooth muscle is found in internal organs such as the walls of arteries and veins, the esophagus, stomach, intestines, bladder, and the airways and is not under voluntary control. Smooth muscle cells are spindle-shaped and smaller than skeletal muscle cells. Cardiac muscle is found in the heart and in the large blood vessels near the heart. It is involuntary like smooth muscle and striated like skeletal muscle. Cardiac muscle has branching fibers and specialized cell junctions called intercalated disks. These characteristics give it the ability to contract in a repetitive, synchronized manner that pumps blood to the lungs and other organs of the body.

An organ is a distinct body part formed from the combination of all four major tissue groups and designed to carry out a more general function than the tissues within it. For example, the stomach performs digestion. It contains epithelial tissue that forms a protective lining and produces digestive juices, acid, and mucus. Connective tissue supports the stomach wall and forms an outer protective layer. Smooth muscle within the stomach wall exerts forces that mix food with the digestive secretions and propel the food toward the small intestine. Nerve tissue conducts signals that coordinate the actions of the epithelial glands and muscle tissue within the stomach and with other parts of the digestive system.

Genes, DNA, and Protein Synthesis

A person's actual genetic makeup is called his or her genotype. The physical expression of the genotype as particular characteristics or traits (e.g., height, strength, hair color) is called the person's phenotype. Success in sports is determined by many factors including motivation, appropriate training, tactics, and nutrition. Perhaps the most important factor, however, is raw talent in terms of the body's phenotype, in other words, the body's physical, physiological, and metabolic characteristics. These characteristics, which in terms of athletic capability might be taken to include muscle fiber type composition, the size of the heart and lungs, body height and mass, are all largely determined by the genotype (or genetic endowment) of the person. Certain physical characteristics are essential for success in many sports at the elite level (for example, in the past 20 years, no male tennis player under 1.75 m in height has won a Grand Slam event and NFL linebackers who weigh less than 90 kg are a rarity).

A person's physical characteristics are determined to a large degree by the genetic information that she or he carries. Only monozygotic twins, individuals who develop from the same fertilized ovum, known as the zygote, as a result of the splitting of the cell mass at a very early stage of embryonic development, carry exactly the same genetic information. Nonidentical (dizygotic) twins result from the fertilization of two different ova and hence have different genotypes.

The Nature of Genetic Information

All the genetic information of every species is contained in its deoxyribonucleic acid (DNA) structure, which determines the type and amount of protein synthesized in each cell of the organism. These proteins are in turn responsible for the synthesis of all other cellular components; the genetic material codes only for proteins and does this by defining their component amino acids. Proteins provide the structural basis of all tissues and organs, and it is largely the protein content of these tissues that gives them their recognizable shape. More important, perhaps, the proteins present in the various tissues confer on each tissue its metabolic capabilities. The presence or absence of a particular enzyme determines whether or not a tissue can carry out a particular function, and the activity (which depends on the amount of enzyme or an isoform) determines how fast that process can proceed. Proteins and amino acids also constitute, or act as precursors for, many of the body's hormones, regulatory peptides, and neurotransmitters as well as act as the receptors for these signaling systems and fulfill a variety of other functions.

Although all somatic cells of the body (that is, all cells except the germ cells, sperm, and ova) contain the same genetic material in their nuclei, not all genes are expressed (i.e., available to be translated into protein). Thus, the structural and functional characteristics of different cell types are determined by selective gene expression. Although all cells in the human body express certain genes (e.g., those that code for the enzymes of glycolysis), only some cells express genes for other specific proteins (e.g., myosin, troponin, hormone receptors, or enzymes of a metabolic pathway specific to a particular tissue type) and other genes will be repressed. This property is what makes a liver cell different from a muscle cell or a nerve cell. Alteration of gene expression is one of the means by which the body develops and adapts. Certain hormones (particularly steroid hormones such as cortisol and testosterone) are known to be important in the regulation of gene expression.

Nucleic Acids and Protein Synthesis

The development of the cell is determined by the chromosomes that are present in its nucleus, which contain the genetic information that defines the characteristics of the mature cell by regulating the synthesis of the many thousands of different proteins that give the cell its structural and functional characteristics. Chromosomes are a compact form of DNA complexed with protein called chromatin and only appear just before cell division. At other times in the cell cycle, DNA in the nucleus is in an uncoiled form, and when freed from contact with chromatin it can be used as a template for ribonucleic acid (RNA) and then protein synthesis.

The parts of the DNA that code for specific proteins are called genes.

All human somatic cells contain 23 pairs of chromosomes, and each cell contains thousands of different proteins. Thus, there are many genes on each chromosome. The chromosomes consist primarily of DNA; the functional unit of DNA, a deoxyribonucleotide, consists of a pentose (five-carbon) sugar molecule called deoxyribose, a phosphate group, and an organic nucleotide base that is either a purine or a pyrimidine. The four bases that are present in DNA are adenine (A), thymine (T), guanine (G), and cytosine (C). Adenine and thymine are purines, whereas guanine and cytosine are pyrimidines. The backbone of the molecule consists of two antiparallel chains of alternating deoxyribose and phosphate groups, and the DNA molecule is typically tens of millions of these units long. The chemistry of the bases in DNA allows bonding to occur between pairs of bases. Strong bonds are formed only between adenine and thymine and between guanine and cytosine, and this accounts for the two parallel strands that effectively run in opposite directions, forming a double helix as illustrated in figure A.20. The hydrogen bonds that are formed are extremely stable, accounting for the stability of the genetic information that these molecules contain, but they can be broken during the process of transcription (see the next section). The order of the nucleotide bases in DNA determines the order of the amino acids in the protein that will be synthesized, and the process is switched on and off by control sequences.

Transcription

Transcription is name given to the process by which a complementary strand of nucleic acids based on the DNA template is formed in the nucleus of the cell. This is needed to transfer the information that they contain to the protein synthetic apparatus, which is located in the cytoplasm of the cell. During the process of transcription, the hydrogen bonds joining the bases are broken and the enzyme ribonucleic acid (RNA) polymerase forms a sequence of ribonucleotides, following the same base-pairing arrangement, with the exception of the presence of uracil (U) in RNA rather than the thymine present in DNA. The sequence of nucleotide bases in the original DNA molecule (or at least in one strand of it—the other strand is not used) thus determines the order of bases on the molecule of RNA, known as messenger

RNA (mRNA), as shown in figure A.20. In other words, the DNA serves as a template from which a complementary RNA molecule is transcribed. The mRNA is translocated from the nucleus of the cell, where it was formed, to the cytoplasm, which is where the ribosomes, the structures on which proteins are synthesized, are located. Although a molecule of mRNA can be quite large, it can pass through the pores in the nuclear membrane.

Translation

The process of translation allows the information contained in the sequence of bases on the mRNA molecule to be used to determine the sequence of amino acids in the polypeptide chain that is synthesised. Each amino acid is denoted by a specific sequence of three base pairs, the genetic code, and each of these sequences is known as a codon. Because there are four different nucleotide bases in RNA (adenine [A], guanine [G], cytosine [C], and uracil [U]), combinations of three bases (triplets) can specify for up to 4^3, or 64, amino acids. In fact, only 20 different amino acids are used in the synthesis of proteins, so the genetic code is said to be degenerate, which means that there is more than one codon for each amino acid. For example, the amino acid valine is coded for by the triplets GUU, GUC, GUA, and GUG; lysine is coded for by AAA and AAG; and methionine is coded for only by the triplet AUG. Certain codons (UAA, UGA, and UAG) act as a code for chain termination, signaling the end of translation of the mRNA information into a polypeptide chain.

Transfer RNA molecules (tRNA) are found in the cytoplasm and contain one specific binding site (an anticodon) that recognizes and binds to the codon and another that binds the appropriate amino acid. Ribosomes contain binding sites for two tRNA molecules and a site just below these along which the mRNA strand can progress. The amino acids

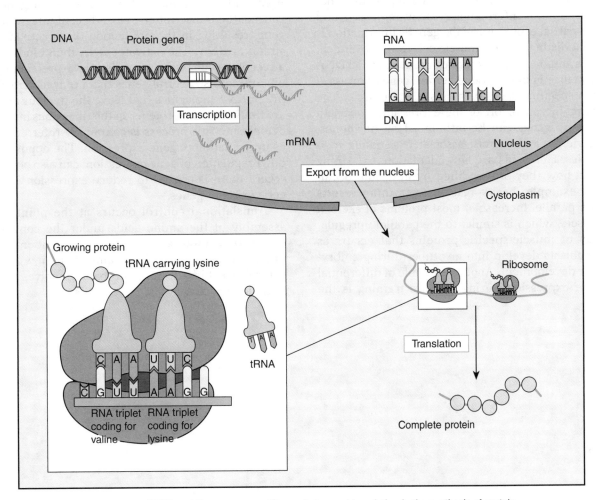

Figure A.20 The structure of DNA and the processes of transcription and translation in the synthesis of protein.

are thus brought into proximity and form peptide bonds in the appropriate sequence, as illustrated in the lower part of figure A.20. The process is initiated when the first tRNA molecule together with its bound amino acid is positioned on the mRNA; this first amino acid is always methionine, and the rate at which this initiation step occurs is probably crucial in the overall control of the rate of protein synthesis. Elongation of the peptide chain is terminated when a sequence of codons that do not correspond to any of the amino acids is encountered. In this way, the sequence of bases in the mRNA determines the sequence of amino acids in the protein, which in turn determines how the protein will fold (i.e., its three-dimensional or tertiary structure). The three-dimensional structure of a protein directly determines its function.

Selective Gene Expression

Each cell in the human body contains all the genetic information necessary to make all the other cells, but this information remains repressed, and this partial expression of the genetic information is what distinguishes a muscle cell from a liver cell. This implies that a unique, tissue-specific DNA sequence is in or around certain genes expressed in a specific tissue, such as skeletal muscle. The switching on or off of the expression of certain specific genes can be influenced by hormones, nutrients, and exercise-associated signaling molecules. This is, in part, how adaptations to training (and how they are modified by nutrition) occur. For example, heavy resistance training results in a parallel increase of most proteins of skeletal muscle, which is similar to the parallel upregulation of muscle-specific proteins that occurs as myoblasts develop into myotubes during embryonic development. Another example of differential gene expression during exercise training is the increase in mitochondrial density without a change in muscle size that occurs because of endurance training. In this situation it is unlikely that the "exercise signal" would interact with the same DNA regulatory sequence that controls contractile protein gene transcription. Rather, the endurance exercise factor would interact with a consensus DNA sequence found uniquely in the regulatory region of the mitochondrial genes. Thus, adaptations that occur in muscle with training reflect a change in the expression of the genetic material.

The control of protein synthesis and the expression of the genetic material can be achieved in a number of ways. Transcriptional control alters the concentration of mRNA, and this control is achieved by regulation of the activity of the mRNA polymerase. Repressor proteins, which are activated or inhibited depending on the availability of specific substrates, allow this control to be exerted. Several hormones exert their effects in this way. The hormone (or a hormone-receptor complex) may bind to a region of DNA on a sensor gene, causing the transcription of an adjacent integrator gene, resulting in the production of an activator strand of RNA. The activator RNA then binds to a receptor gene, which permits the expression of one or more structural genes that are transcribed into mRNA molecules that leave the nucleus and are translated into proteins on the ribosomes in the cytoplasm. This process is commonly referred to as upregulation of gene expression. The opposite, downregulation of gene expression, can also occur where there is a need to reduce expression of a gene or set of genes.

Translational control occurs at the point of assembly of the amino acids under the control of mRNA without any change in the amount of mRNA. There is some uncertainty as to how this control is achieved, but it probably involves the initiation process.

Unit Conversion Tables

To measure energy, volume, weight, and length, a standardized system known as the System Internationale (SI) has been established. The SI units are based on the metric system. In many countries, however, the English system of measures is also used, and in the field of nutrition, both systems are utilized. The following tables define the SI units and provide equivalents that allow the reader to convert between the English system and the SI system.

■ **TABLE B.1** ■

Systeme Internationale (SI) Units

Physical quantity	Name of unit	Symbol	Definition of unit
Length	Meter	m	
Mass	Kilogram	kg	
Time	Second	s	
Temperature	Degrees Kelvin	°K	
	Degrees Celsius	°C	Temperature °K − 273.15
Amount of substance	Mole	mol	
Angle	Radian	rad	
Electric current	Ampere	A	
Potential difference	Volt	V	$kg.m^2.s^{-3}.A^{-1} = J.A^{-1}.s^{-1}$
Electric charge	Coulomb	C	A.s
Resistance	Ohm	Ω	$kg.m^2.s^{-3}.A^{-2} = V.A^{-1}$
Energy	Joule	J	$kg.m^2.s^{-2}$
Force	Newton	N	$kg.m.s^{-2} = J.m^{-1}$
Power	Watt	W	$kg.m^2.s^{-3} = J.s^{-1}$
Pressure	Pascal	Pa	$N.m^{-2}$
Frequency	Hertz	Hz	$cycles.s^{-1}$
Density	Kilogram per cubic meter		$kg.m^{-3}$

■ TABLE B.2 ■
SI Fractions and Multiples

	Prefix	Symbol	Examples
FRACTION			
10^{-1}	Deci	d	Deciliter, dl
10^{-2}	Centi	c	Centimeter, cm
10^{-3}	Milli	m	Millisecond, ms
10^{-6}	Micro	μ	Micromole, μmol
10^{-9}	Nano	n	Nanometer, nm
10^{-12}	Pico	p	Picogram, pg
10^{-15}	Femto	f	Femtoliter, fl
MULTIPLE			
10^3	Kilo	k	Kilogram, kg
10^6	Mega	M	Megajoule, MJ
10^9	Giga	G	Gigaohm, GΩ

TABLE B.3
Derived SI Units and Non-SI Units Used in Biochemistry, Physiology, and Nutrition

Physical quantity	Name of unit	Symbol	Definition of unit
Length	Degree Angstrom Inch Foot	°A in ft	10^{-10} m = 10^{-1} nm 0.0254 m 0.3048 m
Mass	Pound Ounce	lb oz	454 g 28.4 g
Temperature	Degree Fahrenheit	°F	1.8 (°C) + 32
Energy	Erg Calorie Horsepower	erg cal h.p.	10^{-7} J 4.1868 J 745.7 W
Force	Dyne	dyn	10^{-5} N
Velocity		V	$m \cdot s^{-1}$ or $km \cdot h^{-1}$
Acceleration			$m \cdot s^{-2}$

Physical quantity	Name of unit	Symbol	Definition of unit
Pressure	Bar	bar	$105\ N \cdot m^{-2}$
	Atmosphere	atm	$101.325\ kN \cdot m^{-2}$
	Torricelli	torr	$133.322\ N \cdot m^{-2}$
Volume	Liter	l	$10^{-3}\ m^3$
	Pint	pint	$0.473 \times 10^{-3}\ m^3$
	Fluid ounce	fl oz	$29.57 \times 10^{-6}\ m^3$
Density			$g \cdot cm^{-3} = g \cdot ml^{-1}$
Enzyme activity	International unit	IU or U	$\mu mol \cdot min^{-1}$
Concentration	Molar	M	$mol \cdot l^{-1}$
	Weight/volume %	%w/v	$g \cdot dl^{-1}$ or $g \cdot 100\ ml^{-1}$
Viscosity	Poise	P	$10^{-1}\ kg^{-1} \cdot s^{-1} = 10^{-1}\ Pa \cdot s$
Radioactivity	Curie	Ci	$37 \times 10^{9}\ counts \cdot s^{-1}$
	Roentgen	R	$22.58 \times 10^{-4}\ counts \cdot kg^{-1}$

TABLE B.4

Useful Conversion Factors (Equivalents) for Units of Length, Mass (Weight), Temperature, Energy, and Volume

Physical quantity	Name of unit	Symbol	Approximate equivalent
Length	Inch	in	2.54 cm
	Foot	ft	0.3048 m
	Centimeter	cm	0.394 in
	Meter	m	3.28 ft
Mass	Ounce	oz	28.4 g
	Pound	lb	454 g
	Gram	g	0.035 oz
	Kilogram	kg	2.2 lb
Temperature	Degree Fahrenheit	°F	$1.8\ (°C) + 32$
	Degree Celsius	°C	$0.555\ (°F) - 32$
Energy	Calorie	cal	4.1868 J
	Joule	J	0.239 cal
Volume	Fluid ounce	fl oz	29.57 ml
	Pint	pint	473 ml
	Milliliter	ml	0.034 fl oz
	Liter	L	33.8 fl oz or 2.112 pints
	Teaspoon		5 ml or 0.17 fl oz
	Tablespoon		15 ml or 0.51 fl oz
	Glass or cup		240 ml or 8 fl oz

Recommended Daily Allowances for North America

TABLE C.1

Food Components and Daily Values Based on a 2,000-Calorie Diet

Food component	Daily value	Food component	Daily value
Total fat	65 g	Niacin	20 mg
Saturated fat	20 g	Vitamin B_6	2 mg
Cholesterol	300 mg	Folate	400 μg
Sodium	2,400 mg	Vitamin B_{12}	6 μg
Potassium	3,500 mg	Biotin	300 μg
Total carbohydrate	300 g	Pantothenic acid	10 mg
Dietary fiber	25 g	Phosphorus	1,000 mg
Protein	50 g	Iodine	150 μg
Vitamin A	5,000 IU	Magnesium	400 mg
Vitamin C	60 mg	Zinc	15 mg
Calcium	1,000 mg	Selenium	70 μg
Iron	18 mg	Copper	2 mg
Vitamin D	400 IU	Manganese	2 mg
Vitamin E	30 IU	Chromium	120 μg
Vitamin K	80 μg	Molybdenum	75 μg
Thiamin	1.5 mg	Chloride	3,400 mg
Riboflavin	1.7 mg		

TABLE C.2
Recommended Intakes for Minerals

Age	MALES						FEMALES					
	9–13 y	14–18 y	19–30 y	31–50 y	51–70 y	≥70 y	9–13 y	14–18 y	19–30 y	31–50 y	51–70 y	≥70 y
Calcium (mg/day)	1,300	1,300	1,000	1,000	1,200	1,200	1,300	1,300	1,000	1,000	1,200	1,200
Chloride (g/day)	2.3	2.3	2.3	2.3	2.0	1.8	2.3	2.3	2.3	2.3	2.0	1.8
Chromium (mg/day)	25	35	35	35	30	30	21	24	25	25	20	20
Copper (µg/day)	700	890	900	900	900	900	700	890	900	900	900	900
Fluoride (mg/day)	2	3	4	4	4	4	2	3	3	3	3	3
Iodine (µg/day)	120	150	150	150	150	150	120	150	150	150	150	150
Iron (mg/day)	8	11	8	8	8	8	8	15	18	18	8	8
Magnesium (mg/day)	240	410	400	420	420	420	240	360	310	320	320	320
Manganese (mg/day)	1.9	2.2	2.3	2.3	2.3	2.3	1.6	1.6	1.8	1.8	1.8	1.8
Molybdenum (µg/day)	34	43	45	45	45	45	34	43	45	45	45	45
Phosphorus (mg/day)	1,250	1,250	700	700	700	700	1,250	1,250	700	700	700	700
Potassium (g/day)	4.5	4.7	4.7	4.7	4.7	4.5	4.7	4.7	4.7	4.7	4.7	4.7
Selenium (µg/day)	40	55	55	55	55	55	40	55	55	55	55	55
Sodium (g/day)	1.5	1.5	1.5	1.5	1.3	1.2	1.5	1.5	1.5	1.5	1.3	1.2
Zinc (mg/day)	8	11	11	11	11	11	8	9	8	8	8	8

TABLE C.3
Recommended Intakes for Vitamins

Age	MALES						FEMALES					
	9–13 y	14–18 y	19–30 y	31–50 y	51–70 y	≥70 y	9–13 y	14–18 y	19–30 y	31–50 y	51–70 y	≥70 y
Biotin (µg/day)	20	25	30	30	30	30	20	25	30	30	30	30
Choline (mg/day)	375	550	550	550	550	550	375	400	425	425	425	425
Folate (µg/day)	300	400	400	400	400	400	300	400	400	400	400	400
Niacin (mg/day)	12	16	16	16	16	16	12	14	14	14	14	14
Pantothenic Acid (mg/day)	4	5	5	5	5	5	4	5	5	5	5	5
Riboflavin (mg/day)	0.9	1.3	1.3	1.3	1.3	1.3	0.9	1.0	1.1	1.1	1.1	1.1
Thiamin (mg/day)	0.9	1.2	1.2	1.2	1.2	1.2	0.9	1.0	1.1	1.1	1.1	1.1
Vitamin A (µg/day)	600	900	900	900	900	900	600	700	700	700	700	700
Vitamin B_6 (mg/day)	1.0	1.3	1.3	1.3	1.7	1.7	1.0	1.2	1.3	1.3	1.5	1.5
Vitamin B_{12} (µg/day)	1.8	2.4	2.4	2.4	2.4	2.4	1.8	2.4	2.4	2.4	2.4	2.4
Vitamin C (mg/day)	45	75	90	90	90	90	45	65	75	75	75	75
Vitamin D (µg/day)	5	5	5	5	10	15	5	5	5	5	10	15
Vitamin E (mg/day)	11	15	15	15	15	15	11	15	15	15	15	15
Vitamin K (mg/day)	60	75	120	120	120	120	60	75	90	90	90	90

Information in this table is taken from the DRI reports (www.nap.edu) and includes RDAs and AIs.

TABLE C.4

Estimated Average Requirements for Macronutrients

Age	9–13 y	14–18 y	19–30 y	31–50 y	51–70 y	≥70 y	9–13 y	14–18 y	19–30 y	31–50 y	51–70 y	≥70 y
	MALES						FEMALES					
Carbohydrate (g/day)	130	130	130	130	130	130	130	130	130	130	130	130
Fiber (g/day)	31	38	38	38	30	30	26	26	25	25	21	21
α-linolenic acid (g/day)	1.2	1.6	1.6	1.6	1.6	1.6	1.0	1.1	1.1	1.1	1.1	1.1
Linolenic acid (g/day)	12	16	17	17	14	14	10	11	12	12	11	11
Protein (g/day)*	34	52	56	56	56	56	34	46	46	46	46	46
Water (L/day)**	2.4	3.3	3.7	3.7	3.7	3.7	2.1	2.3	2.7	2.7	2.7	2.7

*Using the reference body weight of 0.8 g/kg.

**Total daily water intake for all food and beverages.

Information in this table is taken from the DRI reports (www.nap.edu) and includes RDAs and AIs.

TABLE C.5
Ranges and Recommendations for Macronutrient Distribution

Macronutrient	4–18 y	≥19 y (adults)
	RANGE IN NUTRITIONALLY ADEQUATE DIET (% OF TOTAL ENERGY)	
Carbohydrate	45-65	45-65
Cholesterol	As low as possible	
Fat	25-35	20-35
α-linolenic acid	0.6-1.2	0.6-1.2
Linoleic acid	5-10	5-10
Trans fatty acids	As low as possible	
Saturated fatty acids	As low as possible	
Protein	10-30	10-35
Sugar	<25	

Data from the National Academy of Sciences, Dietary Reference Intakes for Energy, Carbohydrate, Fiber, Fat, Fatty Acids, Cholesterol, Protein, and Amino Acids (2002).

TABLE C.6
DRIs and EERs

Height (meters)	Physical activity level	EER FOR MEN (kcal/day)		EER FOR WOMEN (kcal/day)	
		18.5 BMI	**24.99 BMI**	**18.5 BMI**	**24.99 BMI**
1.5 m		**41.6 kg**	**56.2 kg**	**41.6 kg**	**56.2 kg**
	Sedentary	1,848	2,080	1,625	1,762
	Low active	2,009	2,267	1,803	1,956
	Active	2,215	2,506	2,025	2,198
	Very active	2,554	2,898	2,291	2,489
1.65 m		**50.4 kg**	**68.0 kg**	**50.4 kg**	**68.0 kg**
	Sedentary	2,068	2,349	1,816	1,982
	Low active	2,254	2,566	2,016	2,202
	Active	2,490	2,842	2,267	2,477
	Very active	2,880	3,296	2,567	2,807
1.8 m		**59.5 kg**	**81.0 kg**	**59.5 kg**	**81.0 kg**
	Sedentary	2,301	2,635	2,015	2,211
	Low active	2,513	2,884	2,239	2,459
	Active	2,782	3,200	2,519	2,769
	Very active	3,225	3,720	2,855	3,141

For each year below 30, add 7 kcal/day for women and 10 kcal/day for men. For each year above 30, subtract that amount.

Data from the National Academy of Sciences, Dietary Reference Intakes for Energy, Carbohydrate, Fiber, Fat, Fatty Acids, Cholesterol, Protein, and Amino Acids (2002).

TABLE C.7

Upper Intake Levels for Minerals

Age	9–13 y	14–18 y	19–70 y	≥70 y
	MALES AND FEMALES			
Calcium (mg/day)	2,500	2,500	2,500	2,500
Chloride (g/day)	3.4	3.6	3.6	3.6
Copper (μg/day)	5,000	8,000	10,000	10,000
Fluoride (mg/day)	10	10	10	10
Iodine (μg/day)	600	900	1,100	1,100
Iron (mg/day)	40	45	45	45
Magnesium (mg/day)	350	350	350	350
Manganese (mg/day)	1.9	2.2	2.3	2.3
Molybdenum (μg/day)	34	43	45	45
Phosphorus (mg/day)	4,000	4,000	4,000	3,000
Selenium (μg/day)	280	400	400	400
Sodium (g/day)	2.2	2.3	2.3	2.3
Zinc (mg/day)	23	34	40	40

Upper intake levels (ULs) are considered to be the maximum level of nutrients (from food and supplements together) that is considered to pose no risk of adverse effects. Where data are not available for a particular mineral's UL, caution should be used in consuming more than the recommended daily intake.

Data from the National Academy of Sciences, 2004, www.nap.edu.

TABLE C.8

Upper Intake Levels for Vitamins

Age	9–13 y	14–18 y	19–70 y	≥70 y
	MALES AND FEMALES			
Choline (mg/day)	2,000	3,000	3,500	3,500
Folate (μg/day)	600	800	1,000	1,000
Niacin (mg/day)	20	30	35	35
Vitamin A (μg/day)	1,700	2,800	3,000	3,000
Vitamin B_6 (mg/day)	60	80	100	100
Vitamin C (mg/day)	1,200	1,800	2,000	2,000
Vitamin D (μg/day)	50	50	50	50
Vitamin E (mg/day)	600	800	1,000	1,000

Upper intake levels (ULs) are considered to be the maximum level of nutrients (from food and supplements together) that is considered to pose no risk of adverse effects. Where data are not available for a particular vitamin's UL, caution should be used in consuming more than the recommended daily intake.

Data from the National Academy of Sciences, 2004, www.nap.edu.

Reference Nutrient Intakes for the United Kingdom

TABLE D.1

Reference Nutrient Intake for Protein in the United Kingdom

Age	Reference nutrient intake (g/day)
0–3 mo	12.5
4–6 mo	12.7
7–9 mo	13.7
10–12 mo	14.9
1–3 y	14.5
4–6 y	19.7
7–10 y	28.3
MALES	
11–14 y	42.1
15–18 y	55.2
19–50 y	55.5
≥50 y	53.3
FEMALES	
11–14 y	41.2
15–18 y	55.2
19–50 y	55.5
≥50 y	53.3
Pregnancy	+6
LACTATION	
0–4 mo	+11
≥4 mo	+8

These figures assume complete digestibility

From Report on Health and Social Subjects: no 41. Dietary Reference Values for food energy and nutrients in the United Kingdom. Report of the Panel on Dietary Reference Values of the Committee on Medical Aspects of Food Policy. London: Her Majesty's Stationary Office, 1991. This is the UK's report Table 1.4. These figures assume complete digestibility.

TABLE D.2
Reference Nutrient Intake for Vitamins in the United Kingdom

Age	Thiamin (mg/day)	Riboflavin (mg/day)	Niacin (mg/day)	Vitamin B$_6$ (mg/day)	Vitamin B$_{12}$ (μg/day)	Folate (μg/day)	Vitamin C (μg/day)	Vitamin A (μg/day)	Vitamin D (μg/day)
0–3 mo	0.2	0.4	3	0.2	0.3	50	25	350	8.5
4–6 mo	0.2	0.4	3	0.2	0.3	50	25	350	8.5
7–9 mo	0.2	0.4	4	0.3	0.4	50	25	350	7
10–12 months	0.3	0.4	5	0.4	0.4	50	25	350	7
1–3 y	0.5	0.6	8	0.7	0.5	70	30	400	*
4–6 y	0.7	0.8	11	0.9	0.8	100	30	400	*
7–10 y	0.7	1.0	12	1.0	1	150	30	500	*
MALES									
11–14 y	0.9	1.2	15	1.2	1.2	200	35	600	*
15–18 y	1.1	1.3	18	1.5	1.5	200	40	700	*
19–50 y	1.0	1.3	17	1.4	1.5	200	40	700	*
≥50 y	0.9	1.3	16	1.4	1.5	200	40	700	*
FEMALES									
11–14 y	0.7	1.1	12	1.0	1.2	200	35	600	*
15–18 y	0.8	1.1	14	1.2	1.5	200	40	600	*
19–50 y	0.8	1.1	13	1.2	1.5	200	40	600	*
≥50 y	0.8	1.1	12	1.2	1.5	200	40	600	*
Pregnancy	+0.1	+0.3	*	*	*	*	*	*	*
LACTATION									
0–4 mo	+0.2	+0.5	+2	*	+0.5	+60	+30	+350	10
≥4 mo	+0.2	+0.5	+2	*	+0.5	+60	+30	+350	10

From Report on Health and Social Subjects: no 41. Dietary Reference Values for food energy and nutrients in the United Kingdom. Report of the Panel on Dietary Reference Values of the Committee on Medical Aspects of Food Policy. London: Her Majesty's Stationary Office, 1991. This is the UK's report Table 1.4.

TABLE D.3
Reference Nutrient Intake for Minerals in the United Kingdom

Age	Calcium (mg/day)	Phosphorus (mg/day)	Magnesium (mg/day)	Sodium (mg/day)	Potassium (mg/day)	Chloride (mg/day)	Iron (mg/day)	Zinc (mg/day)	Copper (μg/day)	Selenium (μg/day)	Iodine (μg/day)
0–3 mo	525	400	55	210	800	320	1.7	4.0	0.2	10	50
4–6 mo	525	400	60	280	850	400	4.3	4.0	0.3	13	60
7–9 mo	525	400	75	320	700	500	7.8	5.0	0.3	10	60
10–12 mo	525	400	80	350	700	500	7.8	5.0	0.3	10	60
1–3 y	350	270	85	500	800	800	6.9	5.0	0.4	15	70
4–6 y	450	350	120	700	1100	1100	6.1	6.5	0.6	20	100
7–10 y	550	450	200	1200	2000	1800	8.7	7.0	0.7	30	110
MALES											
11–14 y	1000	775	280	1600	3100	2500	11.3	9.0	0.8	45	130
15–18 y	1000	775	300	1600	3500	2500	11.3	9.5	1.0	70	140
19–50 y	700	550	300	1600	3500	2500	8.7	9.5	1.2	75	140
≥50 y	700	550	300	1600	3500	2500	8.7	9.5	1.2	75	140
FEMALES											
11–14 y	800	625	280	1600	3100	2500	14.8	9.0	0.8	45	130
15–18 y	800	625	300	1600	3500	2500	14.8	7.0	1.0	60	140
19–50 y	700	550	270	1600	3500	2500	14.8	7.0	1.2	60	140
≥50 y	700	550	270	1600	3500	2500	8.7	7.0	1.2	60	140
Pregnancy	*	*	*	*	*	*	*	*	*	*	*
LACTATION											
0–4 mo	+550	+450	+50	*	*	*	*	+6.0	+0.3	+15	*
≥4 mo	+550	+450	+50	*	*	*	*	+2.5	+0.3	+15	*

* No recommendation.

From Report on Health and Social Subjects: no 41. Dietary Reference Values for food energy and nutrients in the United Kingdom. Report of the Panel on Dietary Reference Values of the Committee on Medical Aspects of Food Policy. London: Her Majesty's Stationary Office, 1991. This is the UK's report Table 1.4.

Appendix E

Recommended Dietary Intakes for Australia

TABLE E.1

Recommended Dietary Intakes of Vitamins, Minerals, and Protein for Adults in Australia Expressed as Mean Daily Intake

	MEN		WOMEN			
	19–64 y	≥64 y	19–54 y	≥54 y	Pregnant	Lactating
Vitamin A (µg retinol equivalents)	750	750	750	750	+0	+450
Thiamin (mg)	1.1	0.9	0.8	0.7	+0.2	+0.4
Riboflavin (mg)	1.7	1.3	1.2	1.0	+0.3	+0.5
Niacin (mg niacin equivalents)	19	16	13	11	+2	+5
Vitamin B_6 (mg)	1.3–1.9	10–1.5	0.9–1.4	0.8–1.1	+0.1	+0.7–0.8
Total folate (µg)	200	200	200	200	+200	+150
Vitamin B_{12} (µg)	2.0	2.0	2.0	2.0	+1.0	+0.5
Vitamin C (mg)	40	40	30	30	+30	+45
Vitamin E (mg α-tocopherol equivalents)	10.0	10.0	7.0	7.0	+0	+2.5
Zinc (mg)	12	12	12	12	+4	+6
Iron (mg)	7	7	12–16	5–7	+10–20	+0
Iodine (mg)	150	150	120	120	+30	+50
Magnesium (mg)	320	320	270	270	+30	+70
Calcium (mg)	800	800	800	1,000	+300	+400
Phosphorus (mg)	1,000	1,000	1,000	1,000	+200	+200
Selenium (µg)	85	85	70	70	+10	+15
Sodium (mmol)	40–100	40–100	40–100	40–100	+0	+0
(mg)	920–2,300	920–2,300	920–2,300	920–2,300	+0	+0
Potassium (mmol)	50–140	50–140	50–140	50–140	+0	+0
(mg)	1,950–5,460	1,950–5,460	1,950–5,460	1,950–5,460	+0	+0
Protein (g)	55	55	45	45	+6	+16

National Health and Medical Research Council, Australia 1982-1989.

Glossary

1,3-DPG (1,3-diphosphoglycerate)—An intermediate compound in glycolysis.

2,3-DPG (2,3-diphosphoglycerate)—A highly anionic organic phosphate that is present in human red blood cells at about the same molar ratio as hemoglobin. It binds to deoxyhemoglobin but not the oxygenated form, therefore diminishing the oxygen affinity of hemoglobin. This is essential in enabling hemoglobin to unload oxygen in tissue capillaries.

3-methylhistidine—A metabolite of the amino acid histidine. Its urinary excretion is used as an index of contractile protein breakdown.

5-HT (5-hydroxytryptamine)—A brain neurotransmitter. Also known as serotonin.

absorption—The transport of nutrients from the intestine into the blood or lymph system.

accelerometer—Small piece of equipment that can be attached to the body to register all accelerations that the body makes. The number and the degree of the accelerations give an indication of the person's activity level.

acclimatization—Adaptation of the body to an environmental extreme (e.g., heat, cold, and altitude).

acetyl CoA—The major fuel for the oxidative processes in the body, being derived from the breakdown of glycogen, glucose, and fatty acids.

acid—A substance that tends to lose a proton (hydrogen ion).

acid–base balance—The relative balance of acid and base products in the body.

acidosis—A disturbance of the normal acid–base balance in which excess acids accumulate, causing a fall in pH (e.g., when lactic acid accumulates in muscle and blood during high-intensity exercise).

ACSM—American College of Sports Medicine.

ACTH (adrenocorticotrophic hormone)—Hormone secreted from anterior pituitary gland, which stimulates release of cortisol from adrenal glands.

actin—One of the major contractile proteins in muscle found in the thin filaments.

active transport—The movement or transport across cell membranes by membrane carriers. An expenditure of energy (ATP) is required.

acute-phase proteins—Several proteins released from liver (e.g., C-reactive protein) and leukocytes that aid the body's response to injury or infection.

acyl carrier protein (ACP)—Protein that transports a fatty acyl-carnitine complex (a fatty acid linked to carnitine) across the inner mitochondrial membrane. Also known as the fatty acyl-carnitine translocase.

acyl group—The long hydrocarbon chain of a fatty acid.

adaptogen—A name used for substances that help the body to adapt to stress situations.

adenine (A)—A purine nucleotide found in DNA and several coenzymes.

adequate intake (AI)—Recommended dietary intake comparable to the RDA but based on less scientific evidence.

adipocyte—An adipose tissue cell whose main function is to store triacylglycerol (fat).

adipose tissue—White fatty tissue that stores triacylglycerol.

adipose tissue-free skeletal muscle (ATFSM)—Lean muscle tissue.

ADP (adenosine diphosphate)—Breakdown product of ATP.

adrenaline—A hormone secreted by the adrenal gland. It is a stimulant that prepares the body for fight or flight and an important activator of fat and carbohydrate breakdown during exercise. Also known as epinephrine.

aerobic—Occurring in the presence of free oxygen.

alanine—A nonessential amino acid.

alcohol—A colorless liquid that has depressant and intoxicating effects. Ethyl alcohol or ethanol (C_2H_5OH) is the alcohol found in wines, spirits, and beers.

aldosterone—A steroid hormone secreted by the adrenal cortex. Primarily involved in fluid and electrolyte balance by controlling sodium and potassium excretion by the kidneys.

alimentary tract—See gastrointestinal tract.

alkalinizer—A group of substances with a buffering function (sodium bicarbonate, sodium citrate).

α-amylase or amylase—A digestive enzyme found in saliva that begins the digestion of starches in the mouth (also called ptyalin). It catalyzes the hydrolysis of starch by cleaving the α-1-4-glycosidic linkages between the component glucose molecules. Amylase is also present in pancreatic juice.

α-ketoisocaproate (α-KIC)—A metabolite of the amino acid leucine.

α-tocopherol—The most biologically active alcohol in vitamin E.

amenorrhea—The absence of at least three successive menstrual cycles in females.

amino acid (AA)—The chief structural molecule of protein, consisting of an amino group (NH_2) and a carboxylic acid group (CO_2H) plus another so-called R-group that determines the properties of the amino acid. Twenty different amino acids can be used to make proteins.

ammonia (NH_3)—A metabolic by-product of the oxidation of amino acids. It may be transformed into urea for excretion from the body.

AMP (adenosine monophosphate)—Product of the breakdown of adenosine diphosphate.

amylopectin—A branched-chain starch (polymer of glucose).

amylose—A straight-chain starch that is more resistant to digestion compared with amylopectin.

anabolism—Constructive metabolism, the process whereby simple body compounds are formed into more complex ones.

anaerobic—Occurring in the absence of free oxygen.

androstenediol—A steroid metabolite.

androstenedione—An androgenic steroid produced in the body that is converted to testosterone. Marketed as a dietary supplement.

anemia—A condition defined by an abnormally low blood hemoglobin content resulting in lowered oxygen carrying capacity.

anion—A negatively charged ion or electrolyte (e.g., chloride, Cl^-; phosphate, HPO_4^{2-}).

anorexia athletica—A form of anorexia nervosa observed in athletes who show significant symptoms of eating disorders but do not meet the criteria of the *Diagnostic and Statistical Manual of Mental Disorders* (American Psychiatric Association 1987) for anorexia or bulimia nervosa.

anorexia nervosa—An eating disorder characterized by abnormally small food intake and refusal to maintain a normal body weight (according to what is expected for gender, age, and height), a distorted view of body image, an intense fear of being fat or overweight and gaining weight or "feeling fat" when clearly the person is below normal weight, and the absence of at least three successive menstrual cycles in females (amenorrhea).

anthropometry—Use of body girths and diameters to evaluate body composition.

antibody—Soluble protein produced by B lymphocytes with antimicrobial effects. Also known as immunoglobulin.

antidiuretic hormone (ADH)—A hormone secreted by the posterior pituitary gland that influences water reabsorption by the kidneys.

antioxidant—Molecules that can prevent or limit the actions of free radicals, usually by removing their unpaired electron and thus converting them into something far less reactive.

apoptosis—An internal program that allows damaged or obsolete cells to commit suicide.

appendix—A nonfunctional part of the small intestine that is short, thin, and outpouching from the cecum.

appetite—A desire for food for the purpose of enjoyment that is developed through previous experience. Believed to be controlled in humans by an appetite center in the hypothalamus.

arginine—An essential amino acid.

arteriosclerosis—Hardening of the arteries. See also atherosclerosis.

arteriovenous (AV)—Refers to comparison of arterial and venous blood composition.

ascorbic acid—Vitamin C; major role is as a water-soluble antioxidant.

aspartame—An artificial sweetener made from amino acids.

aspartates—Salts of aspartic acid, an amino acid.

atherosclerosis—A specific form of arteriosclerosis characterized by the formation of fatty plaques on the luminal walls of arteries.

atom—The smallest unit of an element that retains all the properties of the element. The atoms of all elements can be broken down physically into the same subatomic particles: protons, neutrons, and electrons. Hence, the atoms of the various elements differ only in the numbers of protons, neutrons, and electrons that they contain.

ATP (adenosine triphosphate)—A high-energy compound that is the immediate source for muscular contraction and other energy-requiring processes in the cell.

ATPase (adenosine triphosphatase)—An enzyme that breaks down ATP to ADP and inorganic phosphate, releasing energy that can be used to fuel biological work.

atrophy—A wasting away, a diminution in the size of a cell, tissue, organ, or part.

Atwater factor—The average net energy values for carbohydrate, fat, and protein, named after Wilbur Olin Atwater: 16 kJ/g (4 kcal/g) for carbohydrate, 36 kJ/g (9 kcal/g) for fat, and 16 kJ/g (4 kcal/g) for protein.

autosome—Any chromosome occurring in a similar form in males and females and therefore able to pair fully during meiosis and mitosis. Distinguished from the sex chromosomes, which differ in the two sexes.

AV-differences—A difference between arterial and venous concentration of a substance, indicating net uptake or release of that substance.

average daily metabolic rate (ADMR)—The average energy expenditure over 24 hours.

base—A substance that tends to donate an electron pair or coordinate an electron.

BCAA (branched-chain amino acid)—Three essential amino acids that can be oxidized by muscle. Includes leucine, isoleucine, and valine.

β-carotene—A precursor for vitamin A found in plants. Also called provitamin A.

beta-hydroxy beta methylbutyrate (HMB)—Metabolite of the essential amino acid leucine. Marketed as a muscle growth promotor.

β-oxidation—Oxygen-requiring process in the mitochondria whereby two-carbon units are sequentially removed from the hydrocarbon chain of a fatty acid in the form of acetyl-CoA, which can then enter the TCA cycle.

bile—Fluid produced by the liver and stored in the gall bladder that contains bile salts, bile pigments, cholesterol, and other molecules. The bile is secreted into the small intestine.

bile salts—Salts or derivatives of cholesterol in bile that are polar on one end and nonpolar on the other end of the molecule. Bile salts act to emulsify fat in the lumen of the small intestine.

bioavailability—In relation to nutrients in food, the amount that may be absorbed into the body.

bioelectrical impedance analysis (BIA)—A method to calculate percentage of body fat by measuring electrical resistance due to the water content of the body.

biopsy—A small sample of tissue taken for analysis.

b.m.—Body mass in kilograms (kg).

BMI (body mass index)—Body mass in kilograms divided by height in meters squared (kg/m^2). An index used as a measure of obesity.

BMR (basal metabolic rate)—Energy expenditure under basal, postabsorptive conditions representing the energy needed to maintain life under these basal conditions.

bomb calorimeter—An instrument to measure the energy content in which food is oxidized and the resulting heat production is measured.

breath-by-breath system—An automated system to analyze gas exchange to estimate energy expenditure and substrate utilization. These systems are able to measure CO_2 production and oxygen consumption from every breath.

brush border—Where the absorption of nutrients takes place in the intestine. The surface of the epithelial cells that line the intestinal wall is covered with microvilli that form the brush border.

buffer—A substance that, in solution, prevents rapid changes in hydrogen ion concentration (pH).

bulimia nervosa—An eating disorder characterized by repeated episodes of binge eating (consumption of large amounts of usually energy-dense foods) followed by purging of the stomach contents, allowing insufficient time for most of the nutrients from the heavy meal to be absorbed.

bulk flow—The transport of materials by the movement of the gas or liquid in which they are contained.

b.w.—Body weight.

caffeine—A stimulant drug found in many food products such as coffee, tea, and cola drinks. Stimulates the central nervous system and used as an ergogenic aid.

calorie (cal)—Traditional unit of energy. One calorie expresses the quantity of energy (heat) needed to raise the temperature of 1 g (1 ml) of water 1 °C (e.g., from 14.5 °C to 15.5 °C).

calorimeter—An insulated chamber to estimate energy expenditure by measuring heat dissipation from the body. This method is called direct calorimetry.

cAMP (cyclic adenosine monophosphate)—An important intracellular messenger in the action of hormones.

C_aO_2 (content of oxygen in arterial blood)—The amount of oxygen per liter of arterial blood.

capillary—The smallest vessel in the cardiovascular system. Capillary walls are only one cell thick. All exchanges of molecules between the blood and tissue fluid occur across the capillary walls.

carbohydrate (CHO)—A compound composed of carbon, hydrogen, and oxygen in a ratio of 1:2:1 (e.g., CH_2O). Carbohydrates include sugars, starches, and dietary fibers.

carboloading—Eating large quantities of carbohydrate to optimize body glycogen stores. A common practice of endurance athletes.

carboxylation—A reaction involving the addition of CO_2, catalyzed by an enzyme using biotin as its prosthetic group.

carcinogen—A cancer-inducing substance.

carnitine—A compound used to assist the transport of fatty acyl-CoA molecules from the muscle sarcoplasm across the mitochondrial inner membrane into the mitochondria for subsequent oxidation.

catabolism—Destructive metabolism whereby complex chemical compounds in the body are degraded to simpler ones (e.g., glycogen to glucose; proteins to amino acids).

catalyst—A substance that accelerates a chemical reaction, usually by temporarily combining with the substrates and lowering the activation energy, and is recovered unchanged at the end of the reaction (e.g., an enzyme).

cation—A positively charged ion or electrolyte (e.g., sodium, Na^+; calcium, Ca^{2+}).

CD (clusters of differentiation or cluster designators)—Proteins expressed on the cell surface of leukocytes (white blood cells) that can be used to identify different types of leukocyte or subsets of lymphocytes.

cecum—A blind pouch, open only at one end, at the beginning of the large intestine.

cell—The smallest discrete living unit of the body.

cellulose—A major component of plant cell walls and the most abundant nonstarch polysaccharide. Cannot be digested by human digestive enzymes.

cerebrospinal fluid (CSF)—The fluid found in the brain and spinal cord.

ceruloplasmin—A glycoprotein that binds copper and is thought to exert a protective effect against cellular damage caused by free radicals.

CHD (coronary heart disease)—Narrowing of the arteries supplying the heart muscle that can cause heart attacks.

cholecystokinin—A hormone secreted by the duodenum that acts to stimulate the secretion of enzymes in pancreatic juice.

cholesterol—A lipid transported in the blood in high- and low-density lipoproteins (HDL and LDL, respectively). High HDL levels are somewhat protective against coronary heart disease.

choline—Can be found in phospholipids (phosphatidylcholine and sphingomyelin) and is a precursor for the neurotransmitter acetylcholine.

chromium—A trace element that plays a role in glucose metabolism.

chylomicrons—A class of lipoproteins that transport exogenous (dietary) cholesterol and triglycerides from the small intestine to tissues after meals.

chyme—The food in the gastrointestinal tract mixed with various secretions of the gastrointestinal tract, forming a homogenous souplike liquid.

cirrhosis—A degenerative disease of the liver. The most common cause is excessive consumption of alcohol.

cis—A prefix indicating the geometrical isomer in which the two like groups are on the same side of a double bond with restricted rotation (e.g., in unsaturated fatty acids in which the hydrogen ions are on the same side of the double bond).

CK (creatine kinase)—An enzyme that catalyzes the transfer of phosphate from phosphocreatine to ADP to form ATP. Also known as creatine phosphokinase.

closed-circuit spirometry—A method to measure resting energy expenditure in which the subject breathes through a mouthpiece into a closed system (spirometer) prefilled with 100% oxygen.

CO_2 (carbon dioxide)—Gas produced during oxidation of carbohydrates and fats.

CoA (coenzyme A)—A molecule that acts as a carrier for acyl or acetyl groups (A stands for acetylation).

CoA-SH—Free form of coenzyme A.

coefficient of digestibility—The percentage energy of food ingested that is digested, absorbed, and available for metabolic processes in the body.

coenzyme—Small molecules that are essential in stoichiometric amounts for the activity of some enzymes. Examples include nicotinamide adenine dinucleotide (NAD), flavin adenine dinucleotide (FAD), pyridoxal phosphate (PLP), thiamin pyrophosphate (TPP), and biotin.

colon—The large intestine. This part of the intestine is mainly responsible for forming, storing, and expelling feces.

complement—Soluble proteins found in body fluids and produced by the liver. Once activated, they exert several antimicrobial effects.

complex carbohydrates—Foods containing starch and other polysaccharides as found in bread, pasta, cereals, fruits, and vegetables in contrast to simple carbohydrates such as glucose, milk sugar, and table sugar.

concentration gradient—Difference in concentration of a substance on either side of a membrane.

condensation—A reaction involving the union of two or more molecules with the elimination of a simpler group such as H_2O.

conduction—In relation to body temperature, the transfer of heat from one substance to another by direct contact.

conformation—Shape of molecules determined by rotation about single bonds, especially in polypeptide chains about carbon–carbon links.

convection—Heat exchange that occurs between a solid medium (e.g., the human body) and one that moves (e.g., air or water).

COOH or CO_2H (carboxyl group)—Acidic group of amino acids and components of the TCA cycle.

CoQ (Coenzyme Q, Q10, or ubiquinone)—An electron carrier that mediates transfer of electrons from flavoprotein to cytochrome c in the electron-transport chain that is located in the inner mitochondrial membrane.

cortisol—A steroid hormone secreted from the adrenal glands.

covalent bond—A chemical bond in which two or more atoms are held together by the interaction of their outer electrons.

covalent regulation—Control of enzyme activity by covalent bonding of phosphate groups to sites other than the active site of the enzyme.

CPT (carnitine palmitoyl transferase)—Enzyme that links the fatty acid palmitate to carnitine so that it can be transported across the inner mitochondrial membrane for subsequent oxidation. Also known as carnitine acyl transferase (CAT).

creatine (Cr)—Compound synthesized from amino acids that is the precursor of phosphocreatine, an important anaerobic energy source for high-intensity exercise.

creatinine—A product of creatine breakdown that is found in the urine. Can be measured to assess overall kidney function. An abnormally elevated blood creatinine level is seen in people with kidney insufficiency and kidney failure.

CSF (colony-stimulating factor)—A cytokine that stimulates increased production and release of leukocytes (white blood cells) from the bone marrow.

CT (computed tomography)—A method that uses ionizing radiation by an X-ray beam to create images of body segments. The CT scan produces qualitative and quantitative information about the total area of the tissue investigated, and the thickness and volume of tissues within an organ.

cutaneous—In the skin.

$C_{\bar{v}}O_2$ (content of oxygen in venous blood)—The amount of oxygen per liter of venous blood (a bar over the v signifies mixed venous blood).

cytochrome—An iron-containing heme protein of the mitochondrial electron-transport chain that can be alternately oxidized and reduced.

cytokine—Protein released from cells that acts as a chemical messenger by binding to receptors on other cells. Cytokines include interleukins (IL), tumor necrosis factors (TNF), colony-stimulating factors (CSF), and interferons (IFN).

cytosine (C)—A pyrimidine nucleotide found in DNA.

cytotoxic—Ability to kill other cells (e.g., those infected with a virus).

deamination—Reaction involving the loss of an amino (NH_2) group.

decarboxylation—Reaction involving the loss of a CO_2 group.

dehydration—Reaction involving the loss of a water molecule or loss of body water.

dehydrogenation—A form of oxidation in which hydrogen atoms are removed from a molecule.

delta efficiency (DE)—The change in energy expended per minute relative to the change in actual work accomplished per minute.

denaturation—Alteration of the physical properties and three-dimensional structure of a protein by a chemical or physical treatment that does not disrupt the primary structure but generally results in the inactivation of the protein (e.g., the inactivation of enzyme activity by the addition of a strong acid).

dental caries—Erosion or decay of tooth caused by the effects of bacteria in the mouth.

densitometry—Method used to estimate the density (mass per unit volume) of the tissues or the whole body.

DHA (dihydroxyacetone)—When linked to phosphate is a metabolite in glycolysis. In combination with pyruvate, it is marketed as an ergogenic aid.

DHEA (dehydroepiandrosterone)—A steroid hormone produced endogenously by the adrenal gland. May be marketed as a nutritional sports ergogenic as derived from herbal precursors. It is often referred to as the youth hormone.

DHEAS (dehydroepiandrosterone sulphate)—Sulphated form of DHEA, a steroid hormone produced endogenously by the adrenal gland.

diabetes mellitus—A disorder of carbohydrate metabolism caused by disturbances in production or utilization of insulin. Causes high blood glucose levels and loss of sugar in the urine.

diacylglycerol—Glycerol backbone with two fatty acids. Formed by the removal of one fatty acid from triacylglycerol. Also known as diglyceride.

diarrhea—Frequent passage of a watery fecal discharge because of a gastrointestinal disturbance or infection.

diastolic—The time between ventricular contractions (systole) in which ventricular filling occurs.

dietary reference intake (DRI)—The term used to encompass the latest nutrient recommendations by the Food and Nutrition Board of the National Academy of Sciences.

Dietary Supplement Health and Education Act (DSHEA)—Legislation passed by the United States Congress defining a dietary supplement and providing legislation to control advertising and marketing.

diet-induced thermogenesis (DIT)—The energy needed for the digestion, assimilation, and metabolism of food that is consumed (also referred to as thermic effect of food, or TEF).

diffusion—The movement of molecules from a region of high concentration to one of low concentration, brought about by their kinetic energy.

digestion—The process of breaking down food to its smallest components so that it can be absorbed in the intestine.

dihydroxyacetone—An intermediate of glycolysis.

direct calorimetry—A method of determining energy expenditure by measuring heat dissipation from the body, usually using an insulated chamber or suit.

direct calorimetry suit—A suit to estimate energy expenditure by measuring heat dissipation from the body. This method is called direct calorimetry.

disaccharide—Sugars that yield two monosaccharides on hydrolysis. Sucrose, the most common, is composed of glucose and fructose.

diuretics—Drugs that act on the kidney to promote urine formation.

d.m. (dry matter, dry material, or dry mass)—Usually refers to tissue weight after removal of water.

DNA (deoxyribonucleic acid)—The compound that forms genes (i.e., the genetic material).

DOPA (dihydroxyphenylalanine)—A neurotransmitter in the brain.

dopamine—A catecholamine neurotransmitter and hormone formed by decarboxylation of dehydroxyphenylalanine (dopa). A precursor of epinephrine (adrenaline) and norepinephrine (noradrenaline).

Douglas bag—A plastic bag (named after British scientist Claude Douglas) used to collect expired gases for a certain period of time and to measure the volume, the O_2 concentration, and the CO_2 concentration of this gas. From the measurements of inhaled and exhaled air, energy expenditure and substrate utilization can be calculated.

DRV (daily reference value)—Recommended daily intakes for the macronutrients (carbohydrate, fat, and protein) as well as cholesterol, sodium, and potassium. On a food label, the DRV is based on a 2,000 kcal (8.3 MJ) diet.

duodenum—The first 20 to 30 cm of the small intestine.

DV (daily value)—A term used in food labeling that is based on a daily energy intake of 2,000 kcal (8.3 MJ) and for the food labeled. Gives the percentage of the RDI and the DRV recommended for healthy people in the United States.

d.w. (dry weight)—Usually refers to tissue weight after removal of water.

DXA (or DEXA)—Dual-energy X-ray absorptiometry is a high-tech technique that has become the clinical standard to measure bone density. The principle is based on absorption of low-energy X-rays.

eating disorder—A psychological disorder centering on the avoidance or purging of food, such as anorexia nervosa and bulimia nervosa.

eccentric exercise—Types of exercise that involve lengthening of the muscle during activation, which can cause damage to some of the myofibers. Types of exercise that have a significant eccentric component include downhill running, bench stepping, and lowering of weights.

economy—Oxygen uptake needed to exercise at a certain work load or speed.

eicosanoids—Derivatives of fatty acids in the body that act as cell-to-cell signaling molecules. They include prostaglandins, thromboxanes, and leukotrienes.

electrolyte—A substance that, when dissolved in water, conducts an electric current. Electrolytes, which include acids, bases, and salts, usually dissociate into ions carrying either a positive charge (cation) or a negative charge (anion).

electron-transport chain (ETC)—Proteins located on the inner mitochondrial membrane that transfer electrons from reduced coenzymes NADH and $FADH_2$ to oxygen and allow protons to be pumped into the space between the inner and outer mitochondrial membranes. The flow of H^+ ions (protons) back into the inner mitochondrial matrix through the ATP synthase complex is used to drive ATP synthesis.

element—The smallest units into which a substance can be broken down chemically are the elements, each of which has different and unique properties. At least 94 elements are known to exist, but only about 12 are common in living organisms. The most abundant are oxygen, carbon, hydrogen, and nitrogen (in that order). Those four elements constitute 96% of the mass of a human.

emetics—Drugs that promote vomiting.

EMS—Eosinophilia-myalgia syndrome.

endocrine—Ductless glands that secrete hormones into the blood.

endogenous—From within the body.

energy—The ability to perform work. Energy exists in various forms, including mechanical, heat, and chemical energy.

energy balance—The balance between energy intake and energy expenditure.

energy expenditure (EE)—The energy expended per unit of time to produce power.

energy expenditure for activity (EEA)—The energy cost associated with physical activity (exercise).

enzyme—A protein with specific catalytic activity. They are designated by the suffix -ase frequently attached to the type of reaction catalyzed. Virtually all metabolic reactions in the body are dependent on and controlled by enzymes.

ephedrine—An α-adrenergic and β-adrenergic agonist that may also enhance release of norepinephrine. It has been used in the treatment of several disorders, including asthma, heart failure, rhinitis, and urinary incontinence and for its central nervous system stimulatory effects in the treatment of narcolepsy and depression. Ephedrine is on the IOC list of banned substances.

epimerization—A type of asymmetric transformation in organic molecules.

epinephrine—A hormone secreted by the adrenal gland. It is a stimulant, prepares the body for fight or flight, and is an important activator of fat and carbohydrate breakdown during exercise. Also known as adrenaline.

ergogenic—Performance enhancing.

ergogenic aids—Substances that improve exercise performance and are used in attempts to increase athletic or physical performance capacity.

ergolytic—Performance impairing.

erythrocyte—Red blood cell that contains hemoglobin and transports oxygen.

esophageal sphincter—A ringlike band of smooth muscle fibers that act as a valve between the esophagus and the stomach.

esophagus—Part of the intestinal tract located between the mouth and the stomach.

essential amino acids—Amino acids that must be obtained in the diet and cannot be synthesized in the body. Also known as indispensable amino acids.

essential fatty acids—Unsaturated fatty acids that cannot be synthesized in the body and must be obtained in the diet (e.g., linoleic acid and linolenic acid).

estimated average requirement (EAR)—Nutrient intake value estimated to meet the requirements of an average individual in a certain age and gender group.

estimated mineral requirement (EMR)—Part of the RDA pertaining to the minimal daily requirement for sodium, chloride, and potassium.

estradiol—A hormone synthesized mainly in the ovary but also in the placenta, testis, and possibly adrenal cortex.

euhydration—Normal state of body hydration (water content).

eumenorrhea—Occurrence of normal menstrual cycles.

evaporation—The loss of water that occurs when water on a surface changes from a liquid to a gas.

excretion—The removal of metabolic wastes.

exogenous—From outside the body.

exogenous carbohydrate oxidation—Oxidation of carbohydrates that have been ingested or infused but are not from body stores.

extracellular fluid (ECF)—Body fluid that is located outside the cells, including the blood plasma, interstitial fluid, cerebrospinal fluid, synovial fluid, and ocular fluid.

F-6-P (fructose-6-phosphate)—A metabolic intermediate in glycolysis.

FA (fatty acid)—A type of fat having a carboxylic acid group (COOH) at one end of the molecule and a methyl (CH_3) group at the other end, separated by a hydrocarbon chain that can vary in length. A typical structure of a fatty acid is $CH_3(CH_2)_{14}COOH$ (palmitic acid or palmitate).

FABPc (cytosolic fatty acid–binding protein)—A protein found in liver and muscle that binds fatty acids in the cytosol of the cell. Involved in transport from the plasma membrane to mitochondria.

FABPpm (plasma membrane fatty acid–binding protein)—A protein found in liver and muscle involved in transport of fatty acids across the plasma membrane.

FAD (flavin adenine dinucleotide, oxidized form)—A coenzyme important in energy metabolism.

$FADH_2$ (flavin adenine dinucleotide, reduced form)—Reduced form of the coenzyme FAD.

fasting—Starvation; abstinence from eating that may be partial or complete.

fat—Fat molecules contain the same structural elements as carbohydrates, but they have little oxygen relative to carbon and hydrogen and are poorly soluble in water. Fats are also known as lipids (derived from the Greek word *lipos*), and fat is a general name for oils, fats, waxes, and related compounds. Oils are liquid at room temperature, whereas fats are solid.

FAT/CD36—Fatty acid translocator involved in the transport of fatty acids across the plasma membrane

fatty acid–binding protein (FABP)—A protein found in liver and muscle that binds fatty acids to maintain a low intracellular free fatty acid concentration.

FDA—United States Food and Drug Administration.

FDP (fructose-1,6-diphosphate)—A metabolic intermediate in glycolysis.

FDPase (fructose-1,6-diphosphatase)—Enzyme that catalyzes the conversion of fructose-1,6-diphosphate to fructose-6-phosphate, a reaction involved in gluconeogenesis.

feces—The excrement discharged from the intestines, consisting of bacteria, cells from the intestines, secretions, and a small amount of food residue.

female athlete triad—A syndrome characterized by the three conditions prevalent in female athletes: amenorrhea, disordered eating, and osteoporosis.

ferritin—A protein that is used to store iron. Ferritin is mostly found in the liver, spleen, and bone marrow. Soluble ferritin is released from cells into the blood plasma in direct proportion to cellular ferritin content. Hence, the serum ferritin concentration can be used to indicate the status of the body's iron stores.

FFA (free fatty acid)—A fatty acid that is not esterified to glycerol or any other molecule. See FA (fatty acid).

FFM (fat-free mass)—Lean mass of a tissue or the whole body.

fiber—Indigestible carbohydrates.

fish oil—Oils high in unsaturated fats extracted from the bodies of fish or fish parts, especially the livers. The oils are used as dietary supplements.

flux—The rate of flow through a metabolic pathway.

FMN (flavin mononucleotide, oxidized form)—A coenzyme important in energy metabolism.

FMNH$_2$ (flavin mononucleotide, reduced form)—Reduced form of the coenzyme FMN.

folic acid or folate—A water-soluble vitamin required in the synthesis of nucleic acids. It appears to be essential in preventing certain types of anemia.

food diary—A written record of sequential food intake over a period of time. Details associated with the food intake are often recorded as well.

fractional breakdown rate (FBR)—The relative rate of protein breakdown, which is calculated from measurements using isotopic tracers.

fractional synthesis rate (FSR)—The relative rate of protein synthesis, which is calculated from measurements using isotopic tracers.

free radical—An atom or molecule that possess at least one unpaired electron in its outer orbit. Important free radicals include the superoxide ($\cdot O_2^-$), hydroxyl ($\cdot OH$), and nitric oxide ($\cdot NO$) radicals. They are highly reactive and may cause damage to lipid membranes, causing membrane instability and increased permeability. Free radicals can also cause oxidative damage to proteins, including enzymes, and damage to DNA.

fTRP—Free tryptophan (used to distinguish from tryptophan that is bound to protein). Tryptophan is an essential amino acid and a precursor of the neurotransmitter serotonin in the brain.

G-1-P (glucose-1-phosphate)—Compound formed from the breakdown of glycogen.

G-6-P (glucose-6-phosphate)—Compound formed by the addition of a phosphate group to a glucose molecule by the action of hexokinase. Can also be formed from G-1-P by glucose phosphate isomerase. G-6-P is the starting substrate for glycolysis.

GABA (γ-amino butyric acid)—A neurotransmitter in the brain.

gallbladder—A digestive organ that stores bile (produced in the liver), which is used in the digestion and absorption of fats in the duodenum.

gastric emptying—The rate at which substances (food and fluids) leave the stomach into the small intestine. A high gastric emptying rate is desirable for sports drinks.

gastric juice—The secretions by the gastric mucosa. Gastric juice contains water, hydrochloric acid, and pepsinogen as major components.

gastrin—A hormone secreted by the stomach that stimulates gastric secretion of hydrochloric acid and pepsin.

gastrointestinal tract—Gastrointestinal system or alimentary tract. The main sites in the body used for digestion and absorption of nutrients. It consists of the mouth, esophagus, stomach, small intestine, large intestine, rectum, and anus.

GDP (guanosine diphosphate)—Compound formed from the breakdown of guanosine triphosphate (GTP).

gene—A specific sequence in DNA that codes for a particular protein. Genes are located on the chromosomes. Each gene is found in a definite position (locus).

genotype—The genetic composition or assortment of genes that together with environmental influences determines the appearance or phenotype of a person.

geometrical isomerism—A form of stereoisomerism in which the difference arises because of hindered rotation about a double bond. An unsaturated fatty acid containing one carbon double bond has two isomers, depending on whether the hydrogen atoms are on the same (cis) side or the opposite (trans) side of the molecule.

ginseng—A root found in Asia and the United States, although the Asian variety is more easily obtainable. Ginseng has been a popular nutritional supplement and medication in Asia for centuries.

glandulars—Extracts from animal glands (such as the adrenals, thymus, pituitary, and testes) that are claimed to enhance the function of the equivalent gland in the human body. Glandular extracts are degraded during the digestive process, however, and so cannot exert a pharmacological effect.

glomerular filtration rates—Measure of the ability of the kidney to filter and remove waste products.

gluconeogenesis—The synthesis of glucose from noncarbohydrate precursors such as glycerol, ketoacids, or amino acids.

GLUT—Glucose (or other monosaccharide) transporter found in cell membranes, including those of the muscle and liver.

GLUT2—Isoform of the glucose transporter found in the liver and epithelial cell membranes of the gut.

GLUT4—Isoform of the glucose transporter found in sarcolemma of muscle fibers.

GLUT5—Isoform of the glucose transporter found in the epithelial cell membranes of the gut. This one is specific for fructose.

glutamate—Amino acid that acts as a neurotransmitter and a precursor of other neurotransmitters.

glutamine—One of the 20 amino acids commonly found in proteins.

glycemic index (GI)—Increase in blood glucose and insulin in response to a meal. The GI of a food is expressed against a reference food, usually glucose.

glycemic load (GL)—Increase in blood glucose and insulin response to a meal (like glycemic index) but does take into account the amount of that food that is normally consumed.

glycerokinase—Enzyme involved in phosphorylation of glycerol to glycerol-3-phosphate.

glycerol—Three-carbon molecule that is the backbone structure of triglycerides.

glycogen—Polymer of glucose used as a storage form of carbohydrate in the liver and muscles.

glycogenolysis—The breakdown of glycogen into glucose-1-phosphate by the action of phosphorylase.

glycolysis—The sequence of reactions that converts glucose (or glycogen) to pyruvate.

glycoprotein—A protein that is attached to one or more sugar molecules.

glycosidic bond—A chemical bond in which the oxygen atom is the common link between a carbon of one sugar molecule and the carbon of another. Glycogen, the glucose polymer, is a branched-chain polysaccharide consisting of glucose molecules linked by glycosidic bonds.

gonadotrophic hormones—Hormones released from the anterior pituitary gland that promote sex steroid hormone synthesis by the ovaries in females and the testes in males.

gross efficiency (GE)—The ratio of the total work accomplished to the energy expended. Humans are approximately 20% efficient.

gross energy value of food—The amount of energy in food when measured in a bomb calorimeter. This energy is more than the energy that would be available to the human body if the food was eaten.

GTP (guanosine triphosphate)—High-energy phosphate compound similar to ATP.

guanine (G)—A purine nucleotide base found in DNA.

gum—A form of water-soluble dietary fiber found in plants.

H$^+$—Hydrogen ion or proton.

H$_2$O$_2$—Hydrogen peroxide.

half-life—Time in which half the quantity or concentration of a substance is eliminated or removed.

HCl—Hydrochloric acid; part of gastric digestive juices.

HCO$_3^-$—Bicarbonate ion, the principal extracellular buffer.

HDL (high-density lipoprotein)—A protein-lipid complex in the blood plasma that facilitates the transport of triacylglycerols, cholesterol, and phospholipids.

HDL cholesterol (high-density lipoprotein cholesterol)—One way in which lipids are transported in the blood.

heart burn—Indigestion and a burning pain as a result of entering of acidic gastric juices into the esophagus.

heatstroke—Elevated body temperature of 41 °C (105.8 °F) or greater caused by exposure to excessive heat or high levels of heat production and diminished heat loss. May result in tissue damage and is potentially fatal.

heat syncope—Fainting caused by excessive heat exposure.

helix—A spiral having a uniform diameter and a periodic spacing between the coils. A common secondary structure of proteins and DNA.

hematocrit—Proportion of the blood volume that is occupied by the cellular elements (red cells, white cells, and platelets). Also known as the packed cell volume.

hematuria—Red blood cells or hemoglobin in the urine.

heme—Molecular ring structure that is incorporated in the hemoglobin molecule enabling this protein to carry oxygen.

hemicellulose—A form of dietary fiber found in plants. Differs from cellulose in that it can be hydrolyzed by acid outside of the body.

hemochromatosis—Presence of excessive iron in the body resulting in an enlarged liver and liver damage in susceptible people.

hemodilution—Thinning of the blood caused by an expansion of the plasma volume without an equivalent rise in red blood cells.

hemoglobin—The red, iron-containing respiratory pigment found in red blood cells. Hemoglobin is important in the transport of respiratory gases and in the regulation of blood pH.

hemolysis—Destruction of red blood cells within the circulation.

hemorrhage—Damage to blood vessel walls resulting in bleeding.

hemorrheology—Study of the viscous properties of blood.

hepatic glucose output—Liver glucose output; the glucose released from the liver as a result of glycogenolysis or gluconeogenesis.

hexokinase (HK)—Enzyme that catalyzes the phosphorylation of glucose to form glucose-6-phosphate.

HMB (beta-hydroxy-beta-methylbutyrate)—A metabolic by-product of the amino acid leucine.

homeostasis—The tendency to maintain uniformity or stability of the internal environment of the cell or of the body.

hormone—An organic chemical produced in cells of one part of the body (usually an endocrine gland) that diffuses or is transported by the blood circulation to cells in other parts of the body, where it regulates and coordinates their activities.

hormone-sensitive lipase—Enzyme that splits triacylglycerols into fatty acids and glycerol. It is regulated by hormones (mainly by epinephrine and insulin).

humoral—Fluid borne.

hydration—A reaction involving the incorporation of a molecule of water into a compound or a term relating to the state of the body water content.

hydrogen bond—A weak intermolecular or intramolecular attraction resulting from the interaction of a hydrogen atom and an electronegative atom possessing a lone pair of electrons (e.g., oxygen or nitrogen). Hydrogen bonding is important in DNA and RNA and is responsible for much of the tertiary structure of proteins.

hydrolysis—A reaction in which an organic compound is split by interaction with water into simpler compounds.

hydroxylation—A reaction involving the addition of a hydroxyl (OH) group to a molecule.

hyperhydration—Increased body-water content above normal level.

hyperthermia—Elevated body temperature (>37 °C or 98.6 °F).

hypertonic—Having a higher concentration of dissolved particles (osmolality) than that of another solution with which it is being compared (usually blood plasma, which has an osmolality of 290 mOsm/kg).

hyperventilation—A state in which an increased amount of air enters the pulmonary alveoli (increased alveolar ventilation), resulting in reduction of carbon dioxide tension and eventually leading to alkalosis.

hyponatremia—Below-normal serum sodium concentration (<140 mmol/L).

hypothalamus—Region at base of brain responsible for integration of sensory input and effector responses in regulation of body temperature. Also contains centers for control of hunger, appetite, and thirst.

hypothermia—Lower than normal body temperature.

hypotonic—Having a lower concentration of dissolved particles (osmolality) than that of another solution with which it is being compared (usually blood plasma, which has an osmolality of 290 mOsm/kg).

hypovolemia—Reduced blood volume.

Hz—Unit of frequency in cycles per second.

IDL—Intermediate-density lipoproteins.

IFN (interferon)—A type of cytokine. Some interferons inhibit viral replication in infected cells.

Ig (immunoglobulin)—Same as antibody.

IGF—Insulin-like growth factor.

immune system—Cells and soluble molecules involved in tissue repair after injury and in the protection of the body against infection.

immunodepression—Lowered functional activity of the immune system.

IMP—Inosine monophosphate. A breakdown product of AMP.

IMTG (intramuscular triacylglycerol)—Storage form of fat found in muscle fibers.

in vitro—Within a glass, observable in a test tube, in an artificial environment.

in vivo—Within the living body.

incisors—Anterior teeth that are used for cutting food.

indirect calorimetry—A method to measure energy expenditure and substrate utilization on the basis of gas exchange measurements. The term *indirect* refers to the measurement of O_2 uptake and CO_2 production rather than the direct measurement of heat transfer.

inflammation—The body's response to injury, which includes redness (increased blood flow) and swelling (edema) caused by increased capillary permeability.

inosine—The fifth base of nucleic acids. Important because it fails to form specific pair bonds with the other bases. In transfer RNAs, this property is used in the anticodon to allow matching of a single tRNA to several codons.

insoluble fiber—Fiber that does not dissolve in water.

insomnia—Difficulty with sleeping.

insulin—A hormone secreted by the pancreas involved in carbohydrate metabolism, particularly in the control of the blood glucose concentration.

interleukin—Type of cytokine produced by leukocytes and some other tissues. Acts as a chemical messenger, rather like a hormone, but usually with localized effects.

interstitial—Fluid-filled spaces that lie between cells.

IOC—International Olympic Committee.

ion—Any atom or molecule that has an electrical charge due to loss or gain of valency (outer shell) electrons. Ions may carry a positive charge (cation) or a negative charge (anion).

ionic bond—A bond in which valence electrons are either lost or gained, and atoms that are oppositely charged are held together by electrostatic forces.

ischemia—Reduced blood supply to a tissue or organ.

isoform—Chemically distinct forms of an enzyme with identical activities usually coded by different genes. Also called isoenzyme.

isomer—One of two or more substances that have an identical molecular composition and relative molecular mass but different structure because of a different arrangement of atoms within the molecule.

isotonicity—Having the same concentration of dissolved particles (osmolality) as that of another solution with which it is being compared (usually blood plasma, which has an osmolality of 290 mOsm/kg).

isotope—One of a set of chemically identical species of an atom that have the same atomic number but different mass numbers (e.g., 12-isotopes, 13-isotopes, and 14-isotopes of carbon whose atomic number is 12).

IU—International units.

jejunum—The middle and longest part of the small intestine where a lot of the absorption of nutrients takes place. The jejunum is approximately 1 to 2 m long.

joule (J)—Unit of energy according to the Systeme Internationale. One joule is the amount of energy needed to move a mass of 1 g at a velocity of 1 m/s.

Ka—Rate constant of a reaction (e.g., for the dissociation of a weak acid into its conjugate base).

Kerckring, folds of—Folds in the intestinal mucosa of the gastrointestinal tract.

keto-acids—An acid containing a ketone group (-C = O) in addition to the acid group(s).

ketogenesis—The synthesis of ketones such as acetoacetate, 3-hydroxybutyrate, and acetone.

ketone bodies—Acidic organic compounds produced during the incomplete oxidation of fatty acids in the liver. Contain a carboxyl group (-COOH) and a ketone group (-C = O). Examples include acetoacetate and 3-hydroxybutyrate.

KIC—alpha-keto isocaproate; a metabolite of the amino acid leucine.

kinase—An enzyme that regulates a phosphorylation-dephosphorylation reaction (i.e., the addition or removal of a phosphate group). This process is one important way in which enzyme activity can be regulated.

kJ (kilojoule)—Unit of energy ($kJ = 10^3 J$).

KM—A kinetic parameter (called the Michaelis constant) used to characterize an enzyme, defined as the concentration of substrate that permits half maximal rate of reaction.

lactase—Enzyme responsible for the splitting of lactose into galactose and glucose.

lactate dehydrogenase (LDH)—Enzyme that catalyzes the reversible reduction of pyruvate to lactate.

lacteal—Lymphatic vessel that drains the villi in the gut wall.

lactic acid—Metabolic end product of anaerobic glycolysis.

lactose—Milk sugar, a disaccharide linking a molecule of glucose and a molecule of galactose.

lactovegetarian—A vegetarian who includes milk products in the diet.

laxatives—Drugs that act on the gut to promote defecation.

LCAT—Lecithin-cholesterol acyl-transferase.

LDL (low-density lipoproteins)—A protein-lipid complex in the blood plasma that facilitates the transport of triacylglycerols, cholesterol, and phospholipids.

LDL-C (low-density lipoprotein cholesterol)—A way in which cholesterol is transported in the blood. High blood levels are associated with increased incidence of coronary heart disease.

lean body mass (LBM)—All parts of the body, excluding fat.

lecithin—Common name for phosphatidylcholine, the most abundant phospholipid found in cell membranes.

lecithin (phosphatidyl choline)—A phospholipid that occurs naturally in a variety of food items (beans, eggs, and wheat germ).

legume—The high-protein fruit or pod of vegetables, including beans, peas, and lentils.

leptin—Regulatory hormone produced by fat cells. When released into the circulation, it influences the hypothalamus to control appetite.

leucine—An essential amino acid that is alleged to slow the breakdown of muscle protein during strenuous exercise and to improve gains in muscle mass with strength training.

leukocyte—White blood cell. Important in inflammation and immune defense.

leukocytosis—Increased number of leukocytes in the circulation.

lingual lipase—A fat-splitting enzyme secreted by cells at the base of the tongue.

linoleic acid—An essential fatty acid.

linolenic acid—An essential fatty acid.

lipase—An enzyme that catalyzes the hydrolysis of triacylglycerols into fatty acids and glycerol.

lipid—A compound composed of carbon, hydrogen, oxygen, and sometimes other elements. Lipids dissolve in organic solvents but not in water and include triacylglycerol, cholesterol, and phospholipids. Lipids are commonly called fats.

lipid peroxidation—Oxidation of fatty acids in lipid structures (e.g., membranes) caused by the actions of free radicals.

lipolysis—The breakdown of triacylglycerols into fatty acids and glycerol.

lipoprotein lipase (LPL)—Enzyme that catalyzes the breakdown of triacylglycerols in plasma lipoproteins.

LNAA—Large neutral amino acid.

long-chain fatty acid (LCFA)—Part of triacylglycerols. Hydrocarbon chains with 12 or more carbon atoms and the most abundant type of fatty acids. Palmitic acid and oleic acid are the most abundant long-chain fatty acids in humans.

long-chain triacylglycerols—Triacylglycerol consisting of glycerol and three long-chain fatty acids

LRNI—Lower reference nutrient intake.

lymphocyte—Type of white blood cell important in the acquired immune response. Includes both T cells and B cells. The latter produce antibodies.

lysis—The process of disintegration of a cell.

lysosome—A membranous vesicle found in the cell cytoplasm. Lysosomes contain digestive enzymes capable of autodigesting the cell.

lysozymes—Enzymes that break down proteins and attack bacteria.

mol (molar)—Unit of concentration (nmol: nanomolar = 10^{-9} mol; μmol: micromolar = 10^{-6} mol; mmol: millimolar = 10^{-3} mol).

macromineral—Dietary elements essential to life processes that each constitute at least 0.01% of total body mass. The seven macrominerals are potassium, sodium, chloride, calcium, magnesium, phosphorus, and sulfur.

macronutrients—Nutrients ingested in relatively large amounts (carbohydrate, fat, protein, and water).

macrophage or monocyte—Type of white blood cell that can ingest and destroy foreign material and initiate the acquired immune response.

maltodextrin—A glucose polymer (commonly containing 6 to 12 glucose molecules) that exerts lesser osmotic effects compared with glucose and is used in a variety of sports drinks as the main source of carbohydrate.

maltose—A disaccharide that yields two molecules of glucose upon hydrolysis.

masticating—Chewing of food.

McArdle's disease—A glycogen phosphorylase deficiency resulting in an inability to break down glycogen.

mechanical digestion—Breaking down food by chewing.

medium-chain fatty acid (MCFA)—A fatty acid with 8 or 10 carbon atoms.

medium-chain triacylglycerol (MCT)—Triacylglycerol (triglyceride) containing fatty acids with hydrocarbon chain lengths of 6 to 12 carbons.

megadose—An excessive amount of a substance in comparison to a normal dose (such as the RDA). Usually used to refer to vitamin supplements.

menarche—The onset of menstruation in adolescent girls.

menstruation—Monthly bleeding and discharge of the outer uterine wall in healthy females.

metabolic acidosis—A metabolic derangement of acid–base balance where the blood pH is abnormally low.

metabolite—A product of a metabolic reaction.

metalloenzyme—An enzyme that needs a mineral component (e.g., copper, iron, magnesium, and zinc) to function effectively.

METS (metabolic equivalents)—A measurement of energy expenditure expressed as multiples of the resting metabolic rate. One MET equals an oxygen uptake rate of approximately 3.5 ml $O_2 \cdot$ kg b.w. $^{-1} \cdot$ min^{-1}.

micromineral or trace element—Dietary elements essential to life processes that each make up less than 0.01% of total-body mass and are needed in quantities of less than 100 mg a day. Among the 14 trace elements are iron, zinc, copper, chromium, and selenium.

micronutrients—Organic vitamins and inorganic minerals that must be consumed in relatively small amounts in the diet to maintain health.

microvilli—Very small (1 μm) fingerlike projections of a cell membrane. They occur on the luminal surface of the cells in the small intestine.

min (minute)—Unit of time; 60 seconds.

mineral—An inorganic element found in nature though the term is usually reserved for those elements that are solid. In nutrition, the term mineral is usually used to classify dietary elements essential to life processes. Examples are calcium and iron.

mitochondrial matrix—The substance occupying the space enclosed by the inner membrane of a mitochondrion. It contains enzymes, filaments of DNA, ribosomes, granules, and inclusions of protein crystals, glycogen, and lipid.

mitochondrion—Oval or spherical organelle containing the enzymes of the tricarboxylic acid cycle and electron-transport chain. Site of oxidative phosphorylation (resynthesis of ATP involving the use of oxygen).

mitogen—Chemical that can stimulate lymphocytes to proliferate (undergo rapid cell divisions).

mitosis—A type of cell division in which each of the two daughter cells receives exactly the same number of chromosomes present in the nucleus of the parent cell.

mole—The amount of a chemical compound whose mass in grams is equivalent to its molecular weight, which is the sum of the atomic weights of its constituent atoms.

molecule—An aggregation of at least two atoms of the same or different elements held together by special forces (covalent bonds) and having a precise chemical formula (e.g., O_2, $C_6H_{12}O_6$).

monoacylglycerol—Glycerol backbone with one fatty acid. Also known as monoglyceride.

monosaccharide—A simple sugar that cannot be hydrolyzed to smaller units (e.g., glucose, fructose, and galactose).

motility—The movement of food through the gastrointestinal tract by coordinated muscular contractions of the intestine.

motor unit—All the muscle fibers supplied by a single motor neuron.

MRI (magnetic resonance imaging)—An imaging technique that generates pictures of body tissues and compartments. The results are somewhat similar to those obtained by a CT scan, but with MRI electromagnetic radiation is used rather than ionizing radiation.

mucosa—Layer of cells lining the mouth, nasal passages, airways, and gut that present a barrier to pathogen entry into the body.

myofibril—Threadlike 1- to 3-μm-thick structures containing the contractile proteins and continuous from end to end in the muscle fiber.

myoglobin—A protein that functions as an intracellular respiratory pigment that is capable of binding oxygen and releasing it only at very low partial pressures.

myosin—One of the major contractile proteins in muscle found in the thick filaments.

NAD⁺ (nicotinamide adenine dinucleotide, oxidized form)—A coenzyme important in energy metabolism.

NADH (nicotinamide adenine dinucleotide, reduced form)—Reduced form of the coenzyme NAD.

NADP⁺ (nicotinamide adenine dinucleotide phosphate, oxidized form)—A coenzyme important in energy metabolism.

NADPH (nicotinamide adenine dinucleotide phosphate, reduced form)—Reduced form of the coenzyme NAD.

nandrolone—A steroid with androgenic and anabolic properties.

NCAA—National Collegiate Athletic Association (United States).

NEFA—Nonesterified fatty acid. Same as free fatty acid (FFA) or fatty acid (FA).

net efficiency (NE)—The work accomplished divided by the energy expended minus resting energy expenditure.

neurotransmitters—Endogenous signaling molecules that transfer information from one nerve ending to the next.

neutrophil—Type of white blood cell that can ingest and destroy foreign material. Important as a first line of defense against bacteria.

NH_2—Amino group.

NH_4^+—Ammonium ion.

NIDDM—Non-insulin-dependent diabetes mellitus. Also know as type 2 diabetes.

nitrogen balance—A dietary state in which the input and output of nitrogen is balanced so that the body neither gains nor loses tissue protein.

NK (natural killer) cell—A type of lymphocyte important in eliminating viral infections and preventing cancer.

NKCA—Natural killer cytotoxic activity. The ability of NK cells to destroy virally infected cells and tumor cells.

NO—Nitric oxide.

NO·—Nitric oxide radical.

nonessential amino acids—Amino acids that can be synthesized in the body.

norepinephrine—Catecholamine neurohormone, the neurotransmitter of most of the sympathetic nervous system (of so-called adrenergic neurons). Also known as noradrenaline.

nutraceutical—A nutrient that may function as a pharmaceutical (drug) when taken in certain quantities.

nutrient—Substances found in food that provide energy or promote growth and repair of tissues.

nutrition—The total of the processes of ingestion, digestion, absorption, and metabolism of food and the subsequent assimilation of nutrient materials into the tissues.

nutrition density—Amount of essential nutrients expressed per unit of energy in the food.

O_2—Oxygen molecule.

O_2^- (superoxide radical)—A highly reactive free radical.

obesity—An excessive accumulation of body fat. Usually reserved for people who are 20% or more above the average weight for their size.

OH—Hydroxyl group.

OH⁻ (hydroxyl radical)—A highly reactive free radical.

oligosaccharide—A saccharide of a small number of component sugars, either O or N, linked to the next sugar.

osmolality—A measure of the total dissolved particle concentration. Units are mOsm/kg.

osmolarity—A measure of the total concentration of a solution. The number of moles of solute per liter of solvent typically expressed in mOsm/L.

osmoreceptors—Sensory cells in the hypothalamus capable of detecting changes in osmolarity of the blood.

osmosis—The diffusion of water molecules from the lesser to the greater concentration of solute (dissolved substance) when two solutions are separated by a membrane that selectively prevents the passage of solute molecules but is permeable to water molecules.

osteoblasts—Cells responsible for mineralization of bone.

osteoclasts—Cells responsible for breakdown (demineralization) of bone.

osteoporosis—A weakening of the bone structure that occurs when the rate of demineralization exceeds the rate of bone formation.

ovolactovegetarian—A vegetarian who also consumes eggs and milk products.

ovulation—Monthly release of an ova (egg) from the ovaries in females.

oxidation—A reaction involving the loss of electrons from an atom. It is always accompanied by a reduction. For example, pyruvate is reduced by NADH to form lactate. In the reverse reaction, lactate is oxidized by NAD⁺ when pyruvate is reformed.

oxidative phosphorylation—Resynthesis of ATP involving the use of oxygen.

Panax ginseng—Chinese or Korean ginseng.

Panax japonicum—Japanese ginseng from India, southern China, and Japan.

Panax quinquefolium—American ginseng.

pancreas—An organ located below and behind the stomach. It secretes insulin and glucagon (involved in plasma glucose regulation) and pancreatic enzymes involved in the digestion of fats and protein in the small intestine.

pancreatic duct—The connecting tube between pancreas and duodenum through which pancreatic juice is transported into the duodenum.

pancreatic juice—The secretions of the pancreas that are transported by the pancreatic duct to the duodenum. Pancreatic juice contains bicarbonate and the digestive enzymes amylase, lipase, and trypsin.

parathyroid hormone (PTH)—Hormone secreted from the parathyroid glands and involved in regulation of the blood plasma calcium ion concentration.

pathogen—Microorganism that can cause symptoms of disease.

PCO_2—Partial pressure of carbon dioxide.

PCr—Phosphocreatine or creatine phosphate. An important energy source in very high-intensity exercise.

PDH complex—Pyruvate dehydrogenase complex, a complex multienzyme system that catalyzes the conversion of pyruvate to acetyl CoA + CO_2.

pectin—A form of soluble dietary fiber found in some fruits.

PEM (protein energy malnutrition)—Inadequate intake of dietary protein and energy.

pepsin—A protein digestive enzyme secreted in pancreatic juice.

pepsinogen—The inactive form (storage form) of pepsin. Pepsinogen is stored in the cells of the stomach wall.

peptide—Small compound formed by the bonding of two or more amino acids. Larger chains of linked amino acids are called polypeptides or proteins.

peptide bond—The bond formed by the condensation of the amino group and the carboxyl group of a pair of amino acids. Peptides are constructed from a linear array of amino acids joined together by a series of peptide bonds.

peristalsis—Waves of contraction in smooth muscle of the digestive tract. It involves circular and longitudinal muscle fibers at successive locations along the tract and serves to propel the contents of the tract in one direction.

pH—A measure of acidity or alkalinity. $pH = -\log_{10}[H^+]$.

phagocyte—Leukocyte capable of ingesting and digesting microorganisms.

phenotype—The appearance or physiological characteristic of an individual that results from the interaction of the genotype and the environment.

phosphagen—The term given to both high-energy phosphate compounds, adenosine triphosphate and phosphocreatine.

phosphodiesterase—An enzyme that cleaves phosphodiesters to give a phosphomonoester and a free hydroxyl group.

phosphoenol pyruvate (PEP)—A metabolic intermediate in glycolysis.

Phosphofructokinase (PFK)—The rate-limiting enzyme in glycolysis.

phospholipids—Fats containing a phosphate group that on hydrolysis yield fatty acids, glycerol, and a nitrogenous compound. Lecithin is an example. Phospholipids are important components of membranes.

phosphorylase—Enzyme that breaks down the glucose polymer glycogen into molecules of glucose-1-phosphate.

phosphorylation—A reaction that involves the addition of a phosphate (PO_3^{2-}) group to a molecule. Many enzymes are activated by the covalent bonding of a phosphate group. The oxidative phosphorylation of ADP forms ATP.

photosynthesis—Process by which green plants and algae absorb light energy and use it to synthesize organic compounds, including glucose.

Pi—Inorganic phosphate (HPO_4^{2-}).

PKU (phenylketonuria)—Congenital lack of an enzyme that metabolizes phenylalanine, an essential amino acid. This condition may lead to mental retardation if not detected early in life.

plaque—The material that accumulates on the inner layer of arteries and contributes to atherosclerosis. It contains cholesterol, lipids, platelets, and other debris. Plaque on the inner layers of the arterial wall is a cause of coronary heart disease.

plasma—The liquid portion of the blood in which the blood cells are suspended. Typically accounts for 55% to 60% of the total blood volume. Differs from serum in that it contains fibrinogen, the clot-forming protein.

PO₂—Partial pressure of oxygen.

polypeptide—A peptide that, upon hydrolysis, yields more than two amino acids.

polyphenols—A large class of naturally occurring compounds that includes the flavonoids, flavonols, flavonones, and anthocyanidins. These compounds contain a number of phenolic hydroxyl (-OH) groups attached to ring structures, which confers them with powerful antioxidant activity.

polysaccharide—Polymers of (arbitrarily) more than about 10 monosaccharide residues linked glycosidically in branched or unbranched chains. Examples include starch and glycogen.

postabsorptive state—The period after a meal has been absorbed from the gastrointestinal tract.

power—Work performed per unit of time.

precursor—A substance from which another substance, usually more active or mature, is formed.

prohormones—A protein hormone before processing to remove parts of its sequence and thus make it active.

prosthetic group—A coenzyme that is tightly bound to an enzyme.

protease—An enzyme that catalyzes the digestion or cleavage of proteins.

protein—Biological macromolecules composed of a chain of covalently linked amino acids. Proteins may have structural or functional roles.

protein breakdown—See protein degradation.

protein degradation—The process in which the individual amino acids from a protein are disconnected.

protein synthesis—The process in which individual amino acids, whether of exogenous or endogenous origin, are connected to each other in peptide linkage in a specific order dictated by the sequence of nucleotides in DNA.

ptyalin—A digestive enzyme found in saliva that begins the digestion of starches in the mouth (also called α-amylase).

PUFA (polyunsaturated fatty acid)—Fatty acid that contains more than one carbon–carbon double bond.

pyloric sphincter—See pylorus.

pylorus—A circular muscle that controls the entry of stomach contents into the duodenum.

pyrogen—A substance that causes body temperature to be elevated, as in fever, and be regulated at a higher set point.

pyruvate—Three-carbon molecule that is the end product of glycolysis.

pyruvate dehydrogenase (PDH)—The enzyme catalyzing the conversion of pyruvate to acetyl-CoA.

Q—Blood flow rate or cardiac output.

R (group)—Side chain of an amino acid.

R_a (rate of appearance)—Usually referring to the rate at which a substance enters the blood circulation.

radiation—Transfer of energy waves that are emitted by one object and absorbed by another (e.g., solar energy from sunlight).

radiolabeled isotopes—An isotope is a specific form of a chemical element. It differs from atoms of other forms (isotopes) of the same element in the number of neutrons in its nucleus. Radiolabeled isotopes will transmit radiation and are used as tracers.

rate-limiting enzyme—An enzyme in a metabolic pathway that regulates the slowest step in the pathway and hence limits the rate of flux through the pathway.

rating of perceived exertion (RPE)—A subjective rating, on a numerical scale, used to express the perceived difficulty of a given exercise task.

RBC—Red blood cell (erythrocyte).

R_d (rate of disappearance)—Usually refers to the rate at which a substance leaves the blood circulation.

RDA (recommended dietary allowance)—Recommended intake of a particular nutrient that meets the needs of nearly all (97%) healthy individuals of similar age and gender. The RDAs are established by the Food and Nutrition Boards of the National Academy of Sciences.

RDI (reference daily intake)—Nutrient intake standards set by the FDA based on the 1968 RDA for various vitamins and minerals. RDIs have been set for infants, toddlers, people over 4 years of age, and pregnant and lactating women.

reactive hypoglycemia—See rebound hypoglycemia.

rebound hypoglycemia—Reactive hypoglycemia. A decrease in blood glucose concentration to hypoglycemic levels (< 3.5 mmol/L) in response to carbohydrate feeding before exercise.

rectum—Last portion of the colon, connected to the anus.

reduction—A reaction in which a molecule gains electrons.

reesterification—Process during which fatty acids are not released into the circulation, but are used to form new triacylglycerols within the adipose tissue.

relative humidity—The percentage of moisture in the air compared with the amount of moisture needed to cause saturation, which is taken as 100%.

reperfusion—Restoration of the blood supply to a tissue or organ.

RER (respiratory exchange ratio)—The ratio of carbon dioxide produced divided by oxygen consumption, representing a measure of substrate utilization at the whole-body level.

respiration chamber—A chamber in which the exchange of CO_2 and O_2 is measured to estimate energy expenditure and substrate utilization.

ribosome—Extremely small organelle composed of protein and RNA that is either free in the cytoplasm or attached to the membranes of the endoplasmic reticulum of a cell. The site of protein synthesis.

RMR (resting metabolic rate)—Energy expenditure under resting conditions.

RNA (ribonucleic acid)—A nucleic acid essential for protein synthesis (mRNA: messenger RNA; tRNA: transfer RNA; rRNA: ribosomal RNA).

RNI (recommended nutrient intake)—Defined as the level of intake required to meet the known nutritional needs of more than 97.5% of healthy persons. In the United Kingdom the RNI is similar to the original RDA.

ROS (reactive oxygen species)—Collective name for free radicals and other highly reactive molecules derived from molecular oxygen. ROS include superoxide radical ($O_2^-\cdot$), hydroxyl radical ($OH^-\cdot$), hydrogen peroxide (H_2O_2), and perchlorous acid (HOCl).

RQ (respiratory quotient)—The ratio of the rate of carbon dioxide production divided by the rate of oxygen consumption, which can be used to establish the approximate pattern of substrate utilization by an organ or tissue (e.g., muscle).

s (second)—A unit of time.

saccharine—An artificial sweetener made from coal tar.

saponins—One of the characteristic compounds in ginseng. Also referred to as ginsenosides or panaxosides.

sarcolemma—The cell membrane of a muscle fiber.

sarcomere—The smallest contractile unit or segment of a muscle fiber; defined as the region between two Z lines.

sarcoplasm—The cytoplasm or intracellular fluid within a muscle fiber.

sarcoplasmic reticulum—An elaborate baglike membranous structure found within a muscle cell. Its interconnecting membranous tubules lie in the narrow spaces between the myofibrils, surrounding and running parallel to them.

SD **(standard deviation)**—A measure of variability about the mean; 68% of the population is within one standard deviation above and below the mean, and about 95% of the population is within two standard deviations of the mean.

SE **(standard error)**—A measure of variability about the mean.

SEE—Standard error of estimate.

serotonin—A brain neurotransmitter. Also known as 5-hydroxytryptamine (5-HT).

serum—Fluid left after blood has clotted.

SGLT—Sodium-dependent glucose transporter.

short-chain fatty acid (SCFA)—A fatty acid containing six or fewer carbon atoms.

smooth muscle—A specialized type of nonstriated muscle tissue composed of single nucleated fibers. It contracts in an involuntary rhythmic fashion in the walls of visceral organs. Also found in the walls of blood vessels.

sodium glucose transporter (SGLT)—Carrier protein that cotransports sodium and glucose across a cell membrane.

sodium pump—Common name for the sodium–potassium ATPase that helps to establish the resting membrane potential of a cell.

soluble fiber—Fiber that dissolves well in water.

solute—A substance dissolved in a solvent liquid such as water.

solvent—A liquid medium in which particles can dissolve.

specific heat—The amount of energy or heat needed to raise the temperature of a unit of mass, such as 1g of body tissue, by 1 °C. Units are $J \cdot g^{-1} \cdot °C^{-1}$.

sphingomyelin—Type of lipid found in the membranes of Schwann cells that provide an insulating sheath around nerve axons.

spirometry—A method to measure breathing.

stable isotope—An isotope is a specific form of a chemical element. It differs from atoms of other forms (isotopes) of the same element in the number of neutrons in its nucleus. *Stable* refers to the fact that the isotope is not radioactive, in contrast to some other types of isotopes.

starch—A carbohydrate made of multiple units of glucose attached together by bonds that can be broken down by human digestion processes. Starch is also known as a complex carbohydrate.

stereoisomerism—The existence of different substances whose molecules possess an identical connectivity but different arrangements of their atoms in space.

steroid—A complex molecule derived from the lipid cholesterol containing four interlocking carbon rings.

STPD—Standard conditions of temperature (0 °C) and pressure (760 mmHg) and dry.

substrate—The reactant molecule in a reaction catalyzed by an enzyme.

Substrate-level phosphorylation—Synthesis of high-energy phosphate bonds through reaction of inorganic phosphate with an activated (usually) organic substrate.

succinate dehydrogenase (SDH)—An enzyme of the tricarboxylic acid cycle.

sucrose—A disaccharide consisting of a combination of glucose and fructose; table sugar.

suit calorimeter—See direct calorimetry suit.

supercompensation of muscle glycogen—Higher than normal muscle glycogen concentrations that can be achieved with a combination of exercise and diet.

superoxide dismutase (SOD)—An enzyme in body cells that helps neutralize free radicals.

Systeme Internationale (SI)—International Unit System, a worldwide uniform system of units.

systolic—Indicating the maximum arterial pressure during contraction of the left ventricle of the heart.

TBARS (thiobarituric acid-reactive substances)—Stable compounds produced as a consequence of free radical actions on lipid structures, which are commonly used as a measure of oxidative stress.

TCA (tricarboxylic acid)—A compound such as citric acid containing three carboxyl (-COOH) groups.

TCA cycle (tricarboxylic acid cycle)—A series of reactions that are important in energy metabolism and take place in the mitochondrion. Also known as the Krebs cycle (after Hans Krebs, who first described the reactions involved) or the citric acid cycle, because citrate is one of the key intermediates in the process.

testosterone—The male sex hormone responsible for male secondary sex characteristics at puberty. It has anabolic and androgenic effects and is responsible for aggressive behavior.

thermic effect of exercise (TEE)—The energy required for exercise. Increased muscle contraction increases heat production.

thermic effect of food (TEF)—See diet-induced thermogeneisis.

thermogenesis—The production of heat. Metabolic processes in the body generate heat constantly.

thermoreceptors—Sensory cells capable of detecting changes in temperature.

thioester bond—A bond in which the oxygen has been replaced by sulfur. For example, the linking of CoA in acetyl-CoA is through a thioester bond.

thymine (T)—A pyrimidine nucleotide found in DNA.

tissue—An organized association of similar cells that perform a common function (e.g., muscle tissue).

TNF (tumor necrosis factor)—A cytokine that promotes inflammation.

tracee—The compound that is traced.

tracer—An element or compound containing atoms that can be distinguished from their normal counterparts by physical means (e.g., radioactivity assay or mass spectrometry) and can thus be used to follow (trace) the metabolism of the normal substances.

trafficking (of leukocytes)—Movements of leukocytes into or out of the circulation.

trans—A prefix indicating that geometrical isomer in which like groups are on opposite sides of a double bond with restricted rotation.

transamination—Reaction involving the transfer of an amino (NH_2) group from an amino acid to a keto-acid.

transcription—The process by which RNA polymerase produces single-stranded RNA complementary to one strand of the DNA.

transit time—The time that food stays in the gastrointestinal tract.

translation—The process by which ribosomes and tRNA decipher the genetic code in mRNA to synthesize a specific polypeptide or protein.

triacylglycerol—The storage form of fat composed of three fatty acid molecules linked to a three-carbon glycerol molecule. Also known as triglyceride.

triglyceride—The storage form of fat composed of three fatty acid molecules linked to a three-carbon glycerol molecule. Also known as triacylglycerol.

triplet code—The sequences of three nucleotides that compose the codons, the units of genetic information in DNA or RNA that specify the order of amino acids in a peptide or protein.

tRNA (transfer ribonucleic acid)—Transports amino acids to ribosomes where protein synthesis takes place.

TRP (tryptophan)—An essential amino acid.

type 1 diabetes mellitus (insulin-dependent diabetes mellitus)—A chronic condition in which the pancreas makes little or no insulin because the beta cells have been destroyed. The body is then not able to use glucose (blood sugar) for energy.

type I fibers—Small-diameter muscle cells that contain relatively slow-acting myosin ATPases and hence contract slowly. Their red color is caused by the presence of myoglobin. These fibers possess a high capacity for oxidative metabolism, are extremely fatigue resistant, and are specialized for the performance of repeated contractions over prolonged periods.

type 2 diabetes mellitus—Non-insulin-dependent diabetes mellitus.

type II fibers—Muscle cells that are much paler than type I fibers because they contain little myoglobin. They possess rapidly acting myosin ATPases, and so their contraction (and relaxation) time is relatively fast. A high activity of glycogen phosphorylase and glycolytic enzymes endows type II fibers with a high capacity for rapid (but relatively short-lived) ATP production.

UDP (uridine diphosphate)—A coenzyme involved in glycogen synthesis.

UFA (unsaturated fatty acid)—Fatty acid (FA) containing at least one double bond within its hydrocarbon chain.

UK—United Kingdom.

UL—Tolerable upper intake level. The highest level of daily nutrient intake likely not to pose a health problem.

uracil (U)—A pyrimidine nucleotide found in RNA.

urea—End product of protein metabolism. Chemical formula: $CO(NH_2)_2$.

uric acid—A breakdown product of nucleic acids present in small quantity in the urine of man and most mammals.

urine—Fluid produced in the kidney and excreted from the body. Contains urea, ammonia, and other metabolic wastes.

URTI—Upper respiratory tract infections like colds and flu.

USDA—United States Department of Agriculture.

USNDB—United States Nutrient Data Bank.

UTP—Uridine triphosphate.

vanadium—A trace element with a role in glucose metabolism.

VCO$_2$—Rate of carbon dioxide production.

vegan—Vegetarian who eats no animal products.

vegetarian—One whose food is of vegetable or plant origin.

villi—Fingerlike folds (1 mm) of the mucosa of the small intestine.

vitamin—An organic substance necessary in small amounts for the normal metabolic functioning of the body. Must be present in the diet because the body cannot synthesize it (or cannot synthesize an adequate amount of it).

vitamin B$_1$—Thiamin.

vitamin B$_2$—Riboflavin.

vitamin B$_6$—Pyridoxine.

vitamin B$_{12}$—Cyanocobalamin.

vitamin C—Ascorbic acid.

vitamin D—Cholecalciferol, the product of irradiation of 7-dehydrocholesterol found in the skin.

vitamin E—α-tocopherol.

vitamin K—Menoquinone.

VLCD—Very low-calorie diet. Same as VLED.

VLDL (very low-density lipoproteins)—A protein–lipid complex in the blood plasma that transports triacylglycerols, cholesterol, and phospholipids; has a very low density.

VLED—Very low-energy diet.

V$_{max}$—Maximal velocity of an enzymatic reaction when substrate concentration is not limiting.

V̇O$_2$—Rate of oxygen uptake.

V̇O$_2$max—Maximal oxygen uptake. The highest rate of oxygen consumption by the body that can be determined in an incremental exercise test to exhaustion.

W (watt)—Unit of power or work rate (J/s).

water—The universal solvent of life (H_2O). The body is composed of 60% water.

WBC—White blood cell (leukocyte); important cells of the immune system that defend the body against invading microorganisms.

wet-bulb globe thermometer index (WBGT index)—A heat-stress index based on four factors measured by the wet-bulb globe thermometer.

weight cycling—A cycle in which the considerable effort applied to achieve weight loss is exceeded by the effort required to maintain the new lower body weight. After the weight is lost, it is regained in a relatively short period. Also referred to as the yo-yo effect.

work efficiency (WE)—The work accomplished divided by the energy expended minus the energy cost in the unloaded condition.

w.w.—Wet weight.

yohimbine—An alkaloid substance derived from yohimbine bark, which functions as an α$_2$ adrenoreceptor blocker (monamine oxidase inhibitor).

yo-yo effect—See weight cycling.

References

Aarsland, A., D. Chinkes, and R.R. Wolfe. 1997. Hepatic and whole-body fat synthesis in humans during carbohydrate overfeeding. *Am J Clin Nutr* 65 (6): 1774–1782.

Abbott, W.G., B.V. Howard, L. Christin, et al. 1988. Short-term energy balance: Relationship with protein, carbohydrate, and fat balances. *Am J Physiol* 255 (3 pt 1): E332–337.

Achten, J., and A.E. Jeukendrup. 2003. The effect of pre-exercise carbohydrate feedings on the intensity that elicits maximal fat oxidation. *J Sports Sci* 21:1017–1024.

Achten, J., M.C. Venables, and A.E. Jeukendrup. 2003. Fat oxidation rates are higher during running compared to cycling over a wide range of intensities. *Metabolism* 52 (6): 747–752.

Achten, J., M. Gleeson, and A.E. Jeukendrup. 2002. Determination of the exercise intensity that elicits maximal fat oxidation. *Med Sci Sports Exerc* 34 (1): 92–97.

Achten, J., S.L. Halson, L. Moseley, M.P. Rayson, A. Casey, and A.E. Jeukendrup. 2004. Higher dietary carbohydrate content during intensified running training results in better maintenance of performance and mood state. J Appl Physiol 96 (4):1331-1340.

Acker, S.A.B.E., M.N.J.L. Tromp, G.R.M.M. Haenen, J.F. Wim, V. Vijgh, and A. Bast. 1995. Flavonoids as scavengers of nitric oxide radical. *Bio Chem Res Rev* 3:755–757.

Akerstrom, T.C., J.B. Birk, D.K. Klein, C. Erikstrup, P. Plomgaard, B.K. Pedersen, and J. Wojtaszewski. 2006. Oral glucose ingestion attenuates exercise-induced activation of 5'-AMP-activated protein kinase in human skeletal muscle. *Biochem Biophys Res Commun* 342:949–955.

Akerstrom TCA, Fischer CP, Plomgaard P, Thomsen C, van Hall G, Klarlund Pedersen B: Glucose ingestion during endurance training does not alter adaptation. J Appl Physiol 106:1771-1779, 2009.*Allen, J.D., J. McLung, A.G. Nelson, and M. Welsch. 1998. Ginseng supplementation does not enhance healthy young adults' peak aerobic exercise performance. *J Am Coll Nutr* 17 (5): 462–466.

American College of Sports Medicine. 1996. Exercise and fluid replacement. *Med Sci Sports Exerc* 16:i–vii.

American Dietetic Association. 1997. Health Implications of Dietary Fiber. *Am Diet Assoc* 97:1157–1160.

American Psychiatric Association Task Force on DSM-IV. 2000. *Diagnostic and statistical manual of mental disorders: DSM-IV-TR*, 4th text revision. Washington, DC: American Psychaitric Association.

American Psychiatric Association. 1994. *Diagnostic and statistical manual of mental disorders*, 4th ed. Washington, DC: American Psychiatric Association.

American Psychiatric Association. 1987. *Diagnostic and statistical manual of mental disorders*, 3rd ed. Washington, DC: American Psychiatric Association.

Andersen, A.E. 1995. Eating disorders in males. In *Eating disorders and obesity: A comprehensive handbook*, ed. K.D. Brownell and C.G. Fairburn, 177–192. London: Guildford Press.

Andersen, A.E. 1990. Diagnosis and treatment of males with eating disorders. In *Males with eating disorders*, ed. A.E. Andersen, 133–162. New York: Brunner/Mazel.

Anderson, M.J., J.D. Cotter, A.P. Garnham, D.J. Casley, and M.A. Febbraio. 2001. Effect of glycerol-induced hyperhydration on thermoregulation and metabolism during exercise in the heat. *Int J Sport Nutr Exerc Metab* 11 (3): 315–333.

Anderson, R.A., and A.S. Kozlovsky. 1985. Chromium intake, absorption and excretion of subjects consuming self-selected diets. *Am J Clin Nutr* 41 (6): 1177–1183.

Andrews, S., L.A. Balart, M.C. Bethea, et al. 1998. *Sugarbusters.* London: Vermillion.

Angus, D.J., M. Hargreaves, J. Dancey, and M.A. Febbraio. 2000. Effect of carbohydrate or carbohydrate plus medium-chain triglyceride ingestion on cycling time trial performance. *J Appl Physiol* 88 (1): 113–119.

Anonymus. 1998. Hyperthermia and dehydration-related deaths associated with intentional rapid weight loss in three collegiate wrestlers—North Carolina, Wisconsin, and Michigan, November–December 1997. *MMWR Morb Mortal Wkly Rep* 47 (6): 105–108.

Applegate, E. 1999. Effective nutritional ergogenic aids. *Int J Sport Nutr* 9 (2): 229–239.

Applegate, E.A., and L.E. Grivetti. 1997. Search for the competitive edge: A history of dietary fads and supplements. *J Nutr* 127 (5 Suppl): S869S–S873.

Ardawi, M.S.M., and E.A. Newsholme. 1994. *Glutamine metabolism in lymphoid tissues,* ed. D. Haussinger and H. Sies, 235–246. Berlin: Springer-Verlag.

Arkinstall, M.J., C.R. Bruce, V. Nikolopoulos, et al. 2001. Effect of carbohydrate ingestion on metabolism during running and cycling. *J Appl Physiol* 91 (5): 2125–2134.

Armstrong, L.E., D.L. Costill, and W.J. Fink. 1985. Influence of diuretic-induced dehydration on competitive running performance. *Med Sci Sports Exerc* 17:456–461.

Armstrong, L.E. 2002. Caffeine, body fluid-electrolyte balance, and exercise performance. *Int J Sport Nutr Exerc Metab* 12 (2): 189–206.

Armstrong, L., A. Pumerantz, M. Roti, D. Judelson, G. Watson, J. Dias, B. Sokmen, D. Casa, C. Maresh, H. Lieberman, M. Kellogg. 2005. Fluid, electrolyte, and renal indices of hydration during 11 days of controlled caffeine consumption. *Int J Sport Nutr Exerc Metab* 15 (3): 252–265.

Atherton, P.J., J. Babraj, K. Smith, J. Singh, M.J. Rennie, and H. Wackerhage. 2005. Selective activation of AMPK-PGC-1alpha or PKB-TSC2-mTOR signaling can explain specific adaptive responses to endurance or resistance training-like electrical muscle stimulation. *FASEB J* 19:786–788.

Atkins, R.C. 1992. Doctor Atkins' new diet revolution. New York: Avon Books.

Aulin, K.P. 2000. Minerals: Calcium. In *Nutrition in sport,* ed. R.J. Maughan, 318–325. Oxford: Blackwell Science.

Baar, K., A.R. Wende, T.E. Jones, M. Marison, L.A. Nolte, M. Chen, D.P. Kelly, J.O. Holloszy. 2002. Adaptations of skeletal muscle to exercise: Rapid increase in the transcriptional coactivator PGC-1. *FASEB J* 16:1879–1886.

Bach, A.C., and V.K. Babayan. 1982. Medium-chain triglycerides: An update. *Am J Clin Nutr* 36:950–962.

Bagby, G.J., H.J. Green, S.Katsuta, and P.D. Gollnick. 1978. Glycogen depletion in exercising rats infused with glucose, lactate or pyruvate. *J Appl Physiol* 45 (3): 425–429.

Ballantyne, C.S., S.M. Phillips, J.R. MacDonald, M A. Tarnopolsky, and J.D. MacDougall. 2000. The acute effects of androstenedione supplementation in healthy young males. *Can J Appl Physiol* 25 (1): 68–78.

Ballor, D.L., and R.E. Keesey. 1991. A meta-analysis of the factors affecting exercise-induced changes in body mass, fat mass and fat-free mass in males and females. *Int J Obes* 15 (11): 717–726

Balsom, P.D., B. Ekblom, K. Soderlund, B. Sjodin, and E. Hultman. 1993. Creatine supplementation and dynamic high-intensity intermittent exercise. *Scand J Med Sci Sports* 3:143–149.

Balsom, P.D., K. Wood, P. Olsson, and B. Ekblom. 1999. Carbohydrate intake and multiple sprint sports: With special reference to football (soccer). *Int J Sports Med* 20 (1): 48–52.

Balsom, P.D., S.D.R. Harridge, K. Soderlund, B. Sjodin, and B. Ekblom. 1993. Creatine supplementation per se does not enhance endurance exercise performance. *Acta Physiol Scand* 149:521–523.

Banderet, L.E., and H.R. Lieberman. 1989. Treatment with tyrosine, a neurotransmitter precursor, reduces environmental stress in humans. *Brain Res Bull* 22 (4): 759–762.

Barnett, C., D.L. Costill, M.D. Vukovich, K.J. Cole, B.H. Goodpaster, S.W. Trappe, and W.J. Fink. 1994. Effect of L-carnitine supplementation on muscle and blood carnitine content and lactate accumulation during high-intensity sprint cycling. *Int J Sports Nutr* 4 (3): 280–288.

Barron, J.L., T.D. Noakes, W. Levy, C. Smith, and R.P. Millar. 1985. Hypothalamic dysfunction in overtrained athletes. *J Clin Endocrinol Metab*, 60 (4):803–806.

Barrett, B. 2003. Medicinal properties of Echinacea: Critical review. *Phytomedicine* 10:66–86.

Barrett, B.P., R.L. Brown, K. Locken, R. Maberry, J.A. Bobula, and D. D'Alessio. 2002. Treatment of the common cold with unrefined Echinacea. A randomized, double-blind, placebo-controlled trial. *Ann Intern Med* 137:939–946.

Barry, A., T. Cantwell, F. Doherty, J.C. Folan, M. Ingoldsby, J.P. Kevany, J.D. O'Broin, H. O'Connor, B. O'Shea, B.A. Ryan, and J. Vaughan. 1981. A nutritional study of Irish athletes. *Br J Sports Med* 5:99.

Bassit, R.A., L.A. Sawada, R.F.P. Bacurau, F. Navarro, E. Martins, R.V.T. Santos, E.C. Caperuto, P. Rogeri, and L.F.B.P. Costa-Rosa. 2002. Branched-chain amino acid supplementation and the immune response of long-distance athletes. *Nutrition* 18:376–379.

Baumgartner, R.N., W.C. Chumlea, and A.F. Roche. 1990. Bioelectric impedance for body composition. *Exerc Sport Sci Rev* 18:193–224.

Beckers, E.J., A.E. Jeukendrup, F. Brouns, A.J.M. Wagenmakers, and W.H.M. Saris. 1992. Gastric emptying of carbohydrate-medium chain triglyceride suspensions at rest. *Int J Sports Med* 13 (8): 581–584.

Beidleman, B.A., J.L. Puhl, and M.J. De Souza. 1995. Energy balance in female distance runners. *Am J Clin Nutr* 61 (2): 303–311.

Below, P., R. Mora-Rodriguez, J. Gonzalez-Alonso, and E.F. Coyle. 1995. Fluid and carbohydrate ingestion independently improve performance during 1 h of intense cycling. *Med Sci Sports Exerc* 27:200–210.

Bennell, K., G. Matheson, and W. Heevwisse. 1999. Risk factors for stress fractures. *Sports Med* 28:91–122.

Bennet, W.M., A.A. Connacher, C.M. Scrimgeour, and M.J. Rennie. 1990. The effect of amino acid infusion on leg protein turnover assessed by L-[15N]phenylalanine and L-[1-13C]leucine exchange [published erratum appears in *Eur J Clin Invest* 20 (4): 479]. *Eur J Clin Invest* 20 (1): 41–50.

Bennet, W.M., and M.J. Rennie. 1991. Protein anabolic actions of insulin in the human body. *Diabetic Med* 8:199–207.

Bergstrom, J., and E. Hultman. 1966. Muscle glycogen synthesis after exercise: An enhancing factor localized in muscle cells in man. *Nature* 210:309–310.

Bergstrom, J., and E. Hultman. 1967a. A study of glycogen metabolism during exercise in man. *Scand J Clin Invest* 19:218–228.

Bergstrom, J., and E. Hultman. 1967b. Synthesis of muscle glycogen in man after glucose and fructose infusion. *Acta Med Scand* 182 (1): 93–107.

Beumont, P.J.V. 1995. The clinical presentation of anorexia and bulimia nervosa. In *Eating disorders and obesity: A comprehensive handbook,* ed. K.D. Brownelland and C.G. Fairburn, 151–158. London: Guildford Press.

Beumont, P.J.V., B. Arthur, J.D. Russell, and S.W. Touyz. 1994. Excessive physical activity in dieting disorder patients: Proposals for a supervised exercise program. *Int J Eating Disorders* 15:21–36.

Bierkamper, G.G., and A.M. Goldberg. 1980. Release of acetylcholine from the vascular perfused rat phrenic nerve-hemidiaphragm. *Brain Res* 202 (1): 234–237.

Biolo, G., B.D. Williams, R.Y. Fleming, and R.R. Wolfe. 1999. Insulin action on muscle protein kinetics and amino acid transport during recovery after resistance exercise. *Diabetes* 48 (5): 949–957.

Biolo, G., S.P. Maggi, B.D. Williams, K.D. Tipton, and R.R. Wolfe. 1995. Increased rates of muscle protein turnover and amino acid transport after resistance exercise in humans. *Am J Physiol* 268 (3 pt 1): E514–E520.

Biolo, G., K. Tipton, S. Klein, and R. Wolfe. 1997. An abundant supply of amino acids enhances the metabolic effect of exercise on muscle protein. *Am J Physiol* 273 (1 Pt 1): E122–129.

Birch, R., D. Noble, and P.L. Greenhaff. 1994. The influence of dietary creatine supplementation on work output and metabolism during repeated bouts of maximal isokenetic cycling in man. *Eur J Appl Physiol* 69 (3): 268–276.

Bishop, N.C., A.K. Blannin, and M.Gleeson. 2000. Effect of carbohydrate and fluid intake during prolonged exercise on saliva flow and IgA secretion. *Med Sci Sports Exerc* 32:2046–2051

Bishop, N.C., A.K. Blannin, N.P. Walsh, and M. Gleeson. 2001. Effect of dietary carbohydrate status on bacterial lipopolysaccharide-stimulated neutrophil degranulation response following cycling to fatigue. *Int J Sports Med* 22:226–231.

Bishop, N.C., A.K. Blannin, N.P. Walsh, P.J. Robson, and M.Gleeson 1999a. Nutritional aspects of immunosuppression in athletes. *Sports Med* 28:151–176.

Bishop, N.C., A.K. Blannin, P.J. Robson, N.P., Walsh, and M. Gleeson. 1999c. The effects of carbohydrate supplementation on neutrophil degranulation responses to a soccer-specific exercise protocol. *J Sports Sci* 17:787–779.

Bishop, N.C., A.K. Blannin, L. Rand, R. Johnson, and M. Gleeson. 1999b. Effects of carbohydrate and fluid intake on the blood leucocyte response to prolonged exercise. *J Sports Sci* 17:26–27.

Bishop, N.C., C. Fitzgerald, P.J. Porter, G.A. Scanlon, and A.C. Smith. 2005. Effect of caffeine ingestion on lymphocyte counts and subset activation in vivo following strenuous cycling. *Eur J Appl Physiol* 93 (5–6): 606–613.

Bishop, N.C., G.J. Walker, L.A. Bowley, et al. 2005. Lymphocyte responses to influenza and tetanus toxoid in vitro following intensive exercise and carbohydrate ingestion on consecutive days. *J Appl Physiol* 99 (4): 1327–1335.

Blaak, E. 2001.Gender differences in fat metabolism. *Curr Opin Clin Nutr Metab Care* 4 (6): 499–502.

Blom, P.C.S., A.T. Høstmark, O. Vaage, K.R. Kardel, and S. Maehlum. 1987. Effect of different post-exercise sugar diets on the rate of muscle glycogen resynthesis. *Med Sci Sports Exerc* 19:491–496.

Blomstrand, E., S. Andersson, P. Hassmen, B. Ekblom, and E.A. Newsholme. 1995. Effect of branched-chain amino acid and carbohydrate supplementation on the exercise-induced change in plasma and muscle concentration of amino acids in human subjects. *Acta Physiol Scand* 153 (2): 87–96.

Blomstrand, E., P. Hassmen, B. Ekblom, and E.A. Newsholme. 1991. Administration of branched-chain amino acids during sustained exercise—effects on performance and on plasma concentration of some amino acids. *Eur J Appl Physiol* 63 (2): 83–88.

Blomstrand, E., P. Hassmen, S. Ek, B. Ekblom, and E.A. Newsholme. 1997. Influence of ingesting a solution of branched-chain amino acids on perceived exertion during exercise. *Acta Physiol Scand* 159 (1): 41–49.

Bloomfield, S.A. 2001. *Optimizing bone health: Impact of nutrition, exercise and hormones.* Gatorade Sport Science Institute, SSE#82, www.gssiweb.com.

Blot, W. 1997. Vitamin/mineral supplementation and cancer risk: International chemoprevention trials. *Proc Soc Exp Biol Med* 261:291–296.

Blundell, J.E., J.R. Cotton, H. Delargy, S. Green, A. Greenough, N.A. King, and C.L. Lawton. 1995. The fat paradox: Fat-induced satiety signals versus high fat overconsumption. *Int J Obes Relat Metab Disord* 19 (11): 832–835.

Blundell, J.E., C.L. Lawton, J.R. Cotton, and J.I. MacDiarmid. 1996. Control of human appetite: Implications for the intake of dietary fat. *Annu Rev Nutr* 16:285–319.

Blundell, J.E., R.J. Stubbs, D.A. Hughes, S. Whybrow, and N.A. King. 2003. Cross talk between physical activity and appetite control: Does physical activity stimulate appetite? *Proc Nutr Soc,* 62 (3): 651–661.

Boden, G., X. Chen, J. Ruiz, G.D. van Rossum, and S. Turco. 1996. Effects of vanadyl sulfate on carbohydrate and lipid metabolism in patients with non-insulin-dependent diabetes mellitus. *Metabolism* 45 (9): 1130–1135.

Bohe, J., A. Low, R.R. Wolfe, and M.J. Rennie. 2003. Human muscle protein synthesis is modulated by extracellular, not intramuscular amino acid availability: A dose-response study. *J Physiol* 552 (Pt 1): 315–324.

Boirie, Y., M. Dangin, P. Gachon, M.-P. Vasson, J.-L. Maubois, and B. Beaufrere. 1997. Slow and fast dietary proteins differently modulate postprandial protein accretion. *Proc Natl Acad Sci USA* 94 (26): 14930–14935.

Bond, V., R. Adams, B. Balkissoon, J. McRae, E. Knight, S. Robbins, and M. Banks. 1987. Effects of caffeine on cardiorespiratory function and glucose metabolism during rest and graded exercise. *J Sports Med* 27:47–52.

Bonen, A., J.J. Luiken, Y. Arumugam, J.F. Glatz, and N.N. Tandon. 2000. Acute regulation of fatty acid uptake involves the cellular redistribution of fatty acid translocase. *J Biol Chem* 275 (19): 14501–14508.

Bonen, A., D.J. Dyck, A. Ibrahimi, and N.A. Abumrad. 1999. Muscle contractile activity increases fatty acid metabolism and transport and FAT/CD36. *Am J Physiol* 276 (4 Pt 1): E642–649.

Borsheim, E., and R. Bahr. 2003. Effect of exercise intensity, duration and mode on post-exercise oxygen consumption. *Sports Med* 33 (14): 1037–1060.

Borsheim, E., K. Tipton, S. Wolf, and R. Wolfe. 2002. Essential amino acids and muscle protein recovery from resistance exercise. *Am J Physiol Endocrinol Metab* 283 (4): E648–657.

Bosch, A.N., S.C. Dennis, and T.D. Noakes. 1994. Influence of carbohydrate ingestion on fuel substrate turnover and oxidation during prolonged exercise. *J Appl Physiol* 76 (6): 2364–2372.

Bouchard, C. 1994. Genetics of obesity: Overview and research directions. In *The genetics of obesity,* ed. C. Bouchard, 223–233. Boca Raton, FL: CRC Press.

Bouchard, C., A. Tremblay, J.P. Despres, A. Nadeau, P.J. Lupien, G. Theriault, J. Dullault, S. Moorjani, S. Pinault, and G. Fournier. 1990. The response to long-term overfeeding in identical twins. *N Engl J Med* 322 (21):1477–1482.

Bowtell, J.L., K. Gelly, M.L. Jackman, A. Patel, M. Simeoni, and M.J. Rennie. 1999. Effect of oral glutamine on whole body carbohydrate storage during recovery from exhaustive exercise. *J Appl Physiol* 86:1770–1777.

Bray, G.A., and B.M. Popkin. 1998. Dietary fat intake does affect obesity! [see comments]. *Am J Clin Nutr* 68 (6): 1157–1173.

Bredle, D.L., J.M. Stager, W.F. Brechue, and M.O. Farber. 1988. Phosphate supplementation, cardiovascular function, and exercise performance in humans. *J Appl Physiol* 65 (4): 1821–1826.

Bremer, J. 1983. Carnitine-metabolism and functions. *Phys Rev* 63 (4): 1420–1479.

Brewerton, T.D., E.J. Stellefson, N. Hibbs, E.L. Hodges, and C.E. Cochrane. 1995. Comparison of eating disorder patients with and without compulsive exercising. *Int J Eating Disorders* 17:413–416.

Brilla, L.R., and T.E. Landerholm. 1990. Effect of fish oil supplementation on serum lipids and aerobic fitness. *J Sports Med Phys Fitness* 30:173–180.

Broeder, C.E., K.A. Burrhus, L.S. Svanevik, et al. 1997. Assessing body composition before and after resistance or endurance training. *Med Sci Sports Exerc* 29 (5): 705–712.

Brooks, G.A. 1986. The lactate shuttle during exercise and recovery. *Med Sci Sports Exerc* 18 (3): 360–368.

Brouns, F. 1991. Etiology of gastrointestinal disturbances during endurance events. *Scand J Med Sci Sports* 1:66–77.

Brouns, F., and E. Beckers. 1993. Is the gut an athletic organ? Digestion, absorption and exercise. *Sports Med* 15 (4): 242–257.

Brouns, F., J. Senden, E.J. Beckers, and W.H.M. Saris. 1995. Osmolarity does not affect the gastric emptying rate of oral rehydration solutions. *JPEN* 19: 403–406.

Brouns, F., W.H.M. Saris, and N.J. Rehrer. 1987. Abdominal complaints and gastrointestinal function during long-lasting exercise. *Int J Sports Med* 8:175–189.

Brouns, F., W.H.M. Saris, J. Stroecken, E. Beckers, R. Thijssen, N.J. Rehrer, and F. ten Hoor. 1989a. Eating, drinking, and cycling. A controlled Tour de France simulation study, part I. *Int J Sports Med* 10 (suppl 1): S32–S40.

Brouns, F., W.H.M. Saris, J. Stroecken, E. Beckers, R. Thijssen, N.J. Rehrer, and F. ten Hoor. 1989b. Eating, drinking, and cycling. A controlled Tour de France simulation study, part II: Effect of diet manipulation. *Int J Sports Med* 10 (suppl 1): S41–S48.

Brouns, F., W.H. Saris, E. Beckers, H. Adlercreutz, G.J. van der Vusse, H.A. Keizer, H. Kuipers, P. Menheere, A.J. Wagenmakers, and F. ten Hoor. 1989. Metabolic changes induced by sustained exhaustive cycling and diet manipulation. *Int J Sports Med* 10 (suppl 1): S49–S62.

Brown, G.D., and S. Gordon. 2003. Fungal beta-glucans and mammalian immunity. *Immunity* 19:311–315.

Brownell, K.D., S.N. Steen, and J.H. Wilmore. 1987. Weight regulation practices in athletes: Analysis of metabolic and health effects. *Med Sci Sports Exerc* 6:546–560.

Brownlie, T., V. Utermohlen, P.S. Hinton, C. Giordano, and J.D. Haas. 2002. Marginal iron deficiency without anemia impairs aerobic adaptation among previously untrained women. *Am J Clin Nutr* 75:734–742.

Brune, M., B. Magnusson, H. Persson, and L. Hallberg. 1986. Iron losses in sweat. *Am J Clin Nutr* 43:438-443.

Brutsaert, T.D., S. Hernandez-Cordero, J. Rivera, T. Viola, G. Hughes, and J.D. Haas. 2003. Iron supplementation improves progressive fatigue resistance during dynamic knee extensor exercise in iron-depleted, nonanemic women. *Am J Clin Nutr* 77:441-448.

Bucci, L.R., J.F. Hickson, Jr., I. Wolinsky, and J.M. Pivarnik. 1992. Ornithine supplementation and insulin release in bodybuilders. *Int J Sport Nutr* 2 (3): 287-291.

Burckes-Miller, M.E., and D.R. Black. 1988. Male and female college athletes: Prevalence of anorexia nervosa and bulimia nervosa. *Athletic Training* 2:137-140.

Burke, L.M., B. Kiens, and J.L. Ivy. 2004. Carbohydrates and fat for training and recovery. *J Sports Sci* 22:15-30.

Burke, L.M. 2001. Nutritional practices of male and female endurance cyclists. *Sports Med* 31 (7): 521-532.

Burke, L.M., A. Claassen, J.A. Hawley, and T.D. Noakes. 1998. Carbohydrate intake during prolonged cycling minimizes effect of glycemic index of preexercise meal. *J Appl Physiol* 85:2220-2226.

Burke, L.M., and V. Deakin. 2000. *Clinical sports nutrition*, 2nd ed. McGraw-Hill: New York.

Burke, L.M., and R.S.D. Read. 1993. Dietary supplements in sport. *Sports Med* 15 (1): 43-65.

Burke, L.M., D.B. Pyne, and R.D. Telford. 1996. Effect of oral creatine supplementation on single-effort sprint performance in elite swimmers. *Int J Sport Nutr* 6 (3): 222-233.

Burke, L.M., D.J. Angus, G.R. Cox, K.M. Gawthorn, J.A. Hawley, M.A. Febbraio, and M. Hargreaves. 1999. Fat adaptation with carbohydrate recovery promotes metabolic adaptation during prolonged cycling. *Med Sci Sports Exerc* 31 (5): 297.

Burke, L.M., G.R. Collier, and M. Hargreaves. 1993. Muscle glycogen storage after prolonged exercise: Effect of glycemic index of carbohydrate feedings. *J Appl Physiol* 75 (2): 1019-1023.

Burns, J.M., D.L. Costill, W.J. Fink, J.B. Mitchell, and J.A. Hol. 1988. Effects of choline on endurance performance. *Med Sci Sports Exerc* 20 (2): S25.

Bussau, V.A., T.J. Fairchild, A. Rao, P. Steele, and P.A. Fournier. 2002. Carbohydrate loading in human muscle: An improved 1 day protocol. *Eur J Appl Physiol* 87 (3): 290-295.

Butterfield, G.E., and D.H. Calloway. 1984. Physical activity improves protein utilization in young men. *Br J Nutr* 51 (2): 171-184.

Byrne, A., and D.G. Byrne. 1993. The effect of exercise on depression, anxiety, and other mood states: A review. *J Psychosomatic Res* 37:565-574.

Byrne, S., and N. McLean. 2002. Elite athletes: Effects of pressure to be thin. *J Sci Med Sport* 5:80-94.

Cade, R., M. Conte, C. Zauner, D. Mars, J. Peterson, D. Lunne, N. Hommen, and D. Packer. 1984. Effects of phosphate loading on 2,3-diphosphoglycerate and maximal oxygen uptake. *Med Sci Sports Exerc* 16 (3): 263-268.

Calle, E.E., M.J. Thun, J.M. Petrelli, et al. 1999. Body-mass index and mortality in a prospective cohort of U.S. adults. *N Engl J Med* 341 (15): 1097-1105

Cannon, J.G., S.F. Orencole, R.A. Fielding, M. Meydani, S.N. Meydani, M.A. Fiatarone, et al. 1990. Acute phase response in exercise: Interaction of age and vitamin E on neutrophils and muscle enzyme release. *Am J Physiol* 259:R1214-R1219.

Carter, J.M., A.E. Jeukendrup, and D.A. Jones. 2004. The effect of carbohydrate mouth rinse on 1-h cycle time trial performance. *Med Sci Sports Exerc* 36 (12): 2107-2111.

Carvalho, J.J., R.G. Baruzzi, P.F. Howard, N. Poulter, M.P. Alpers, L.J. Franco, L.F. Marcopito, V.J. Spooner, A.R. Dyer, P. Elliott, et al. 1989. Blood pressure in four remote populations in the intersalt study. *Hypertension* 14 (3): 238-246.

Casey, A., and P.L. Greenhaff. 2000. Does dietary creatine supplementation play a role in skeletal muscle metabolism and performance? *Am J Clin Nutr* 72 (2 suppl): 607S-617S.

Casey, A., D. Constantin-Teodosiu, S. Howell, E. Hultman, and P.L. Greenhaff. 1996. Creatine ingestion favorably affects performance and muscle metabolism during maximal exercise in humans. *Am J Physiol* 271 (1 pt 1): E31-E37.

Casey, Mann, Banister, Fox, Morris, Macdonald, and Greenhaff. 2000. Effect of carbohydrate ingestion on glycogen resynthesis in human liver and skeletal muscle, measured by (13)C MRS. *Am J Physiol Endocrinol Metab* 278 (1): E65-75.

Castell, L.M., and E.A. Newsholme. 1996. Does glutamine have a role in reducing infections in athletes? *Eur J Appl Physiol* 73:488-490.

Castell, L.M., J.R. Poortmans, and E.A. Newsholme. 1996. Does glutamine have a role in reducing infections in athletes? *Eur J Appl Physiol* 73:488-490.

Castell, L.M., J.R. Poortmans, R. Leclercq, M. Brasseur, J. Duchateau, and E.A. Newsholme. 1997. Some aspects of the acute phase response after a marathon race, and effect of glutamine supplementation. *Eur J Appl Physiol* 75:47-53.

Ceesay, S.M., A.M. Prentice, K.C. Day, P.R. Murgatroyd, G.R. Goldberg, W. Scott, and G.B. Spurr. 1989. The use of heart rate monitoring in the estimation of energy expenditure: A validation study using indirect whole-body calorimetry. *Br J Nutr* 61:175-186.

Chan, J.L., and C.S. Mantzoros. 2005. Role of leptin in enrgy-deprivation states: Normal human physiology and clinical implications for hypothalamic amenorrhea and anorexia nervosa. *Lancet* 366 (9479): 74-85.

Chandler, J., and J. Hawkins. 1984. The effect of bee pollen on physiological performance. *Int J Biosci Res* 6:107.

Chaouloff, F., G.A. Kennett, B. Serrurier, D. Merino, and G. Curzon. 1986. Amino acid analysis demonstrates that increased plasma free tryptophan causes the increase of brain tryptophan during exercise in the rat. *J Neurochem* 46 (5): 1647-1650.

Chasiotis, D. 1983. The regulation of glycogen phosphorylase and glycogen breakdown in human skeletal muscle. *Acta Physiol Scand Suppl* 518:1-68.

Chilibeck, P.D., C. Magnus, and M. Anderson. 2007. Effect of in-season creatine supplementation on body composition and performance in rugby union football players. *Appl Physiol Nutr Metab* 32 (6): 1052-1057.

Christensen, E.H. 1932. Der Stoffwechsel und die Respiratorischen Funktionen bei schwerer körperlicher Arbeit. *Skand Arch Physiol* 81:160-171.

Christensen, E.H., and O. Hansen. 1939. Arbeitsfahigkeit Und Ernahrung. *Skand Arch Physiol* 81:160-171.

Civitarese, A.E., M.K. Hesselink, A.P. Russell, E. Ravussin, P. Schrauwen. 2005. Glucose ingestion during exercise blunts exercise-induced gene expression of skeletal muscle fat oxidative genes. *Am J Physiol Endocrinol Metab* 289:E1023-1029.

Clancy, R.L., M. Gleeson, A. Cox, et al. 2006. Reversal in fatigued athletes of a defect in interferon gamma secretion after administration of *Lactobacillus acidophilus*. *Br J Sports Med* 40:351-354.

Clancy, S.P., P.M. Clarkson, M.E. DeCheke, K. Nosaka, P.S. Freedson, J.J. Cunningham, and B. Valentine. 1994. Effects of chromium picolinate supplementation on body composition, strength, and urinary chromium loss in football players. *Int J Sport Nutr* 4 (2): 142-153.

Close, G.L., T. Ashton, T. Cable, D. Doran, C. Holloway, F. McArdle, and D.P. MacLaren. 2006. Ascorbic acid supplementation does not attenuate post-exercise muscle soreness following muscle-damaging exercise but may delay the recovery process, *Brit J Nutr* 95:976–981.

Cluberton, L.J., S.L. McGee, R.M. Murphy, and M. Hargreaves. 2005. Effect of carbohydrate ingestion on exercise-induced alterations in metabolic gene expression. *J Appl Physiol* 99:1359–1363.

Coffey, V.G., Z. Zhong, A. Shield, B.J. Canny, A.V. Chibalin, J.R. Zierath, J.A. Hawley. 2006. Early signaling responses to divergent exercise stimuli in skeletal muscle from well-trained humans. *FASEB J* 20:190–192.

Cohen, N., M. Halberstam, P. Shlimovich, C.J. Chang, H. Shamoon, and L. Rossetti. 1995. Oral vanadyl sulfate improves hepatic and peripheral insulin sensitivity in patients with non-insulin-dependent-diabetis-mellitus. *J Clin Invest* 95:2501–2509.

Collins, M.A., M.L. Millard-Stafford, P.B. Sparling, et al. 1999. Evaluation of the BOD POD for assessing body fat in collegiate football players. *Med Sci Sports Exerc* 31 (9): 1350–1356.

Collomp, K., S. Ahmaidi, M. Audran, et al. 1991. Effects of caffeine ingestion on performance and anaerobic metabolism during the wingate test. *Int J Sports Med* 12 (5): 439–443.

Conlay, L.A., R.J. Wurtman, K. Blusztajn, I.L. Coviella, T.J. Maher, and G.E. Evoniuk. 1986. Decreased plasma choline concentrations in marathon runners [letter]. *N Engl J Med* 315 (14): 892.

Conlee, R.K., R.L. Hammer, W.W. Winder, M.L. Bracken, A.G. Nelson, and D.W. Barnett. 1990. Glycogen repletion and exercise endurance in rats adapted to a high fat diet. *Metabolism* 39 (3): 289–294.

Constantin-Teodosiu, D., J.I. Carlin, G. Cederblad, R.C. Harris, and E. Hultman. 1991. Acetyl group accumulation and pyruvate dehydrogenase activity in human muscle during incremental exercise. *Acta Physiol Scand* 143 (4): 367–372.

Coris, E.E., A.M. Ramirez, and D.J. Van Durme. 2004. Heat illness in athletes: The dangerous combination of heat, humidity and exercise. *Sports Medicine* 34 (1): 9–16.

Costill, D.L., R. Bowers, G. Branam, and K. Sparks. 1971. Muscle glycogen utilization during prolonged exercise on successive days. J Appl Physiol 31:834–838.

Costill, D.L., and W.J. Fink. 1974. Plasma volume changes following exercise and thermal dehydration. *J Appl Physiol* 37:521–525.

Costill, D.L., M.G. Flynn, J.P. Kirwan, J.A. Houmard, J.B. Mitchell, R. Thomas, and S.H. Park. 1988. Effects of repeated days of intensified training on muscle glycogen and swimming performance. *Med Sci Sports Exerc* 20:249–254.

Costill, D.L., and J.M. Miller. 1980. Nutrition for endurance sport: Carbohydrate and fluid balance. *Int J Sports Med* 1:2–14.

Costill, D.L., A. Bennett, G. Branam, and D. Eddy. 1973. Glucose ingestion at rest and during prolonged exercise. *J Appl Physiol* 34 (6): 764–769.

Costill, D.L., and B. Saltin. 1974. Factors limiting gastric emptying during rest and exercise. *J Appl Physiol* 37 (5): 679–683.

Costill, D.L., E. Coyle, G. Dalsky, W. Evans, W. Fink, and D. Hoopes. 1977. Effects of elevated plasma FFA and insulin on muscle glycogen usage during exercise. *J Appl Physiol* 43 (4): 695–699.

Costill, D.L., G.P. Dalsky, and W.J. Fink. 1978. Effects of caffeine ingestion on metabolism and exercise performance. *Med Sci Sports Exerc* 10 (3): 155–158.

Costill, D.L., R. Bowers, G. Branam, and K. Sparks. 1971. Muscle glycogen utilization during prolonged exercise on successive days. *J Appl Physiol* 31:834–838.

Costill, D.L., W.M. Sherman, W.J. Fink, C. Maresh, M. Witten, and J.M. Miller. 1981. The role of dietary carbohydrates in muscle glycogen resynthesis after strenuous running. *Am J Clin Nutr* 34:1831–1836.

Cox, A.J., D.B. Pyne, P.U. Saunders, and P.A. Fricker. 2008. Oral administration of the probiotic *Lactobacillus fermentum* VRI-003 and mucosal immunity in endurance athletes. *Br J Sports Med* doi: 10.1136/bjsm.2007.044628.

Cox, G.R., B. Desbrow, P.G. Montgomery, M.E. Anderson, C.R. Bruce, T.A. Macrides, D.T. Martin, A. Moquin, A. Roberts, J.A. Hawley, and L.M. Burke. 2002. Effect of different protocols of caffeine intake on metabolism and endurance performance. *J Appl Physiol* 93 (3): 990–999.

Coyle, E.F., A.E. Jeukendrup, A.J.M. Wagenmakers, and W.H.M. Saris. 1997. Fatty acid oxidation is directly regulated by carbohydrate metabolism during exercise. *Am J Physiol* 273:E268–E275.

Coyle, E.F., A.E. Jeukendrup, M.C. Oseto, B.J. Hodgkinson, and T.W. Zderic. 2001. Low-fat diet alters intramuscular substrates and reduces lipolysis and fat oxidation during exercise. *Am J Physiol Endocrinol Metab* 280 (3): E391–E398.

Coyle, E.F., A.R. Coggan, M.K. Hemmert, and J.L. Ivy. 1986. Muscle glycogen utilization during prolonged strenuous exercise when fed carbohydrate. *J Appl Physiol* 61 (1): 165–172.

Coyle, E.F., A.R. Coggan, M.K. Hemmert, R.C. Lowe, and T.J. Walters. 1985. Substrate usage during prolonged exercise following a preexercise meal. *J Appl Physiol* 59 (2): 429–433.

Coyle, E.F., and A.R. Coggan. 1984. Effectiveness of carbohydrate feeding in delaying fatigue during prolonged exercise. *Sports Med* 1:446–458.

Coyle, E.F., J.M. Hagberg, B.F. Hurley, W.H. Martin, A.A. Ehsani, and J.O. Holloszy. 1983. Carbohydrate feeding during prolonged strenuous exercise. *J Appl Physiol* 55 (1): 230–235.

Craig, E.N., and E.G. Cummings. 1966. Dehydration and muscular work. *J Appl Physiol* 21:670–674.

Crook, T.H., J. Tinklenberg, J. Yesavage, W. Petrie, M.G. Nunzi, and D.C. Massari. 1991. Effects of phosphatidylserine in age-associated memory impairment. *Neurology* 41 (5): 644–649.

Crooks, C.V., C.R .Wall, M.L. Cross, et al. 2006. The effect of bovine colstrum supplementation on salivary IgA in distance runners. *Int J Sport Nutr Exerc Metabol* 16: 47–64.

Cumming, D. 1996. Exercise-associated amenorrhoea, low bone density and oestradiol replacement therapy. *Arch Intern Med* 156:2193–2195.

Curatolo, P.W., and D. Robertson. 1983. The health consequences of caffeine. *Ann Intern Med* 98 (5 pt 1): 641–653.

Currell, K., and A.E. Jeukendrup. 2008. Superior endurance performance with ingestion of multiple transportable carbohydrates. *Med Sci Sports Exerc* 40 (2): 275–281.

Currell, K., and A.E. Jeukendrup. 2008. Validity, reliability and sensitivity of measures of sporting performance. *Sports Med* 38 (4): 297–316.

DaCosta, M., and K.A. Halmi. 1992. Classification of anorexia nervosa: Question of subtypes. *Int J Eating Disorders* 11:305–314.

Dahlstrom, M., E. Jansson, E. Nordevang, and L. Kaijser. 1990. Discrepancy between estimated energy intake and requirement in female dancers. *Clin Physiol* 10 (1): 11–25.

Davies, K.J.A., A.T. Quintanilha, G.A. Brooks, and L. Packer. 1982. Free radicals and tissue damage produced by exercise. *Biochem Physiol Res Communications* 107:1198–1205.

Davis, C. 1992. Body image, dieting behaviours and personality factors: A study of high performance female athletes. *Int J Sport Psychol* 23:179–192.

Davis, C., S.H. Kennedy, E. Ralevski, and M. Dionne. 1994. The role of physical activity in the development and maintenance of eating disorders. *Psycholog Med* 24:957–967.

Davis, J.M., E.A. Murphy, A.S. Brown, M.D. Carmichael, A. Ghaffar, and E.P. Mayer. 2004. Effects of oat beta-glucan on innate immunity and infection after exercise stress. *Med Sci Sports Exerc* 36:1321–1327.

Davis, S.E., G.B. Dwyer, K. Reed, et al. 2002. Preliminary investigation: The impact of the NCAA Wrestling Weight Certification Program on weight cutting. *J Strength Cond Res* 16 (2): 305–307.

Davison, G., M. Gleeson, and S. Phillips. 2007. Antioxidant supplementation and immunoendocrine responses to prolonged exercise. *Med Sci Sports Exerc* 39 (4): 645–652.

Deakin, V. 2000. Iron depletion in athletes. In *Clinical sports nutrition,* ed. V. Deakin, 273–311. New York: McGraw-Hill.

De Bock, K., W. Derave, B.O. Eijnde, M.K. Hesselink, E. Koninckx, A.J. Rose, P. Schrauwen, A. Bonen, E.A. Richter, and P. Hespel. 2008. Effect of training in the fasted state on metabolic responses during exercise with carbohydrate intake. *J Appl Physiol* 104:1045–1055.

de Castro, J.M., and D.K. Elmore. 1988. Subjective hunger relationships with meal patterns in the spontaneous feeding behavior of humans: Evidence for a causal connection. *Physiol Behav* 43 (2): 159–165.

de Castro, J.M. 1987. Macronutrient relationships with meal patterns and mood in the spontaneous feeding behavior of humans. *Physiol Behav* 39 (5): 561–569.

De Luca, L., and S. Ross. 1996. Beta-carotene increases lung cancer incidence in cigarette smokers. *Nutr Rev* 54:178–180.

DeFronzo, R.A., D. Thorin, J.P. Felber, D.C. Simonson, D. Thiebaud, E. Jequier, and A. Golay. 1984. Effect of beta and alpha adrenergic blockade on glucose-induced thermogenesis in man. *J Clin Invest* 73 (3): 633–639.

Depaola, D.P., M.P. Faine, and C.A. Pamer. 1999. Nutrition in relation to dental medicine. In *Modern nutrition in health and disease,* ed. M.E. Shils, J.A. Olson, M. Shike, and A.C. Ross, 1099–1124. Baltimore: Williams & Wilkins.

Derave, W., M.S. Ozdemir, R. Harris, A. Pottier, H. Reyngoudt, K. Koppo, J.A. Wise, and E. Achten. 2007. beta-Alanine supplementation augments muscle carnosine content and attenuates fatigue during repeated isokinetic contraction bouts in trained sprinters. *J Appl Physiol* 103 (5): 1736–1743.

DeSilva, P., and S.B.G. Eysenck. 1987. Personality and addictiveness in anorexic and bulimic patients. *Pers Indiv Differ* 8:749–751.

Devries, M.C., S.A. Lowther, A.W. Glover, M.J. Hamadeh, and M.A. Tarnopolsky. 2007. IMCL area density, but not IMCL utilization, is higher in women during moderate-intensity endurance exercise, compared with men. *Am J Physiol Regul Integr Comp Physiol* 293 (6): R2336–2342.

Dietary guidelines for Americans. 2005. U.S. Department of Health and Human Services. www.health.gov/dietary-guidelines/.

Dietary Supplement Health and Education Act of 1994. 1994. Public law. 103-417, 103rd Congress. Available at www.fda.gov/opacom/laws/dshea.html.

Dill, D.B., H.T. Edwards, and J.H. Talbott. 1932. Factors limiting the capacity for work. *J Physiol* 1932:49–62.

Dodd, S.L., E. Brooks, S.K. Powers, and R. Tulley. 1991. The effects of caffeine on graded exercise performance in caffeine naive versus habituated subjects. *Eur J Appl Physiol* 62:424–429.

Doherty, M., and P.M. Smith. 2004. Effects of caffeine ingestion on exercise testing: A meta-analysis. *Int J Sport Nutr Exerc Metab* 14 (6): 626–646.

Doherty, M., and P.M. Smith. 2005. Effects of caffeine ingestion on rating of perceived exertion during and after exercise: A meta-analysis. *Scand J Med Sci Sports* 15 (2): 69–78.

Dohm, G.L., E.B. Tapscott, H.A. Barakat, and G.J. Kasperek. 1983. Influence of fasting on glycogen depletion in rats during exercise. *J Appl Physiol* 55 (3): 830–833.

Dohm, G.L., R.T. Beeker, R.G. Israel, and E.B. Tapscott. 1986. Metabolic responses after fasting. *J Appl Physiol* 61 (4): 1363–1368.

Douglas R.M., H. Hemila, E. Chalker, and B. Treacy. 2007. Vitamin C for preventing and treating the common cold. *Cochrane DB Syst Rev,* Issue 3: CD000980.

Drinkwater, B.L., K. Nilson, C.H. Chesnut, 3rd, et al. 1984. Bone mineral content of amenorrheic and eumenorrheic athletes. *N Engl J Med* 311 (5): 277–281.

Duchman, S.M., A.J. Ryan, H.P. Schedl, R.W. Summers, T.L. Bleiler, and C.V. Gisolfi. 1997. Upper limit for intestinal absorption of a dilute glucose solution in men at rest. *Med Sci Sports Exerc* 29 (4): 482–488.

Duffy, D.J., and R.K. Conlee. 1986. Effects of phosphate loading on leg power and high intensity treadmill exercise. *Med Sci Sports Exerc* 18 (6): 674–677.

Dulloo, A.G., and J. Jacquet. 1998. Adaptive reduction in basal metabolic rate in response to food deprivation in humans: A role for feedback signals from fat stores. *Am J Clin Nutr* 68 (3): 599–606.

Dummer, G.M., L.W. Rosen, and W.W. Heusner. 1987. Pathogenic weight-control behaviors of young competitive swimmers. *Physician Sports Med* 5:75–86.

Dupre, J., J.D. Curtis, R.W. Waddell, and J.C. Beck. 1968. Alimentary factors in the endocrine response to administration of arginine in man. *Lancet* 2 (7558): 28–29.

Durnin, J.V., and J. Womersley. 1974. Body fat assessed from total body density and its estimation from skin fold thickness: Measurements on 481 men and women aged from 16 to 72 years. *Br J Nutr* 32 (1): 77–97.

Duthie, G.G. 1999. Determination of activity of antioxidants in human subjects. *Pro Nutr Soc* 58:1015–1024.

Dyck, D.J., C.T. Putman, G.J.F. Heigenhauser, E. Hultman, and L.L. Spriet. 1993. Regulation of fat-carbohydrate interaction in skeletal muscle during intense aerobic cycling. *Am J Physiol* 265: E852–859.

Dyck, D.J., S.A. Peters, P.S. Wendling, A. Chesley, E. Hultman, and L.L. Spriet. 1996. Regulation of muscle glycogen phosphorylase activity during intense aerobic cycling with elevated FFA. *Am J Physiol* 265:E116–E125.

Edwards, H.T., R. Margaria, and D.B. Dill. 1934. Metabolic rate, blood sugar and the utilization of carbohydrate. *Am J Physiol* 108:203–209.

Eichner, E.R. 2000. Minerals: Iron. In *Nutrition in sport,* ed. R.J. Maughan, 326–338. Oxford: Blackwell Science.

Elliot, T.A., M.G. Cree, A.P. Sanford, R.R. Wolfe, and K.D. Tipton. 2006. Milk ingestion stimulates net muscle protein synthesis following resistance exercise. *Med Sci Sports Exerc* 38 (4): 667–674.

Elowsson, P., A.H. Forslund, H. Mallmin, et al. 1998. An evaluation of dual-energy X-ray absorptiometry and underwater weighing to estimate body composition by means of carcass analysis in piglets. *J Nutr* 128 (9): 1543–1549.

Engels, H.J., and J.C. Wirth. 1997. No ergogenic effects of ginseng (*Panax ginseng* C.A. Meyer) during graded maximal aerobic exercise. *J Am Diet Assoc* 97 (10): 1110–1115.

Epling, W.F., and W.D. Pierce. 1988. Activity based anorexia: A biobehavioural perspective. *Int J Eating Disorders* 7:475–485.

Erickson, M.A., R.J. Schwarzkopf, and R.D. McKenzie. 1987. Effects of caffeine, fructose, and glucose ingestion on muscle glycogen utilization during exercise. *Med Sci Sports Exerc* 19 (6): 579–583.

Espinosa, A., A. Leiva, M. Pena, M. Muller, A. Debandi, C. Hidalgo, M.A. Carrasco, and E. Jaimovich. 2006. Myotube depolarization generates reactive oxygen species through NAD(P)H oxidase: ROS-elicited Ca^{2+} stimulates ERK, CREB, early genes. *J Cell Physiol* 209:379–388.

Essig, D., D.L. Costill, and P.J. Van Handel. 1980. Effects of caffeine ingestion on utilization of muscle glycogen and lipid during leg ergometer cycling. *Int J Sports Med* 1:86–90.

Evain-Brion, D., M. Donnadieu, M. Roger, and J.C. Job. 1982. Simultaneous study of somatotrophic and corticotrophic pituitary secretions during ornithine infusion test. *Clin Endocrinol* 17 (2): 119–122.

Evans, G.W. 1989. The effect of chromium picolinate on insulin controlled parameters in humans. *Int J Biosoc Med Res* 11:163–180.

Fahey, T.D., J.D. Larsen, G.A. Brooks, W. Colvin, S. Henderson, and D. Lary. 1991. The effects of ingesting polylactate or glucose polymer drinks during prolonged exercise. *Int J Sport Nutr* 1 (3): 249–256.

Fairchild, T.J., S. Fletcher, P. Steele, C. Goodman, B. Dawson, and P. Fournier. 2002. Rapid carbohydrate loading after a short bout of near maximal-intensity exercise. *Med Sci Sports Exerc* 34 (6): 980–986.

Falk, B., R. Burstein, I. Ashkenazi, et al. 1989. The effect of caffeine ingestion on physical performance after prolonged exercise. *Eur J Appl Physiol* 59:168–173.

Fallowfield, J.L., C. Williams, J. Booth, B.H. Choo, and S. Growns. 1996. Effect of water ingestion on endurance capacity during prolonged running. *J Sports Sci* 14:497–502.

Fery, F., and E.O. Balasse. 1983. Ketone body turnover during and after exercise in overnight-fasted and starved humans. *Am J Physiol* 245:E18–E25.

Field, A.E., T. Byers, D.J. Hunter, et al. 1999. Weight cycling, weight gain, and risk of hypertension in women. *Am J Epidemiol* 150 (6): 573–579.

Fielding, R.A., T.J. Manfredi, W. Ding, M.A. Fiatarone, W.J. Evans, and J.G. Cannon. 1993. Acute phase response in exercise III. Neutrophil and IL-1β accumulation in skeletal muscle. *Am J Physiol* 265:R166–R172.

Fischer, C.P., N.J. Hiscock, M. Penkowa, et al. 2004. Supplementation with vitamins C and E inhibits the release of interleukin-6 from contracting human skeletal muscle. *J Physiol* 558:633–645.

Flatt J-P. 1995. Use and storage of carbohydrate and fat. *Am J Clin Nutr* 61:952S–959S.

Floyd, J.C., Jr., S.S. Fajans, J.W. Conn, R.F. Knopf, and J. Rull. 1966. Stimulation of insulin secretion by amino acids. *J Clin Invest* 45 (9): 1487–1502.

Fogelholm, G.M., H.K. Naveri, K.T. Kiilavuori, and M.H. Harkonen. 1993a. Low dose amino acid supplementation: No effects on serum growth hormone and insulin in male weightlifters. *Int J Sports Nutr* 3:290–297.

Fogelholm, M. 1994a. Vitamins, minerals and supplementation in soccer. *J Sports Sci* 12:S23–S27.

Fogelholm, M. 1994b. Effects of body weight reduction on sports performance. *Sports Med* 4:249–267.

Fogelholm, M., R. Koskinen, and J. Laasko. 1993b. Gradual and rapid weight loss: Effects on nutrition and performance in male athletes. *Med Sci Sports Exerc* 25:371–377.

Food and Nutrition Board. 2005. *Dietary reference intakes for energy, carbohydrate, fiber, fat, fatty acids, cholesterol, protein, and amino acids (macronutrients)*. Washington, DC: National Academies Press.

Food and Nutrition Board. 1989. *Recommended daily allowances*, 52–77. Washington, DC: National Research Council.

Foster, C., D.L. Costill, and W.J. Fink. 1979. Effects of preexercise feedings on endurance performance. *Med Sci Sports* 11 (1): 1–5.

Frexes-Steed, M., D.B. Lacy, J. Collins, and N.N. Abumrad. 1992. Role of leucine and other amino acids in regulating protein metabolism in vivo. *Am J Physiol* 262 (6 pt 1): E925–E935.

Fujii, N., T. Hayashi, M.F. Hirshman, J.T. Smith, S.A. Habinowski, L. Kaijser, J. Mu, O. Ljungqvist, M.J. Birnbaum, L.A. Witters, A. Thorell, L.J. Goodyear. 2000. Exercise induces isoform-specific increase in 5'AMP-activated protein kinase activity in human skeletal muscle. *Biochem Biophys Res Commun* 273:1150–1155.

Gadpalle, W.J., C.F. Sandborn, and W.W. Wagner. 1987. Athletic ammenorhea, major affective disorders and eating disorders. *Am J Psychiatry* 144:939–943.

Galbo, H., J.J. Holst, and H.J. Christensen. 1979. The effect of different diets and of insulin on the hormonal response to prolonged exercise. *Acta Physiologica Scandanavica* 107:19–32

Galbo, H. 1983. *Hormonal and metabolic adaptation to exercise*. New York: Verlag.

Galbo, H. 1992. Exercise physiology: Humoral function. *Sport Sci Rev* 1:65–93.

Galloway, S.D., M.S. Tremblay, J.R. Sexsmith, and C.J. Roberts. 1996. The effects of acute phosphate supplementation in subjects of different aerobic fitness levels. *Eur J Appl Physiol* 72 (3): 224–230.

Galloway, S.D.R., and R.J. Maughan. 2000. The effects of fluid and substrate provision on thermoregulatory and metabolic responses to prolonged exercise in a hot environment. *J Sports Sci* 18:339–351.

Gardiner, J.E., and M.C. Gwee. 1974. The distribution in the rabbit of choline administered by injection or infusion. *J Physiol (Lond)* 239 (3): 459–476.

Garner, M.D., P.E. Garfinkel, W. Rockert, and M.P. Olmsted. 1987. A prospective study of eating disturbances in the ballet. *Psychother Psychosomat* 48:170–175.

Gibson, S.A. 1996. Are high-fat, high-sugar foods and diets conducive to obesity? *Int J Food Sci Nutr* 47 (5): 405–415.

Gill, H.S., and M.L. Cross. 2002. Probiotics and immune function. In *Nutrition and immune function*, ed P.C. Calder, C.J. Field, and H.S. Gill, 251–272. Oxford: CABI.

Girandola, R.N., R.A. Wiswell, and R. Bulbulian. 1980. Effects of pangamic acid (B-15) ingestion on metabolic response to exercise. *Biochem Med* 24 (2): 218–222.

Gleeson, M. 1998. Temperature regulation during exercise. *Int J Sports Med* 19 (suppl 2): S96–S99.

Gleeson, M. 2000. Minerals and exercise immunology. In *Nutrition and exercise immunology*, ed. D.C. Nieman and B.K. Pedersen, 137–154. Boca Raton, FL: CRC Press.

Gleeson, M., A.K. Blannin, N.P. Walsh, N.C. Bishop, and A.M. Clark. 1998. Effect of low and high carbohydrate diets on the plasma glutamine and circulating leukocyte responses to exercise. *Int J Sport Nutr* 8:49–59.

Gleeson, M., and N.C. Bishop. 1999. Immunology. In *Basic and applied sciences for sports medicine*, ed. R.J. Maughan, 199–236. Oxford: Butterworth Heinemann.

Gleeson, M., and N.C. Bishop. 2000a. Elite athlete immunology: Importance of nutrition. *Int J Sports Med* 21 (suppl 1): S44–S50.

Gleeson, M., and N.C. Bishop. 2000b. Modification of immune responses to exercise by carbohydrate, glutamine and antioxidant supplements. *Immunol Cell Biol* 78:554–561.

Gleeson, M., J.D. Robertson, and R.J. Maughan. 1987. Influence of exercise on ascorbic acid status in man. *Clin Sci* 73:501-505.

Gleeson, M., R.J. Maughan, and P.L. Greenhaff. 1986. Comparison of the effects of pre-exercise feeding of glucose, glycerol and placebo on endurance and fuel homeostasis in man. *Eur J Appl Physiol* 55 (6): 645-653.

Gleeson, M. 2008. Dosing and efficacy of glutamine supplementation in human exercise and sport training. *J Nutr* 138 (10): 2045S-2049S.

Godek, S.F., A.R. Bartolozzi, and J.J. Godek. 2005. Sweat rate and fluid turnover in American football players compared with runners in a hot and humid environment. *Br J Sports Med* 39:205-211.

Goedecke, J.H., R. Elmer-English, S.C. Dennis, I. Schloss, T.D. Noakes, and E.V. Lambert. 1999. Effects of medium chain triacylglycerol ingested with carbohydrate on metabolism and exercise performance. *Int J Sports Nutr* 9 (1): 35-47.

Going, S.B., M.P. Massett, M.C. Hall, et al. 1993. Detection of small changes in body composition by dual-energy x-ray absorptiometry. *Am J Clin Nutr* 57 (6): 845-850.

Golay, A., and E. Bobbioni. 1997. The role of dietary fat in obesity. *Int J Obes Relat Metab Disord* 21 (suppl 3): S2-S11.

Goldberg, A.L., and T.W. Chang. 1978. Regulation and significance of amino acid metabolism in skeletal muscle. *Fed Proc* 37:2301-2307.

Golden, N.H. 2002. A review of the female athlete triad (amenorrhea, osteoporosis and disordered eating). *Int J Adolesc Med Health* 14:9-17.

Gomez-Cabrera, M.C., C. Borras, F.V. Pallardo, J. Sastre, L.L. Ji, and J. Vina. 2005. Decreasing xanthine oxidase-mediated oxidative stress prevents useful cellular adaptations to exercise in rats. *J Physiol* 567:113-120.

Gomez-Cabrera, M.C., E. Domenech, M. Romagnoli, A. Arduini, C. Borras, F.V. Pallardo, J. Sastre, and J. Vina. 2008. Oral administration of vitamin C decreases muscle mitochondrial biogenesis and hampers training-induced adaptations in endurance performance. *Am J Clin Nutr* 87 (1): 142-149.

Gontzea, I., R. Sutzeescu, and S. Dumitrache. 1975. The influence of adaptation to physical effort on nitrogen balance in man. *Nutr Rep Internat* 11 (3): 231-236.

Gonzalez-Alonso, J., J.A.L. Calbet, and B. Nielsen. 1998. Muscle blood flow is reduced with dehydration during prolonged exercise in humans. *J Physiol* 513:895-905.

Goodpaster, B.H., D.E. Kelley, F.L. Thaete, et al. 2000. Skeletal muscle attenuation determined by computed tomography is associated with skeletal muscle lipid content. *J Appl Physiol* 89 (1): 104-110.

Gordon, D.J. 1995a. Cholesterol and mortality: What can meta-analysis tell us? In *Cardiovascular disease 2*, ed. L.L. Gallo, 333-340. New York: Plenum Press.

Gordon, D.J. 1995b. Cholesterol lowering and mortality. In *Lowering cholestrol in high risk individuals and populations*, ed. B.M. Rifkind, 33-48. New York: Marcel Dekker.

Gould, A.L., J.E. Rossouw, N.C. Santanello, J.F. Heyse, and C.D. Furberg. 1998. Cholesterol reduction yields clinical benefit: Impact of statin trials. *Circulation* 97 (10): 946-952.

Graham, T.E., E. Hibbert, and P. Sathasivam. 1998. Metabolic and exercise endurance effects of coffee and caffeine ingestion. *J Appl Physiol* 85 (3): 883-889.

Graham, T.E., and L.L. Spriet. 1991. Performance and metabolic responses to a high caffeine dose during prolonged exercise. *J Appl Physiol* 71 (6): 2292-2298.

Graham, T.E., and L.L. Spriet. 1995. Metabolic, catecholamine, and exercise performance responses to various doses of caffeine. *J Appl Physiol* 78 (3): 867-874.

Graham, T.E., J.W. Rush, and M.H. van Soeren. 1994. Caffeine and exercise: Metabolism and performance. *Can J Appl Physiol* 19 (2): 111-138.

Graham, T.E., P.K. Pedersen, and B. Saltin. 1987. Muscle and blood ammonia and lactate responses to prolonged exercise with hyperoxia. *J Appl Physiol* 63 (4): 1457-1462.

Graudal, N.A., A.M. Galloe, and P. Garred. 1998. Effects of sodium restriction on blood pressure, renin, aldosterone, catecholamines, cholesterols, and triglyceride: A meta-analysis. JAMA 279 (17): 1383-1391.

Gray, M.E., and L.W. Titlow. 1982. The effect of pangamic acid on maximal treadmill performance. *Med Sci Sports Exerc* 14 (6): 424-427.

Green, A.L., D.A. Sewell, L. Simpson, E. Hultman, and P.L. Greenhaff. 1995. Carbohydrate ingestion stimulates creatine uptake in human skeletal muscle. *J Physiol* 489:27P.

Green, A.L., E.J. Simpson, J.J. Littlewood, I.A. MacDonald, and P.L. Greenhaff. 1996. Carbohydrate ingestion augments creatine retention during creatine feeding in humans. *Acta Physiol Scand* 158:195-202.

Green, H.J. 1995. Metabolic determinants of activity induced muscular fatigue. In *Exercise metabolism*, ed. M. Hargreaves, 211-256. Champaign, IL: Human Kinetics.

Green, N.R., and A.A. Ferrando. 1994. Plasma boron and the effects of boron supplementation in males. *Environ Health Perspect* 102 (suppl 7): 73-77.

Greenhaff, P.L., and J.A. Timmons. 1998. Interaction between aerobic and anaerobic metabolism during intense muscle contraction. *Exerc Sport Sci Rev* 26:1-30.

Greenhaff, P.L., K. Bodin, R.C. Harris, D.A. Jones, D.B. McIntyre, K. Soderlund, and D.L. Turner. 1993. The influence of oral creatine supplementation on muscle phosphocreatine resynthesis following intense contraction in man. *J Physiol* 467:75P.

Greenhaff, P.L. 1998. The nutritional biochemistry of creatine. *Nutr Biochem* 11:1610-1618.

Greenhaff, P.L., A. Casey, A.H. Short, R. Harris, K. Soderlund, and E. Hultman. 1993. Influence of oral creatine supplementation of muscle torque during repeated bouts of maximal voluntary exercise in man. *Clin Sci* 84:565-571.

Greenhaff, P.L., and J.A. Timmons. 1998. Pyruvate dehydrogenase complex activation status and acetyl group availability as a site of interchange between anaerobic and oxidative metabolism during intense exercise. *Adv Exp Med Biol* 441:287-298.

Greenhaff, P.L., K. Bodin, K. Soderlund, and E. Hultman. 1994. Effect of oral creatine supplementation on skeletal muscle phosphocreatine resynthesis. *Am J Physiol* 266:E725-E730.

Greenleaf, J.E. 1979. Hyperthermia in exercise. In *International review of physiology: Environmental physiology III*, Vol. 20, ed. D. Robertshaw, 1-50. Baltimore: University Park Press.

Greer, F., C. McLean, and T.E. Graham. 1998. Caffeine, performance, and metabolism during repeated wingate exercise tests. *J Appl Physiol* 85 (4): 1502-1508.

Guezennec, C.Y., J.F. Nadaud, P. Satabin, F. Léger, and P. Lafargue. 1989. Influence of polyunsaturated fatty acid diet on the hemorrheological response to physical exercise in hypoxia. *Int J Sports Med* 10 (4): 286-291.

Guthrie, J.F., and Morton, J.F. 2000. Food sources of added sweeteners in the diets of Americans. *J Am Diet Assoc* 100 (1): 43-51.

Halberstam, M., N. Cohen, P. Shlimovich, L. Rossetti, and H. Shamoon. 1996. Oral vanadyl sulfate improves insulin sensitivity in NIDDM but not in obese nondiabetic subjects. *Diabetes* 45:659-666.

Hall, J.N., S. Moore, S.B. Harper, and J.W. Lynch. 2009. Global variability in fruit and vegetable consumption. *Am J Prev Med* 36 (5): 402–409, e405.

Hallmark, M.A., T.H. Reynolds, C.A. DeSouza, C.O. Dotson, R.A. Anderson, and M.A. Rogers. 1996. Effects of chromium and resistive training on muscle strength and body composition. *Med Sci Sports Exerc* 28 (1): 139–144.

Halson, S.L., G.I. Lancaster, J. Achten, M. Gleeson, and A.E. Jeukendrup. 2004. Effects of carbohydrate supplementation on performance and carbohydrate oxidation after intensified cycling training. J Appl Physiol, 97 (4):1245–1253.

Hambraeus, L., A. Sjodin, P. Webb, A. Forslund, K. Hambraeus, and T. Hambraeus. 1994. A suit calorimeter for energy balance studies on humans during heavy exercise. *Eur J Appl Physiol* 68 (1): 68–73.

Hansen, A.K., C.P. Fischer, P. Plomgaard, J.L. Andersen, B. Saltin, B.K. Pedersen. 2005. Skeletal muscle adaptation: Training twice every second day vs. training once daily. *J Appl Physiol* 98:93–99.

Hargreaves, K.M., J.A. Hawley, and A.E. Jeukendrup. 2004. Pre-exercise carbohydrate and fat ingestion: Effects on metabolism and performance. *J Sports Sci* 22:31–38.

Hargreaves, K.M., and W.M. Pardridge. 1988. Neutral amino acid transport at the human blood-brain barrier. *J Biol Chem* 263 (36): 19392–19397.

Hargreaves, M. 1995. *Exercise metabolism.* Champaign, IL: Human Kinetics.

Hargreaves, M., and L. Spriet. 2006. *Exercise metabolism,* 2nd ed. Champaign, IL: Human Kinetics.

Harper, A.E. 1999. Nutritional essentiality: Evolution of the concept. *Nutr Today* 36:216–222.

Harris, R.C., K. Soderlund, and E. Hultman. 1992. Elevation of creatine in resting and exercised muscle of normal subjects by creatine supplementation. *Clin Sci* 83:367–374.

Harris, R.C., M.J. Tallon, M. Dunnett, L. Boobis, J. Coakley, H.J. Kim, J.L. Fallowfield, C.A. Hill, C. Sale, and J.A. Wise. 2006. The absorption of orally supplied beta-alanine and its effect on muscle carnosine synthesis in human vastus lateralis. *Amino Acids* 30 (3): 279–289.

Hartman, J.W., J.E. Tang, S.B. Wilkinson, M.A. Tarnopolsky, R.L. Lawrence, A.V. Fullerton, and S.M. Phillips. 2007. Consumption of fat-free fluid milk after resistance exercise promotes greater lean mass accretion than does consumption of soy or carbohydrate in young, novice, male weightlifters. *Am J Clin Nutr* 86 (2): 373–381.

Haskell, W.L., I.M. Lee, R.R. Pate, et al. 2007. Physical activity and public health: Updated recommendation for adults from the American College of Sports Medicine and the American Heart Association. *Med Sci Sports Exerc* 39:1423–34.

Hasten, D.L., E.P. Rome, B.D. Franks, and M. Hegsted. 1992. Effects of chromium picolinate on beginning weight training students. *Int J Sport Nutr* 2 (4): 343–350.

Haubrich, D.R., P.F. Wang, D.E. Clody, and P.W. Wedeking. 1975. Increase in rat brain acetylcholine induced by choline or deanol. *Life Sci* 17 (6): 975–980.

Havel, R.J., B. Pernow, and N.L. Jones. 1967. Uptake and release of free fatty acids and other metabolites in the legs of exercising men. *J Appl Physiol* 23 (1): 90–99.

Hawley, J.A., A.N. Bosch, S.M. Weltan, S.C. Dennis, and T.D. Noakes. 1994. Glucose kinetics during prolonged exercise in euglycemic and hyperglycemic subjects. *Pflügers Arch* 426:378–386.

Hawley, J.A., E.J. Schabort., T.D. Noakes, and S.C. Dennis. 1997. Carbohydrate loading and exercise performance. *Sports Med* 24 (1): 1–10.

Heinonen, O.J. 1996. Carnitine and physical exercise. *Sports Med* 22 (2): 109–132.

Helge, J.W., B. Wulff, and B. Kiens. 1998. Impact of a fat-rich diet on endurance in man role of the dietary period. *Med Sci Sports Exerc* 30:456–461.

Henson, D.A., D.C. Nieman, J.C.D. Parker, M.K. Rainwater, D.E. Butterworth, B.J. Warren, A. Utter, J.M. Davis, O.R. Fagoaga, and S.L. Nehlsen-Cannarella. 1998. Carbohydrate supplementation and the lymphocyte proliferative response to long endurance running. *Int J Sports Med* 19:574–580.

Herbert, V. 1979. Pangamic acid ("vitamin B_{15}"). *Am J Clin Nutr* 32 (7): 1534–1540.

Hertog, M.C.L., E.M. Feskens, P.C.H. Hollman, and M.B. Katan. 1993. Dietary antioxidant flavonoids and risk of coronary heart disease: The Zutphen elderly study. *Lancet* 342:1007–1011.

Heymsfield, S.B., R. Smith, M. Aulet, et al. 1990. Appendicular skeletal muscle mass: Measurement by dual-photon absorptiometry. *Am J Clin Nutr* 52 (2): 214–218.

Hill, C.A., R.C. Harris, H.J. Kim, B.D. Harris, C. Sale, L.H. Boobis, C.K. Kim, and J.A. Wise. 2007. Influence of beta-alanine supplementation on skeletal muscle carnosine concentrations and high intensity cycling capacity. *Amino Acids* 32 (2): 225–233.

Hinton, P.S., C. Giordano, T. Brownlie, and J.D. Haas. 2000. Iron supplementation improves endurance after training in iron-depleted, nonanemic women. *J Appl Physiol* 88:1103–1111.

Hiscock, N., and B.K. Pedersen. 2002. Exercise-induced immunosuppression—plasma glutamine is not the link. *J Appl Physiol* 93:813–822.

Hogervorst, E., S. Bandelow, J. Schmitt, R. Jentjens, M. Oliveira, J. Allgrove, T. Carter, and M. Gleeson. 2008. Caffeine improves physical and cognitive performance during exhaustive exercise. *Med Sci Sports Exerc* 40 (10): 1841–1851.

Hogervorst, E., W.J. Riedel, E. Kovacs, F. Brouns, and J. Jolles. 1999. Caffeine improves cognitive performance after strenuous physical exercise. *Int J Sports Med* 20 (6): 354–361.

Holloszy, J.O., and E.F. Coyle. 1984. Adaptations of skeletal muscle to endurance exercise and their metabolic consequences. *J Appl Physiol* 56 (4): 831–838.

Holloszy, J.O., and W. Booth. 1976. Biochemical adaptations to endurance exercise in muscle. *Ann Rev Physiol* 38:273–291.

Holt, P.R. 1968. Medium chain triglycerides: Their absorption, metabolism and clinical applications. In *Progress in gastroenterology,* ed. B. George and J. Glass, 277–298. New York: Grune & Stratton, Inc.

Hopkins, W.G., J.A. Hawley, and L.M. Burke. 1999. Design and analysis of research on sport performance enhancement. *Med Sci Sports Exerc* 31 (3): 472–485.

Hopkins, W.G. 2000. Measures of reliability in sports medicine and science. *Sports Med* 30 (1): 1–15.

Hoppeler, H., and M. Fluck. 2003. Plasticity of skeletal muscle mitochondria: Structure and function. *Med Sci Sports Exerc* 35:95–104.

Horowitz, J.F., R. Mora-Rodriguez, L.O. Byerley, and E.F. Coyle. 2000. Preexercise medium-chain triglyceride ingestion does not alter muscle glycogen use during exercise. *J Appl Physiol* 88 (1): 219–225.

Horowitz, J.F., R. Mora-Rodriguez, L.O. Byerley, and E.F. Coyle. 1997. Lipolytic suppression following carbohydrate ingestion limits fat oxidation during exercise. *Am J Physiol* 273:E768–E775.

Horswill, C.A. 1995. Effects of bicarbonate, citrate, and phosphate loading on performance. *Int J Sports Nutr* 5:S111–S119.

Houmard, J.A., D.L. Costill, J.A. Davis, J.B. Mitchell, D.D. Pascoe, and R.A. Robergs. 1990. The influence of exercise intensity on heat acclimation in trained subjects. *Med Sci Sports Exerc* 22 (5): 615-620.

Houmard, J.A., P.C. Egan, R.A. Johns, et al. 1991. Gastric emptying during 1 h of cycling and running at 75% V\od\ O$_2$max. *Med Sci Sports Exerc* 23 (3): 320-325.

Hu, F.B., M.J. Stampfer, J.E. Manson, E. Rimm, G.A. Colditz, B.A. Rosner, C.H. Hennekens, and W.C. Willett. 1997. Dietary fat intake and the risk of coronary heart disease in women [see comments]. *N Engl J Med* 337 (21): 1491-1499.

Hubert, P., N.A. King, and J.E. Blundell. 1998. Uncoupling the effects of energy expenditure and energy intake: Appetite response to short-term energy deficit induced by meal omission and physical activity. *Appetite* 31:9-19.

Hulston, C.J., and A.E. Jeukendrup. 2008. Substrate metabolism and exercise performance with caffeine and carbohydrate intake. *Med Sci Sports Exerc* 40 (12): 2096-2104.

Hultman, E. 1967. Physiological role of muscle glycogen in man, with special reference to exercise. *Circ Res* 10:I99-I114.

Hultman, E., and L.H. Nilsson. 1971. Liver glycogen in man: Effects of different diets and muscular exercise. In *Muscle metabolism during exercise, II,* ed. B. Pernow and B. Saltin, 143-151. New York: Plenum.

Hultman, E., K. Soderlund, J.A. Timmons, G. Cederblad, and P.L. Greenhaff. 1996. Muscle creatine loading in men. *J Appl Physiol* 81 (1): 232-237.

Hultman, E., P.L. Greenhaff, J.M. Ren, and K. Soderlund. 1991. Energy metabolism and fatigue during intense muscle contraction. *Biochem Soc Trans* 19 (2): 347-353.

Hunt, C., N.K. Chakaravorty, G. Annan, N. Habibzadeh, and C.J. Schorah. 1994. The clinical effects of vitamin C supplementation in elderly hospitalized with acute respiratory infections. *Int J Vit Nutr Res* 64:202-207.

Hunt, J.N., and I. Donald. 1954.The influence of volume on gastric emptying. *J Physiol* 126:459-474.

Inder, W.J., M.P. Swanney, R.A. Donald, T.C.R. Prickett, and J. Hellemans. 1998. The effect of glycerol and desmopressin on exercise performance and hydration in triathletes. *Med Sci Sports Exerc* 30:1263-1269.

Issekutz, B., H.I. Miller, P. Paul, and K. Rodahl. 1964. Source of fat in exercising dogs. *Am J Physiol* 207 (3): 583-589.

Isselbacher, K.J. 1968. Mechanisms of absorption of long and medium chain triglycerides. In *Medium chain triglycerides,* ed. J.R. Senior, 21-37. Philadelphia: University of Pensylvania Press.

Ivy, J.L. 1998. Glycogen resynthesis after exercise: Effect of carbohydrate intake. *Int J Sports Med* 19:S142-S145.

Ivy, J.L., A.L. Katz, C.L. Cutler, W.M. Sherman, and E.F. Coyle. 1988b. Muscle glycogen synthesis after exercise: Effect of time of carbohydrate ingestion. *J Appl Physiol* 64:1480-1485.

Ivy, J.L., and C.-H. Kuo. 1998. Regulation of GLUT4 protein and glycogen synthase during musle glycogen synthesis after exercise. *Acta Physiol Scand* 162:295-304.

Ivy, J.L., D.L. Costill, W.J. Fink, and R.W. Lower. 1979. Influence of caffeine and carbohydrate feedings on endurance performance. *Med Sci Sports* 11:6-11.

Ivy, J.L., M.C. Lee, J.T. Brozinick, and M.J. Reed. 1988a. Muscle glycogen storage after different amounts of carbohydrate ingestion. *J Appl Physiol* 65:2018-2023.

Ivy, J.L., P.T. Res, R.C. Sprague, and M.O. Widzer. 2003. Effect of a carbohydrate-protein supplement on endurance performance during exercise of varying intensity. *Int J Sport Nutr Exerc Metab* 13 (3): 382-395.

Jackman, M., P. Wendling, D. Friars, and T.E. Graham. 1996. Metabolic catecholamine, and endurance responses to caffeine during intense exercise. *J Appl Physiol* 81 (4): 1658-1663.

Jackson, A.S., and M.L. Pollock. 1978. Generalized equations for predicting body density of men. *Br J Nutr* 40 (3): 497-504.

Jackson, M.J. 2000. Exercise and oxygen radical production by muscle. In *Handbook of oxidants and antioxidants in exercise,* ed. C.K. Sen, L. Packer, and O.P. Hanninnen Osmo, 297-321. Amsterdam: Elsevier.

Jackson, M.J. 2007. Free radicals generated by contracting muscle: By-products of metabolism or key regulators of muscle function? *Free Radical Bio Med* 44 (2): 132-141.

Jagetia, G.C., and B.B. Aggarwal. 2007. "Spicing up" of the immune system by curcumin. *J Clin Immunol* 27 (1): 19-35.

Jakubowicz, D., N. Beer, and R. Rengifo. 1995. Effect of dehydroepiandrosterone on cyclic-guanosine monophosphate in men of advancing age. *Ann N Y Acad Sci* 774:312-315.

Jansson, E., and L. Kaijser. 1982. Effect of diet on the utilization of blood-borne and intramuscular substrates during exercise in man. *Acta Physiol Scand* 115:19-30.

Jeffery, R.W., W.L. Hellerstedt, S.A. French, et al. 1995. A randomized trial of counseling for fat restriction versus calorie restriction in the treatment of obesity. *Int J Obes Relat Metab Disord* 19 (2): 132-137.

Jentjens, R.L., and A.E. Jeukendrup. 2002. Effect of acute and short-term administration of vanadyl sulphate on insulin sensitivity in healthy active humans. *Int J Sport Nutr Exerc Metab* 12 (4): 470-479.

Jentjens, R.L., and A.E. Jeukendrup. 2005a. High rates of exogenous carbohydrate oxidation from a mixture of glucose and fructose ingested during prolonged cycling exercise. *Br J Nutr* 93 (4): 485-492.

Jentjens, R.L., L. Moseley, R.H. Waring, L.K. Harding, and A.E. Jeukendrup. 2004a. Oxidation of combined ingestion of glucose and fructose during exercise. *J Appl Physiol* 96 (4): 1277-1284.

Jentjens, R.L., and A.E. Jeukendrup. 2003b. Determinants of post-exercise glycogen synthesis during short-term recovery. *Sports Med* 33 (2): 117-144.

Jentjens, R.L., L. Moseley, R.H. Waring, L.K. Harding, and A.E. Jeukendrup. 2003. Oxidation of combined ingestion of glucose and fructose during exercise. *J Appl Physiol* [online]. Available at DOI, 10.1152/japplphysiol.00974.

Jentjens, R.L., and A.E. Jeukendrup. 2002. Effect of acute and short-term administration of vanadyl sulphate on insulin sensitivity in healthy active humans. *Int J Sports Nutr Exerc Metab* 12:434-443.

Jentjens, R.L., and A.E. Jeukendrup. 2003a. Effects of pre-exercise ingestion of trehalose, galactose and glucose on subsequent metabolism and cycling performance. *Eur J Appl Physiol* 88 (4-5): 459-465.

Jentjens, R.L., C. Cale, C. Gutch, and A.E. Jeukendrup. 2003. Effects of pre-exercise ingestion of differing amounts of carbohydrate on subsequent metabolism and cycling performance. *Eur J Appl Physiol* 88 (4-5): 444-452.

Jentjens, R.L., L.J. van Loon, C.H. Mann, A.J. Wagenmakers, and A.E. Jeukendrup. 2001. Addition of protein and amino acids to carbohydrates does not enhance postexercise muscle glycogen synthesis. *J Appl Physiol* 91 (2): 839-846.

Jentjens, R.L., C. Shaw, T. Birtles, R.H. Waring, L.K. Harding, and A.E. Jeukendrup. 2005b. Oxidation of combined ingestion of glucose and sucrose during exercise. *Metabolism* 54 (5): 610-618.

Jentjens, R.L., K. Underwood, J. Achten, K. Currell, C.H. Mann, and A.E. Jeukendrup. 2006. Exogenous carbohydrate oxidation rates are elevated after combined ingestion of glucose and fructose during exercise in the heat. *J Appl Physiol* 100 (3): 807-816.

Jentjens, R.L., M.C. Venables, and A.E. Jeukendrup. 2004b. Oxidation of exogenous glucose, sucrose, and maltose during prolonged cycling exercise. *J Appl Physiol* 96 (4): 1285-1291.

Jeukendrup, A.E., and G.A. Wallis. 2005. Measurement of substrate oxidation during exercise by means of gas exchange measurements. *Int J Sports Med* 26 (Suppl 1): S28-37.

Jeukendrup, A.E., A.J. Wagenmakers, J.H. Stegen, A.P. Gijsen, F. Brouns, and W.H. Saris. 1999. Carbohydrate ingestion can completely suppress endogenous glucose production during exercise. *Am J Physiol* 276 (4 pt 1): E672-E683.

Jeukendrup, A.E., A.J.M. Wagenmakers, L.M.L.A. Van Etten, R.L.P. Jentjens, G.J. Oomen, J.H.C.H. Stegen, P.F. Schoffelen, and W.H.M. Saris. 2000c. Negative fat balance in weight stable physically active humans on a low-fat diet. *J Physiol* 523:223P.

Jeukendrup, A.E., and R.L. Jentjens. 2000. Oxidation of carbohydrate feedings during prolonged exercise: Current thoughts, guidelines and directions for future research. *Sports Med* 29 (6): 407-424.

Jeukendrup, A.E., F. Brouns, A.J.M. Wagenmakers, and W.H.M. Saris. 1997. Carbohydrate-electrolyte feedings improve 1 h time trial cycling performance. *Int J Sports Med* 18 (2): 125-129.

Jeukendrup, A.E., J.J.H.C. Thielen, A.J.M. Wagenmakers, F. Brouns, and W.H.M. Saris. 1998. Effect of MCT and carbohydrate ingestion on substrate utilization and cycling performance. *Am J Clin Nutr* 67:397-404.

Jeukendrup, A.E., K. Vet-Joop, A. Sturk, J.H. Stegen, J. Senden, W.H. Saris, and A.J. Wagenmakers. 2000a. Relationship between gastro-intestinal complaints and endotoxaemia, cytokine release and the acute-phase reaction during and after a long-distance triathlon in highly trained men. *Clin Sci (Colch)* 98 (1): 47-55.

Jeukendrup, A.E., N.P. Craig, and J.A. Hawley. 2000b. The bioenergetics of world class cycling. *J Sci Med Sport* 3 (4): 414-433.

Jeukendrup, A.E., N.P. Craig, and J.A. Hawley. 2000. The bioenergetics of world class cycling. *J Sci Med Sport* 3 (4): 414-433.

Jeukendrup, A.E., M.K.C. Hesselink, A.C. Snyder, H. Kuipers, and H.A. Keizer. 1992. Physiological changes in male competitive cyclists after two weeks of intensified training. Int J Sports Med, 13:534-541.

Jeukendrup, A.E., L. Moseley, G.I. Mainwaring, S. Samuels, S. Perry, and C.H. Mann. 2006. Exogenous carbohydrate oxidation during ultraendurance exercise. *J Appl Physiol* 100 (4): 1134-1141.

Jeukendrup, A.E., W.H.M. Saris, F. Brouns, and A.D.M. Kester. 1996. A new validated endurance performance test. *Med Sci Sport Exerc* 28 (2): 266-270.

Jeukendrup, A.E., W.H.M. Saris, P. Schrauwen, F. Brouns, and A.J.M. Wagenmakers. 1995. Metabolic availability of medium chain triglycerides co-ingested with carbohydrates during prolonged exercise. *J Appl Physiol* 79 (3): 756-762.

Jeukendrup, A.E. 2004. Carbohydrate intake during exercise and performance. *Nutrition* 20 (7-8): 669-677.

Jeukendrup, A.E. 2008. Carbohydrate feeding during exercise. *Eur J Sport Sci* 8 (2): 77-86.

Ji, L.L. 2007. Antioxidant signaling in skeletal muscle: A brief review. *Experimental Gerontology* 42 (7): 582-593.

Johannes, C.B., R.K. Stellato, H.A. Feldman, C. Longcope, and J.B. McKinlay. 1999. Relation of dehydroepiandrosterone and dehydroepiandrosterone sulfate with cardiovascular disease risk factors in women: Longitudinal results from the Massachusetts Women's Health Study. *J Clin Epidemiol* 52 (2): 95-103.

Johansson, L., K. Solvoll, G.E. Bjorneboe, and C.A. Drevon. 1998. Under- and overreporting of energy intake related to weight status and lifestyle in a nationwide sample. *Am J Clin Nutr* 68 (2): 266-274.

Jones, D.A., and O.M. Rutherford. 1987. Human muscle strength training: The effects of three different regimens and the nature of the resultant changes. *J Physiol (Lond)* 391:1-11.

Jowko, E., P. Ostaszewski, M. Jank, J. Sacharuk, A. Zieniewicz, J. Wilczak, and S. Nissen. 2001. Creatine and beta-hydroxy-beta-methylbutyrate (HMB) additively increase lean body mass and muscle strength during a weight-training program. *Nutrition* 17 (7-8): 558-566.

Jozsi, A.C., T.A. Trappe, R.D. Starling, B. Goodpaster, S.W. Trappe, W.J. Fink, D.L. Costill. 1996. The influence of starch structure on glycogen resynthesis and subsequent cycling performance. *Int J Sports Med* 17 (5): 373-378.

Judelson, D.A., C.M. Maresh, J.M. Anderson, et al. 2007. Hydration and muscular performance: Does fluid balance affect strength, power and high-intensity endurance? *Sports Medicine* 37 (10): 907-921.

Kagan, A., B.R. Harris, W. Winkelstein, Jr., K.G. Johnson, H. Kato, S.L. Syme, G.G. Rhoads, M.L. Gay, M.Z. Nichaman, H.B. Hamilton, and J. Tillotson. 1974. Epidemiologic studies of coronary heart disease and stroke in Japanese men living in Japan, Hawaii and California: Demographic, physical, dietary and biochemical characteristics. *J Chronic Dis* 27 (7-8): 345-364.

Kamada, T., S. Tokuda, S.-I. Aozaki, and S. Otsuji. 1993. Higher levels of erethrocyte membrane fluidity in sprinters and long-distance runners. *J Appl Physiol* 74 (1): 354-358.

Kaminski, M., and R. Boal. 1992. An effect of ascorbic acid on delayed-onset muscle soreness. *Pain* 50:317-321.

Kandelman, D. 1997. Sugar, alternative sweeteners and meal frequency in relation to caries prevention: New perspectives. *Br J Nutr* 77 (suppl 1): S121-S128.

Kantamala, D., M. Vongsakul, and J. Satayavivad. 1990. The in vivo and in vitro effects of caffeine on rat immune cell activities: B, T and NK cells. *Asian Pac J Allergy Immunol* 8:77-82

Karlsson, J., and B. Saltin. 1970. Lactate, ATP, and CP in working muscles during exhaustive exercise in man. *J Appl Physiol* 29 (5): 596-602.

Kasperek, G.J., and R.D. Snider. 1989. Total and myofibrillar protein degradation in isolated soleus muscles after exercise. *Am J Physiol* 257 (1 pt 1): E1-E5.

Kazis, K., and E. Iglesias. 2003. The female athlete triad. *Adolesc Med* 14:87-95.

Keeffe, E.B., D.K. Lowe, J.R. Goss, and R. Wayne. 1984. Gastrointestinal symptoms of marathon runners. *West J Med* 141:481-484.

Keesey, R.E., and M.D. Hirvonen. 1997. Body weight set-points: Determination and adjustment. *J Nutr* 127 (9): 1875S-1883S

Keizer, H., H. Kuipers, and G. van Kranenburg. 1987. Influence of liquid and solid meals on muscle glycogen resynthesis, plasma fuel hormone response, and maximal physical working capacity. *Int J Sports Med* 8:99-104.

Keizer, H., H. Kuipers, G. van Kranenburg, and P. Geurten. 1987b. Influence of liquid and solid meals on glycogen resynthesis, plasma fuel hormone response, and maximal physical working capacity. *Int J Sports Med* 8 (2): 99–104.

Kekkonen, R.A., T.J. Vasankari, T. Vuorimaa, et al. 2007. The effects of probiotics on respiratory infections and gastrointestinal symptoms during training in marathon runners. *Int J Sport Nutr Exerc Metabol* 17:352–363.

Kelly, J.M., B.A. Gorney, and K.K. Kalm. 1978. The effects of a collegiate wrestling season on body composition, cardiovascular fitness and muscular strength and endurance. *Med Sci Sports* 10 (2): 119–124

Khatta, M., B.S. Alexander, C.M. Krichten, M.L. Fisher, R. Freudenberger, S.W. Robinson, and S.S. Gottlieb. 2000. The effect of coenzyme Q10 in patients with congestive heart failure. *Ann Intern Med* 132 (8): 636–640.

King, N.A., V.J. Burley, and J.E. Blundell. 1994. Exercise-induced suppression of appetite: Effects on food intake and implications for energy balance. *Eur J Clin Nutr* 48 (10): 715–724.

King, D.S., R.L. Sharp, M.D. Vukovich, G.A. Brown, T.A. Reifenrath, N.L. Uhl, and K.A. Parsons. 1999. Effect of oral androstenedione on serum testosterone and adaptations to resistance training in young men: A randomized controlled trial [see comments]. *JAMA* 281 (21): 2020–2028.

Kjaer, M. et al. 1988. Hormonal response to exercise in humans: Influence of hypoxia and physical training. *American Journal of Physiology* 254:R197–203.

Kleessen, B., W. Schroedl, M. Stueck, et al. 2005. Microbial and immunological responses relative to high altitude exposure in mountaineers. *Med Sci Sports Exerc* 37:1313–1318.

Klein, S., E.F. Coyle, and R.R. Wolfe. 1994. Fat metabolism during low-intensity exercise in endurance trained and untrained men. *Am J Physiol* 267:E934–E940.

Klein, S., J.-M. Weber, E.F. Coyle, and R.R. Wolfe. 1996. Effect of endurance training on glycerol kinetics during strenuous exercise in humans. *Metabolism* 45 (3): 357–361.

Knapik, J., C. Meredith, B. Jones, R. Fielding, V. Young, and W. Evans. 1991. Leucine metabolism during fasting and exercise. *J Appl Physiol* 70 (1): 43–47.

Knapik, J.J., B.H. Jones, M.M. Toner, W.L. Daniels, and W.J. Evans. 1983. Influence of caffeine on serum substrate changes during running in trained and untrained individuals. *Bioch Exerc* 13:514–519.

Knapik, J.J., C.N. Meredith, B.H. Jones, L. Suek, V.R. Young, and W.J. Evans. 1988. Influence of fasting on carbohydrate and fat metabolism during rest and exercise in men. *J Appl Physiol* 64 (5): 1923–1929.

Knopf, R.F., J.W. Conn, J.C. Floyd, Jr., S.S. Fajans, J.A. Rull, E.M. Guntsche, and C.A. Thiffault. 1966. The normal endocrine response to ingestion of protein and infusions of amino acids: Sequential secretion of insulin and growth hormone. *Trans Assoc Am Physicians* 79:312–321.

Kochan, R.G., D.R. Lamb, S.A. Lutz, C.V. Perrill, E.M. Reimann, and K.K. Schlender. 1979. Glycogen synthase activation in human skeletal muscle: Effects of diet and exercise. *Am J Physiol* 5 (6): E660–E666.

Koenigsberg, P.S., K.K. Martin, H.R. Hlava, and M.L. Riedesel. 1995. Sustained hyperhydration with glycerol ingestion. *Life Sci* 57 (7): 645–653.

Kohrt, W.M. 1995. Body composition by DXA: Tried and true? *Med Sci Sports Exerc* 27 (10): 1349–1353.

Konig, D., A. Berg, C. Weinstock, J. Keul, and H. Northoff. 1997. Essential fatty acids, immune function and exercise. *Exercise and Immunology Review* 3:1–31.

Koopman, R., D.L. Pannemans, A.E. Jeukendrup, A. Gijsen, J.M.G. Senden, D. Halliday, W.H.M. Saris, L.J.C. van Loon, and A.J.M. Wagenmakers. 2004. Combined ingestion of protein and carbohydrate improves protein balance during ultra-endurance exercise. *Am J Physiol Endocrinol Metab* 287 (4): E712–720.

Koopman, R., A.J.M. Wagenmakers, R.J.F. Manders, A.H.G. Zorenc, J.M.G. Senden, M. Gorselink, H.A. Keizer, and L.J.C. van Loon. 2005. Combined ingestion of protein and free leucine with carbohydrate increases postexercise muscle protein synthesis in vivo in male subjects. *Am J Physiol Endocrinol Metab* 288 (4): E645–653.

Kopp-Hoolihan, L. 2001. Prophylactic and therapeutic uses of probiotics: A review. *J Am Diet Assoc* 101:229–238.

Koubi, H.E., D. Desplanches, C. Gabrielle, J.M. Cottet-Emard, B. Sempore, and R.J. Favier. 1991. Exercise endurance and fuel utilization: A reevaluation of the effects of fasting. *J Appl Physiol* 70 (3): 1337–1343.

Koulmann, N., C. Jimenez, D. Regal, et al. 2000. Use of bioelectrical impedance analysis to estimate body fluid compartments after acute variations of the body hydration level. *Med Sci Sports Exerc* 32 (4): 857–864.

Kovacs, E.M.R., J.H.C.H. Stegen, and F. Brouns. 1998. Effect of caffeinated drinks on substrate metabolism, caffeine excretion, and performance. *J Appl Physiol* 85:709–715.

Kraemer, W.J., J.F. Patton, S.E. Gordon, et al. 1995. Compatibility of high-intensity strength and endurance training on hormonal and skeletal muscle adaptations. *J Appl Physiol* 78 (3): 976–989.

Kreider, R.B., M. Ferreira, M. Wilson, P. Grindstaff, S. Plisk, J. Reinardy, E. Cantler, and A.L. Almada. 1998. Effects of creatine supplementation on body composition, strength, and sprint performance. *Med Sci Sports Exerc* 30 (1): 73–82.

Kreider, R.B., G.W. Miller, D. Schenck, C.W. Cortes, V. Miriel, C.T. Somma, P. Rowland, C. Turner, and D. Hill. 1992. Effects of phosphate loading on metabolic and myocardial responses to maximal and endurance exercise. *Int J Sport Nutr* 2 (1): 20–47.

Kreider, R.B., G.W. Miller, M.H. Williams, C.T. Somma, and T.A. Nasser. 1990. Effects of phosphate loading on oxygen uptake, ventilatory anaerobic threshold, and run performance. *Med Sci Sports Exerc* 22 (2): 250–256.

Krogh, A., and J. Lindhard. 1920. The relative value of fat and carbohydrate as sources of muscular energy. *Biochem J* 14:290–363.

Kromhout, D., A. Menotti, B. Bloemberg, C. Aravanis, H. Blackburn, R. Buzina, A.S. Dontas, F. Fidanza, S. Giampaoli, A. Jansen, et al. 1995. Dietary saturated and *trans* fatty acids and cholesterol and 25-year mortality from coronary heart disease: The Seven Countries study. *Prev Med* 24 (3): 308–315.

Kromhout, D., and C. de Lezenne Coulander. 1984. Diet, prevalence and 10-year mortality from coronary heart disease in 871 middle-aged men: The Zutphen study. *Am J Epidemiol* 119 (5): 733–741.

Kron, L., J.L. Katz, G. Gorzynski, and H. Weiner. 1978. Hyperactivity in anorexia nervosa: A fundamental clinical feature. *Comp Psych* 19:433–440.

Kuipers, H., D.L. Costill, D.A. Porter, W.J. Fink, and W.M. Morse. 1986. Glucose feeding and exercise in trained rats: Mechanisms for glycogen sparing. *J Appl Physiol* 61 (3): 859–863.

Kuipers, H., W.H.M. Saris, F. Brouns, H.A. Keizer, and C. ten Bosch. 1989. Glycogen synthesis during exercise and rest with carbohydrate feeding in males and females. *Int J Sports Med* 10 (suppl 1): S63–S67.

Kumanyika, S.K., and J.A. Cutler. 1997. Dietary sodium reduction: Is there cause for concern? *J Am Coll Nutr* 16 (3): 192–203.

Lambert, C.P., D. Ball, J.B. Leiper, and R.J. Maughan. 1999. The use of a deuterium tracer technique to follow the fate of fluids ingested by human subjects: Effects of drink volume and tracer concentration and content. *Exp Physiol* 84 (2): 391–399.

Lambert, M.I., J.A. Hefer, R.P. Millar, and P.W. Macfarlane. 1993. Failure of commercial oral amino acid supplements to increase serum growth hormone concentrations in male body-builders. *Int J Sport Nutr* 3 (3): 298–305.

Lamont, L.S., A.J. McCullough, and S.C. Kalhan. 1999. Comparison of leucine kinetics in endurance-trained and sedentary humans. *J Appl Physiol* 86 (1): 320–325.

Lancaster, G.I., Q. Khan, P.T. Drysdale, et al. 2005. Effect of prolonged exercise and carbohydrate ingestion on type 1 and type 2 lymphocyte distribution and intracellular cytokine production in humans. *J Appl Physiol* 98:565–571.

Lang, F., G.L. Busch, M. Ritter, H. Volkl, S. Waldegger, E. Gulbins, and D. Haussinger. 1998. Functional significance of cell volume regulatory mechanisms. *Physiol Rev* 78 (1): 247–306.

Lanou, A.J., and N.D. Barnard. 2008. Dairy and weight loss hypothesis: An evaluation of the clinical trials. *Nutr Rev* 66 (5): 272–279.

Latzka, W.A., M.N. Sawka, S.J. Montain, G.S. Skrinar, R.A. Fielding, R.P. Matott, and K.B. Pandolf. 1997. Hyperhydration: Thermoregulatory effects during compensable exercise-heat stress. *J Appl Physiol* 83 (3): 860–866.

Latzka, W.A., M.N. Sawka, S.J. Montain, G.S. Skrinar, R.A. Fielding, R.P. Matott, and K.B. Pandolf. 1998. Hyperhydration: Tolerance and cardiovascular effects during uncompensable exercise-heat stress. *J Appl Physiol* 84:1858–1864.

Layman, D., and D. Walker. 2006. Potential importance of leucine in treatment of obesity and the metabolic syndrome. *J Nutr* 136 (1 Suppl): 319S–323S.

Lebenstedt, M., P. Platte, and K.M. Pirke. 1999. Reduced resting metabolic rate in athletes with menstrual disorders. *Med Sci Sports Exerc* 31 (9): 1250–1256.

Leenders, N.M., D.R. Lamb, and T.E. Nelson. 1999. Creatine supplementation and swimming performance. *Int J Sport Nutr* 9 (3): 251–262.

Lee-Young, R.S., M.J. Palmer, K.C. Linden, K. LePlastrier, B.J. Canny, M. Hargreaves, G.D. Wadley, B.E. Kemp, and G.K. McConell. 2006. Carbohydrate ingestion does not alter skeletal muscle AMPK signaling during exercise in humans. *Am J Physiol Endocrinol Metab* 291:E566–573.

Leibel, R.L., M. Rosenbaum, and J. Hirsch. 1995. Changes in energy expenditure resulting from altered body weight. *N Engl J Med* 332 (10): 621–628.

Leiper, J.B., A.S. Prentice, C. Wrightson, and R.J. Maughan. 2001a. Gastric emptying of a carbohydrate-electrolyte drink during a soccer match. *Med Sci Sports Exerc* 33 (11): 1932–1938.

Leiper, J.B., N.P. Broad, and R.J. Maughan. 2001b. Effect of intermittent high-intensity exercise on gastric emptying in man. *Med Sci Sports Exerc* 33 (8): 1270–1278.

Levine, S.A., B. Gordon, and C.L. Derick. 1924. Some changes in chemical constituents of blood following a marathon race. *JAMA* 82:1778–1779.

Lichtenstein, A.H., L.M. Ausman, S.M. Jalbert, and E.J. Schaefer. 1999. Effects of different forms of dietary hydrogenated fats on serum lipoprotein cholesterol levels [see comments] [published erratum appears in *N Engl J Med* 341 (11): 856]. *N Engl J Med* 340 (25): 1933–1940.

Lieberman, H.R. 2003. Nutrition, brain function and cognitive performance. *Appetite* 40 (3): 245–254.

Linde, K., B. Barrett, K. Wolkart, R. Bauer, and D. Melcahrt. 2006. Echinacea for preventing and treating the common cold. *Cochrane Database Syst Rev*. Issue 1: CD000530.

Linderman, J.K., and K.L. Gosselink. 1994. The effects of sodium bicarbonate ingestion on exercise performance. *Sports Med* 18 (2): 75–80.

Lohman, T.G., and S.B. Going. 1993. Multicomponent models in body composition research: Opportunities and pitfalls. *Basic Life Sci* 60:53–58.

Louard, R.J., E.J. Barrett, and R.A. Gelfand. 1990. Effect of infused branched-chain amino acids on muscle and whole-body amino acid metabolism in man. *Clin Sci (Colch)* 79 (5): 457–466.

Loucks, A. 2006. The evolution of the female athlete triad. In *Clinical sports nutrition*, 3rd ed. ed. L. Burke and V. Deakin, 227–235. New York: McGraw-Hill.

Loucks, A.B., and J.R. Thuma. 2003. Luteinizing hormone pulsatility is disrupted at a threshold of energy availability in regularly menstruating women. *J Clin Endocr Metab* 88:297–311.

Loy, S.F., R.K. Conlee, W.W. Winder, A.G. Nelson, D.A. Arnall, and A.G. Fisher. 1986. Effect of 24-hour fast on cycling endurance time at two different intensities. *J Appl Physiol* 61 (2): 654–659.

Lukaski, H.C., W.W. Bolonchuk, W.A. Siders, and D.B. Milne. 1996. Chromium supplementation and resistance training: Effects on body composition, strength, and trace element status of men. *Am J Clin Nutr* 63 (6): 954–965.

Luke, A., K.C. Maki, N. Barkey, R. Cooper, and D. McGee. 1997. Simultaneous monitoring of heart rate and motion to assess energy expenditure. *Med Sci Sports Exerc* 29 (1): 144–148.

Lyons, T.P., M.L. Riedesel, L.E. Meuli, and T.W. Chick. 1990. Effects of glycerol-induced hyperhydration prior to exercise in the heat on sweating and core temperature. *Med Sci Sports Exerc* 22 (4): 477–483.

Mackinnon, L.T. 1999. *Advances in exercise and immunology.* Champaign, IL: Human Kinetics.

Macknin, M.L. 1999. Zinc lozenges for the common cold. *Cleveland Clin J Med* 66:27–32.

MacLean, D.A., T.E. Graham, and B. Saltin. 1994. Branched-chain amino acids augment ammonia metabolism while attenuating protein breakdown during exercise. *Am J Physiol* 267 (6 Pt 1): E1010–1022.

Madsen, K., D.A. MacLean, B. Kiens, and D. Christensen. 1996. Effects of glucose, glucose plus branched-chain amino acids, or placebo on bike performance over 100 km. *J Appl Physiol* 81 (6): 2644–2650.

Malm, C., M. Svensson, B. Ekblom, and B. Sjodin. 1997. Effects of ubiquinone-10 supplementation and high intensity training on physical performance in humans. *Acta Physiol Scand* 161 (3): 379–384.

Mannix, E.T., J.M. Stager, A. Harris, and M.O. Farber. 1990. Oxygen delivery and cardiac output during exercise following oral phosphate-glucose. *Med Sci Sports Exerc* 22 (3): 341–347.

Manore, M.M. 2002. Dietary recommendations and athletic menstrual dysfunction. *Sports Med* 32:887–901.

Marmy-Conus, N., S. Fabris, J. Proietto, and M. Hargreaves. 1996. Preexercise glucose ingestion and glucose kinetics during exercise. *J Appl Physiol* 81 (2): 853–857.

Marshall, I. 2000. Zinc for the common cold. *Cochrane Database Syst Rev*, CD001364.

Martin, W.H., III, G.P. Dalsky, B.F. Hurley, D.E. Matthews, D.M. Bier, J.M. Hagberg, M.A. Rogers, D.S. King, and J.O. Holloszy. 1993. Effect of endurance training on plasma free fatty acid turnover and oxidation during exercise. *Am J Physiol* 265:E708–E714.

Martin, B., S. Robinson, and D. Robertshaw. 1978. Influence of diet on leg uptake of glucose during heavy exercise. *Am J Clin Nutr* 31:62–67.

Martin, C.K., L.K. Heilbronn, L. de Jonge, J.P. DeLany, J. Volaufova, S.D. Anton, L.M. Redman, S.R. Smith, and E. Ravussin. 2007. Effect of calorie restriction on resting metabolic rate and spontaneous physical activity. *Obesity (Silver Spring)* 15 (12): 2964–2973.

Matson, L.G., and Z. Vu Tran. 1993. Effects of sodium bicarbonate ingestion on anaerobic performance: A meta-analytic review. *Int J Sport Nutrition* 3:2–28.

Matthews, C.E., I.S. Ockene, P.S. Freedson, M.C. Rosal, P.A. Merriam, and J.R. Hebert. 2002. Moderate to vigorous physical activity and the risk of upper-respiratory tract infection. *Med Sci Sports Exerc* 34:1242–1248.

Matthews, D.E. 1999. Proteins and amino acids. In *Modern nutrition in health and disease,* ed. M.E. Shils, J.A. Olson, M. Shike, and A.C. Ross, 11–30. Baltimore: Williams & Wilkins.

Maughan, R.J. 1985. Thermoregulation and fluid balance in marathon competition at low ambient temperature. *Int J Sports Med* 6:15–19.

Maughan, R.J. 1991. Fluid and electrolyte loss and replacement in exercise. *J Sports Sci* 9:117–142.

Maughan, R.J., A.E. Donnelly, M. Gleeson, P.H. Whiting, K.A. Walker, and P.J. Clough. 1989. Delayed-onset muscle damage and lipid peroxidation in man after a downhill run. *Muscle Nerve* 12:332–336.

Maughan, R.J., and R. Murray, eds. 2000. *Sports drinks: Basic science and practical aspects.* Boca Raton, FL: CRC Press.

Maughan, R.J., C.E. Fenn, M. Gleeson, and J.B. Leiper. 1987. Metabolic and circulatory responses to the ingestion of glucose polymer and glucose/electrolyte solutions during exercise in man. *Eur J Appl Physiol* 56:356–362.

Maughan, R.J., J.B. Leiper, and S.M. Shirreffs. 1996. Restoration of fluid balance after exercise-induced dehydration: Effects of food and fluid intake. *Eur J Appl Physiol* 73:317–325.

Maughan, R.J., L. Bethell, and J.B. Leiper. 1996. Effects of ingested fluids on homeostasis and exercise performance in man. *Exper Physiol* 81:847–859.

Maughan, R.J., M. Gleeson, P.L. Greenhaff. 1997a. *Biochemistry of exercise and training.* Oxford: Oxford University Press.

Maughan, R.J., and D.J. Sadler. 1983. The effects of oral administration of salts of aspartic acid on the metabolic response to prolonged exhausting exercise in man. *Int J Sports Med* 4 (2): 119–123.

Maughan, R.J., and M. Gleeson. 1988. Influence of a 36 h fast followed by refeeding with glucose, glycerol or placebo on metabolism and performance during prolonged exercise in man. *Eur J Appl Physiol* 57 (5): 570–576.

Maughan, R.J., and M. Gleeson. 2004. *The biochemical basis of sports performance.* Oxford: Oxford University Press.

Maughan, R.J., C. Williams, D.M. Campbell, and D. Hepburn. 1978. Fat and carbohydrate metabolism during low intensity exercise: Effects of the availability of muscle glycogen. *Eur J Appl Physiol* 39:7–16.

Maughan, R.J., P.L. Greenhaff, J.B. Leiper, D. Ball, C.P. Lambert, and M. Gleeson. 1997b. Diet composition and the performance of high-intensity exercise. *J Sports Sci* 15 (3): 265–275.

McCarty, M.F. 1996. Chromium (III) picolinate (letter). *FASEB J* 10 (2): 365–369.

McCrory, M.A., P.A. Mole, L.A. Nommsen-Rvers, and K.G. Dewey. 1997. Between-day and within-day variation in the relation between heart rate and oxygen consumption: Effect on the estimation of energy expenditure by heart-rate monitoring. *Am J Clin Nutr* 66:18–25.

McElroy, B.H., and S.P. Miller. 2002. Effectiveness of zinc gluconate glycine lozenges (Cold-Eeze) against the common cold in school-aged subjects: A retrospective chart review. *Am J Ther* 9:472–475.

McGee, S.L., K.F. Howlett, R.L. Starkie, D. Cameron-Smith, B.E. Kemp, and M. Hargreaves. 2003. Exercise increases nuclear AMPK alpha2 in human skeletal muscle. *Diabetes* 52:926–928.

McGinnis, J.M., and W.H. Foege. 1993. Actual causes of death in the United States. *JAMA* 270 (18): 2207–2212.

McLay, R.T., C.D. Thomson, S.M. Williams, and N.J. Rehrer. 2007. Carbohydrate loading and female endurance athletes: Effect of menstrual-cycle phase. *Int J Sport Nutr Exerc Metab* 17 (2): 189–205.

McLellan, T.M., and D.G. Bell. 2004. The impact of prior coffee consumption on the subsequent ergogenic effect of anhydrous caffeine. *Int J Sport Nutr Exerc Metab* 14 (6): 698–708.

McMurray, R.G., V. Ben-Ezra, W.A. Forsythe, et al. 1985. Responses of endurance-trained subjects to caloric deficits induced by diet or exercise. *Med Sci Sports Exerc* 17 (5): 574–579.

McNaughton, L., and R. Cedaro. 1992. Sodium citrate ingestion and its effects on maximal anaerobic exercise of different durations. *Eur J Appl Physiol* 64 (1): 36–41.

McNaughton, L., B. Dalton, and G. Palmer. 1999a. Sodium bicarbonate can be used as an ergogenic aid in high-intensity, competitive cycle ergometry of 1 h duration. *Eur J Appl Physiol* 80 (1): 64–69.

McNaughton, L., B. Dalton, and J. Tarr. 1999b. Inosine supplementation has no effect on aerobic or anaerobic cycling performance. *Int J Sport Nutr* 9:333–344.

McNaughton, L.R. 1990. Sodium citrate and anaerobic performance: Implications of dosage. *Eur J Appl Physiol* 61 (5–6): 392–397.

Mensink, R.P., and M.B. Katan. 1990. Effect of dietary *trans* fatty acids on high-density and low-density lipoprotein cholesterol levels in healthy subjects. *N Engl J Med* 323 (7): 439–445.

Merimee, T.J., D.A. Lillicrap, and D. Rabinowitz. 1965. Effect of arginine on serum-levels of human growth-hormone. *Lancet* 2 (7414): 668–670.

Meydani, M., W.J. Evans, A. Handleman, R.A. Biddle, R.A. Fielding, S.N. Meydani, et al. 1993. Protective effect of vitamin E on exercise-induced oxidative damage in young and older adults. *Am J Physiol* 264:R992–R998.

Mikkelsen, P.B., S. Toubro, and A. Astrup. 2000. Effect of fat-reduced diets on 24-h energy expenditure: Comparisons between animal protein, vegetable protein, and carbohydrate. *Am J Clin Nutr* 72 (5): 1135–1141.

Miller, S.L., K.D. Tipton, D.L. Chinkes, S.E. Wolf, and R.R. Wolfe. 2003. Independent and combined effects of amino acids and glucose after resistance exercise. *Med Sci Sports Exerc* 35 (3): 449–455.

Miller, W.C., R. Bryce, and R.K. Conlee. 1984. Adaptation to a high-fat diet that increase exercise endurance in male rats. *J Appl Physiol* 56 (1): 78–83.

Mishell, D.R. 1993. Non-contraceptive benefits of oral contraceptives. *J Reprod Med* 38:1021–1029.

Mitchell, J.B., F.X. Pizza, A. Paquet, J.B. Davis, M.B. Forrest, and W.A. Braun. 1998. Influence of carbohydrate status on immune responses before and after endurance exercise. *J Appl Physiol* 84:1917-1925.

Mitsiopoulos, N., R.N. Baumgartner, S.B. Heymsfield, et al. 1998. Cadaver validation of skeletal muscle measurement by magnetic resonance imaging and computerized tomography. *J Appl Physiol* 85 (1): 115-122.

Modlesky, C.M., K.J. Cureton, R.D. Lewis, et al. 1996. Density of the fat-free mass and estimates of body composition in male weight trainers. *J Appl Physiol* 80 (6): 2085-2096.

Montagnani, G.F., B. Arena, and N. Maffulli. 1992. Oestradiol and progesterone during exercise in healthy untrained women. *Med Sci Sports Exerc* 24:764-768.

Montain, S.J., M.K. Hopper, A.R. Coggan, and E.F. Coyle. 1991. Exercise metabolism at different time intervals after a meal. *J Appl Physiol* 70 (2): 882-888.

Monteleone, P., L. Beinat, C. Tanzillo, M. Maj, and D. Kemali. 1990. Effects of phosphatidylserine on the neuroendocrine response to physical stress in humans. *Neuroendocrinology* 52 (3): 243-248.

Monteleone, P., M. Maj, L. Beinat, M. Natale, and D. Kemali. 1992. Blunting by chronic phosphatidylserine administration of the stress-induced activation of the hypothalamo-pituitary-adrenal axis in healthy men. *Eur J Clin Pharmacol* 42 (4): 385-388.

Moore, D.R., M.J. Robinson, J.L. Fry, J.E. Tang, E.I. Glover, S.B. Wilkinson, T. Prior, M.A. Tarnopolsky, and S.M. Phillips. 2009. Ingested protein dose response of muscle and albumin protein synthesis after resistance exercise in young men. *Am J Clin Nutr,* in press.

Morrison, M.A., L.L. Spriet, and D.J. Dyck. 2000. Pyruvate ingestion for 7 days does not improve aerobic performance in well-trained individuals. *J Appl Physiol* 89:549-556.

Mortola, J.F., and S.S. Yen. 1990. The effects of oral dehydroepiandrosterone on endocrine-metabolic parameters in postmenopausal women. *J Clin Endocrinol Metab* 71 (3): 696-704.

Morton, J.F., and J.F. Guthrie. 1998. Changes in children's total fat intakes and their group sources of fat, 1989-91 versus 1994-95: Implications for diet quality. *Fam Econ Nutr Rev* 11:44-57.

Moseley, L., and A.E. Jeukendrup. 2001. The reliability of cycling efficiency. *Med Sci Sports Exerc* 33 (4): 621-627.

Moseley, L., G.I. Lancaster, R.L.P.G. Jentjens, J. Achten, and A.E. Jeukendrup. 2001. The effect of timing of pre-exercise carbohydrate feedings on metabolism and cycling performance. *Med Sci Sports Exerc* 34 (5): S203.

Moseley, L., G.I. Lancaster, and A.E. Jeukendrup. 2003. Effects of timing of pre-exercise ingestion of carbohydrate on subsequent metabolism and cycling performance. *Eur J Appl Physiol* 88 (4-5): 453-458.

Mourier, A., A.X. Bigard, E. de Kerviler, B. Roger, H. Legrand, and C.Y. Guezennec. 1997. Combined effects of caloric restriction and branched-chain amino acid supplementation on body composition and exercise performance in elite wrestlers. *Int J Sports Med* 18 (1): 47-55.

Mujika, I., J.C. Chatard, L. Lacoste, F. Barale, and A. Geyssant. 1996. Creatine supplementation does not improve sprint performance in competitive swimmers. *Med Sci Sports Exerc* 28 (11): 1435-1441.

Murray, R., D.E. Eddy, G.L. Paul, J.G. Seifert, and G.A. Halaby. 1991. Physiological responses to glycerol ingestion during exercise. *J Appl Physiol* 71 (1): 144-149.

Myburgh, K.H., L.K. Bachrach, and B. Lewis, 1993. Low bone mineral density at axial and appendicular sites in amenorrhoeic athletes. *Med Sci Sports Exerc* 25:1197-1202.

Myerson, M., B. Gutin, M.P. Warren, et al. 1991. Resting metabolic rate and energy balance in amenorrheic and eumenorrheic runners. *Med Sci Sports Exerc* 23 (1): 15-22.

Nachtigall, D., P. Nielsen, R. Fischer, R. Engelgardt, and E.E. Gabbe. 1996. Iron deficiency in distance runners: A reinvestigation using 59Fe-labelling and non-invasive liver iron quantification. *Int J Sports Med* 17:473-479.

Nadel, E.R., E. Cafarelli, M.F. Roberts, and C.B. Wenger. 1979. Circulatory regulation during exercise in different ambient temperatures. *J Appl Physiol* 46:430-437.

Nadel, E.R., S.M. Fortney, and C.B. Wenger. 1980. Effect of hydration state on circulatory and thermal regulations. *J Appl Physiol* 49:715-721.

Nair, K.S., D.E. Matthews, S.L. Welle, and T. Braiman. 1992. Effect of leucine on amino acid and glucose metabolism in humans. *Metabolism* 41 (6): 643-648.

Narkar ,V.A., M. Downes, R.T. Yu, E. Embler, Y.X. Wang, E. Banayo, M.M. Mihaylova, M.C. Nelson, Y. Zou, H. Juguilon, H. Kang, R.J. Shaw, and R.M. Evans. 2008. AMPK and PPARdelta agonists are exercise mimetics. *Cell* 134:405-415.

National Research Council. 2001. *Recommended daily allowances,* 10th ed. Washington, DC: National Academy Press.

Nehlsen-Cannarella, S.L., O.R. Fagoaga, D.C. Nieman, D.A. Henson, D.E. Butterworth, R.L. Schmitt, E.M. Bailey, B.J. Warren, A. Utter, and J.M. Davis. 1997. Carbohydrate and the cytokine response to 2.5 h of running. *J Appl Physiol* 82:1662-1667.

Nelson, J.L., and R.A. Rogbergs. 2007. Exploring the potential ergogenic effects of glycerol hyperhydration. *Sports Medicine* 37 (11): 981-1000.

Nestler, J.E., C.O. Barlascini, J.N. Clore, and W.G. Blackard. 1988. Dehydroepiandrosterone reduces serum low density lipoprotein levels and body fat but does not alter insulin sensitivity in normal men. *J Clin Endocrinol Metab* 66 (1): 57-61.

Newsholme, E.A., M. Parry-Billings, N. McAndrew, and R. Budgett. 1991. A biochemical mechanism to explain some mechanisms of overtraining. In Advances in nutrition and topsport, Vol. 32, ed. F. Brouns, 79-93. Basel: Karger.

Neufer, P.D., D.L. Costill, M.G. Flynn, J.P. Kirwan, J.B. Mitchell, and J. Houmard. 1987. Improvements in exercise performance: Effects of carbohydrate feedings and diet. *J Appl Physiol* 62 (3): 983-988.

Neufer, P.D., A.J. Young, and M.N. Sawka. 1989. Gastric emptying during exercise: Effects of heat stress and hypohydration. *Eur J Appl Physiol* 58:433-439.

Neville, V., M. Gleeson, and J.P. Folland. 2008. Salivary IgA as a risk factor for upper respiratory infection: A longitudinal prospective study in athletes. *Med Sci Sports Exerc* (in press).

Newsholme, E.A., E. Blomstrand, and B. Ekblom. 1992. Physical and mental fatigue: Metabolic mechanisms and importance of plasma amino acids. *Brit Med Bull* 48 (3): 477-495.

Newsholme, E.A., I.N. Acworth, and E. Blomstrand. 1987. Amino acids, brain neurotransmitters and a functional link between muscle and brain that is important in sustained exercise. In *Advances in myochemistry,* ed. G. Benzi, 127-147. London: John Libby Eurotext.

NHANES 2003-2004. www.cdc.gov/nchs/about/major/nhanes/nhanes2003-2004/nhanes03_04.htm.

Nielsen, F.H. 1996. Other trace elements. In *Present knowledge of nutrition,* ed. E.E. Ziegler and L.J. Filer, 355-358. Washington, DC: ILSI Press.

Nielsen, F.H., C.D. Hunt, L.M. Mullen, and J.R. Hunt. 1987. Effect of dietary boron on mineral, estrogen, and testosterone metabolism in postmenopausal women. *FASEB J* 1 (5): 394–397.

Nieman, D.C. 1994. Exercise, infection, and immunity. *Int J Sports Med* 15 (suppl 3): S131–S141.

Nieman, D.C., S.L. Nehlsen-Cannarella, O.R. Fagoaga, D.A. Henson, M. Shannon, J.M. Davis, M.D. Austin, C.L. Hisey, J.C. Holbeck, J.M. Hjertman, M.R. Bolton, and B.K. Schilling. 1999. Immune response to two hours of rowing in elite female rowers. *Int J Sports Med* 20:476–481.

Nieman, D.C., A.R. Miller, D.A. Henson, B.J. Warren, G. Gusewitch, R.L. Johnson, J.M. Davis, D.E. Butterworth, and S.L. Nehlsen-Cannarella. 1993. Effects of high- versus moderate-intensity exercise on natural killer activity. *Med Sci Sports Exerc* 25:1126–1134.

Nieman, D.C., and B.K. Pedersen, eds. 2000. *Nutrition and exercise immunology.* Boca Raton, FL: CRC Press.

Nieman, D.C., D.A. Henson, O.R. Fagoaga, et al. 2002. Change in salivary IgA following a competitive marathon race. *Int J Sports Med* 23:69–75.

Nieman, D.C., D.A. Henson, S.J. Gross, et al. 2007. Quercetin reduces illness but not immune perturbations after intensive exercise. *Med Sci Sports Exerc* 39:1561–1569.

Nieman, D.C., D.A. Henson, S.R. McAnulty, et al. 2002. Influence of vitamin C supplementation on oxidative and immune changes after an ultramarathon. *J Appl Physiol* 92:1970–1977.

Nieman, D.C., L.M. Johansen, J.W. Lee, and K. Arabatzis. 1990. Infectious episodes in runners before and after the Los Angeles Marathon. *J Sports Med Phys Fitness* 30:316–328

Nieman, D.C., S.L. Nehlsen-Cannarella, O.R. Fagoaga, et al. 1998a. Effects of mode and carbohydrate on the granulocyte and monocyte response to intensive, prolonged exercise. *J Appl Physiol* 84 (4): 1252–1259.

Nieman, D.C., S.L. Nehlsen-Cannarella, O.R. Fagoaga, et al. 1998b. Influence of mode and carbohydrate on the cytokine response to heavy exertion. *Med Sci Sports Exerc* 30 (5): 671–678.

Nilsson, L.H., and E Hultman. 1973. Liver glycogen in man; the effects of total starvation or a carbohydrate-poor diet followed by carbohydrate feeding. *Scand J Clin Lab Invest* 32:325–330.

Nissen, S.L., R. Sharp, M. Ray, J.A. Rathmacher, D. Rice, J.C. Fuller, Jr., A.S. Connelly, and N. Abumrad. 1996. Effect of leucine metabolite beta-hydroxy-beta-methylbutyrate on muscle metabolism during resistance-exercise training. *J Appl Physiol* 81 (5): 2095–2104.

Nissen, S.L., R.L. Sharp, L. Panton, M. Vukovich, S. Trappe, and J.C. Fuller, Jr. 2000. Beta-hydroxy-beta-methylbutyrate (HMB) supplementation in humans is safe and may decrease cardiovascular risk factors. *J Nutr* 130 (8): 1937–1945.

Nissen, S.L., and R.L. Sharp. 2003. (Online in 2002). Effect of dietary supplements on lean mass and strength gains with resistance exercise: A meta-analysis. *J Appl Physiol* 94 (2): 651–659.

Nitzke et al. 2007. Position of the American Dietetic Association: Total diet approach to communicating food and nutrition information. *J Am Dietetic Assoc* 107 (7): 1224–32.

Noakes, T.D. 1986. *Lore of running.* Cape Town: Oxford University Press.

Noakes, T.D., N. Goodwin, B.L. Rayner, T. Branken, and R.K.N. Taylor. 1985. Water intoxication: A possible complication during endurance exercise. *Med Sci Sports Exerc* 17:370–375.

Noakes, T.D. 2007. The limits of human endurance: What is the greatest endurance performance of all time? Which factors regulate performance at extreme altitude? *Adv Exp Med Biol* 618:255–276.

Nose, H., G.W. Mack, X. Shi, and E.R. Nadel. 1988. Role of osmolality and plasma volume during rehydration in humans. *J Appl Physiol* 65:325–331.

Notivol, R., I. Carrio, L. Cano, M. Estorch, and F. Vilardell. 1984. Gastric emptying of solid and liquid meals in healthy young subjects. *Scand J Gastroenterol* 19 (8): 1107–1113.

Odland, L.M., G.J.F. Heigenhauser, G.D. Lopaschuk, and L.L. Spriet. 1996. Human skeletal muscle malonyl-COA at rest and during prolonged submaximal exercise. *Am J Physiol* 270:E541–E44.

Odland, L.M., R.A. Howlett, G.J. Heigenhauser, E. Hultman, and L.L. Spriet. 1998. Skeletal muscle malonyl-COA content at the onset of exercise at varying power outputs in humans. *Am J Physiol* 274 (6 pt 1): E1080–E1085.

Oostenbrug, G.S., R.P. Mensink, T. De Vries, M.R. Hardeman, F. Brouns, and G. Hornstra. 1997. Exercise performance, red blood cell characteristics and lipid peroxidation: Effect of fish oil and vitamin E. *J Appl Physiol* 83 (3): 746–752.

Oppliger, R.A., D.H. Nielsen, C.G. Vance. 1991. Wrestlers' minimal weight: Anthropometry, bioimpedance, and hydrostatic weighing compared. *Med Sci Sports Exerc* 23 (2): 247–253.

Oppliger, R.A., H.S. Case, C.A. Horswill, et al. 1996. American College of Sports Medicine position stand. Weight loss in wrestlers. *Med Sci Sports Exerc* 28 (6): ix–xii.

Oscai, L.B., D.A. Essig, and W.K. Palmer. 1990. Lipase regulation of muscle triglyceride hydrolysis. *J Appl Physiol* 69 (5): 1571–1577.

Packer, L. 1997. Oxidants, antioxidant nutrients and the athlete. *J Sports Sci* 15:353–363.

Paddon-Jones, D., A. Keech, and D. Jenkins. 2001. Short-term beta-hydroxy-beta-methylbutyrate supplementation does not reduce symptoms of eccentric muscle damage. *Int J Sport Nutr Exerc Metab* 11 (4): 442–450.

Paddon-Jones, D., E. Westman, R.D. Mattes, R.R. Wolfe, A. Astrup, and M. Westerterp-Plantenga. 2008. Protein, weight management, and satiety. *Am J Clin Nutr* 87 (5): 1558S–1561S.

Pagala, M.K., T. Namba, and D. Grob. 1984. Failure of neuromuscular transmission and contractility during muscle fatigue. *Muscle Nerve* 7 (6): 454–464.

Pan, D.A., S. Lillioja, A.D. Kriketos, M.R. Milner, L.A. Baur, C. Bogardus, A.B. Jenkins, and L.H. Storlien. 1997. Skeletal muscle triglyceride levels are inversely related to insulin action. *Diabetes* 46:983–988.

Pannemans, D.L.E., A.J.M. Wagenmakers, K.R. Westerterp, G. Schaafsma, and D. Halliday. 1998. Effect of protein source and quantity on protein metabolism in elderly women. *Am J Clin Nutr* 68 (6): 1228–1235.

Panton, L.B., J.A. Rathmacher, S. Baier, and S. Nissen. 2000. Nutritional supplementation of the leucine metabolite beta-hydroxy-beta-methylbutyrate (Hmb) during resistance training. *Nutrition* 16 (9): 734–739.

Papet, I., P. Ostaszewski, F. Glomot, C. Obled, M. Faure, G. Bayle, S. Nissen, M. Arnal, and J. Grizard. 1997. The effect of a high dose of 3-hydroxy-3-methylbutyrate on protein metabolism in growing lambs. *Br J Nutr* 77 (6): 885–896.

Parry-Billings, M., R. Budgett, Y. Koutedakis, E. Blomstrand, S. Brooks, C. Williams, P.C. Calder, S. Pilling, R. Baigrie, and E.A. Newsholme. 1992. Plasma amino acid concentrations in the overtraining syndrome: Possible effects on the immune system. *Med Sci Sports Exerc* 24 (12): 1353–1358.

Pasman, W.J., M.A. van Baak, A.E. Jeukendrup, and A. deHaan. 1995. The effect of varied dosages of caffeine on endurance performance time. *Int J Sports Med* 16 (4): 225–230.

Patton, G.C., R. Selzer, C. Coffey, J.B. Carlin, and R.Wolfe. 1999. Onset of adolescent eating disorders: population based cohort study over 3 years. *Br Med J* 318 (7186):765-768.

Pedersen, B.K., and H. Bruunsgaard. 1995. How physical exercise influences the establishment of infections. *Sports Med* 19:393–400.

Pedersen, B.K., J. Helge, E. Richter, T. Rhode, K. Ostrowski, and B. Kiens. 2000. Training and natural immunity: Effects of diets rich in fat or carbohydrate. *Eur J Appl Physiol* 82:98–102.

Pedersen, D.J., S.J. Lessard, V.G. Coffey, E.G. Churchley, A.M. Wootton, T. Ng, M.J. Watt, and J.A. Hawley. 2008. High rates of muscle glycogen resynthesis after exhaustive exercise when carbohydrate is coingested with caffeine. *J Appl Physiol* 105 (1): 7–13.

Pendergast, D.R., P.J. Horvath, J.J. Leddy, and J.T. Venkatraman. 1996. The role of dietary fat on performance, metabolism and health. *Am J Sports Med* 24 (6): S53–S58.

Perusse, L., and C. Bouchard. 2000. Gene-diet interactions in obesity. *Am J Clin Nutr* 72 (5 suppl): 1285S–1290S.

Peters, E.M., J.M. Goetzsche, B. Grobbelaar, and T.D. Noakes. 1993. Vitamin C supplementation reduces the incidence of post-race symptoms of upper respiratory tract in ultramarathon runners. *Am J Clin Nutr* 57:170–174.

Peters, E.M., and E.D. Bateman. 1983. Ultramarathon running and URTI: An epidemiological survey. *S Afr Med J* 64:582–584.

Peters, E.M., and J.M. Goetzsche. 1997. Dietary practices of South African ultradistance athletes. *Int J Sport Nutr* 7:80–103.

Peters, E.M., J.M. Goetzsche, L.E. Joseph, and T.D. Noakes. 1996. Vitamin C as effective as combinations of anti-oxidant nutrients in reducing symptoms of upper respiratory tract infections in ultramarathon runners. *S Afr J Sports Med* 11:23–27.

Peyrebrune, M.C., M.E. Nevill, F.J. Donaldson, and D.J. Cosford. 1998. The effects of oral creatine supplementation on performance in single and repeated sprint swimming. *J Sports Sci* 16 (3): 271–279.

Phillips, S.M., K.D. Tipton, A. Aarsland, S.E. Wolf, and R.R. Wolfe. 1997. Mixed muscle protein synthesis and breakdown after resistance exercise in humans. *Am J Physiol* 273 (1 pt 1): E99–E107.

Phillips, S.M., K.D. Tipton, A.A. Ferrando, and R.R. Wolfe. 1999. Resistance training reduces the acute exercise-induced increase in muscle protein turnover. *Am J Physiol* 276 (1 pt 1): E118–E124.

Phinney, S.D., B.R. Bistrian, R.R. Wolfe, and G.L. Blackburn. 1983a. The human metabolic response to chronic ketosis without caloric restriction: Physical and biochemical adaptation. *Metabolism* 32 (8): 757–768.

Phinney, S.D., B.R. Bistrian, W.J. Evans, E. Gervino, and G.L. Blackburn. 1983b. The human metabolic response to chronic ketosis without caloric restriction: Preservation of submaximal exercise capability with reduced carbohydrate oxidation. *Metabolism* 32 (9): 769–776.

Phinney, S.D., E.S. Horton, E.A.H. Sims, J.S. Hanson, E. Danforth, and B.M. LaGrange. 1980. Capacity for moderate exercise in obese subjects after adaptation to a hypocaloric, ketogenic diet. *J Clin Invest* 66:1152–1161.

Phoenix, J., R.H. Edwards, and M.J. Jackson. 1991. The effect of vitamin E analogues and long hydrocarbon chain compounds on calcium-induced muscle damage: A novel role for alpha-tocopherol? *Biochimica Biophysica Acta* 1097:212–218.

Pilegaard, H., C. Keller, A. Steensberg, J.W. Helge, B.K. Pedersen, B. Saltin, and P.D. Neufer. 2002. Influence of pre-exercise muscle glycogen content on exercise-induced transcriptional regulation of metabolic genes. *J Physiol* 541:261–271.

Pilegaard, H., B. Saltin, and P.D. Neufer. 2003. Exercise induces transient transcriptional activation of the PGC-1alpha gene in human skeletal muscle. *J Physiol* 546:851–858.

Pinchan, G., R.K. Gauttam, O.S. Tomar, and A.C. Babaj. 1988. Effects of primary hypohydration on physical work capacity. *Int J Biometeorol* 32:176–180.

Pirnay, F., A.J. Scheen, J.F. Gautier, M. Lacroix, and P.J. Lefèbvre. 1995. Exogenous glucose oxidation during exercise in relation to the power output. *Int J Sports Med* 16 (7): 456–460.

Pirnay, F., J.M. Crielaard, N. Pallikarakis, M. Lacroix, F. Mosora, G. Krzentowski, A.S. Luyckx, and P.J. Lefebvre. 1982. Fate of exogenous glucose during exercise of different intensities in humans. *J Appl Physiol* 53:1620–1624.

Pizza, F.X., J.M. Peterson, J.H. Baas, and T.J. Koh. 2005. Neutrophils contribute to muscle injury and impair its resolution after lengthening contractions in mice. *J Physiol* 562(3):899-913.

Polivy, J., and C.P. Herman. 1995. Dieting and its relation to eating disorders. In *Eating disorders and obesity: A comprehensive handbook,* ed. K.D. Brownell and C.G. Fairburn, 83–86. London: Guildford Press.

Pomeroy, C., and S.F. Mitchell. 1992. Medical issues in the eating disorders. In *Eating, body weight and performance in athletes: Disorders of modern society,* ed. K.D. Brownell, J. Rodin, and J.H. Wilmore, 202–221. Philadelphia: Lea & Febiger.

Poppitt, S.D., and A.M. Prentice. 1996. Energy density and its role in the control of food intake: Evidence from metabolic and community studies. *Appetite* 26 (2), 153–174.

Posner, B.M., L.A. Cupples, M.M. Franz, and D.R. Gagnon. 1993. Diet and heart disease risk factors in adult American men and women: The Framingham offspring-spouse nutrition studies. *Int J Epidemiol* 22 (6): 1014–1025.

Potteiger, J.A., G.L. Nickel, M.J. Webster, M.D. Haub, and R.J. Palmer. 1996. Sodium citrate ingestion enhances 30 km cycling performance. *Int J Sports Med* 17 (1): 7–11.

Pottier, A., J. Bouckaert, W. Gilis, T. Roels, and W. Derave. 2008. Mouth rinse but not ingestion of a carbohydrate solution improves 1-h cycle time trial performance. *Scand J Med Sci Sports,* Nov. 3.

Powers, S.K., and M.J. Jackson. 2008. Exercise-induced oxidative stress: Cellular mechanisms and impact on muscle force production. *Physiol Rev* 88:1243–1276.

Powers, S.K., A.N. Kavazis, and J.M. McClung. 2007. Oxidative stress and muscle disuse atrophy. *Journal of Applied Physiology* 102:2389–2397.

Powers, S.K., R.J. Byrd, R. Tulley, and T. Callender. 1983. Effects of caffeine ingestion on metabolism and performance during graded exercise. *Eur J Appl Physiol* 50:301–307.

Pujol, P., J. Huguet, F. Drobnic, et al. 2000. The effect of fermented milk containing *Lactobacillus casei* on the immune response to exercise. *Sports Med Train Rehab* 9:209–223.

Quadrilatero, J., and L. Hoffman-Goetz. 2004. N-acetyl-L-cysteine prevents exercise-induced intestinal lymphocyte apoptosis by maintaining intracellular glutathione levels and reducing mitochondrial membrane depolarization. *Biochem Biophys Res Comm* 319:894–901.

Randle, P.J., P.B. Garland, C.N. Hales, and E.A. Newsholme. 1963. The glucose fatty acid cycle: Its role in insulin sensitivity and the metabolic disturbances of diabetes mellitus. *Lancet* 1:786–789.

Rankinen, T., L. Perusse, S.J. Weisnagel, et al. 2002. The human obesity gene map: The 2001 update. *Obes Res* 10 (3): 196–243.

Rasmussen, B.B., E. Volpi, D.C. Gore, and R.R. Wolfe. 2000a. Androstenedione does not stimulate muscle protein anabolism in young healthy men. *J Clin Endocrinol Metab* 85 (1): 55–59.

Rasmussen, B.B., K.D. Tipton, S.L. Miller, S.E. Wolf, and R.R. Wolfe. 2000b. An oral essential amino acid-carbohydrate supplement enhances muscle protein anabolism after resistance exercise. *J Appl Physiol* 88 (2): 386–392.

Rehrer, N.J., A.J.M. Wagenmakers, E.J. Beckers, D. Halliday, J.B. Leiper, F. Brouns, R.J. Maugham, K. Westerterp, and W.H.M. Saris. 1992. Gastric emptying, absorption and carbohydrate oxidation during prolonged exercise. *J Appl Physiol* 72 (2): 468–475.

Rehrer, N.J., E.J. Beckers, F. Brouns, F. ten Hoor, and W.H. Saris. 1990. Effects of dehydration on gastric emptying and gastrointestinal distress while running. *Med Sci Sports Exerc* 22 (6): 790–795.

Rehrer, N.J., M. van Kemenade, W. Meester, F. Brouns, and W.H.M. Saris. 1992. Gastrointestinal complaints in relation to dietary intake in triathletes. *Int J Sport Nutr* 2:48–59.

Ren, J.M., C.F. Semenkovich, E.A. Gulve, J. Gao, and J.O. Holloszy. 1994. Exercise induces rapid increases in GLUT4 expression, glucose transport capacity, and insulin-stimulated glycogen storage in muscle. *J Biol Chem* 269 (20): 14396–14401.

Rennie, M.J., and K.D. Tipton. 2000. Protein and amino acid metabolism during and after exercise and the effects of nutrition. *Annu Rev Nutr* 20:457–483.

Rennie, M.J., P.A. MacLellan, H.S. Hundal, B. Weryl, K. Smith, P.M. Taylor, C. Egan, and P.W. Watt. 1989. Skeletal muscle glutamine concentration and muscle protein turnover. *Clin Exp* 38:47–51.

Riley, M.L., R.G. Israel, D. Holbert, E.B. Tapscott, and G.L. Dohm. 1988. Effect of carbohydrate ingestion on exercise endurance and metabolism after 1-day fast. *Int J Sports Med* 9:320–324.

Robson, P.J., A.K. Blannin, N.P. Walsh, L.M. Castell, and M. Gleeson. 1999. Effects of exercise intensity, duration and recovery on in vitro neutrophil function in male athletes. *Int J Sports Med* 20:128–135.

Rohde, T., S. Asp, D. Maclean, and B.K. Pedersen. 1998. Competitive sustained exercise in humans, and lymphokine activated killer cell activity—an intervention study. *Eur J Appl Physiol* 78:448–453.

Rolls, B.J., and E.A. Bell. 1999. Intake of fat and carbohydrate: Role of energy density. *Eur J Clin Nutr* 53 (suppl 1): S166–S173.

Rolls, B.J., E.A. Bell, V.H. Castellanos, M. Chow, C.L. Pelkman, and M.L. Thorwart. 1999. Energy density but not fat content of foods affected energy intake in lean and obese women. *Am J Clin Nutr* 69 (5): 863–871.

Romeo, J., J. Warnberg J, E. Nova, et al. 2007. Moderate alcohol consumption and the immune system. A review. *Br J Nut* 98 (1): S111–S116.

Romer, L.M., J.P. Barrington, and A.E. Jeukendrup. 2001. Effects of oral creatine supplementation on high intensity, intermittent exercise performance in competitive squash players. *Int J Sports Med* 22 (8): 546–552.

Romijn, J.A., E.F. Coyle, L.S. Sidossis, X.-J. Zhang, and R.R. Wolfe. 1995. Relationship between fatty acid delivery and fatty acid oxidation during strenuous exercise. *J Appl Physiol* 79 (6): 1939–1945.

Romijn, J.A., E.F. Coyle, L.S. Sidossis, A. Gastaldelli, J.F. Horowitz, E. Endert, and R.R. Wolfe. 1993. Regulation of endogenous fat and carbohydrate metabolism in relation to exercise intensity. *Am J Physiol* 265:E380–E391.

Rontoyannis, G.P., T. Skoulis, and K.N. Pavlou. 1989. Energy balance in ultramarathon running. *Am J Clin Nutr* 49 (5 suppl): 976–979.

Rosen, L.W., and D.O. Hough. 1988. Pathogenic weight control behaviors of female college gymnasts. *Physician Sports Med* 9:141–144.

Rosenthal, L.A., D.D. Taub, M.A. Moors, and K.J. Blank. 1992. Methylxanthine-induced inhibition of the antigen- and superantigen-specific activation of T and B lymphocytes. *Immunopharmacol* 24:302–217

Ross, S. 2000. Functional foods: The Food and Drug Administration perspective. *Am J Clin Nutr* 71 (6 suppl): 1735S–1738S; discussion 1739S-1742S.

Rossiter, H.B., E.R. Cannell, and P.M. Jakeman. 1996. The effect of oral creatine supplementation on the 1000-m performance of competitive rowers. *J Sports Sci* 14 (2): 175–179.

Roth, A., and G. Fonagy. 1998. *What works for whom?* New York: Guildford Press.

Rucinski, A. 1989. Relationship of body image and dietary intake of competitive ice skaters. *J Am Dietetic Assoc* 89:98–100.

Rueda, R. 2007. The role of dietary gangliosides on immunity and the prevention of infection. *Br J Nutr* 98:S68–S73.

Sabatini, S. 2001. The female athlete triad. *Am J Med Sci* 322:193–195.

Saltin, B. 1973. Metabolic fundamentals in exercise. *Med Sci Sports Exerc* 5:137–146.

Saltin, B., A.P. Gagge, and J.A.J. Stolwijk. 1968. Muscle temperature during submaximal exercise in man. *J Appl Physiol* 25:679–688.

Sandage, B.W., R.N. Sabounjian, R. White, and R.J. Wurtman. 1992. Choline citrate may enhance athletic performance. *Physiologist* 35:236A.

Saris, W.H.M., B.H. Goodpaster, A.E. Jeukendrup, F. Brouns, D. Halliday, and A.J.M. Wagenmakers. 1993. Exogenous carbohydrate oxidation from different carbohydrate sources during exercise. *J Appl Physiol* 755:2168–2172.

Saris, W.H.M., M.A. van Erp-Baart, F. Brouns, K.R. Westerterp, and F. ten Hoor. 1989. Study on food intake and energy expenditure during extreme sustained exercise: The Tour de France. *Int J Sports Med* 10 (1 suppl): S26–S31.

Sarna, S., and J. Kaprio. 1994. Life expectancy of former elite athletes. *Sports Med* 17 (3): 49–51.

Sasaki, H., J. Maeda, S. Usui, and T. Ishiko. 1987. Effect of sucrose and caffeine ingestion on performance of prolonged strenuous running. *Int J Sports Med* 8:261–265.

Saunders, M.J., M.D. Kane, and M.K. Todd. 2004. Effects of a carbohydrate-protein beverage on cycling endurance and muscle damage. *Med Sci Sports Exerc* 36 (7): 1233–1238.

Saunders, M.J., N.D. Luden, and J.E. Herrick. 2007. Consumption of an oral carbohydrate-protein gel improves cycling endurance and prevents postexercise muscle damage. *J Strength Cond Res* 21 (3): 678–684.

Saunders, M.J., J.E. Blevins, and C.E. Broeder. 1998. Effects of hydration changes on bioelectrical impedance in endurance trained individuals. *Med Sci Sports Exerc* 30 (6): 885–892.

Sawka, M.N., A.J. Young, B.S. Cadarette, L. Levine, and K.B. Pandolf. 1985a. Influence of heat stress and acclimation on maximal aerobic power. *Eur J Appl Physiol* 53:294-298.

Sawka, M.N., A.J. Young, R.P. Francesconi, S.R. Muza, and K.B. Pandolf. 1985b. Thermoregulatory and blood responses during exercise at graded hypohydration levels. *J Appl Physiol* 59:1394-1401.

Sawka, M.N., A.J. Young, W.A. Latzka, P.D. Neufer, M.D. Quigley, and K.B. Pandolf. 1992. Human tolerance to heat strain during exercise: Influence of hydration. *J Appl Physiol* 73:368-375.

Sawka, M.N., and C.B. Wenger. 1988. Physiological responses to acute-exercise heat stress. In *Human performance physiology and environmental medicine at terrestrial extremes*, ed. K. Pandolf. 1-38. Indianapolis, IN: Benchmark Press.

Sawka, M.N., and K.B. Pandolf. 1990. Effects of body water loss on physiological function and exercise performance. In *Perspectives in exercise science and sports medicine*, Vol. 3, ed. C.V. Gisolfi and D.R. Lamb, 1-38. Benchmark Press: Carmel, IN.

Sawka, M.N., and S.J. Montain. 2000. Fluid and electrolyte supplementation for exercise heat stress. *Am J Clin Nutr* 72 (2): 564S-572s.

Schlundt, D.G., J.O. Hill, J. Pope-Cordle, et al. 1993. Randomized evaluation of a low fat ad libitum carbohydrate diet for weight reduction. *Int J Obes Relat Metab Disord* 17 (11): 623-629.

Schoeller, D.A., E. Ravussin, Y. Schutz, K.J. Acheson, P. Baertschi, and E. Jequier. 1986. Energy expenditure by doubly labeled water: Validation in humans and proposed calculation. *Am J Physiol* 250 (5 pt 2): R823-R830.

Schoffelen, P.F., K.R. Westerterp, W.H.M. Saris, and F. ten Hoor. 1997. A dual respiration chamber system with automated calibration. *J Appl Physiol* 83:2064-2072.

Scott, J.W., F.A. Ross, J.K. Liu, and D.G. Hardie. 2007. Regulation of AMP-activated protein kinase by a pseudosubstrate sequence on the gamma subunit. *EMBO J* 26:806-815.

Sears, B. 1995. *The zone: A dietary road map*. New York: Harper Collins.

Segura, R., and J.L. Ventura. 1988. Effect of L-tryptophan supplementation on exercise performance. *Int J Sports Med* 9:301-305.

Seidell, J.C. 1997. Time trends in obesity: An epidemiological perspective. *Horm Metab Res* 29 (4): 155-158.

Seidell, J.C. 1998. Dietary fat and obesity: An epidemiologic perspective. *Am J Clin Nutr* 67 (3 suppl): 546S-550S.

Senate Select Committee on Nutrition and Human Needs. 1977. *Dietary goals for the United States*. Washington: U.S. Government Printing Office.

Shephard, R.J. 1997. *Physical activity, training and the immune response*. Carmel, IN: Cooper.

Sheppard, L., A.R. Kristal, and L.H. Kushi. 1991. Weight loss in women participating in a randomized trial of low-fat diets. *Am J Clin Nutr* 54 (5): 821-828.

Sherman, W.M., and D.L. Costill. 1984. The marathon: Dietary manipulation to optimize performance. *Am J Sports Med* 12 (1): 44-51.

Sherman, W.M., D.L. Costill, W.J. Fink, and J.M. Miller. 1981. The effect of exercise and diet manipulation on muscle glycogen and its subsequent utilization during performance. *Int J Sports Med* 2:114-118.

Sherman, W.M., J.A. Doyle, D.R. Lamb, and R.H. Strauss. 1993. Dietary carbohydrate, muscle glycogen, and exercise performance during 7 d of training. *Am J Clin Nutr* 57:27-31.

Shi, X., R.W. Summers, H.P. Schedl, S.W. Flanagan, R. Chang, and C.V. Gisolfi. 1995. Effects of carbohydrate type and concentration and solution osmolality on water absorption. *Med Sci Sports Exerc* 27 (12): 1607-1615.

Shils, M.E., J.A. Olson, M. Shike, and A.C. Ross. 1999. *Modern nutrition in health and disease*, 9th ed. Baltimore: Williams & Wilkins.

Shirreffs, S.M., A.J. Taylor, J.B. Leiper, and R.J. Maughan. 1996. Post-exercise rehydration in man: Effects of volume consumed and drink sodium content. *Med Sci Sports Exerc* 28:1260-1271.

Shirreffs, S.M., and R.J. Maughan. 1998. Volume repletion following exercise-induced volume depletion in man: Replacement of water and sodium losses. *Am J Physiol* 274:F868-F875.

Shirreffs, S.M., and R.J. Maughan. 2000. Rehydration and recovery of fluid balance after exercise. *Exer Sports Sci Rev* 28:27-32.

Shirreffs, S.M., and R.J. Maughan. 1997. Restoration of fluid balance after exercise-induced dehydration: Effects of alcohol consumption. *J Appl Physiol* 83:1152-1157.

Sidossis, L.S., A. Gastaldelli, S. Klein, and R.R. Wolfe. 1997. Regulation of plasma fatty acid oxidation during low- and high-intensity exercise. *Am J Physiol* 272:E1065-1070.

Silva, A.C., M.S. Santos-Neto, A.M. Soares, M.C. Fonteles, R.L. Guerrant, and A.A. Lima. 1998. Efficacy of a glutamine-based oral rehydration solution on the electrolyte and water absorption in a rabbit model of secretory diarrhea induced by cholera toxin [see comments]. *J Pediatr Gastroenterol Nutr* 26 (5): 513-519.

Simi, B., B. Sempore, M.-H. Mayet, and R.J. Favier. 1991. Additive effects of training and high-fat diet on energy metabolism during exercise. *J Appl Physiol* 71 (1): 197-203.

Simonsen, J.C., W.M. Sherman, D.R. Lamb, A.R. Dernbach, J.A. Doyle, and R. Strauss. 1991. Dietary carbohydrate, muscle glycogen, and power output during rowing training. *J Appl Physiol* 70:1500-1505.

Singh, A., M.L. Failla, and, P.A. Deuster. 1994. Exercise-induced changes in immune function: Effects of zinc supplementation. *J Appl Physiol* 76:2298-2301.

Singh, R.B., M.A. Niaz, S. Ghosh, R. Beegom, P. Agarwal, S. Nangia, M. Moshiri, and E.D. Janus. 1998. Low fat intake and coronary artery disease in a population with higher prevalence of coronary artery disease: The Indian paradox. *J Am Coll Nutr* 17 (4): 342-350.

Siri, W.E. 1956. The gross composition of the body. *Adv Biol Med Physiol* 4:239-280.

Sirrs, S.M., and R.A. Bebb. 1999. DHEA: Panacea or snake oil? *Can Fam Physician* 45:1723-1728.

Sjodin, A.M., A.B. Andersson, J.M. Hogberg, and K.R. Westerterp. 1994. Energy balance in cross-country skiers: A study using doubly labeled water. *Med Sci Sports Exerc* 26 (6): 720-724.

Slater, G., D. Jenkins, P. Logan, H. Lee, M. Vukovich, J.A. Rathmacher, and A.G. Hahn. 2001. Beta-hydroxy-beta-methylbutyrate (hmb) supplementation does not affect changes in strength or body composition during resistance training in trained men. *Int J Sport Nutr Exerc Metab* 11 (3): 384-396.

Snow-Harter, C.M. 1994. Bone health and prevention of osteoporosis in active and athletic women. *Clin Sport Med* 13:389-404.

Snyder, A.C., H. Kuipers, B. Cheng, R. Servais, and E. Fransen. 1995. Overtraining following intensified training with normal muscle glycogen. *Med Sci Sports Exerc* 27:1063-1070.

Snyder, A.C., K.P. O'Hagan, P.S. Clifford, et al. 1993. Exercise responses to in-line skating: Comparisons to running and cycling. *Int J Sports Med* 14 (1): 38-42.

Sole, C.C., and T.D. Noakes. 1989. Faster gastric emptying for glucose-polymer and fructose solutions than for glucose in humans. *Eur J Appl Physiol* 58:605-612.

Spector, S.A., M.R. Jackman, L.A. Sabounjian, C. Sakkas, D.M. Landers, and W.T. Willis. 1995. Effect of choline supplementation on fatigue in trained cyclists. *Med Sci Sports Exerc* 27 (5): 668-673.

Spriet, L.L. 1991. Phosphofructokinase activity and acidosis during short-term tetanic contractions. *Can J Physiol Pharmacol* 69:298-304.

Spriet, L.L. 1995. Anaerobic metabolism during high-intensity exercise. In *Exercise metabolism,* ed. M. Hargreaves, 1-39. Champaign, IL: Human Kinetics.

Spriet, L.L. 1995. Caffeine and performance. *Int J Sports Nutr* 5:S84-S99.

Spriet, L.L., D.A. MacLean, D.J. Dyck, E. Hultman, G. Cederblad, and T.E. Graham. 1992. Caffeine ingestion and muscle metabolism during prolonged exercise in humans. *Am J Physiol* 262, E891-E898.

Spurr, G.B., A.M. Prentice, P.R. Murgatroyd, G.R. Goldberg, J.C. Reina, and N.T. Christman. 1988. Energy expenditure from minute-by-minute heart-rate recording: Comparison with indirect calorimetry. *Am J Clin Nutr* 48:552-559.

St-Pierre, J., J.A. Buckingham, S.J. Roebuck, and M.D. Brand. 2002. Topology of superoxide production from different sites in the mitochondrial electron transport chain. *J Biol Chem* 277: 44784-44790.

Stanko, R.T., R.J. Robertson, R.J. Spina, J.J. Reilly, Jr., K.D. Greenawalt, and F.L. Goss. 1990a. Enhancement of arm exercise endurance capacity with dihydroxyacetone and pyruvate. *J Appl Physiol* 68 (1): 119-124.

Stanko, R.T., R.J. Robertson, R.W. Galbreath, J.J. Reilly, K.D. Greenawalt, and F.L. Goss. 1990b. Enhanced leg exercise endurance with a high-carbohydrate diet and dihydroxyacetone and pyruvate. *J Appl Physiol* 69 (5): 1651-1656.

Starling, R.D., T.A. Trappe, K.R. Short, M. Sheffield-Moore, A.C. Jozsi, W.J. Fink, and D.L. Costill. 1996. Effect of inosine supplementation on aerobic and anaerobic cycling performance. *Med Sci Sports Exerc* 28 (9): 1193-1198.

Starritt, E.C., R.A. Howlett, G.J. Heigenhauser, and L.L. Spriet. 2000. Sensitivity of CPT I tomalonyl-COA in trained and untrained human skeletal muscle. *Am J Physiol Endocrinol Metab* 278 (3): E462-E468.

Stearns, D.M., J.J. Belbruno, and K.E. Wetterhahn. 1995. A prediction of chromium (III) accumulation in humans from chromium dietary supplements. *FASEB J* 9 (15): 1650-1657.

Stearns, D.M., Sr., J.P. Wise, S.R. Patierno, and K.E. Wetterhahn. 1995. Chromium (III) picolinate produces chromosome damage in Chinese hamster ovary cells. *FASEB J* 9 (15): 1643-1648.

Steensberg, A., C. Keller, T. Hillig, C. Fresig, J.F. Wojtaszewski, B.K. Pedersen, H. Pilegaard, and M. Sander. 2007. Nitric oxide production is a proximal signalling event controlling exercise-induced mRNA expression in human skeletal muscle. *FASEB J* 21 (11): 2683-2694.

Stellingwerff, T., L.L. Spriet, M.J. Watt, N.E. Kimber, M. Hargreaves, J.A. Hawley, and L.M. Burke. 2006. Decreased PDH activation and glycogenolysis during exercise following fat adaptation with carbohydrate restoration. *Am J Physiol Endocrinol Metab* 290 (2): E380-388.

Stensrud, T., F. Ingjer, H. Holm, and S.B. Strømme. 1992. L-tryptophan supplementation does not improve running performance. *Int J Sports Med* 13 (6): 481-485.

Stephens, F.B., D. Constantin-Teodosiu, and P.L. Greenhaff. 2007a. New insights concerning the role of carnitine in the regulation of fuel metabolism in skeletal muscle. *J Physiol* 581 (Pt 2): 431-444.

Stephens, F.B., D. Constantin-Teodosiu, D. Laithwaite, E.J. Simpson, and P.L. Greenhaff. 2006. Insulin stimulates L-carnitine accumulation in human skeletal muscle. *FASEB J* 20 (2): 377-379.

Stephens, F.B., D. Constantin-Teodosiu, D. Laithwaite, E.J. Simpson, and P.L. Greenhaff. 2007b. A threshold exists for the stimulatory effect of insulin on plasma L-carnitine clearance in humans. *Am J Physiol Endocrinol Metab* 292 (2): E637-641.

Stephens, F.B., C.E. Evans, D. Constantin-Teodosiu, and P.L. Greenhaff. 2007c. Carbohydrate ingestion augments L-carnitine retention in humans. *J Appl Physiol* 102 (3): 1065-1070.

Stewart, I., L. McNaughton, P. Davies, and S. Tristram. 1990. Phosphate loading and the effects on V\od\O$_2$max in trained cyclists. *Res Q Exerc Sport* 61 (1): 80-84.

Stoecker, B.J. 1996. Chromium. In *Present knowledge in nutrition,* ed. E.E. Ziegler and L.J. Filer, 344-353. Washington, DC: ILSI Press.

Stolarczyk, L.M., V.H. Heyward, M.D. Van Loan, et al. 1997. The fatness-specific bioelectrical impedance analysis equations of Segal et al.: Are they generalizable and practical? *Am J Clin Nutr* 66 (1): 8-17.

Stubbs, R.J., C.J. Habron, P.R. Murcatroyd, and A.M. Prentice. 1995a. Covert manipulation of dietary fat and energy density: Effect on substrate flux and food intake in men eating ad libitum. *Am J Clin Nutr* 62:316-329.

Stubbs, R.J., C.J. Harbron, and A.M. Prentice. 1996. Covert manipulation of the dietary fat to carbohydrate ratio of isoenergetically dense diets: Effect on food intake in feeding men ad libitum. *Int J Obes Relat Metab Disord* 20 (7): 651-660.

Stubbs, R.J., P. Ritz, W.A. Coward, and A.M. Prentice. 1995b. Covert manipulation of the ratio of dietary fat to carbohydrate and energy density: Effect on food intake and energy balance in free-living men eating ad libitum. *Am J Clin Nutr* 62 (2): 330-337.

Sundgot-Borgen, J. 2000. Eating disorders in athletes. In *Nutrition in sport,* ed. R.J. Maughan, 510-522. Oxford: Blackwell Science.

Sundgot-Borgen, J. 1994a. Eating disorders in female athletes. *Sports Med* 3:176-188.

Sundgot-Borgen, J. 1994b. Risk and trigger factors for the development of eating disorders in female elite athletes. *Med Sci Sports Exerc* 4:414-419.

Sundgot-Borgen, J., and S. Larsen. 1993. Pathogenic weight-control methods and self-reported eating disorders in female elite athletes and controls. *Scand J Med Sci Sports* 3:150-155.

Sutton, J.R., and O. Bar-Or. 1980. Thermal illness in fun running. *Am Heart J* 100:778-781.

Svensson, M., C. Malm, M. Tonkonogi, B. Ekblom, B. Sjodin, and K. Sahlin. 1999. Effect of Q10 supplementation on tissue Q10 levels and adenine nucleotide catabolism during high-intensity exercise. *Int J Sport Nutr* 9 (2): 166-180.

Swensen, T., G. Crater, D.R. Bassett, Jr., and E.T. Howley. 1994. Adding polylactate to a glucose polymer solution does not improve endurance. *Int J Sports Med* 15 (7): 430-434.

Tang, J.E., J.W. Hartman, and S.M. Phillips. 2006. Increased muscle oxidative potential following resistance training induced fibre hypertrophy in young men. *Appl Physiol Nutr Metab* 31 (5): 495-501.

Tappy, L. 1996. Thermic effect of food and sympathetic nervous system activity in humans. *Reprod Nutr Dev* 36 (4): 391-397.

Tarnopolsky, M.A., S.A. Atkinson, S.M. Phillips, and J.D. MacDougall. 1995. Carbohydrate loading and metabolism during exercise in men and women. *J Appl Physiol* 78 (4): 1360–1368.

Tarnopolsky, M.A., M. Bosman, J.R. MacDonald, D. Vandeputte, J. Martin, and B.D. Roy. 1997. Post-exercise protein-carbohydrate and carbohydrate supplements increase muscle glycogen in men and women. *J Appl Physiol* 83 (6): 1877–1883.

Tarnopolsky, M.A., S.A. Atkinson, J.D. McDoughall, D.G. Sale, and J.R. Sutton. 1989. Physiological responses to caffeine during endurance running in habitual caffeine users. *Med Sci Sports Exerc* 21 (4): 418–424.

Terada, S., M. Goto, M. Kato, K. Kawanaka, T. Shimokawa, and I. Tabata. 2002. Effects of low-intensity prolonged exercise on PGC-1 mRNA expression in rat epitrochlearis muscle. *Biochem Biophys Res Commun* 296:350–354.

Terada, S., K. Kawanaka, M. Goto, T. Shimokawa, and I. Tabata. 2005. Effects of high-intensity intermittent swimming on PGC-1alpha protein expression in rat skeletal muscle. *Acta Physiol Scand* 184:59–65.

Terjung, R.L., P. Clarkson, E.R. Eichner, P.L. Greenhaff, P.J. Hespel, R.G. Israel, W.J. Kraemer, R.A. Meyer, L.L. Spriet, M.A. Tarnopolsky, A.J. Wagenmakers, and M.H. Williams. 2000. American College of Sports Medicine roundtable. The physiological and health effects of oral creatine supplementation. *Med Sci Sports Exerc* 32 (3): 706–717.

Thompson, R.A., and R. Trattner-Sherman. 1993. *Helping athletes with eating disorders.* Champaign, IL: Human Kinetics.

Timmons, J.A., S.M. Poucher, D. Constantin-Teodosiu, V. Worrall, I.A. Macdonald, and P.L. Greenhaff. 1996. Increased acetyl group availability enhances contractile function of canine skeletal muscle during ischemia. *J Clin Invest* 97:879–883.

Tiollier, E., C.D.T.M. Chennaoui, D. Gomez-Merino, et al. 2007. Effect of a probiotics supplementation on respiratory infections and immune and hormonal parameters during intense military training. *Military Med* 172:1006–1011.

Tippett, K.S., and L.E. Cleveland., eds. 1999. How current diets stack up: Comparison with dietary guidelines. Agriculture Information Bulletin no. 750, 51–70. Washington, DC: United States Department of Agriculture, Economic Research Service.

Tipton, C.M., and R.A. Oppliger. 1993. Nutritional and fitness considerations for competitive wrestlers. *World Rev Nutr Diet* 71:84–96.

Tipton, K.D., T.A. Elliott, M.G. Cree, A.A. Aarsland, A.P. Sanford, and R.R. Wolfe. 2007. Stimulation of net muscle protein synthesis by whey protein ingestion before and after exercise. *Am J Physiol Endocrinol Metab* 292 (1): E71–76.

Tipton, K.D., A.A. Ferrando, S.M. Phillips, D. Doyle, Jr., and R.R. Wolfe. 1999. Postexercise net protein synthesis in human muscle from orally administered amino acids. *Am J Physiol* 276 (4 pt 1): E628–634.

Tipton, K.D., B.B. Rasmussen, S.L. Miller, S.E. Wolf, S.K. Owens-Stovall, B.E. Petrini, and R.R. Wolfe. 2001. Timing of amino acid-carbohydrate ingestion alters anabolic response of muscle to resistance exercise. *Am J Physiol Endocrinol Metab* 281 (2): E197–206.

Toner, M.M., D.T. Kirkendall, D.J. Delio, J.M. Chase, P.A. Cleary, and E.L. Fox. 1982. Metabolic and cardiovascular responses to exercise with caffeine. *Ergonomics* 25:1175–1183.

Touyz, S.W., P.J.V. Beumont, and S. Hook. 1987. Exercise anorexia: A new dimension in anorexia nervosa? *Handbook of Eating Disorders* 1:143–157.

Trappe, T.A., F. White, C.P. Lambert, D. Cesar, M. Hellerstein, and W.J. Evans. 2002. Effect of ibuprofen and acetaminophen on postexercise muscle protein synthesis. *Am J Physiol Endocrinol Metab* 282:E551–556.

Tremblay, M.S., S.D. Galloway, and J.R. Sexsmith. 1994. Ergogenic effects of phosphate loading: Physiological fact or methodological fiction? *Can J Appl Physiol* 19 (1): 1–11.

Tsintzas, K., and C. Williams. 1998. Human muscle glycogen metabolism during exercise: Effect of carbohydrate supplementation. *Sports Med* 25 (1): 7–23.

Tsintzas, O.K., C. Williams, L. Boobis, and P. Greenhaff. 1995. Carbohydrate ingestion and glycogen utilisation in different muscle fibre types in man. *J Physiol* 489 (1): 243–250.

Turcotte, L.P., E.A. Richter, and B. Kiens. 1995. Lipid metabolism during exercise. In *Exercise metabolism*, ed. M. Hargreaves, 99–130. Champaign, IL: Human Kinetics.

U.S. Department of Agriculture, Agricultural Research Service. 2007. *Nutrient intakes from food: Mean amounts and percentages of calories from protein, carbohydrate, fat, and alcohol, one day, 2003–2004.* Available: www.ars.usda.gov/ba/bhnrc/fsrg.

U.S. Department of Agriculture. 1991. United States Nutrition Labeling and Education Act of 1990. *Nutr Rev* 49:273–276.

U.S. Department of Agriculture. 2000. *Dietary guidelines for Americans, 2000.* Available: www.usda.gov/cnpp/Pubs/DG2000/Index.htm.

U.S. Department of Agriculture. 2003. *USDA national nutrient database for standard reference* (release 16). Available: www.nal.usda.gov/fnic/foodcomp/Data/index.html.

Van der Meulen, J.H., A. McArdle, M.J. Jackson, and J.A. Faulkner. 1997. Contraction-induced injury to the extensor digitorum longus muscles of rats: The role of vitamin E. *J Appl Physiol* 83:817–823.

van Erp-Baart, A.M.J., W.H.M. Saris, R.A. Binkhorst, J.A. Vos, and J.W.H. Elvers. 1989a. Nationwide survey on nutritional habits in elite athletes. Part I: Energy carbohydrate, protein. *Int J Sports Med* 10 (suppl 1): S3–S10.

van Erp-Baart, A.M.J., W.H.M. Saris, R.A. Binkhorst, J.A. Vos, and J.W.H. Elvers. 1989b. Nationwide survey on nutritional habits in elite athletes. Part II: Mineral and vitamin intake. *Int J Sports Med* 10 (1): S11–S16.

van Essen, M.J., and M.J. Gibala. 2006. Failure of protein to improve time trial performance when added to a sports drink. *Med Sci Sports Exerc* 38 (8): 1476–1483.

Van Etten, L.M., F.T. Verstappen, and K.R. Westerterp. 1994. Effect of body build on weight-training-induced adaptations in body composition and muscular strength. *Med Sci Sports Exerc* 26 (4): 515–521.

Van Hall, G., J.S.H. Raaymakers, W.H.M. Saris, and A.J.M. Wagenmakers. 1995. Ingestion of branched-chain amino acids and tryptophan during sustained exercise in man: Failure to affect performance. *J Physiol* 486 (3): 789–794.

Van Loan, M.D., N.L. Keim, K. Berg, et al. 1995. Evaluation of body composition by dual energy X-ray absorptiometry and two different software packages. *Med Sci Sports Exerc* 27 (4): 587–591.

van Loon, L.J., P. Greenhaff, D. Constantin-Teodosiu, W.H. Saris, and A.J. Wagenmakers. 2001. The effects of increasing exercise intensity on muscle fuel utilisation in humans. *J Physio* 536 (Pt 1): 295–304.

van Loon, L.J., W.H. Saris, M. Kruijshoop, and A.J. Wagenmakers. 2000. Maximizing postexercise muscle glycogen synthesis: Carbohydrate supplementation and the application of amino acid or protein hydrolysate mixtures. *Am J Clin Nutr* 72 (1): 106–111.

Van Nieuwenhoven, M.A., R.-J.M. Brummer, and F. Brouns. 2000. Gastrointestinal function during exercise: Comparison of water, sports drink, and sports drink with caffeine. *J Appl Physiol* 89 (3): 1079–1085.

van Oort, M.M., J.M. van Doorn, A. Bonen, J.F.C. Glatz, D.J. van der Horst, K.W. Rodenburg, and J.J.F.P. Luiken. 2008. Insulin-induced translocation of CD36 to the plasma membrane is reversible and shows similarity to that of GLUT4. *Biochim Biophys Acta* 1781 (1-2): 61-71.

Van Soeren, M.H., and T.E. Graham. 1998. Effect of caffeine on metabolism, exercise endurance, and catecholamine responses after withdrawal. *J Appl Physiol* 85 (4): 1493-501.

Van Soeren, M.H., P. Sathasivam, L.L. Spriet, and T.E. Graham. 1993. Caffeine metabolism and epinephrine responses during exercise in users and nonusers. *J Appl Physiol* 75 (2): 805-812.

Van Thienen, R., K. Van Proeyen, B. Vanden Eynde, J. Puype, T. Lefere, and P. Hespel. 2009. Beta-alanine improves sprint performance in endurance cycling. *Med Sci Sports Exerc* 41 (4): 898-903.

Van Zeyl, C.G., E.V. Lambert, J.A. Hawley, T.D. Noakes, and S.C. Dennis. 1996. Effects of medium-chain triglyceride ingestion on carbohydrate metabolism and cycling performance. *J Appl Physiol* 80:2217-2225.

Vandenberghe, K., M. Goris, P. Van Hecke, M. Van Leemputte, L. Vangerven, and P. Hespel. 1997. Long-term creatine intake is beneficial to muscle performance during resistance training. *J Appl Physiol* 83 (6): 2055-2063.

Varnier, M., P. Sarto, D. Martines, L. Lora, F. Carmignoto, G.P. Leese, and R. Naccarato. 1994. Effect of infusing branched-chain amino acid during incremental exercise with reduced muscle glycogen content. *Eur J Appl Physiol* 69 (1): 26-31.

Venables, M.C., L. Shaw, A.E. Jeukendrup, A. Roedig-Penman, M. Finke, R.G. Newcombe, J. Parry, and A.J. Smith. 2005. Erosive effect of a new sports drink on dental enamel during exercise. *Med Sci Sports Exerc* 37 (1): 39-44.

Vergauwen, L., F. Brouns, and P. Hespel. 1998. Carbohydrate supplementation improves stroke performance in tennis. *Med Sci Sports Exerc* 30 (8): 1289-1295.

Verma, S., M.C. Cam, and J.H. McNeill. 1998. Nutritional factors that can favorably influence the glucose/insulin system: Vanadium. *J Am Coll Nutr* 17:11-18.

Vist, G.E., and R.J. Maughan. 1994. Gastric emptying of ingested solutions in man: Effect of beverage glucose concentration. *Med Sci Sports Exerc* 26 (10): 1269-1273.

Vist, G.E., and R.J. Maughan. 1995. The effect of osmolality and carbohydrate content on the rate of gastric emptying of liquids in man. *J Physiol* 486 (pt 2): 523-531.

Volek, J.S., W.J. Kraemer, J.A. Bush, M. Boetes, T. Incledon, K.L. Clark, and J.M. Lynch. 1997. Creatine supplementation enhances muscular performance during high-intensity resistance exercise. *J Am Diet Assoc* 97 (7): 765-770.

Volek, J.S., R. Silvestre, J.P. Kirwan, M.J. Sharman, D.A. Judelson, B.A. Spiering, J.L. Vingren, C.M. Maresh, J.L. Vanheest, and W.J. Kraemer. 2006. Effects of chromium supplementation on glycogen synthesis after high-intensity exercise. *Med Sci Sports Exerc* 38 (12): 2102-2109.

Volman, J.J., J.D. Ramakers, and J. Plat. 2008. Dietary modulation of immune function by β-glucans. *Physiol Behav* 94 (2): 276-284.

Volpe, S.L., L.J. Taper, and S. Meacham. 1993. The relationship between boron and magnesium status and bone mineral density in the human: A review. *Magnes Res* 6 (3): 291-296.

von Allworden, H.N., S. Horn, J. Kahl, and W. Feldheim. 1993. The influence of lecithin on plasma choline concentrations in triathletes and adolescent runners during exercise. *Eur J Appl Physiol* 67 (1): 87-91.

Vukovich, M.D., D.L. Costill, M.S. Hickey, S.W. Trappe, K.J. Cole, and W.J. Fink. 1993. Effect of fat emulsion infusion and fat feeding on muscle glycogen utilization during cycle exercise. *J Appl Physiol* 75 (4): 1513-1518.

Vukovich, M.D., D.L. Costill, and W.J. Fink. 1994. Carnitine supplementation: Effect on muscle carnitine and glycogen content during exercise. *J Appl Physiol* 26 (9): 1122-1129.

Wachter, S., M. Vogt, R. Kreis, C. Boesch, P. Bigler, H. Hoppeler, and S. Krahenbuhl. 2002. Long-term administration of L-carnitine to humans: Effect on skeletal muscle carnitine content and physical performance. *Clin Chim Acta* 318 (1-2): 51-61.

Wagenmakers, A.J. 1999. Amino acid supplements to improve athletic performance. *Curr Opin Clin Nutr Metab Care* 2 (6): 539-544.

Wagenmakers, A.J.M. 1999. Nutritional supplements: Effects on exercise performance and metabolism. In *The metabolic basis of performance in exercise and sport,* ed. D.R. Lamb and R. Murray, 209-220. Carmel, IN: Cooper.

Wagenmakers, A.J.M., E.J. Beckers, F. Brouns, H. Kuipers, P.B. Soeters, G.J. van der Vusse, and W.H.M. Saris. 1991. Carbohydrate supplementation, glycogen depletion, and amino acid metabolism during exercise. *Am J Physiol* 260 (6): E883-E890.

Wagenmakers, A.J.M., J.H. Brookes, J.H. Coakley, T. Reilly, and R.H.T. Edwards. 1989. Exercise-induced activation of branched-chain 2-oxo acid dehydrogenase in human muscle. *Eur J Appl Physiol* 59:159-167.

Wagenmakers, A.J.M. 1991. L-carnitine supplementation and performance in man. In *Advances in nutrition and top sport,* ed. F. Brouns, Vol. 32, 110-127. Basel: Karger.

Wagner, D.R., V.H. Heyward, A.L. Gibson. 2000. Validation of air displacement plethysmography for assessing body composition. *Med Sci Sports Exerc* 32 (7): 1339-1344.

Wahrenberg, H., J. Bolinder, P. Arner. 1991. Adrenergic regulation of lipolysis in human fat cells during exercise. *Eur J Clin Invest* 21:534-541.

Walberg, J.L., M.K. Leidy, D.J. Sturgill, D.E. Hinkle, S.J. Ritchey, and D.R. Sebolt. 1988. Macronutrient content of a hypoenergy diet affects nitrogen retention and muscle function in weight lifters. *Int J Sports Med* 9 (4): 261-266.

Walker, G.J., P. Caudwell, N. Dixon, and N.C. Bishop. 2006. The effect of caffeine ingestion on neutrophil oxidative burst responses following prolonged exercise. *Int J Sport Nutr Exerc Metab* 16 (1): 24-35.

Wallace, M.B., J. Lim, A. Cutler, and L. Bucci. 1999. Effects of dehydroepiandrosterone vs androstenedione supplementation in men. *Med Sci Sports Exerc* 31 (12): 1788-1792.

Waller, M.F., and E.M. Haymes. 1996. The effects of heat and exercise on sweat iron loss. *Med Sci Sports Exer* 28:197-203.

Wallis, G.A., D.S. Rowlands, C. Shaw, R.L.P.G. Jentjens, and A.E. Jeukendrup. 2005. Oxidation of combined ingestion of maltodextrins and fructose during exercise. *Med Sci Sports Exerc* 37 (3): 426-432.

Walsh, N.P., A.K. Blannin, N.C. Bishop, P.J. Robson, and M.Gleeson. 2000. Oral glutamine supplementation does not attenuate the fall in human neutrophil lipopolysaccharide-stimulated degranulation following prolonged exercise. *Int J Sport Nutr* 10:39-50.

Walsh, N.P., A.K. Blannin, P.J. Robson, and M. Gleeson. 1998. Glutamine, exercise and immune function: Links and possible mechanisms. *Sports Med* 26:177-191.

Wannamethee, S.G., A.G. Shaper, and M. Walker. 2002. Weight change, weight fluctuation, and mortality. *Arch Intern Med* 162 (22): 2575-2580.

Wapnir, R.A., M.C. Sia, and S.E. Fisher. 1996. Enhancement of intestinal water absorption and sodium transport by glycerol in rats. *J Appl Physiol* 81 (6): 2523-2527.

Warren, B.J., A.L. Stanton, and D.L. Blessing. 1990. Disordered eating patterns in competitive female athletes. *Int J Eating Disorders* 5:565-569.

Warren, J.A., R.R. Jenkins, L. Packer, E.H. Witt, and R.B. Armstrong. 1992. Elevated muscle vitamin E does not attenuate eccentric exercise-induced muscle injury. *J Appl Physiol* 72:2168-2175.

Weaver, C., and S. Rajaram. 1992. Exercise and iron status. *J Nutrition* 122:782-787.

Webb, P., W.H.M. Saris, P.F.M. Schoffelen, G.J. van Ingen Schenau, and F. ten Hoor. 1988. The work of walking: A calorimetric study. *Med Sci Sports Exerc* 20:331-337.

Wee, S.L., C. Williams, S. Gray, and J. Horabin. 1999. Influence of high and low glycemic index meals on endurance running capacity. *Med Sci Sports Exerc* 31 (3): 393-399.

Weigle, D.S., P.A. Breen, C.C. Matthys, H.S. Callahan, K.E. Meeuws, V.R. Burden, and J.Q. Purnell. 2005. A high-protein diet induces sustained reductions in appetite, ad libitum caloric intake, and body weight despite compensatory changes in diurnal plasma leptin and ghrelin concentrations. *Am J Clin Nutr* 82 (1): 41-48.

Welle, S., R. Jozefowicz, and M. Statt. 1990. Failure of dehydro-epiandrosterone to influence energy and protein metabolism in humans. *J Clin Endocrinol Metab* 71 (5): 1259-1264.

Wemple, R.D., D.R. Lamb, and K.H. McKeever. 1997. Caffeine vs caffeine-free sports drinks: Effects on urine production at rest and during prolonged exercise. *Int J Sports Med* 18 (1): 40-46.

Westerterp, K.R. 1993. Food quotient, respiratory quotient, and energy balance. *Am J Clin Nutr* 57 (5 suppl): 759S-764S; discussion 764S-765S.

Westerterp, K.R., J.H.H.L.M. Donkers, E.E.H.M. Fredrix, et al. 1995. Energy intake, physical activity and body weight: A simulation model. *Br J Nutr* 73:337-347.

Westerterp, K.R., W.H. Saris, M. van Es, and F. ten Hoor. 1986. Use of the doubly labeled water technique in humans during heavy sustained exercise. *J Appl Physiol* 61 (6): 2162-2167.

Weyers, A.M., S.A. Mazzetti, D.M. Love, et al. 2002. Comparison of methods for assessing body composition changes during weight loss. *Med Sci Sports Exerc* 34 (3): 497-502.

WHO. 1996. *Trace elements in human nutrition and health.* WHO Press: Geneva.

Wiles, J.D., S.R. Bird, J. Hopkins, and M. Riley. 1992. Effect of caffeinated coffee on running speed, respiratory factors, blood lactate and perceived exertion during 1500-m treadmill running. *Br J Sports Med* 26 (2): 116-191.

Wilkinson, S.B., S.M. Phillips, P.J. Atherton, R. Patel, K.E. Yarasheski, M.A. Tarnopolsky, M.J. Rennie. 2008. Differential effects of resistance and endurance exercise in the fed state on signaling molecule phosphorylation and protein synthesis in human muscle. *J Physiol* 586:3701-3717.

Wilkinson, S.B., P.L. Kim, D. Armstrong, and S.M. Phillips. 2006. Addition of glutamine to essential amino acids and carbohydrate does not enhance anabolism in young human males following exercise. *Appl Physiol Nutr Metab* 31 (5): 518-529.

Wilkinson, S.B., M.A. Tarnopolsky, M.J. Macdonald, J.R. Macdonald, D. Armstrong, and S.M. Phillips. 2007. Consumption of fluid skim milk promotes greater muscle protein accretion after resistance exercise than does consumption of an isonitrogenous and isoenergetic soy-protein beverage. *Am J Clin Nutr* 85 (4): 1031-1040.

Willett, W.C. 2000. Diet and cancer. *Oncologist* 5:393-404.

Williams, J.H., J.F. Signorile, W.F. Barnes, and T.W. Henrich. 1988. Caffeine, maximal power output and fatigue. *Br J Sports Med* 22 (4): 132-134.

Williams, M.H. 1993. Nutritional supplements for strength trained athletes. *Sports Sci Exch* 6 (6): 1-4.

Williams, M.H., R.B. Kreider, and J.D. Branch. 1999. *Creatine the power supplement.* Champaign, IL: Human Kinetics.

Williams, M.H., R.B. Kreider, D.W. Hunter, et al. 1990. Effect of inosine supplementation on 3-mile treadmill run performance and V\od\O$_2$ peak. *Med Sci Sports Exerc* 22 (4): 517-522.

Wilmore, J.H., K.C. Wambsgans, M. Brenner, et al. 1992. Is there energy conservation in amenorrheic compared with eumenorrheic distance runners? *J Appl Physiol* 72 (1): 15-22.

Wilson, J.G., J.M. Wilson, and A.H. Manninen. 2008. Effects of beta-hydroxy-beta-methylbutyrate (HMB) on exercise performance and body composition across varying levels of age, sex, and training experience: A review. *Nutr Metab (Lond)* 5:1.

Winder, W.W., and D.G. Hardie. 1996. Inactivation of acetyl-CoA carboxylase and activation of AMP-activated protein kinase in muscle during exercise. *Am J Physiol* 270:E299-304.

Winder, W.W. 1986. Effect of intravenous caffeine on liver glycogenolysis during prolonged exercise. *Med Sci Sports Exerc* 18 (2): 192-196.

Wojtaszewski, J.F., C. MacDonald, J.N. Nielsen, Y. Hellsten, D.G. Hardie, B.E. Kemp, B. Kiens, and E.A. Richter. 2003. Regulation of 5'AMP-activated protein kinase activity and substrate utilization in exercising human skeletal muscle. *Am J Physiol Endocrinol Metab* 284:E813-822.

Wolfe, R.R. 1992. *Radioactive and stable isotope tracers in biomedicine.* New York: Wiley-Liss.

Wolfe, R.R., R.D. Goodenough, M.H. Wolfe, G.T. Royle, and E.R. Nadel. 1982. Isotopic analysis of leucine and urea metabolism in exercising humans. *J Appl Physiol* 52 (2): 458-466.

Wolfe, R.R., S. Klein, F. Carraro, and J.-M. Weber. 1990. Role of triglyceride-fatty acid cycle in controlling fat metabolism in humans during and after exercise. *Am J Physiol* 258:E382-E389.

Wright, D.C., D.H. Han, P.M. Garcia-Roves, P.C. Geiger, T.E. Jones, J.O. Holloszy. 2007. Exercise-induced mitochondrial biogenesis begins before the increase in muscle PGC-1alpha expression. *J Biol Chem* 282:194-199.

Wurtman, R.J., and M.C. Lewis. 1991. Exercise, plasma composition and neurotransmission. *Med Sport Sci* 32:94-109.

Wyss, M., and R. Kaddurah-Daouk. 2000. Creatine and creatinine metabolism. *Physiol Rev* 80 (3): 1107-1213.

Xia, R., J.A. Webb, L.L. Gnall, K. Cutler, and J.J. Abramson. 2003. Skeletal muscle sarcoplasmic reticulum contains a NADH-dependent oxidase that generates superoxide. *American Journal of Physiology* 285:C215-C221.

Yang, Y., A. Creer, B. Jemiolo, S. Trappe. 2005. Time course of myogenic and metabolic gene expression in response to acute exercise in human skeletal muscle. *J Appl Physiol* 98:1745-1752.

Yaspelkis, B.B., J.G. Patterson, P.A. Anderla, Z. Ding, and J.L. Ivy. 1993. Carbohydrate supplementation spares muscle glycogen during variable-intensity exercise. *J Appl Physiol* 75 (4): 1477-1485.

Yeo, W.K., C.D. Paton, A.P. Garnham, L.M. Burke, A.L. Carey, J.A. Hawley. 2008. Skeletal muscle adaptation and performance responses to once a day versus twice every second day endurance training regimens. *J Appl Physiol* 105:1462-1470.

Yeo, S.E., R.L.P.G. Jentjens, G.A. Wallis, and A.E. Jeukendrup. 2005. Caffeine increases exogenous carbohydrate oxidation during exercise. *J Appl Physiol* 99:844-850.

Zawadzki, K.M., B.B. Yaspelkis III, and J.L. Ivy. 1992. Carbohydrate-protein complex increases the rate of muscle glycogen storage after exercise. *J Appl Physiol* 72 (5): 1854-1859.

Zeisel, S.H. 1998. *Choline and phosphatidylcholine.* Washington, DC: ILSI Press.

Zeisel, S.H., K.A. Da Costa, P.D. Franklin, E.A. Alexander, J.T. Lamont, N.F. Sheard, and A. Beiser. 1991. Choline, an essential nutrient for humans [see comments]. *FASEB J* 5 (7): 2093-2098.

Zemel, M.B., J. Richards, S. Mathis, A. Milstead, L. Gebhardt, and E. Silva. 2005. Dairy augmentation of total and central fat loss in obese subjects. *Int J Obes (Lond)* 29 (4): 391-397.

Zemel, M.B., H. Shi, B. Greer, D. Dirienzo, and P.C. Zemel. 2000. Regulation of adiposity by dietary calcium. *FASEB J* 14 (9): 1132-1138.

Zemel, M.B. 2004. Role of calcium and dairy products in energy partitioning and weight management. *Am J Clin Nutr* 79 (5): 907S-912S.

Zerba, E., T.E. Komorowski, and J.A. Faulkner. 1990. Free radical injury to skeletal muscles of young, adult, and old mice. *Am J Physiol* 258:C429-C435.

Zinker, B.A., K. Britz, and G.A. Brooks. 1990. Effects of a 36-hour fast on human endurance and substrate utilization. *J Appl Physiol* 69 (5): 1849-1855.

Index

Note: Page numbers followed by an italicized *f* or *t* refer to the figure or table on that page.

A

accelerometry 90
acesulfame potassium 39*t*
acetyl-CoA 52*f*
achlorhydria 113
ACTH (adrenocorticotrophic hormone) 68
actin 170
action potential 49
active transport 109
additives 37-38
adipocyte 151
adipose tissue 6
    availability in body 150
    lipolysis 59*f*
    and resting metabolic rate 91
ADP
    and ATP resynthesis 52
    and energy storage 48
    and metabolism regulation 64
adrenaline
    and lipolysis in adipocytes 151
    and metabolism regulation 67*f*, 68
aerobic metabolism
    carbohydrate oxidation 56-58
    and fat oxidation 158
    using fatty acids 58-61
    using protein 61-62
AI (adequate intake) 28, 29
albumin 153
alcohol 20, 34-35, 216, 380-381
α-amylase 104
alpha-carotene 21
α-linolenic acid 10*f*
alpha-linoleic acid 34
amenorrhea 349
amino acids
    absorption 110, 111*f*
    and central fatigue hypothesis 187
    degradation pathways 173*t*
    as ergogenic aids 184-191
    essential and nonessential 15
    as glucogenic precursors 171
    and immune function 379-380
    incorporation into protein 174
    intake and protein synthesis 183
    as lipogenic precursors 171
    metabolism 170-171
    products synthesized from 175*t*
    as source of ATP 52*f*
    structure 15, 16*f*
    as supplements 184-195
    synthesis 174
    and TCA cycle 172*f*
    transamination 172
    transport 170

aminotransferase reactions 172
AMP 64
amylopectin 3, 4*f*
amylose 4*f*
anaerobic activity
    and ATP production 53*t*
    and fatigue 69-71
    and glycolysis 53-56
    and muscle fiber type 50
    role of phosphocreatine 51-53
    and sodium bicarbonate 289-290
anemia 240*t*, 241-242
anorexia nervosa 247, 348-350
anthocyanins 21
anthropometry 314, 317
antibodies 367-368, 369*f*, 370*f*
antigens 364, 366, 370*f*
antioxidants 222
    and immune function 381-384
    mechanisms 235-236
    micronutrients 232-239
    as supplements 238-239
    and training adaptation 306-307
apolipoproteins 12
apoprotein 12
appetite 332-333
arachidonic acid 10
Archimedes' principle 319
arginine 184-185
artificial sweeteners 38, 39*t*, 339, 341
aspartame 38
aspartate 185-186
ATP
    anaerobic production 53*t*
    anaerobic resynthesis rates 70*f*
    chemical breakdown 51
    and energy storage 48
    and metabolism regulation 64
    in resting muscle 51
    resynthesis mechanisms 51, 53*t*, 59
    sources for muscle force generation 52
    transport mechanism 280*f*
Atwater, Wilbur Olin 82

B

basal metabolic rate 90-91
bee pollen 263
β alanine 263
beta-carotene 21
beta-cryoxanthin 21
betaglucans 5, 391
beta-hydroxy beta methylbutyrate 264-265
beta-lymphocytes 367
beta-oxidation 52*f*, 60-61, 155
bile 103, 110

bioelectric impedance analysis 322-323, 324
blood 125, 247
blood glucose
    availability in body 150
    and carbohydrate intake 122-123
    control 125
    normalization by fiber 7
    regulation of concentration 126
body composition
    component models 315-316
    genetic influence 330-331
    optimal 314
    and sports differences 330
body composition measurement
    air displacement plethysmography 326
    bioelectric impedance analysis 322-323, 324
    body density calculation 322*t*
    computed tomography 325
    densitometry (underwater weighing) 319-320
    dual-energy x-ray absorptiometry 325
    MRI (magnetic resonance imaging 325-326
    multicomponent models 326
    skinfold measurement tables 323
    skinfolds 321-322
    techniques 317*t*
    waist-to-hip ratio 318
body fat 316
body mass 314-315, 330
body mass index 317, 318
body temperature
    and energy efficiency 80
    regulation 18-19, 198, 200
body weight 314, 316, 330
bomb calorimeter 81-82
bone formation 231*f*
boron 232, 265
branched chain amino acids (BCAA) 170, 186-187, 259, 305-306, 310
bulimia nervosa 348-350
B vitamins 242, 247

C

caffeine
    and carbohydrate absorption 269
    and carbohydrate oxidation 142
    chemical structure 265
    and coffee 269-270
    and cognitive functioning 268
    dosage 268
    and endurance exercise 267

About the Authors

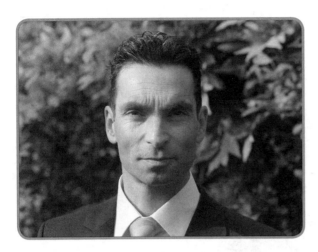

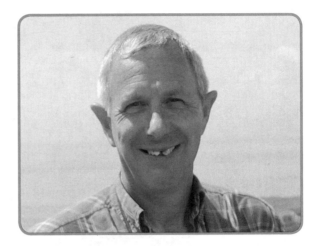

Asker Jeukendrup, PhD, is a professor of exercise metabolism in the School of Sport and Exercise Sciences at the University of Birmingham in Edgbaston, Birmingham, United Kingdom. He is an active researcher credited with many of the new findings in sport nutrition in the past decade. He is a registered sport and exercise nutritionist, having worked with many elite athletes and clubs, including the professional cycling team Rabobank, the Chelsea Football Club, UK Athletics, the British Olympic Association, African runners, and several Olympic and world champions.

Jeukendrup has published extensively in sport nutrition and was an invited delegate to the IOC Consensus Conference on Sports Nutrition in Lausanne in 2003. He is a fellow of the American College of Sports Medicine and the European College of Sport Sciences, the Physiological Society, the Nutrition Society, BASES, the New York Academy of Sciences, and the American Diabetic Association. He is also the editor of the *European Journal of Sport Sciences*. In his leisure time, he enjoys running, cycling, and competing in triathlons. He has completed more than 17 Ironman-distance races, including the Ironman Hawaii four times.

Michael Gleeson, PhD, is a professor of exercise biochemistry in the School of Sport, Exercise and Health Sciences at Loughborough University in Loughborough, Leicestershire, United Kingdom. Gleeson is an active researcher in sport nutrition and has worked with numerous world-class athletes and professional football clubs. He has taught sport nutrition at the university level and has published extensively in scientific and medical journals. He also was an invited delegate to the IOC Consensus Conference on Sports Nutrition in Lausanne in 2003. He has a particular interest and expertise in the effects of exercise, training, and nutrition on immune function and has been both vice president and president of the International Society of Exercise and Immunology.

Gleeson is also a fellow of the European College of Sport Sciences and a member of the American College of Sports Medicine, the Physiological Society, and the British Association of Sport and Exercise Sciences. He enjoys playing tennis, hill walking, and watching football and films.

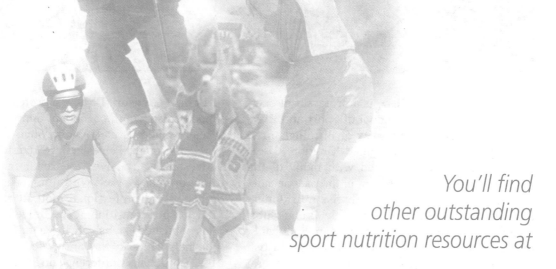

*You'll find
other outstanding
sport nutrition resources at*

www.HumanKinetics.com

In the U.S. call

1-800-747-4457

Australia..08 8372 0999
Canada 1-800-465-7301
Europe..+44 (0) 113 255 5665
New Zealand...0800 222 062

 HUMAN KINETICS
The Information Leader in Physical Activity
P.O. Box 5076 • Champaign, IL 61825-5076 USA